NUTRITION ESSENTIALS *for* NURSING PRACTICE

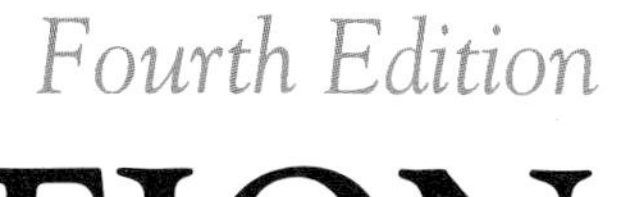

Fourth Edition

NUTRITION ESSENTIALS *for* NURSING PRACTICE

Susan G. Dudek, RD, CDN, BS
Consultant Dietitian in Private Practice
Salem, Virginia

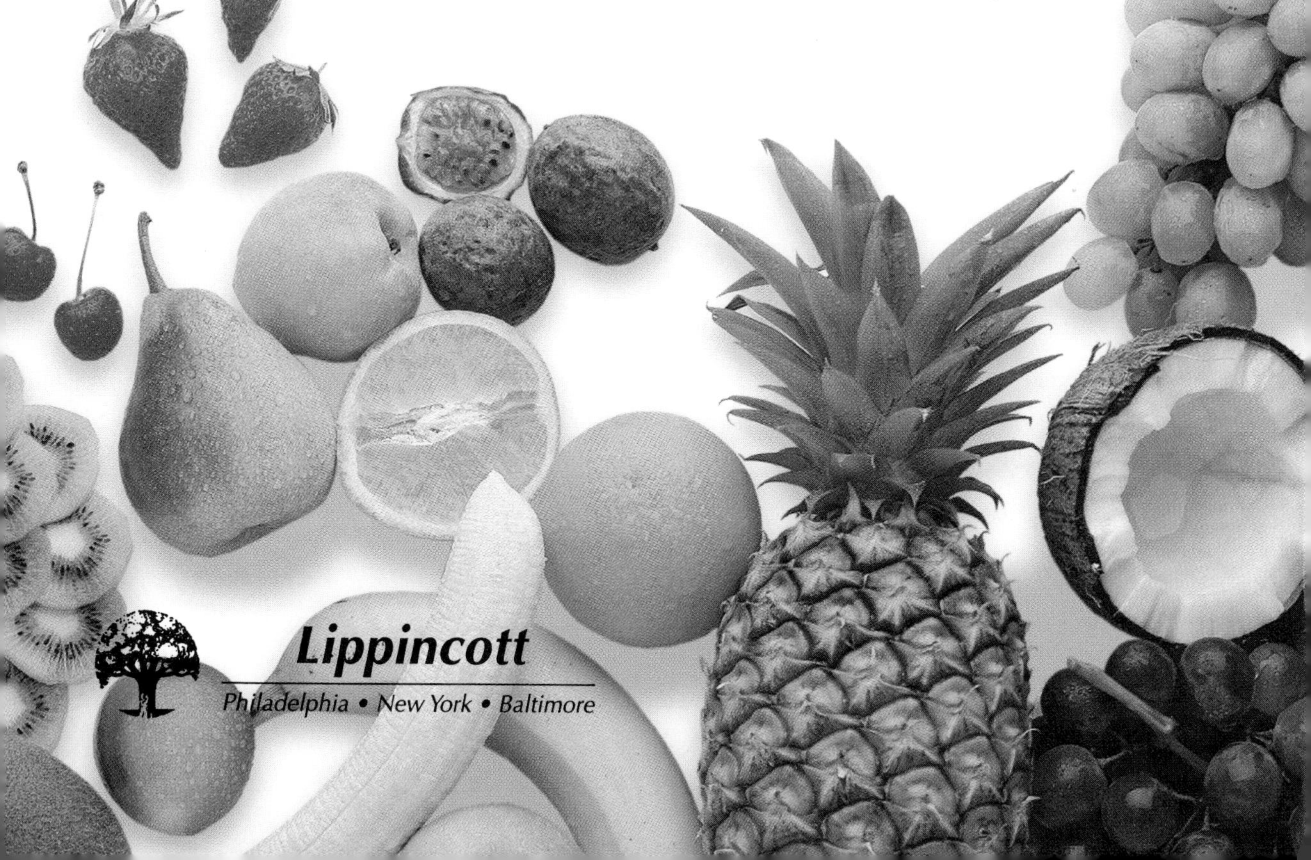

Lippincott
Philadelphia • New York • Baltimore

Acquisitions Editor: Ilze Rader
Managing Editor: Jane Velker
Developmental Editors: Danielle DiPalma/Carol Loyd
Project Editor: Nicole Walz
Senior Production Manager: Helen Ewan
Production Coordinator: Mike Carcel
Art Director: Doug Smock
Manufacturing Manager: William Alberti
Indexer: Kathy Pitcoff
Compositor: Pine Tree Composition
Printer: R.R. Donnelley & Sons

4th Edition

9 8 7 6 5 4 3 2 1

Library of Congress Cataloging-in-Publication Data

Dudek, Susan G.
Nutrition essentials for nursing practice / Susan G. Dudek.—4th ed.
p. ; cm.
Includes bibliographical references and index.
ISBN 0-7817-2344-2 (alk. paper)
1. Diet therapy. 2. Nutrition. 3. Nursing. I. Title.
[DNLM: 1. Diet Therapy—Handbooks. 2. Diet Therapy—Nurses' Instruction. 3. Nutrition—Handbooks. 4. Nutrition—Nurses' Instruction. WB 39 D845n 2001]
RM216 .D863 2001
615.8'54—dc21

00-041261

Care has been taken to confirm the accuracy of the information presented and to describe generally accepted practices. However, the authors, editors, and publisher are not responsible for errors or omissions or for any consequences from application of the information in this book and make no warranty, expressed or implied, with respect to the content of the publication.

The authors, editors, and publisher have exerted every effort to ensure that drug selection and dosage set forth in this text are in accordance with current recommendations and practice at the time of publication. However, in view of ongoing research, changes in government regulations, and the constant flow of information relating to drug therapy and drug reactions, the reader is urged to check the package insert for each drug for any change in indications and dosage and for added warnings and precautions. This is particularly important when the recommended agent is a new or infrequently employed drug.

Some drugs and medical devices presented in this publication have Food and Drug Administration (FDA) clearance for limited use in restricted research settings. It is the responsibility of the health care provider to ascertain the FDA status of each drug or device planned for use in his or her clinical practice.

To my husband, Joe,
who has faced
the challenge of a lifetime
with courage, dignity,
and even humor.
You are my hero.

Reviewers

We thank the many instructors and clinical specialists who gave us feedback on students' needs and shared their clinical expertise.

Donna Arcadipane, RN, MSN, OCRN
Professor of Nursing
Charles Community College
Laplata, Maryland

Joan W. Conklin, RNC, EdD
Professor of Nursing
Bloomfield College
Bloomfield, New Jersey

Linda Carman Copell, PhD, RNCS, DAPA, ACFE, CFLE
Associate Professor
Villanova University
Villanova, Pennsylvania

Loree Crain, PhD, RNC
Level Coordinator for PN & ASN/Bridge Nursing Program
Santa Fe Community College
Gainesville, Florida

Joan Webb Dresh, RN, MSN
Professor
Widener University School of Nursing
Chester, Pennsylvania

Mary Engberg, BSN, MA
Nursing Instructor/Student Coordinator
Southeastern Community College
West Burlington, Iowa

Geralyn Frandsen, MSN, RN
Assistant Professor of Nursing
Maryville University
St. Louis, Missouri

Kathleen Furniss, RNC, MSN
Women's Health Initiative
University of M&D–New Jersey
Mahwah, New Jersey

Janet Goshorn, ARNP, MSN, CCRN, CS
Nurse Practitioner
Nemours Children's Clinic
Orlando, Florida

Randy Gross, MS, RN, CS, AOCN
Clinical Nurse Specialist
Memorial Sloan-Kettering Cancer Center
New York, New York

Sandra Jean Hartranft, RN, BSN, CDE
Diabetes Educator
Abington Hospital Diabetes Center
Willow Grove, Pennsylvania

Connie S. Heflin, MSN, RN
Professor
Paducah Community College
Paducah, Kentucky

Jette R. Hogenmiller, RN, MN, CFNP
Assistant Professor
Creighten University
Omaha, Nebraska

Sharon Jensen, RN, MN
Instructor
Seattle University
Seattle, Washington

Lynell Johnson, RN
Instructor
Poway ROP Vocational Program
Poway, California

Sharon Kallam, BSN, RN, MSN
Chairperson Allied Health Division
Surry Community College
Dobson, North Carolina

Launa Martindale, RN, MSN
Associate Professor
University of Arkansas at Little Rock
Little Rock, Arkansas

Susan B. Quinn, MS, RD
Instructor
Southeastern Louisiana University
Hammond, Louisiana

Sherrie L. Underwood, MSN, RN, CNS
Assistant Professor
Walsh Unviersity
North Canton, Ohio

Preface

Nutrition is a basic human need, ever-changing throughout the life cycle and along the wellness–illness continuum. It is a vital and integral component of nursing care. Knowledge of nutrition principles and the ability to apply that knowledge are required of nurses, whether they are involved in home health, community wellness, outpatient settings, or acute or long-term care.

Today, more than ever, health care providers are expected to do more with less. Often the constraints of time and resources challenge nurses to be all things to all people. With the movement of health care toward wellness and primary prevention, the significance of nutrition becomes more evident.

The fourth edition of *Nutrition Handbook for Nursing Practice* has a new identity. It has a new title, *Nutrition Essentials for Nursing Practice*, and, as that title implies, the book is more focused than its predecessor. Its scope has evolved from "anything you ever wanted to know about nutrition" to "what you need to know about nutrition and how you can use that knowledge to your client's advantage."

Updated terminology (eg, "eating style") eliminates the negative connotations inherent in that previously used (eg, "diet"). The authoritative manner is replaced with a conversational tone, and the importance of fitting nutrition into the client's lifestyle, rather than altering the client's lifestyle to fit nutrition, is a recurrent theme.

Section One is entitled "Principles of Nutrition." It begins with a new chapter, "Nutrition in Nursing," which focuses on why and how nutrition is important to nurses in all settings. Chapters that address carbohydrates, protein, lipids, vitamins, fluids and minerals, and energy metabolism and expenditure highlight basic nutrition information under the heading of "Keys to Understanding...." The second part of each chapter presents health promotion topics and demonstrates practical application of essential information. Examples of topics covered include criteria to consider when buying a vitamin supplement, the advantages/disadvantages of fat replacers, and fat-burning supplements promoted to increase performance among athletes.

Section Two, "Nutrition in Health Promotion," presents guidelines for healthy eating, such as the Dietary Guidelines for Americans, Canada's Guidelines for Healthy Eating, and the American Cancer Society's nutrition recommendations to reduce the risk of cancer. Criteria used to assess nutritional status and needs are introduced. Information on cultural influences on food choices has been expanded into its own chapter. Nutritional needs associated with the life cycle are discussed in chapters devoted to pregnant and lactating women, children and adolescents, and adults and older adults.

Section Three, "Nutrition in Clinical Practice," presents nutrition therapy for obesity and eating disorders, enteral and parenteral nutrition, protein-calorie malnutrition and stress, gastrointestinal disorders, cardiovascular disorders, diabetes, renal disorders, and cancer and HIV/AIDS. The fact that every disorder is not presented within the framework of the nursing process is a major organizational change in this edition. Although pathophysiology is downplayed somewhat in this edition, it has been tightly focused within the context of nutrition.

My bias as a dietitian and nutrition educator leads me to believe that all information presented in this edition is equally important. Yet, from a nursing perspective, some topics will be more meaningful than others, simply because they facilitate patient care or behavior change. As such, the student may find that some sections are particularly useful, including:

- "Tips on . . . ," which are featured throughout the book. Examples include Tips on Eating Out (Chapter 18), Tips for Reducing Calories (Chapter 7), and Tips for Healthy Eating During Pregnancy (Chapter 11).
- Nutrition-focused assessment criteria in each clinical chapter
- Criteria presented in a question form, which challenges students to understand the interrelationship between nutrition and laboratory values, physical findings, eating habits, and medical–socioeconomic status
- Nursing process cases that illustrate assessment and teaching points
- Internet addresses that enable the student to gather more detailed information or direct the client to valuable resources
- The recurring use of the Food Guide Pyramid as a teaching/assessment tool for a variety of clients, such as pregnant women, older adults, and obese people

Certain topics are new to this edition, including a discussion of herbs and supplements to maintain or improve health and the DASH diet for the prevention and treatment of hypertension. The old Recommended Dietary Allowances are evolving into new reference standards, which are discussed throughout the text. In addition, the text includes:

- The fifth revision of the Dietary Guidelines for Americans
- An emphasis on the health benefits of activity even if and when weight loss is not desired
- The new guidelines for the treatment of obesity

Acknowledgments

This book is the product of combined efforts by many dedicated and creative professionals at Lippincott Williams & Wilkins: Ilze Rader, Claudia Vaughn, Jane Velker, Danielle DiPalma, Carol Loyd, Nicole Walz, and Brett MacNaughton. I humbly acknowledge that because of their support and talents, I am able to do what I love—write, create, teach, and learn. On a personal level, I am thankful for the extra time and space they gave me to complete this project during a difficult time in my life. They have my utmost respect and gratitude.

I especially thank:

Ilze Rader, who provided the vision and impetus to overhaul the content, style, and design of this book. From the new title to the expansion of color, Ilze was the change-agent, challenging me to step outside of my comfort zone to rethink and redo.

The reviewers of the third and fourth editions, whose thoughtful comments and suggestions helped guide the evolution of this text into a new and improved edition.

My friends, parents, and family for their support and encouragement, particularly my children, Chris, Kait, and Kara, for the sacrifices they made so I could "work on the book."

Contents

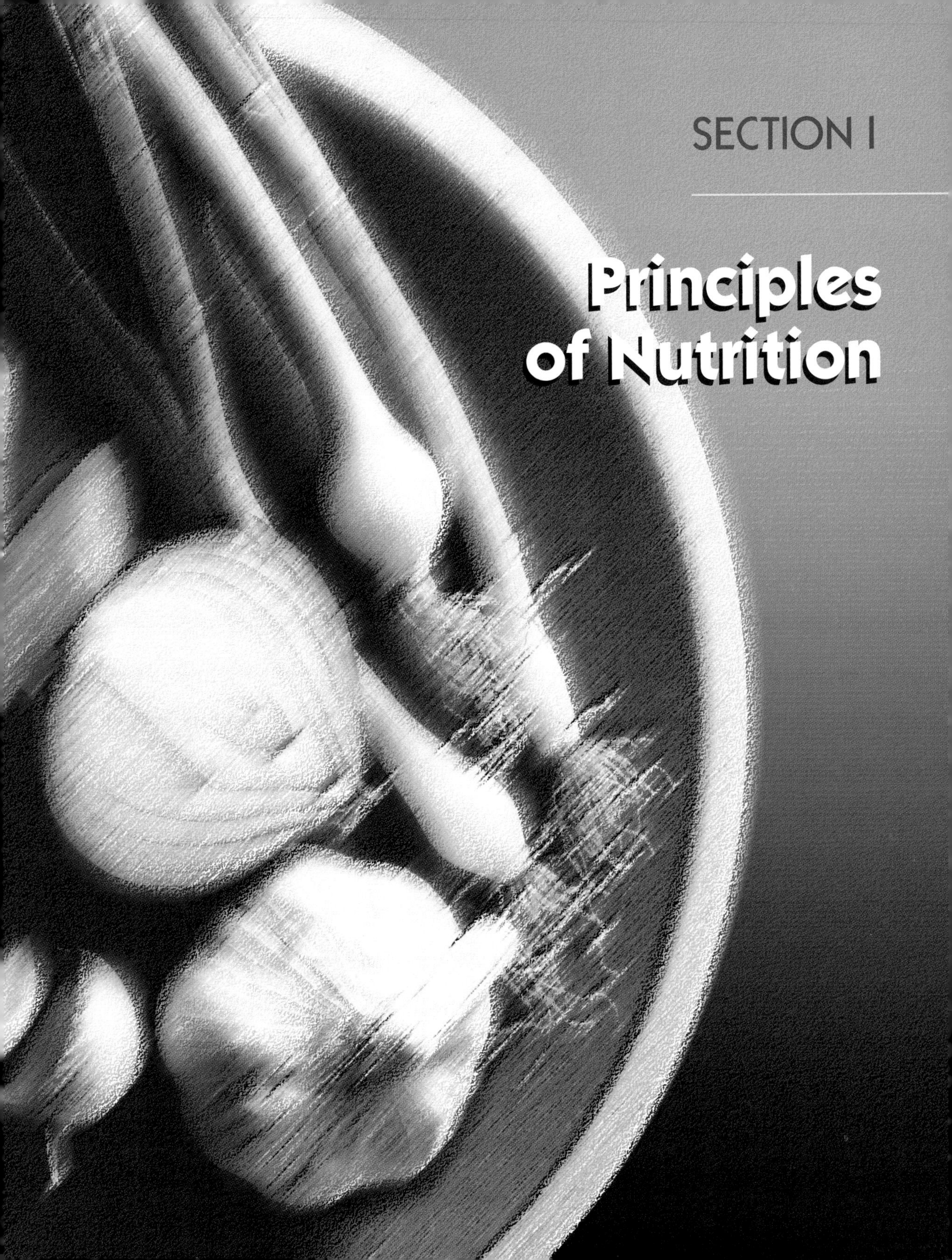

SECTION I

Principles of Nutrition

CHAPTER 1

Nutrition in Nursing

TRUE	FALSE	Check your knowledge of nutrition in nursing.
☐	☐	1 The nurse's role in nutrition is to call the dietitian.
☐	☐	2 For most people, the most important consideration when choosing foods is nutritional value.
☐	☐	3 The first three letters of diet are "die," and that's what people feel like doing when they hear they're going to be on a diet.
☐	☐	4 Written handouts that list "foods to avoid" and "foods to choose" are valuable teaching tools because they provide explicit do's and don'ts.
☐	☐	5 If a food misconception is harmless, it should be respected.

Upon completion of this chapter, you will be able to

- Discuss why clients are often confused about nutrition messages.
- Describe how nutritional care can be approached using the nursing care process.
- Discuss alternatives to the term "diet" and why they should be used.
- Describe questions to consider to discern the reliability and validity of nutrition information.
- List six warning signals that may indicate a nutrition or health claim is not credible.
- Explain the qualities of sensitivity, objectivity, and creativity in debunking nutrition misinformation.

Introduction

It is a new age in nutrition. The proliferation of cyberspace information—and misinformation—gives millions of Americans ready access to nutritional concepts. Advances in food technology have brought us food irradiation, "functional foods," and the discovery of phytochemicals, as well as new questions about food safety and optimal nutrition. The ever-evolving science of nutrition has taken us from three square meals a day and a well-rounded diet to the Food Guide Pyramid. A baby boomer–inspired quest for health and eternal youth has thrust nutrition into the spotlight, not only as a means to prevent chronic health problems but as a way to enhance quality of life. It is an age that presents both old and new challenges for health professionals.

Today, people know more and more about nutrition but less and less about food. Consider the issue of reducing fat intake. Over the last 20 years and from every direction, Americans have gotten the message to eat less fat, but they're unsure how to do that in terms of food choices, serving sizes, and recipes. In their black-or-white view, fat is "bad" rather than a shade of gray that varies with what kind, how much, and how often it is eaten. They are confused about which is better: butter or margarine, olive oil or canola. They misapply the guideline of "30% of calories from fat" to individual foods rather than the total day's intake as intended. To many, "fat free" on the label gives them leave to eat the whole package. They are unaware that low fat is only one aspect of healthy eating, or that eating more fruits, vegetables, and whole grains may be as important as cutting fat. They are hopeful that the supplement advertised to block fat absorption from food will let them enjoy cheesecake without guilt. In short, Americans recognize that nutrition is important but are baffled about what to eat.

Some of the confusion stems from the fact that nutritional considerations are not the primary factor in making food choices—taste is. To many people, "low fat" is synonymous with "no taste," and perceived lack of taste is the biggest obstacle to healthy eating. Convenience is another important consideration in food choices. People who believe fast food is more convenient than fruits and vegetables eat fast food more often. To many people, choices are absolute: tasty or healthy, convenient or time-consuming. People need to understand that tasty and healthy are not mutually exclusive food traits; they need to learn quick and easy ways to add healthy foods to an eating plan.

Although its not as simple as "one diet fits all," nutrition guidelines issued by leading health authorities to promote wellness are remarkably similar: eat less fat, saturated fat, and sodium; avoid obesity; eat more complex carbohydrates and fiber; use alcohol moderately, if at all. It's not *what* to do, but *how* to do it that is the problem. How do I avoid sodium when I rely on boxes, mixes, and cans to prepare quick and easy meals? How do I get enough calcium if I don't like milk? How can I eat healthy when I eat out? Which is more important for weight control: calories or fat grams? If I don't like vegetables, can I just eat more fruit? How can I get enough fiber if the only bread I eat is white? Although nutrition guidelines are consistent, they generate an abundance of diverse questions.

Compared with "well" clients, patients in a clinical setting may be more motivated to follow nutritional advice, especially if they feel better by doing so or are fearful of a relapse or complications. But hospitalized patients are also prone to confusion about nutrition messages. Time spent with a dietitian or diet technician learning about a "diet" may be brief or interrupted. Even if the "diet" represents a whole new eating style that is best achieved by making sequential changes, nutrition counseling in the hospital is often limited to one or two sessions with the dietitian. The patient may not even know what questions to ask until long after the dietitian is gone. The patient's ability to assimilate new information may be compromised by pain, medication, anxiety, or a distracting setting. Hospital menus or diets that differ from discharge orders add to the confusion. Because the nurse is the team member who has the greatest contact with the patient, family, and other team members, he or she is an ideal candidate to provide ongoing tidbits of nutrition information to fill in knowledge gaps and sustain the patient's motivation.

This chapter focuses on the importance of nutrition in nursing practice. The *nursing process* is used to illustrate how nutrition is integrated into nursing in the real world. The nurse's credibility in regard to nutrition is enhanced when he or she is well informed, discriminates between nutrition fact and fiction, and combats misinformation. Real-life situations are described to show practical application.

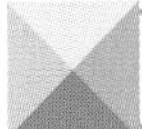

Nutritional Care Process

What does the client need? What can you or others do to effectively and efficiently help the client meet his or her needs? What criteria will you use to judge success? These and similar questions are the foundation of the decision-making process, whether the focus is on general nursing or specifically on nutrition.

ASSESSMENT

Assessment is a two-step process of gathering and interpreting data to determine the client's nutritional status and identify problems. Accurate assessment is essential so that appropriate interventions can be implemented and later evaluated for their effectiveness. The extent of assessment varies widely among settings and clients. Assessment is quick and specific at a worksite cholesterol screening but methodical and thorough in a hospital burn unit. Nursing histories and physical examinations provide a variety of data to assess nutritional status and needs. Laboratory data add more information. Keep in mind that it is not necessary to examine all data for every client. For instance, it is not necessary to assess abdominal girth in a hospice client with terminal cancer. Chapter 9 discusses nutritional assessment.

Historical Data

Historical data with nutritional implications include current and past health history, intake information, weight history, medication use, and other pertinent information.

Current and past health history that may affect intake or nutritional status includes such things as whether the client:

- Has a medical condition that may benefit from nutrition therapy, such as diabetes or hypertension
- Has physical complaints that interfere with intake or nutrient use, such as difficulty chewing and swallowing, heartburn, nausea, vomiting, or diarrhea

Intake information examines the client's usual intake to help identify potential and actual conditions related to intake. The client interview can reveal whether the client:

- Has a poor appetite
- Eats alone
- Tries to follow a special diet
- Does not have enough food to eat each day
- Skips meals
- Does the shopping and cooking
- Frequently eats out
- Eliminates one or more food groups from the diet
- Has food allergies or intolerances
- Uses nutritional supplements
- Has difficulty chewing or swallowing
- Drinks alcohol daily (more than one drink for women, more than two drinks for men)
- Has an understanding of what he or she should be eating
- Is willing to make changes in eating habits

Weight history reveals whether the client has experienced significant unintentional weight loss.

Investigating medication use includes assessing prescribed, over-the-counter, and dietary supplements for their impact on nutritional status.

Other pertinent information that may affect nutritional status includes the following:

- Advanced age
- Use of tobacco or recreational drugs
- Frequency and intensity of physical activity
- Cultural, religious, or ethnic influences on food choices
- Adequacy of food budget
- Adequacy of food storage and preparation facilities
- Social support

Physical Findings

Body measurements, such as height and weight, indirectly assess protein and calorie stores in adults.

Physical signs and symptoms of malnutrition that may be apparent on inspection include:

- Hair that is dull, brittle, dry, or falls out easily
- Swollen glands of the neck and cheeks
- Dry, rough, or spotty skin, which may have a sandpaper feel
- Poor or delayed wound healing or sores
- Thin appearance with lack of subcutaneous fat
- Muscle wasting (decreased size and strength)
- Edema of the lower extremities
- Weakened hand grasp
- Depressed mood
- Abnormal heart rate, heart rhythm, or blood pressure

- Enlarged liver or spleen
- Loss of balance and coordination

Laboratory Data

Biochemical data measure the body internally. Some laboratory data, such as the concentration of albumin, the major protein in the blood, are routinely evaluated to give a snapshot view of nutritional status. Other data are looked at on a case-specific basis. For instance, people with type 2 diabetes tend to have altered levels of fat in their blood, so for them it is important to check serum triglyceride and cholesterol levels. All abnormal values should be examined for their potential nutritional significance.

Evaluation

After the data have been collected, they are evaluated according to established normal standards (eg, laboratory values) so that goals can be formulated. For instance, body mass index can be calculated from the client's weight and height to evaluate whether the client is underweight, within a healthy weight range, or overweight. Interpretation of subjective data, such as the client's level of interest and motivation to change, relies on your experience and perception of verbal and nonverbal cues.

To make your assessments most effective, keep the following points in mind:

- **Focus is everything.** If your aim is to investigate inadequate weight gain during the third trimester of pregnancy, it is irrelevant and distracting to ask questions about whether the client uses white bread or wheat bread or drinks calcium-fortified orange juice. Know what you are looking for and formulate questions accordingly.
- **Keep your mind open and your questions open-ended.** A client may interpret the question "What do you eat for breakfast?" as "Breakfast is normal. You should eat breakfast. Tell me something breakfasty because nobody actually eats soup when they get up in the morning." A better question would be, "What is usually the first thing you eat during the day, and when do you eat it?" Even the term "meal" may elicit a stereotypical mental picture. Just as laboratory normal standards are not appropriate for all ages, races, and individuals, accepted "normal" eating plans may not be appropriate for all clients. Not everyone eats meat, and not everyone drinks milk, yet neither scenario inevitably means a deficient intake. Eating styles that deviate from the typical American intake should not be automatically deemed inadequate or in need of repair. Keep an open mind. Open-ended questions provide much more information than those that can be answered with a simple yes or no. The answer to the question "What kind of milk do you drink?" tells you much more than the answer to "Do you drink milk?" Allow the client to elaborate whenever possible.
- **The client's perception of need may differ from yours.** In matters that do not involve life or death, it is best to first address the client's concerns. Your primary consideration may be the patient's significant weight loss during the last 6 months of chemotherapy; the patient's major concern may be fatigue. The two is-

sues are undoubtedly related, but your effectiveness as a change agent is greater if you approach the problem from the client's perspective.

- **Avoid making assumptions.** Not all obese people are getting enough of all essential nutrients. Not all people with high serum cholesterol levels eat a high-fat diet. Not all people with long-standing diabetes know all there is to know about diet and exercise.

NURSING DIAGNOSIS

Based on the data collected and interpreted, actual or potential nutritional problems are stated in nursing diagnoses. Nursing diagnoses in hospitals and long-term care facilities provide written documentation of the client's status and serve as a framework for the plan of care that follows. The diagnoses relate directly to nutrition when altered nutrition is the problem, or indirectly when a change in intake will help manage a nonnutritional problem.

Some nursing diagnoses with nutritional relevance are the following:

- Altered nutrition: more than body requirements
- Altered nutrition: less than body requirements
- Altered nutrition: risk for more than body requirements
- Constipation
- Diarrhea
- Fluid volume excess
- Fluid volume deficit
- Risk for aspiration
- Altered oral mucous membrane
- Altered dentition
- Impaired skin integrity
- Noncompliance (with prescribed diet)
- Impaired swallowing
- Knowledge deficit (about nutrition therapy)
- Pain
- Nausea

In wellness settings, documentation may be informal, or, in the case of a one-time-only opportunity such as a community health fair, documentation may be nonexistent. In those instances, nursing diagnoses may be mentally noted but physically unwritten.

PLANNING AND IMPLEMENTATION

The steps in planning and implementation include setting priorities, formulating goals, and determining what nursing actions are needed to help the client achieve those goals. Although planning for high-risk clients is the dietitian's responsibility, the nurse may plan for healthy clients and for those at low or mild risk for nutritional problems.

Setting Priorities

Based on Maslow's Hierarchy of Needs, food and nutrition rank on the same level as air as basic necessities of life. Obviously, without food, death eventually occurs. Less intense nutritional inadequacies have less intense outcomes. In the hospital setting, clients with poor nutritional status experience prolonged or complicated recovery from illness, and their responses to medical treatments and drug therapies are diminished. Among well clients, suboptimal nutrition can lead to fatigue, weakness, and other nonspecific complaints. Therefore, a priority for all clients is to consume or obtain adequate calories and nutrients based on their own individual needs. Sometimes it is necessary to prioritize among nutrients. The priority for a nursing home resident with heart disease who is experiencing significant weight loss is not to maintain a low-fat diet but to increase calories (even with more fat) so as to halt or reverse the weight loss. Equally important is that those calories and nutrients must be in a usable form: clients get little benefit from food they cannot digest and absorb. Finally, because food nourishes the soul as well as the body, it is a priority to provide calories and nutrients through foods that are familiar to and liked by the client, whenever possible.

It is also essential to prioritize what the client needs to learn about nutrition. The client who is a newly diagnosed type 2 diabetic with irregular eating habits, a high cholesterol level, obesity, and osteoporosis has many nutritional concerns. Rather than suggest that he or she avoid sugar, time meals consistently, cut fat, limit red meat intake, switch to soft margarine, eat more vegetables, use canola oil, eat oatmeal, and drink more milk, it is better to prioritize: establishing a regular eating pattern and simply reducing portions are the most important first steps.

Formulating Goals

Goals should be measurable, attainable, specific, and client-centered. How do you measure success against a vague goal of "gain weight by eating better"? Is "eating better" achieved by adding butter to foods to increase calories or by substituting 1% milk for whole milk because it is heart-healthy? Is a 1-pound weight gain in 1 month acceptable, or is 1 pound/week preferable? Is 1 pound/week attainable if the client has accelerated metabolism and catabolism caused by third-degree burns?

Client-centered goals place the focus on the client, not the health care provider; they specify where the client is heading. Whenever possible, give the client the opportunity to actively participate in goal setting. This allows the client to "own" the goal, which greatly increases the commitment to achieving it.

Keep in mind that for all clients the goal is to maintain or restore optimal nutritional status using foods they like and tolerate, as appropriate. Additional short-term goals may be to alleviate symptoms or side effects of disease or treatments, if possible, and to prevent complications or recurrences, if appropriate. After short-term goals are met, attention can center on promoting healthy eating to reduce the risk of chronic diet-related diseases such as obesity, diabetes, hypertension, and atherosclerosis.

Examples of client-centered goals in a community-based weight management program are:

- Eat breakfast every day.
- On 3 days/week, replace the usual mid-morning snack of soda and a doughnut with sugar-free soda and a piece of fruit.
- Switch from regular margarine to diet margarine.
- Switch from whole milk to 2% milk.

Nursing Interventions

What can you or others do to effectively and efficiently help the client achieve his or her goals? Interventions may take the form of promoting an adequate and appropriate intake, teaching the client about nutrition, and monitoring the client's response.

Promoting an Adequate and Appropriate Intake

Throughout this book, the heading Nutrition Therapy is used in place of Diet Management, which was used in previous editions. To nurses and dietitians the change is subtle, because the definition of *diet* is "usual intake" or "normal eating pattern." But among clients, *diet* is a four-letter word with negative connotations such as counting calories, deprivation, sacrifice, and misery. A diet is viewed as a short-term punishment to endure until a normal pattern of eating can resume. Whether nutrition therapy recommendations are short- or long-term, clients respond better to newer terminology that is less emotionally charged. Use terms such as *eating pattern*, *food intake*, *eating style*, or *the food you eat* to keep the lines of communication open.

Nutrition therapy recommendations are usually general suggestions to increase/decrease, limit/avoid, reduce/encourage, or modify/maintain aspects of the diet, because exact nutrient requirements are determined on an individual basis. Where more precise amounts of nutrients are specified, consider them as a starting point and monitor the client's response.

Keep in mind that nutrition theory may not apply to practice. Factors such as the client's prognosis, outside support systems, level of intelligence and motivation, willingness to comply, emotional health, financial status, religious or ethnic background, and other medical conditions may cause the optimal diet to be impractical in either the clinical or the home setting. Generalizations do not apply to all individuals at all times. Also, comfort foods (eg, chicken soup, peanut butter, ice cream) are valuable for their emotional benefits if not nutritional ones. Honor clients' requests for individual comfort foods whenever possible.

Some nursing interventions to facilitate intake are:

- Encourage a big breakfast if appetite deteriorates throughout the day.
- Advocate discontinuation of intravenous therapy as soon as feasible.
- Replace meals withheld for diagnostic tests.
- Promote congregate dining if appropriate.
- Question diet orders that appear inappropriate.

- Display a positive attitude when serving food or discussing nutrition.
- Order snacks and nutritional supplements.
- Request assistance with feeding or meal setup.
- Get the patient out of bed to eat if possible.
- Encourage good oral hygiene.
- Solicit information on food preferences.

Client Teaching

Teaching involves not only imparting knowledge but also counseling the client to help bring about a change in eating behaviors. A client with newly diagnosed type 1 diabetes needs to know (be taught) that three meals plus two planned snacks must be eaten daily to match the peaks in insulin action. If such a client dislikes typical breakfast food and is pressed for time in the morning, he or she needs help to figure out (through counseling) what types and amounts of quick and easy foods can be eaten and are appealing. The counselor provides an adequate knowledge base and then "brainstorms" with the client on how to translate knowledge into behaviors that will work for that individual.

Nutrition counseling by nurses *and* dietitians is more effective and efficient than that done by nurses *or* dietitians. First of all, nurses are often available as a nutrition resource when dietitians are not, such as when trays are passed, during the evening, on weekends, and when the client is sitting on the edge of the bed fully dressed and waiting for transport home. In home care and wellness settings, dietitians may be available only on a consultative basis. Secondly, nurses reinforce nutrition counseling performed by dietitians: the more the message is repeated and the more people tell it, the more likely the message will stick. Finally, nurses initiate basic nutrition counseling for hospitalized clients with low to mild risk who otherwise may not be given such information. The nurse has greatest contact with the client, family, and other members of the health care team; the dietitian has nutrition and food expertise. Together, the nurse and dietitian form a strong alliance.

As an example, consider a male client of normal weight who is admitted to the hospital because of difficulty breathing. According to nutritional screening data, he is not at nutritional risk. You find that although his weight is within the normal range, he experienced progressive weight loss before admission because of shortness of breath and fatigue that interfered with eating. You seize the opportunity to suggest protein- and calorie-dense foods that are easy to prepare and consume, such as instant breakfast made with whole milk, yogurt with cereal, whole-milk fruit smoothies, and cottage cheese with canned fruit. You also suggest that the client eat or drink every 2 hours. He admits that he considered this idea before but rejected it because he thought it would interfere with his appetite. You reassure him that planned nutritious snacks will add to rather than detract from his eating plan. You ask the dietitian to see the client in case there are other concerns or misconceptions. Without your intervention, his weight loss probably would have continued, increasing the risk of future health problems.

Some nursing interventions to facilitate client and family teaching are:

- Listen to the client's concerns and ideas.
- Encourage family involvement if appropriate.

- Reinforce the importance of obtaining adequate nutrition.
- Reassure clients who are apprehensive about eating.
- Help the client select appropriate foods.
- Counsel the client about drug-nutrient interactions.
- Avoid using the term "diet."
- Emphasize things "to do" instead of things "not to do."
- Keep the message simple.
- Review written handouts with the client.
- Advise the client to avoid any foods that are not tolerated.

Monitoring

Think of monitoring as a precursor to evaluation in which you watch and document the impact of interventions on the client on an ongoing basis so that immediate concerns can be quickly addressed.

For example, after counseling a female employee at a worksite on how to manage mild hypertension through food choices and exercise, you suggest she stop by the health office every day during her lunch break so that you can take her blood pressure. During those visits you ask her specific questions: How many meatballs did you eat with your spaghetti last night? Was the sauce labeled "reduced sodium"? Did you double your normal portion of vegetables? What kind of milk are you drinking? How much exercise did you do yesterday? Her answers help you determine how well she understands the counseling information and how successfully she is implementing the strategies to achieve her goals. Talking about specific foods is likely to stimulate discussion that provides the client with more information, more options, or revised goals.

Ideally, behavior change occurs gradually and sequentially to become part of the client's new normal way of eating. In a less than perfect, time-challenged world, it is necessary to prioritize the client's needs and address the most important ones.

Nurses are in an ideal position to:

- Monitor intake.
- Document appetite and take action when the client does not eat.
- Assess tolerance (ie, absence of side effects).
- Monitor progress (eg, weight gain).
- Monitor progression of restrictive diets.
- Monitor the client's grasp of the information and motivation to change.

EVALUATION

The optimal outcome of interventions is that the client's goals are completely met on a timely basis. But goals may be only partially met or not achieved at all, and in those instances it is important to determine why the outcome was less than ideal. Were the goals realistic for this particular client? Were the interventions appropriate and consistently implemented? Evaluation includes deciding whether to continue, change, or abolish the plan.

Consider a male client admitted to the hospital for chronic diarrhea. During the 3 weeks before admission, the client experienced significant weight loss due to malabsorption secondary to diarrhea. Your goal is for the client to maintain his admission weight. Your interventions are to provide small meals of low-residue foods as ordered, to eliminate lactose because of the likelihood of intolerance, to increase protein and calories with appropriate nutrient-dense supplements, and to explain the nutrition therapy recommendations to the client to ease his concerns about eating. You find that the client's intake is poor because of lack of appetite and a fear that consumption of foods and fluids will promote diarrhea. You notify the dietitian, who counsels the client about low-residue foods, obtains likes and dislikes, and urges the client to think of the supplements as part of the medical treatment, not as a food eaten for taste or pleasure. You document intake and diligently encourage the client to eat and drink everything served. However, the client's weight continues to drop. You attribute this to his reluctance to eat and to the slow resolution of diarrhea due to inflammation. You determine that the goal is still realistic and appropriate but that the client is not willing or able to consume foods orally. You consult with the physician and dietitian about the client's refusal to eat, and the plan changes from an oral diet to tube feeding.

As team players, nurses can:

- Communicate with the registered dietitian (RD).
- Serve as a liaison between the physician and the RD.
- Identify clients who may benefit from programs such as Meals on Wheels.
- Request a referral to a speech therapist.
- Confer with the discharge planner, social services worker, and physical or occupational therapist.

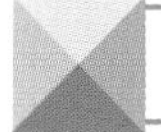

Nutrition in Health Promotion

BEING WELL INFORMED

Nutrition is a hot topic that sells. It is featured on radio talk shows and television news programs. Controversial results from new "studies" claim headlines in newspapers and magazines and lend themselves to best-selling books. The World Wide Web provides instant access to both reliable and junk science. Americans spend billions of dollars each year on nutritional supplements, and tens of billions annually on weight loss products. Everyone from celebrities to next-door neighbors knows something about nutrition—and probably knows more fallacies than facts.

It is said that the half-life of nutrition information is 3 years. In other words, 3 years from now, half of what we know about nutrition today will be out of date. Some "facts" are relatively solid but are disproved after years of studies. For instance, it was long believed that monounsaturated fats had neither a positive nor a negative effect on heart disease. Today we know that monounsaturated fats are heart-healthy and should provide the majority of fat calories in a person's diet. Other "facts" come and go more quickly, like the oat bran craze of the early 1980s. It is important to stay current, because today's facts may be tomorrow's fiction.

DISCRIMINATING BETWEEN FACT AND FICTION

To protect yourself and your clients from misinformation, be cautious and skeptical about what you hear and read about nutrition (Box 1–1). Resist jumping on the latest bandwagon until all the evidence is critically examined. Keep in mind that headlines sell, but the bottom line, which is usually less sensational, may be buried deep in the article, the part least likely to be read. Ask yourself the age-old questions—who, what, when, where, and why—to test the validity and reliability of nutrition "news."

- **Who?** Who is promoting the message? The name may or may not be important. A celebrity attracts more attention than an unknown spokesperson but may be equally unfit to summarize nutrition reports or provide nutrition advice. Investigate the validity of the author's or web site's credentials. A "doctor" with a scientific breakthrough on how to combine foods to speed metabolism may be a doctor of education, theology, or economics. A supplement manufacturer whose web site promotes the anti-aging effects of vitamin E is not the best authority on the subject. Look for ethical conflicts of interest. Anyone who stands to benefit economically by promoting a food, supplement, or diet is not likely to be an objective resource.
- **What?** What is the message? Box 1–1 lists the Food and Nutrition Science Alliance (FANSA) warning signals that may indicate a study or nutrition report is less than credible.

BOX 1.1

Ten Warning Signs That What You Read or Hear May Not Be Credible

1. Promise of a quick fix
2. Warnings of imminent danger from a product or regimen
3. It sounds too good to be true
4. Simple conclusions from a complex study
5. Makes recommendations based on a single study
6. Makes statements that are refuted by reputable scientific organizations
7. Promotes the idea of "good" and "bad" foods
8. Recommendations help sell a product
9. Recommendations are from published studies that were not peer-reviewed
10. Recommendations are from studies that ignore individual and group differences

Source: Food and Nutrition Science Alliance (FANSA). (1995). *Junk science: Scientists issue 10 red flags for consumers*. www.lft.org/resource/news/news_rel/ FANSA/sc_h03.shtml.

- **When?** When was the study conducted, the results published, the web site updated? Even seemingly legitimate information can become quickly outdated. As previously stated, 3 years is a long time in the life of nutrition data.
- **Where?** Where was the study conducted? Was the site a reputable research institution or an impressive-sounding but unknown facility? Internet addresses ending in .edu (educational institutions), .org (organizations), or .gov (government agencies) are more credible than those ending in .com (commercial), whose main objective may be to sell a product.
- **Why?** Is the purpose of the article or web site to further the reader's awareness and knowledge or to sell or promote a product? Freedom of speech guarantees Americans the right to express opinions about nutrition, but fraudulent claims cannot be used to advertise a product. Magazines and newsletters that blur the lines between articles and advertisements are misleading but legal. Question objectivity when the author or site has a financial interest in a supposed "breakthrough."

COMBATING NUTRITION MISINFORMATION

Determining whether information is valid and reliable may be easier than persuading a client that he or she has been a victim of hype. Many people assume that anything that appears in print form (eg, in a book, magazine, or newspaper) is accurate. Not everyone recognizes the shortcomings of the World Wide Web. Smaller still is the number of people who acknowledge their susceptibility to nutrition fraud. Battling misinformation in a client convinced he or she has the facts requires objectivity, sensitivity, and creativity.

- **Objectivity.** First of all, the motto is "Do no harm." If clients' beliefs are unsupported but harmless, you may risk alienating them for no reason by waging a war to convince them they're misinformed. For instance, a male client who believes that using wheat germ will increase his libido nevertheless gets risk-free benefits from the fiber, vitamin E, and other nutrients in the wheat germ he consumes. Even though wheat germ does not objectively enhance sexual performance, the placebo effect may accomplish the same result. Respect harmless food beliefs that do not financially exploit the client.
- **Sensitivity.** Be sensitive to the client's perspective. Determine how much of an emotional investment the client has in believing the misinformation. Casual or judgmental dismissal of misinformation can cause clients to become defensive and distrustful. They may conclude that you are not as up-to-date as they are about nutrition and reject you as a credible reference. Use reputable facts, be brief, and keep the message simple.
- **Creativity.** Provide verbal or written documentation about the true facts. Furnish a list of reputable nutrition resources. Box 1–2 lists web sites that are sources of reliable nutrition information. Refer the client to the American Dietetic Association hot line or local dietetic association.

BOX 1.2

Internet Addresses of Some Reliable Nutrition Resources

American Cancer Society
www.cancer.org

American Diabetes Association
www.diabetes.org

American Dietetic Association
www.eatright.org

Cancer Net, National Cancer Institute, National Institutes of Health
www.nci.nih.gov

Center for Nutrition Policy and Promotion, U.S. Department of Agriculture
www.usda.gov/cnpp/

U.S. Department of Health and Human Services Healthfinder
www.healthfinder.gov

U.S. Food and Drug Administration
www.fda.gov

Food and Nutrition Information Center, National Agricultural Center, U.S. Department of Agriculture
www.nal.usda.gov/fnic

Health On the Net Foundation
www.hon.ch

International Food Information Council
www.ificinfo.health.org

Mayo Clinic
www.mayohealth.org

National Council Against Health Fraud, Inc.
www.ncahf.org

National Heart, Lung, and Blood Institute, National Institutes of Health
www.nhlbi.nih.gov

Office of Disease Prevention and Health Promotion, U.S. Department of Health and Human Services
www.odphp.osophs.dhhs.gov

PubMed, National Library of Medicine
www.ncbi.nlm.nih.gov/Pubmed/

Tufts Nutrition Navigator
www.navigator.tufts.edu

World Health Organization
www.who.int

Questions You May Hear

Should I save my menus from the hospital to help me plan meals at home? This is not a bad idea if the in-house and discharge food plans are the same, but the menus should serve as a guide not a gospel. Just because shrimp was never on the menu doesn't mean it is taboo. Likewise, if the client hated the orange juice that was served every morning, he or she shouldn't feel compelled to continue drinking it. By necessity, hospital menus are more rigid than at-home eating plans.

Can you just tell me what to eat and I'll do it? A black-and-white approach should be used only when absolutely necessary, such as for food allergies or for clients who prefer to be told what to eat instead of being responsible for making their own decisions. In most cases, advice should be as flexible as possible, even if the client insists it is not necessary to individualize the eating plan for his or her particular eating pattern. Individualization requires more work, but it is worth the effort for the flexibility it provides. Impress on the client that, except in special conditions, foods are not inherently good or bad. What matters more is how much, what kind, and how often a food is eaten.

KEY CONCEPTS

- Nutrition is a field that is rapidly changing and growing. New challenges in nutrition stem from advances in food technology, the explosion of information available on the World Wide Web, and the aging baby-boom generation's quest for quality of life.
- Americans make food choices based on several factors, with taste primary. Cost, convenience, and nutritional considerations are less important. People who believe that a "good diet" is tasteless are not likely to make healthy changes in their food choices, at least not in the long term.
- All clients need "how-to" information to help them make better food choices that become part of their normal way of eating. Nurses are in an ideal position to offer clients and their families ongoing nutritional advice and support.
- Ask focused questions when gathering assessment data. An eating pattern that deviates from the typical American diet is not necessarily deficient or excessive.
- Be attuned to what the client's nutrition or food concerns are; they may be completely different from yours.
- Nursing diagnoses relate directly to nutrition when the client's intake of nutrients is too much or too little for body requirements. Many other nursing diagnoses, including constipation, impaired skin integrity, health-seeking behaviors, noncompliance, and risk for infection, relate indirectly to nutrition because nutrition contributes to the problem or solution.
- A nutrition priority for all clients is to obtain adequate calories and nutrients based on individual needs. Sometimes it is necessary to prioritize nutrient needs. Other priorities are to provide calories and nutrients in a form the client can use and, if possible, through foods that are familiar to and liked by the client.
- Short-term nutrition goals are to attain or maintain adequate weight and nutritional status and (as appropriate) to avoid nutrition-related symptoms and complications of illness. Long-term goals are to promote healthy eating so as to avoid chronic diet-

related diseases such as heart disease, hypertension, obesity, and type 2 diabetes. Help the client formulate nutrition goals that are measurable, attainable, and specific.

- The term *diet* inspires negative feelings in most people. Replace it with *eating pattern*, *eating style*, or *foods you normally eat* to avoid negative connotations.
- Keep in mind that intake recommendations are not always appropriate for all persons, that clients' needs change, that what is recommended in theory may not work for an individual, and that clients may revert to comfort foods during periods of illness or stress.
- The term *counseling* means teaching plus brainstorming to help the client understand *and implement* intake recommendations. Nurses can reinforce nutrition counseling done by the dietitian and initiate counseling for clients with low or mild risk.
- Use preprinted lists of "do's and don'ts" only if absolutely necessary, such as in the case of celiac disease. For most people, actual food choices should be considered in view of how much and how often they are eaten, rather than as foods that "must" or "must not" be consumed.
- Ask who, what, when, where, and why to judge the validity and reliability of nutrition "news." Mental alarms should ring when claims sound too good to be true, when foods are listed as "good" or "bad," when the recommendations promise a quick fix, and when the recommendations are intended to help sell a product.
- Nutrition misinformation is everywhere and can be difficult to refute in a client who is convinced that what he or she knows is accurate. Use objectivity, sensitivity, and creativity.

ANSWER KEY

1. **FALSE** The nurse is in an ideal position to provide nutrition information to patients and their families since he or she is the one with the greatest client contact.
2. **FALSE** Nutrition is not the primary consideration in making food choices; taste is.
3. **TRUE** The term "diet" has negative connotations for many people.
4. **FALSE** Specific lists of foods to choose and foods to avoid should be used only if absolutely necessary. It is important to focus on the quantity and frequency of foods consumed rather than absolute "do's" and "don'ts."
5. **TRUE** If a patient's misconception about food is harmless, it is important to respect that belief.

REFERENCES

American Dietetic Association. (1995). Position of the American Dietetic Association: Food and nutrition misinformation. *J Am Diet Assoc*, 95(6), 705–707.

The American Dietetic Association's complete food and nutrition guide. (1998). Minneapolis, MN: Chronimed Publishing.

Kratina K. King & N. Hayes D. (1996). *Moving away from diets*. Lake Dallas, TX: Helm Seminars Publishing.

Maslow, A. (1968). *Toward a psychology of being* (2nd ed.). New York: Von Nostrand.

Robbers J., & Tyler V. (1999). *Herbs of choice*. Binghamton, NY: The Haworth Press.

Vozenilek G. (1998). The wheat from the chaff: Sorting out nutrition information on the Internet. *J Am Diet Assoc*, 98(11), 1270–1272.

CHAPTER 2

Carbohydrates

TRUE	FALSE	Check your knowledge of carbohydrates.
		1 Bread is just as likely as candy to cause cavities.
		2 Artifically sweetened mints are less likely to cause cavities than sugar sweetened mints.
		3 A high sugar intake is worse than a high fat intake.
		4 The fibers in wheat bran help lower serum cholesterol levels.
		5 The predominate fibers in oats and fruit help slow glucose absorption.
		6 Carbonated beverages contribute more added sugars to the typical American diet than any other food or beverage.
		7 The sugar in fruit is better for you than the sugar in candy.
		8 The sugar content on food labels refers to added sugars only, not those that are naturally present in the food.
		9 Cornflakes have a greater effect on blood glucose levels than ice cream.
		10 When carbohydrate intake is inadequate, protein from the diet or body tissue is broken down for energy.

Upon completion of this chapter, you will be able to

- Name the types of carbohydrates and sources of each.
- Discuss the differences between refined and whole grains.
- Discuss the Nutrition Facts label as it applies to carbohydrates.
- Explain ways to limit sugar intake.
- Describe ways to increase fiber intake.
- Discuss the benefits and disadvantages of using nonnutritive sweeteners.
- Explain guidelines to help clients consume 50% to 60% of their calories from carbohydrates.

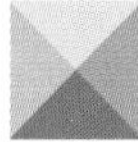

Keys to Understanding Carbohydrates

Carbohydrates are a family of compounds that consists of **simple carbohydrates** and **complex carbohydrates**, commonly referred to as "sugars" and "starches," respectively. Simple carbohydrates include *monosaccharides* (one sugar molecule) and *disaccharides* (two sugar molecules). Starch, glycogen, and fiber are examples of complex carbohydrates, or *polysaccharides* (many sugar molecules).

MONOSACCHARIDES

Glucose, fructose, and galactose are the most common monosaccharides, or single-sugar units. Each molecule contains 6 carbon atoms, 12 hydrogen atoms, and 6 oxygen atoms. The differences in how their atoms are arranged account for their differences in sweetness. Fructose is the sweetest of all sugars, glucose is mildly sweet, and galactose is not sweet. Monosaccharides are absorbed without undergoing digestion.

- **Glucose** (dextrose) is found naturally in fruits, vegetables, honey, and corn syrup and is made commercially from the hydrolysis of cornstarch. Glucose is extremely important in that it is a component of all disaccharides and is virtually the sole component of complex carbohydrates. The liver converts fructose and galactose to glucose.
- **Fructose** ("fruit sugar") is found naturally in fruit and honey and is added to many foods in the form of crystalline (granulated) fructose or high-fructose corn syrup (HFCS). Crystalline fructose, which looks and tastes like regular table sugar, is made commercially from cornstarch. HFCS is a blend of glucose and fructose; it is made commercially from the dextrose in cornstarch. When used together, fructose synergistically increases the sweetness of sucrose and artificial sweeteners. Because fructose is used extensively in soft drinks, fruit drinks, baked foods, and other products, the intake of fructose as a proportion of total sugars is rising.
- **Galactose** does not occur in appreciable amounts in foods. The significance of galactose is that it combines with glucose to form the disaccharide lactose.

DISACCHARIDES

Sucrose, maltose, and lactose are *disaccharides* ("double sugars"); each is composed of two monosaccharides, at least one of which is glucose. Disaccharides are digested into their component monosaccharides before being absorbed.

- **Sucrose,** formed from glucose and fructose, is what is commonly called "sugar" or table sugar; small amounts occur naturally in some fruits and vegetables. Sugar is produced when sucrose from sugarcane and sugar beets is refined and granulated. The differences among brown, white, confectioner's, and turbinado sugars have to do with the degree of refining. Sucrose is sweeter than glucose but not as sweet as fructose.

- **Maltose** is composed of two glucose molecules joined together. Maltose is not found naturally in foods, but it occurs as an intermediate in starch digestion.
- **Lactose** ("milk sugar") is composed of glucose and galactose. It is found naturally in milk and is used as an additive in many foods and drugs. Lactose enhances the absorption of calcium and promotes the growth of friendly intestinal bacteria that produce vitamin K. Lactose is not sweet.

POLYSACCHARIDES

Complex carbohydrates, also known as polysaccharides, include starch, glycogen, and fiber. Polysaccharides do not taste sweet because their molecules are too large to fit on the tongue's taste bud receptors that sense sweetness.

- **Starch,** the storage form of glucose in plants, is composed of hundreds to thousands of glucose molecules joined together. Starch is found only in plant foods, and it is most abundant in grains, legumes, and starchy vegetables such as corn and potatoes. Fruit provides only small amounts of starch: starch is converted to sugar as fruit ripens, which is why fruit tastes sweeter as it matures. The opposite is true of vegetables: mature vegetables taste less sweet than young vegetables because sugars have been converted to starches.
- **Glycogen.** Animals and humans store a limited amount of excess glucose in the form of glycogen located in the liver and muscles. Liver glycogen breaks down and releases glucose into the bloodstream between meals to maintain normal blood glucose levels and provide fuel for tissues. Muscles do not share their supply of glycogen but use it for their own energy needs. There is virtually no dietary source of glycogen, because any glycogen stored in animal tissue is quickly converted to lactic acid at the time of slaughter.
- **Fiber,** commonly referred to as "roughage" or "residue," is a generic term for a diverse group of polysaccharides that provide structure to plants. Unlike starch, the chains of sugar molecules that make up fibers cannot be broken down into monosaccharides by human enzymes. Despite being indigestible, fibers have important physiologic functions and provide significant health benefits. All sources of fiber provide a blend of both water-insoluble and water-soluble fibers.
  - **Insoluble fibers** include cellulose, many hemicelluloses, and lignins. They give texture to plant foods; they are found in the skin of fruits, the shell of corn kernels, the covering of seeds, and the bran (outer layer) of grains. Insoluble fibers increase fecal weight, speed transit time through the intestines, and prevent or relieve constipation. The richest sources of insoluble fiber are wheat bran, whole grains, dried peas and beans (legumes), and vegetables.
  - **Soluble fibers** include gums, pectins, some hemicelluloses, and mucilages. They dissolve to a gummy, viscous texture. Soluble fibers slow gastric emptying and the movement of chyme through the intestines, delay the absorption of

glucose from the small intestine, and lower elevated blood cholesterol concentrations. Fruits, oats, barley, and legumes are the best sources of soluble fibers.

HOW THE BODY HANDLES CARBOHYDRATES

Digestion

Monosaccharides are the only form of carbohydrates the body is able to absorb intact; all other digestible carbohydrates must be broken down to monosaccharides before they can be absorbed (Fig. 2–1). For disaccharides, digestion is accomplished by simply splitting the double sugars into single molecules. For starches, digestion proceeds step by step as the long glucose chains are ultimately reduced to single glucose units. The human gastrointestinal tract lacks the enzymes needed to digest fibers.

Cooked starch begins to undergo digestion in the mouth by the action of salivary amylase, but the overall effect is small because food is not held in the mouth for long. The stomach serves to churn and mix its contents, but its acid medium halts any residual effect of the swallowed amylase. Most carbohydrate digestion occurs in the small intestine, where pancreatic amylase works to reduce complex carbohydrates into shorter chains and disaccharides. Disaccharidase enzymes (maltase, sucrase, and lactase) on the surface of the cells of the small intestine finish the process of digestion by splitting maltose, sucrose, and lactose, respectively, into monosaccharides. Normally 95% of starch is digested, usually within 1 to 4 hours after eating.

Fibers are not digested but influence the speed of digestion. Soluble fibers delay gastric emptying, which contributes to a feeling of satiety or fullness. Although they are not truly digested by enzymes, most fibers are fermented by bacteria in the colon to produce water, gas, other compounds, and short-chain fatty acids. These short-chain fatty acids are a source of energy for the mucosal lining of the colon.

Absorption

Glucose, fructose, and galactose are absorbed through intestinal mucosa cells and travel to the liver via the portal vein. Small amounts of starch that have not been fully digested pass into the colon with fiber and are excreted in the stools. Fibers may impair the absorption of some minerals—namely calcium, zinc, and iron—by binding with them in the small intestine. Soluble fiber slows the absorption of glucose, thereby delaying and stifling the rise in serum glucose that occurs after eating.

Metabolism

Glucose, fructose, and galactose arrive at the liver via the portal vein; fructose and galactose are converted to glucose. The liver releases glucose into the bloodstream, where its level is held fairly constant by the action of hormones. A rise in blood glucose

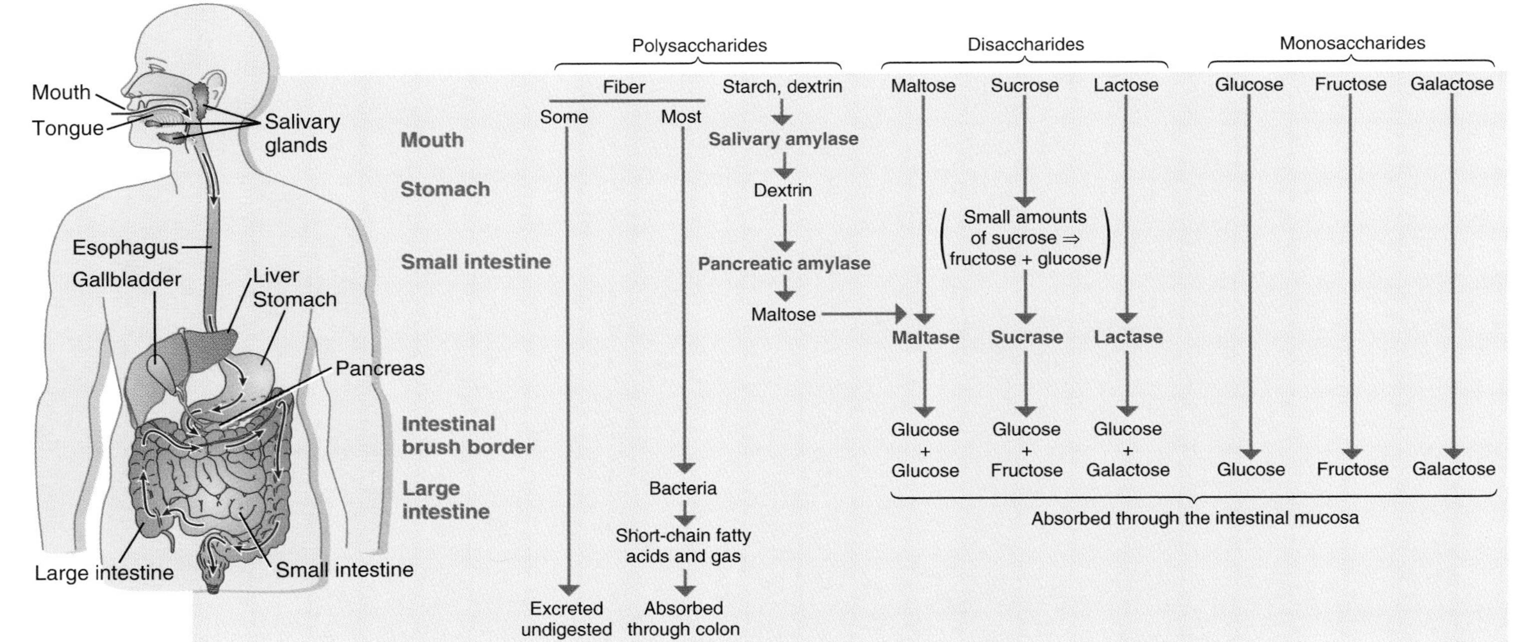

FIGURE 2-1 Carbohydrate digestion. Dietary carbohydrates include the polysaccharides or complex carbohydrates (fiber, starch, dextrin), the disaccharides (maltose, sucrose, lactose), and the monosaccharides (glucose, fructose, and galactose). Digestion begins in the *mouth,* where food is chewed into pieces and salivary amylase begins the process of chemical digestion. The *stomach* churns and mixes the carbohydrate, but stomach acids halt residual action of the salivary amylase. The *small intestine* is the site of most carbohydrate digestion, and pancreatic amylase reduces complex carbohydrates into disaccharides. Disaccharide enzymes (maltase, sucrase, and lactase) on the surface of the small intestine cells split maltose, sucrose, and lactose into monosaccharides, thus completing the process of carbohydrate digestion. Fiber is not digested per se, but most is fermented by bacteria in the *large intestine* to yield gas, water, and short-chain fatty acids.

concentration after eating causes the pancreas to secrete insulin, which moves glucose out of the bloodstream and into the cells. Most cells take only as much glucose as they need for immediate energy needs; muscle and liver cells take extra glucose to store as glycogen. The release of insulin lowers blood glucose to normal levels.

After a while, as the body uses up the energy from the last meal, the blood glucose concentration begin to drop. Even a slight fall in blood glucose stimulates the pancreas to release glucagon, which causes the liver to release glucose from its supply of glycogen. The result is that blood glucose levels increase to normal.

Insulin and glucagon are the major hormones responsible for regulation of blood glucose levels. When the blood glucose concentration rises after eating, the pancreas secretes insulin, which enables glucose to move from the bloodstream into cells. Glucagon is secreted by the pancreas in response to low blood glucose levels. It stimulates the breakdown of glycogen to release glucose into the blood.

Another hormone that influences blood glucose concentration is epinephrine, the "stress hormone" secreted by the adrenal gland. Epinephrine is quickly released during times of stress to make extra energy available for the "fight or flight" response. It works by stimulating the release of glucose from glycogen and inhibiting the secretion of insulin.

FUNCTIONS OF GLUCOSE

Glucose metabolism is a dynamic state of balance between burning glucose for energy (*catabolism*) and using glucose to build other compounds (*anabolism*). This process is a continuous response to the supply of glucose from food and the demand for glucose for energy needs.

Burning Glucose for Energy

First and foremost, glucose circulates in the bloodstream to serve as a ready source of energy for cells. Within the cell, the six-carbon glucose molecule is partially broken down into two three-carbon molecules (pyruvate) to yield energy in the form of adenosine triphosphate (ATP). This process is known as glycolysis; it produces only a fraction of the total energy available from glucose.

If more energy is needed and oxygen is available, catabolism continues as the pyruvate molecules lose a carbon atom to become the two-carbon compound acetate. (Although two pyruvate molecules can be reassembled to form glucose, the body cannot recreate glucose from acetate molecules; excess acetate molecules are made into fat.) Acetate continues through a series of complex reactions, such as the tricarboxylic acid cycle and the electron transport chain, to ultimately produce energy, carbon dioxide, and water. All digestible carbohydrates provide 4 cal/g consumed.

Glucose is the body's preferred fuel. It is burned more efficiently and more completely than either protein or fat, and it does not leave an end product that the body must excrete. Although muscles use a mixture of fat and glucose for energy, the brain, nervous tissue, and developing red blood cells rely exclusively on glucose for energy.

As part of its catabolic function, glucose plays a role in sparing protein and preventing ketosis.

Sparing Protein

The body's first priority when allocating calories is to meet its need for energy, preferably from glucose and fat (although not all body cells are able to use fat for energy). If adequate glucose is not available, the body uses dietary protein for energy. Protein used for energy is not available to do what only protein can do, such as replenish enzymes, hormones, blood cells, and hair. If still more calories are needed, typically because a very low-calorie, low-carbohydrate fad diet is consumed, the body resorts to breaking down its own protein tissue, both (1) to supply energy and (2) to reduce energy needs (muscle tissue is metabolically active and needs a steady supply of calories for maintenance). Conversely, an adequate carbohydrate intake "spares protein" from being used for energy. An adequate carbohydrate intake is especially important whenever protein needs are high, such as for wound healing and during pregnancy and lactation.

Preventing Ketosis

To efficiently and completely burn fat for energy, glucose fragments are needed. Without adequate glucose, fat oxidation prematurely stops at the intermediate step of ketone body formation. Although muscles and other tissues can use ketone bodies for energy, they are normally produced only in small quantities. An increased production of ketone bodies and their accumulation in the bloodstream causes nausea, fatigue, loss of appetite, and ketoacidosis. Dehydration and sodium depletion may follow as the body tries to excrete ketones in the urine. The rapid weight loss that is a characteristic result of low-carbohydrate fad diets is related to the loss of body fluids that occurs secondary to increased urinary excretion of ketones (from fat burning) and nitrogen (from use of protein for energy).

Using Glucose to Make Other Compounds

After energy needs are met, excess glucose can be converted to glycogen, used to make nonessential amino acids and specific body compounds, or converted to fat and stored.

Converted to Glycogen

The body's backup supply of glucose is liver glycogen. Liver and muscle cells pick up extra glucose molecules during times of plenty and join them together to form glycogen, which can quickly release glucose in time of need. Typically, one third of the body's glycogen reserve is in the liver and can be released into circulation for all body cells to use, and two thirds is in muscle, which is available only for use by muscles. Unlike fat, glycogen storage is limited and may provide only enough calories for about half a day of moderate activity.

Used to Make Nonessential Amino Acids

If an adequate supply of essential amino acids is available, the body can use them and glucose to make nonessential amino acids.

Used to Make Body Compounds That Contain Carbohydrates

The body can convert glucose to other essential carbohydrates, such as ribose, a component of ribonucleic acid (RNA) and deoxyribonucleic acid (DNA), keratan sulfate (in fingernails), and hyaluronic acid (found in the fluid that lubricates the joints and vitreous humor of the eyeball).

Converted to Fat

Any glucose remaining at this point—after energy needs are met, glycogen stores are saturated, and other specific compounds are made—is converted by liver cells to triglycerides and stored in the body's fat tissue. The body does this by combining acetate molecules to form fatty acids, which then are combined with glycerol to make triglycerides. Although it sounds easy for excess carbohydrates to be converted to fat, it is not a primary pathway; the body prefers to make body fat from dietary fat, not carbohydrates.

SOURCES OF CARBOHYDRATES

Carbohydrates are found in every one of the Food Guide Pyramid food groups (see Chapter 8). The amounts and types of carbohydrates vary considerably between food groups and among selections within each group. The inverted-triangle icons depicted in the Food Guide Pyramid represent added sugars, which are present to varying degrees in all groups except the Vegetable group and the Meat, Poultry, Fish, Dry Beans, Eggs, and Nuts group.

Bread, Cereal, Rice, and Pasta Group

The title of this group is synonymous with *grains*, the dietary staple in most civilizations throughout history: wheat, barley, oats, and rye in Europe; maize in North America; quinoa in South America; rice in Eastern cultures; and millet in Africa. This group provides complex carbohydrates together with some protein, and some selections contain fat. Fiber content is low in refined products, moderate in whole grains, and highest in bran products. This group represents the foundation of a healthy diet.

For many selections from this group, it is generally accepted that 1 serving provides approximately 15 g of carbohydrate. One serving is equal to 1 slice of bread; ½ cup cooked cereal, rice, or pasta; 1 ounce of ready-to-eat cereal; or ½ hamburger roll, bagel, or English muffin. This standard can be used to estimate carbohydrate intake, but it is not a precise measure. Some examples of the actual carbohydrate content of common selections from this group are

Grain Product	Portion	Carbohydrate (g)	Fiber (g)	Calories
White bread	1 slice	12.4	0.6	67
Whole wheat bread	1 slice	12.9	1.9	69
White rice	½ cup	22.3	0.3	104
Brown rice	½ cup	22.4	1.8	108
Egg noodles	½ cup	19.9	0.9	107
Whole wheat macaroni	½ cup	18.6	2.0	87
Cream of Wheat	½ cup	14.3	3.3	68
Wheatena	½ cup	13.8	0.9	67
Puffed wheat	1 oz	22.2	1.2	101
All-Bran cereal	1 oz	23.0	10.0	81

Surprisingly, this group also contains foods commonly considered "sweets," such as doughnuts, Danish pastries, cookies, cakes, and pies. Generally, these foods are made with refined flour, sugar, and fat; compared to the complex carbohydrates, they provide less fiber and micronutrients, more sugar, and more fat.

"Sweet" Grain Product	Portion	Carbohydrate (g)	Fiber (g)	Calories
Doughnut	½ medium	11.7	0.4	99
Danish pastry	½ medium	14.5	0.4	131
Chocolate cake (from mix)	One-twelfth of a 9-in. diameter cake (approximately 2 oz)	31.9	1.4	198
Cookies (peanut butter)	2 medium	17.6	0.6	142

Vegetable Group

The majority of calories in vegetables are from starch, with some sugars, insignificant amounts of fat, and varying quantities of protein. Although all vegetables technically belong to this group, dried peas and beans (legumes) are usually classified with the starches or grains, because they are higher in carbohydrates than other vegetables, or with the meats, because they are a significant source of protein. Likewise, food group exchange plans, such as those used by the American Diabetes Association, group potatoes, corn, peas, and other *starchy vegetables* in the same category as grains. Some examples of the difference in carbohydrate content between starchy and "watery" vegetables are

Vegetable Product	Classification	Portion	Carbohydrate (g)	Calories
Potatoes	Starchy	½ cup	12.2	54
Lettuce	Watery	1 cup	1.4	8
Winter squash (acorn)	Starchy	½ cup	14.9	57
Summer squash (zucchini)	Watery	½ cup	3.5	14
Peas	Starchy	½ cup	11.4	62
Mung bean sprouts	Watery	½ cup	3.1	16

Fruit Group

Fruits contain mostly sugars, with small amounts of starch and minute quantities of protein and fat. Dried fruits are higher in sugar than fresh fruits because removal of the water increases the sugar concentration. Canned fruits may have added sugar.

Fruit Product	Portion	Carbohydrate (g)	Calories
Fresh plum	1 medium	8.6	36
Canned plum (in heavy syrup)	3 plums	30.9	118
Dried prune	5 medium	26.4	100

Because fiber is located in the skin of fruits, fresh whole fruits provide more fiber than do fresh peeled fruits or canned fruits.

Fruit Product	Portion	Total Fiber (g)
Unpeeled fresh apple	1	3.0
Peeled fresh apple	1	1.9
Applesauce	½ cup	1.5
Apple juice	6 oz	Negligible

Milk, Yogurt, and Cheese Group

Lactose is the carbohydrate found naturally in milk. Flavored milk and yogurt have added sugars, as do ice cream, ice milk, and frozen yogurt. Cheese is generally low in lactose because much of it is converted to lactic acid during production. Because fiber is found only in plants, all items in this group are fiber free.

Milk Product	Portion	Carbohydrate (g)	Calories
Milk (1%)	8 oz	11.0	102
Chocolate milk (1%)	8 oz	26.1	158
Plain yogurt (1.5% milk fat)	8 oz	15.0	130
Strawberry yogurt (1% milk fat)	8 oz	48.5	251
Ice cream (regular vanilla)	½ cup	15.6	133
Swiss cheese	1 oz	1.0	107

Meat, Poultry, Fish, Dry Beans, Eggs, and Nuts Group

Although this group is synonymous with *protein*, the plants in this group also provide carbohydrates. (Lactose is the only animal source of carbohydrate.) The majority of calories in nuts are from fat, but most varieties of nuts have 4 to 8 g of carbohydrates per 1-ounce serving. Dry beans are high in starch and rich in fibers.

Legume or Nut Product	Portion	Carbohydrate (g)	Fiber (g)	Calories
Kidney beans	½ cup cooked	19.0	4.5	104
Lentils	½ cup cooked	20.0	2.0	115
Great northern beans	½ cup cooked	27.5	8.2	150
Peanut butter, chunky	2 tbsp	6.9	2.1	188
Pecans, dry-roasted	1 oz	6.3	2.6	187
Walnuts	1 oz	4.0	1.0	190

Fats, Oils, and Sweets Group

This is a catchall group for the "extras" that add flavor, interest, and calories to meal plans but provide few nutrients; hence the recommendation is to use these items sparingly.

Products at the Apex of the Food Guide Pyramid	Portion	Carbohydrate (g)	Calories
White sugar	1 tsp	4.0	15
Brown sugar	1 tsp	4.5	17
Jelly	1 tsp	4.5	17
Gelatin	½ cup	19.0	80
Cola drink	12 oz	40.0	160

INTAKE RECOMMENDATIONS

Because the body can make glucose from amino acids (protein) and from the glycerol backbone of triglycerides (fat), a Recommended Dietary Allowance (RDA) for carbohydrate has not been set. However, as the body's major energy source, carbohydrates represent an essential and major component of the diet. In addition, complex carbohydrates (grains, legumes, and vegetables) and natural sugars (fruits) are major sources of vitamins, minerals, fiber, and phytochemicals ("plant chemicals") that are important for good health. They are also generally low in fat, depending on the selection. And although sugar provides *empty calories* (calories with few or no nutrients), it satisfies the inborn preference for sweets.

As little as 50 to 100 g of carbohydrate is actually needed to prevent ketoacidosis, muscle protein breakdown, and the side effects associated with a low carbohydrate intake. This is a bare minimum, not an optimal level for health and well-being. In most human diets, carbohydrates provide the majority of calories.

The method used to design or evaluate a meal plan for optimal carbohydrate content is based on the total number of calories consumed. Leading health authorities recommend the following:

- Carbohydrates should provide 50% to 60% of total calories, mostly in the form of complex carbohydrates.
- Added sugars should be limited to 10% or less of total calories.
- Adults should consume 20 to 35 g of fiber daily, or 10 to 13 g/1000 cal.

For example, someone consuming 1600 cal daily should:

- Consume 200 g of carbohydrate (50% × 1600 cal = 800 cal, and 800 cal ÷ 4 cal/g = 200 g of carbohydrate, much more than the minimum of 50 to 100 g).
- Limit sugar to 40 g/day (10% × 1600 cal = 160 cal, and 160 cal ÷ 4 cal/g = 40 g of sugar); at 4 g/teaspoon, 40 g is the equivalent of 10 teaspoons of added sugar. The Food Guide Pyramid suggests limiting added sugars to 6 teaspoons/day in a 1600 calorie meal plan.
- Eat approximately 21 g of fiber, using the upper-end recommendation of 13 g of fiber per 1000 cal consumed.

However, except for some diabetics and some people on calorie-controlled diets, few people count carbohydrate grams or know how much they should eat.

Less precise guidelines to achieve an adequate and appropriate carbohydrate intake appear in *Dietary Guidelines for Americans* (see Chapter 8), which suggests that people should "Choose a variety of grains daily, especially whole grains," "Choose a variety of fruits and vegetables daily," and "Choose beverages and foods to moderate your intake of sugars." Unfortunately, *variety* and *moderate* mean different things to different people and are vague guidelines for implementation. Fewer than one third of American adults think it is very important to choose a diet with plenty of grain products. Although most adults think it is important to use sugars only in moderation, the average intake of added sugars is approximately double the recommended level. Because food is eaten in servings, not percentages or grams, the suggestions for implementation given here use the Food Guide Pyramid (see Chapter 8) to translate recommendations into daily food choices.

- **Choose 6 to 11 servings from the Bread, Cereal, Rice, and Pasta group.** Eat several servings of various whole-grain breads and cereals daily, such as whole-grain products made from wheat, rice, oats, corn, and barley. Prepare and serve grain products with little or no fats and sugars.
- **Eat 3 to 5 servings from the Vegetable group.** Choose dark green leafy and deep yellow vegetables often. Eat dry beans, peas, and lentils often. Eat starchy vegetables, such as potatoes and corn. Prepare and serve vegetables with little or no fats.
- **Choose 2 to 4 servings from the Fruit group.** Choose citrus fruits or juices, melons, or berries regularly. Eat fruits as desserts or snacks. Drink fruit juices. Prepare and serve fruits with little or no added sugars.

But does this really translate into 50% to 60% of total calories from carbohydrates? According to the Food Guide Pyramid, limiting the number of servings to the lowest number listed for each group provides about 1600 calories. The low-end serving suggestions are

Food Group	No. Servings	g of Carbohydrate per Serving	Carbohydrates (g)	
			per Group	Total
Bread, cereal, rice, and pasta	6	15	90	
Vegetable	3	5–15	15–45	
Fruit	2	15	30	
				135–165
plus				
Milk	2	12	24	
				159–189
plus				
Dry beans	1	15	15	
				174–204

However, because the grams of carbohydrate for each food group above are *estimates*, not *actual* figures, the day's actual total carbohydrate consumption could be much different depending on individual food choices and serving sizes. For instance, if 2 cups of flavored yogurt were consumed instead of 2 cups of milk, the carbohydrate contribution from the Milk, Yogurt, and Cheese group would jump from 24 to 97 g—an increase of 73 g, all from added sugars. In addition, consumption of foods containing sugar selected from the Fats, Oils, and Sweets group would boost total carbohydrate intake.

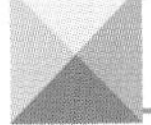

Carbohydrates in Health Promotion

GETTING ENOUGH FIBER

The most consistent benefit of consuming adequate fiber, specifically insoluble fiber, is to relieve or prevent constipation. Insoluble fibers may also be protective against colon and rectal cancers and may help prevent diverticulitis in people with diverticula. Soluble fibers are credited with lowering high cholesterol levels, and they help delay and reduce the rise in blood glucose concentration in diabetics by slowing the absorption of glucose from the small intestine. Generally, foods that are high in fiber are lower in calories than refined and processed foods. Because of their bulk and the feeling of fullness they provide, high-fiber foods may aid weight management. High-fiber foods such as whole grains, legumes, vegetables, and fruits are also major sources of micronutrients and phytochemicals. Clearly there are benefits to consuming adequate amounts of fiber.

The recommendation to eat more fiber—20 to 35 g/day—is not qualified as to how much of which types of fiber. In the first place, fiber does not fit the definition of an essential nutrient that must be consumed through food in order to prevent a deficiency disease; the need for fiber is based on its physiologic effects in the body. For instance, people who are prone to constipation benefit from eating more fiber, whereas people with rapid transit times do not "need" more fiber. Likewise, someone with a high blood cholesterol concentration may experience a drop in the cholesterol level from eating more foods that are high in soluble fiber, whereas a person with a normal level may see no change from eating more soluble fiber. Secondly, fiber is the carbohydrate that remains after digestion, and because digestion is difficult to replicate in a laboratory, methods for measuring dietary fiber may not be valid. It is difficult to calculate fiber intake because (1) current data on fiber content may not be accurate, (2) data on total fiber content are not available for all food sources, and (3) data on the amount of specific types of fiber (eg, cellulose, hemicellulose, pectin) are even more scarce. Therefore, inherent in the general recommendation to eat more fiber are the following points: individual tolerance to fiber must be considered, and it is important to consume a variety of fiber sources, because different sources provide different types and proportions of specific fibers.

Currently, the usual intake of fiber among Americans is 13.7 g/day for women and 18.5 g/day for men, far less than the recommended level. That is because most popular American foods are not high in fiber. According to food consumption data from the 1989–1991 *Continuing Survey of Food Intakes by Individuals*, the top five sources of fiber in the typical adult American diet in descending order are yeast bread, ready-to-eat cereal, dried beans/lentils, white potatoes, and tomatoes (Subar, Krebs-Smith, Cook, et al., 1998).

Tips for Eating More Fiber

Eat a Variety of Plant Foods

The types and amounts of fiber in strawberries differ from those in kidney beans, which differ from those in bran cereal, which differ from those in oatmeal. However, there do not seem to be differences in fiber content among different varieties of the same foodstuff; for instance, the fiber content of apples is consistent among Granny Smith, Macintosh, Cortland, and Delicious varieties. Eating a variety of plant foods means choosing different foods, not different varieties of the same food.

Eat at Least Two to Three Servings of Whole Grains Daily

As part of their daily 6 to 11 servings of bread, cereal, rice, and pasta, people should eat 2 to 3 servings of whole grains. Items from this group are generally classified as either "refined/processed" or "whole grain/wholesome."

Refined grains and flours are made from the endosperm (inner part) of the grain seed only; this is the part that contains most of the protein and starch, together with small amounts of vitamins and trace minerals. Refined grains are artificially enriched with certain B vitamins and iron that are lost through processing. However, enriched flour is not equivalent to whole-grain flour in fiber content or in the levels of other nutrients, such as protein, magnesium, potassium, and zinc. Examples of refined grains include:

- Wheat—white flour, wheat flour (except "whole wheat" flour), white pasta, Cream of Wheat, puffed wheat
- Oats—oat flour
- Corn—cornstarch, cornflakes, grits
- Rice—white rice, Rice Krispies, Cream of Rice
- Barley—pearl barley

Whole grains and flours (Fig. 2–2) contain the entire grain, or seed, which includes the endosperm portion plus the following components:

- The **bran**, or outer layer, which is rich in B vitamins and fiber. Technically, bran cereals are not truly whole-grain products, because the endosperm and germ are

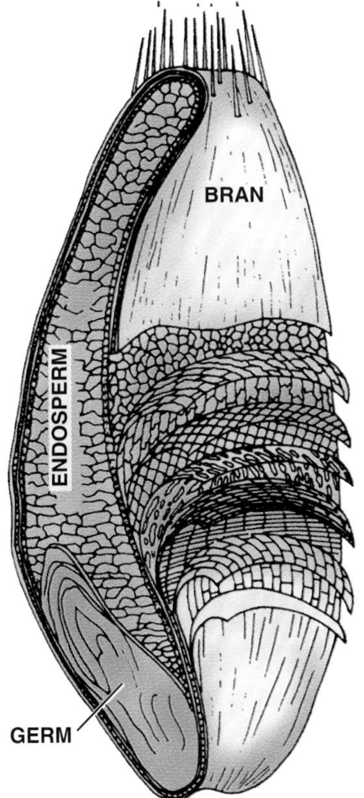

COMPONENT	RICHEST IN:
BRAN	Fiber Vitamin B_6 Pantothenic acid Niacin Selenium
GERM	Fat Thiamine Vitamin E Potassium Phosphorus Iron Selenium
ENDOSPERM	Protein Starch

FIGURE 2-2 Whole wheat kernel. The components of the whole wheat kernel are the *bran*, the *germ*, and the *endosperm*.

missing, but they are a concentrated source of fiber. Bran can be derived from wheat, oats, corn, or rice.
- The **germ,** the small embryo or sprouting portion of the seed. Some B vitamins, minerals, and some protein are found in the germ. Because the germ also contains fat, it is usually not included in flours, because fat limits the keeping quality of flours. Technically, wheat germ is not a whole grain because the bran and endosperm portions are removed.

Examples of whole grains include:

- Wheat—whole wheat flour, Wheatena, Shredded Wheat, Wheaties, wheat berries, bulgur, cracked wheat
- Oats—oatmeal, Cheerios
- Whole-grain barley
- Rye
- Corn
- Brown rice
- Millet
- Quinoa
- Triticale flour

Eat at Least Five Servings of Fruits and Vegetables Daily

Do not peel fruits or vegetables. Peeling cuts the fiber content of potatoes in half and reduces fiber from fruits by 25%. Edible seeds, such as those found in strawberries, kiwifruit, tomatoes, and cucumbers, contribute significant fiber. Whole and fresh fruits and vegetables have more fiber than canned ones. Juices have negligible fiber.

Eat Legumes Two to Three Times per Week

Legumes are excellent sources of both insoluble and soluble fibers and are a fat-free alternative to meat. Try meatless entrees featuring beans, such as bean burritos, minestrone soup, hummus on pita bread, or meatless chili.

Choose a Breakfast Cereal With Five Grams of Fiber or More per Serving

Cooked and ready-to-eat bran and whole-grain cereals offer variety, convenience, fiber, and lots of nutrition in a low-fat package.

Estimating Fiber Intake

Adequacy of fiber intake is usually overlooked or only superficially considered during the process of nutritional screening or assessment. Questions about the types of breads and cereals consumed and whether legumes are regularly eaten may represent the extent of fiber assessment; fiber may not even be addressed unless the client has problems with elimination or hypercholesterolemia. There has been no quick, easy, and valid tool to assess fiber intake.

The following method may provide a relatively accurate estimate of total fiber intake using a 24-hour recall or usual food pattern. Because the fiber contents of fruits, veg-

TABLE 2.1 ***Estimating Fiber Intake***

Food Group	Number of Servings Eaten		Mean Fiber Content per Serving (g)		Total Grams of Fiber
Fruit (except juice)	__	×	1.5	=	__
Vegetables	__	×	1.5	=	__
Refined grains	__	×	1.0	=	__
Whole grains	__	×	2.5	=	__
Other foods*	__	×	__[†]	=	__
Total					__

*Such as high-fiber grains, nuts and seeds, and legumes.
[†]Use specific values.

etables, refined grains, and whole grains are relatively similar within each group, multiplying the servings consumed from each of these groups by the mean fiber content provides a fairly accurate measurement. For other sources of fiber in the diet—specifically high-fiber grains, nuts and seeds, and legumes—there is a large range of fiber content among the individual choices within each group. Therefore, mean values are not valid, and any foods eaten from these categories must have the actual fiber content added to the total from the other groups. The quick method is shown in Table 2–1.

Notice that without several servings of whole grains or some high-fiber choices from "Other foods," obtaining 20 to 35 g of fiber is unlikely. Consider a pattern based on the low-end serving recommendations from the Food Guide Pyramid.

Food Item	No. Servings		Fiber Content per Serving (g)		Total Fiber (g)
Fruits	2	×	1.5	=	3.0
Vegetables	3	×	1.5	=	4.5
Refined grains	6	×	1.0	=	6.0
Total					13.5

The total is an amount consistent with the average adult American intake.

By simply substituting a couple of servings of whole grains and a serving of high-fiber cereal for three of the servings of refined grains, the day's total would be within the recommended range. A revised plan is

Food Item	No. Servings		Fiber Content per Serving (g)		Total Fiber (g)
Fruits	2	×	1.5	=	3.0
Vegetables	3	×	1.5	=	4.5
Refined grains	3	×	1.0	=	3.0
Whole grains	2	×	2.5	=	5.0
All-Bran cereal	1	×	10.0	=	10.0
Total					25.5

SUGAR: TOO MUCH OF A GOOD THING

In foods, sugar adds flavor and interest. Few would question the value brown sugar adds to a bowl of hot oatmeal. Besides its sweet taste, sugar has important functions in baked goods. In yeast breads, sugar promotes fermentation by serving as food for the yeast. Sugar in cakes promotes tenderness and a smooth crumb texture. Cookies owe their crisp texture and light-brown color to sugar. In jams and jellies sugar inhibits the growth of mold, and in candy it influences texture. Sugar has many functional roles in foods, including taste, physical properties, antimicrobial purposes, and chemical properties.

In the body, sugar is frequently blamed for a variety of health problems, including:

- **Behavioral problems in children.** However, evidence that sugar causes hyperactivity is lacking, even among children who are reported to be sensitive to sugar.
- **Obesity.** Obesity is a complex problem that cannot simply be blamed on one factor. Total calorie intake is important, as are activity patterns, reasons for eating, fat grams, and sugar grams. In fact, there appears to be an inverse relationship between sugar intake and obesity, as well as between sugar intake and fat intake: meal plans low in sugar tend to have a greater proportion of calories from fat. The potential risks of eating too much fat are greater than of eating too much sugar.
- **Diabetes mellitus.** For type 2 diabetes, too many calories and too much body weight are the problem, not specifically too much sugar.

Drawbacks of Sugar

Even though sugar is not an independent risk factor for any particular disease, avoiding too much sugar is prudent. High sugar intakes are linked to increased triglyceride and insulin levels. The most notable drawbacks of sugar are that it promotes dental caries and provides empty calories.

Dental Caries

Feeding off of sugars and starches, bacteria residing in the mouth produce an acid that erodes tooth enamel. Although whole-grain crackers and orange juice are more nutritious than doughnuts and soft drinks, their potential damage to teeth is the same. How often carbohydrates are consumed, what they are eaten with, and how long after eating brushing occurs may be more important than whether they are "sticky." Anticavity strategies include the following:

- Choose between-meal snacks that are healthy and teeth-friendly, such as fresh vegetables, apples, cheese, and popcorn.
- Limit between-meal carbohydrate snacking, including drinking soft drinks.
- Avoid high-sugar items that stay in the mouth a long time, such as hard candy, suckers, and cough drops.
- Brush promptly after eating.
- After eating, chew gum sweetened with sugar alcohols (eg, sorbitol, mannitol, xylitol) or with nonnutritive sweeteners. This may cut the risk of cavities by stim-

ulating the production of saliva, which helps rinse the teeth and neutralize plaque acids. Unlike sucrose and other nutritive sweeteners, sugar alcohols and artificial sweeteners are not fermented by bacteria in the mouth, so they do not promote cavities.
- Use fluoridated toothpaste.

Empty Calories

Empty-calorie foods provide calories with few or no other nutrients. Consumption of empty-calorie foods *in place of* nutrient-dense foods results in lower levels of nutrients per total calorie intake. People who eat diets high in sugar consume less calcium, fiber, zinc, iron, folate and vitamins A, C, and E than people with low intakes of added sugar. Empty-calorie foods *added to* a meal plan cause calories to increase while the nutrient intake remains unchanged. With either scenario, the ratio of nutrients to calories decreases; that is, the meal plan becomes less nutrient-dense. For instance, the calorie values of cola and 1% milk are similar, but the nutrient values differ significantly.

Nutrient	1% Milk (8 oz)	Cola (8 oz)
Calories	102.0	97
Protein (g)	8.0	0
Vitamin A (RE)	144.0	0
Vitamin B_2 (mg)	0.41	0
Potassium (mg)	381.0	0
Calcium (mg)	300.0	0

RE, retinol equivalents.

The nutrient most significantly affected by the use of soft drinks in place of milk is calcium. If the soft drink replaces milk, calories remain constant but the level of calcium (and other nutrients) drops. If the soft drink is consumed in addition to the normal food plan, nutrients are not sacrificed but calorie intake increases. In either case, nutrient density decreases, increasing the risk of consuming inadequate amounts of nutrients, too many calories, or both.

How Much is Enough?

The *Dietary Guidelines for Americans* (see Chapter 8) recommends that people choose sensibly to moderate their intake of beverages and foods that are high in sugar. As stated in the Food Guide Pyramid (see Chapter 8), added sugars should be limited to 6 teaspoons daily in a 1600-calorie meal plan, 12 teaspoons for 2200 calories, 18 teaspoons for 2800 calories, or 6% to 10% of the total calorie intake.

According to data from the U.S. Department of Agriculture, enough sugar was produced in the United States during 1996 to provide every citizen with 152 pounds. Granted, that figure overestimates the amount of sugar actually eaten, but data show a 30% increase in the intake of added sugars since 1983. A typical American consumes

16% of total calories from added sugars. Soft drinks contribute the most added sugars; average annual consumption is 55 gallons per person, or 19 ounces/day (63 g of sugar).

Tips for Eating Less Sugar

- **Replace soft drinks with 100% fruit juice or low-fat milk.** Total calorie intake may not change significantly, but the intake of vitamins, minerals, and phytochemicals will increase. It is the total package that is important, not just the amount of calories.
- **Rely on natural sugars in fruit to satisfy a "sweet tooth."** Besides being less concentrated in sugars than candy, cookies, pastries, and cakes, fruits boost nutrient and fiber intake.
- **Cut sugar in home-baked products, if possible.** Although in some foods reducing the amount of sugar does not appreciably alter taste or other qualities, in others it can be disastrous. For instance, because sugar in jams and jellies inhibits the growth of mold, less sugar results in a product that supports mold growth.

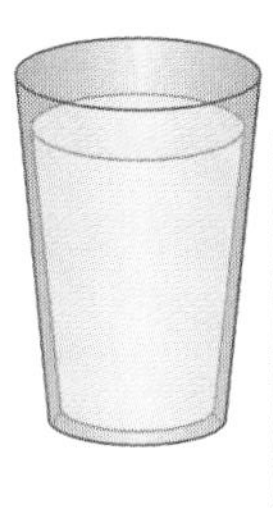

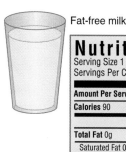

Fat-free milk

Nutrition Facts
Serving Size 1 Cup (240mL)
Servings Per Container 16

Amount Per Serving	
Calories 90	Calories from Fat 0
	% Daily Value*
Total Fat 0g	**0%**
Saturated Fat 0g	**0%**
Cholesterol 5mg	**2%**
Sodium 125mg	**5%**
Total Carbohydrate 12g	**4%**
Dietary Fiber 0g	**0%**
Sugars 11g	
Protein 8g	

Vitamin A 10% • Vitamin C 4%
Calcium 30% • Iron 0% • Vitamin D 25%

* Percent Daily Values are based on a 2,000 calorie diet. Your daily values may be higher or lower depending on your calorie needs:

	Calories	2,000	2,500
Total Fat	Less than	65g	80g
Sat Fat	Less than	20g	25g
Cholesterol	Less than	300mg	300mg
Sodium	Less than	2,400mg	2,400mg
Total Carbohydrate		300g	375g
Dietary Fiber		25g	30g

Calories per gram:
Fat 9 • Carbohydrate 4 • Protein 4

INGREDIENTS: FAT FREE MILK, VITAMIN A PALMITATE, VITAMIN D_3.

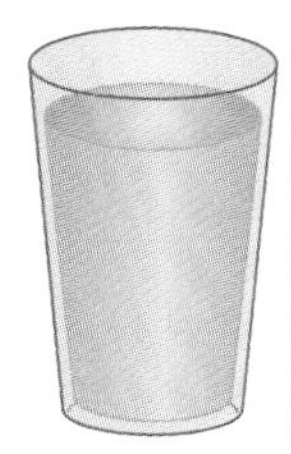

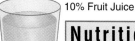

10% Fruit Juice

Nutrition Facts
Serving Size 8 oz.
Servings Per Container 10

Amount Per Serving	
Calories 107	Calories from Fat 0
	% Daily Value *
Total Fat 0g	**0%**
Saturated Fat 0g	**0%**
Cholesterol 0mg	**0%**
Sodium 24mg	**1%**
Total Carbohydrate 30g	**10%**
Dietary Fiber 0g	**0%**
Sugars 30g	
Protein 0g	

* Percent Daily Values are based on a 2,000 calorie diet. Your daily values may be higher or lower depending on your calorie needs:

	Calories	2,000	2,500
Total Fat	Less than	65g	80g
Sat Fat	Less than	20g	25g
Cholesterol	Less than	300mg	300mg
Sodium	Less than	2,400mg	2,400mg
Total Carbohydrate		300g	375g
Dietary Fiber		25g	30g

Calories per gram:
Fat 9 • Carbohydrate 4 • Protein 4

INGREDIENTS: WATER; HIGH FRUCTOSE CORN SYRUP; RED GRAPE, PEAR, AND PEACH JUICE CONCENTRATES; CITRIC ACID; STRAWBERRY JUICE CONCENTRATE; NATURAL FLAVOR.

FIGURE 2-3 Nutrition Facts labels for fat-free milk and a 10% fruit drink. Compare the nutrients provided and the amounts in which they are present.

- **Check labels.** Although Nutrition Facts labels (see Chapter 8) list the amount of total carbohydrates and sugars per serving, they do not include sugar alcohols and do not distinguish between natural and added sugars. People concerned with limiting sugar who restrict their focus to the grams of sugar per serving may inappropriately conclude that foods high in natural sugars, such as milk and fruit juice, should be avoided. When judging the value of a food high in sugar, it is important to look beyond sugar grams to the whole package. What other nutrients are provided, and are they present in significant amounts? Are the sugars naturally present, or are they added? Consider the difference between skim milk and a fruit drink (Fig. 2–3). Eight ounces of skim milk provides 11 g of sugar (lactose), 10% of the Daily Value for vitamin A, 25% for vitamin D, and 30% for calcium. The ingredients are pasteurized nonfat milk, vitamin A, and vitamin D_3. Analysis: Milk provides significant amounts of several nutrients with no added sugar. Eight ounces of the fruit drink contains 30 g of sugar and no other nutrients. The ingredients in the fruit drink are water; HFCS; red grape, pear, and peach juice concentrates; citric acid; strawberry juice concentrate; and natural flavor. Analysis: The fruit drink's only nutrient is sugar, and the ingredient list indicates more added sugars than natural sugars (from the fruit juices). Box 2–1 lists sources of added sugars. The more of these on the ingredient label and the closer to the beginning of the list they appear, the higher the content of added sugar.
- **Consider using sugar alternatives such as sugar alcohols or nonnutritive sweeteners.** Sugar alternatives may help reduce sugar intake. They do not produce a rise in blood glucose as nutritive sweeteners do. They are not fermented by bacteria in the mouth and therefore do not promote tooth decay. On the downside, the use of sugar alternatives may not affect total calorie intake, nor does it ensure a nutritious meal plan. Sugar alternatives are discussed in the next section.

ALTERNATIVES TO SUGAR

Alternatives to sugar arise from Americans' desire to "have their cake and eat it too." People want the taste of sweetness without feeling guilty about the calories. The food in-

BOX 2.1

Sources of Added Sugars

Brown sugar	High-fructose corn syrup
Confectioner's sugar	Honey
Corn sweetener	Invert sugar
Corn syrup	Lactose
Crystallized cane sugar	Maltose
Dextrose	Molasses
Fructose	Raw sugar
Fruit juice concentrate	Sucrose
Glucose	Turbinado sugar

dustry has responded to this demand by developing numerous low-calorie and calorie-free (nonnutritive) sweeteners.

- **Low-calorie sweeteners.** Sugar alcohols (eg, sorbitol, mannitol, xylitol) are natural sweeteners derived from monosaccharides. Sorbitol and mannitol are 50% to 70% as sweet as sucrose; xylitol has the same sweetness as sucrose. Although small amounts of sugar alcohols are found in some fruits and berries, most are commercially synthesized and used as sugar replacements. They are considered low-calorie sweeteners because they are incompletely absorbed, so that their calorie value ranges from 1.6 to 2.6 cal/g. This slow and incomplete absorption causes them to produce a smaller effect on blood glucose levels and insulin secretion than sucrose does. They are not fermented by mouth bacteria. Sugar alcohols are approved for use in a variety of products, including candies, chewing gum, jams and jellies, baked goods, and frozen confections. Some people experience a laxative effect (abdominal gas, discomfort, osmotic diarrhea) after consuming sorbitol or mannitol. In small amounts and in products that stay in the mouth a long time, such as chewing gum and breath mints, sugar alcohols offer sweetness without promoting cavities.
- **Nonnutritive sweeteners** provide sweetness with negligible or no calories. They are considered high-intensity sweeteners because they are hundreds of times sweeter than sugar and small amounts can be used to sweeten foods. Blending high-intensity sweeteners together produces a synergistically sweeter taste, decreases the amount of sweetener needed, and minimizes aftertaste. Because they have little effect on serum glucose levels, nonnutritive sweeteners appeal to diabetics. They also do not promote dental decay. The nonnutritive sweeteners approved for use in the United States are saccharin, aspartame, acesulfame-K, and sucralose.
  - **Saccharin,** used for more than 100 years and in more than 100 countries, is found in soft drinks and in the tabletop sweeteners Sweet 'N Low and Sweet 10. Saccharin is 200% to 700% sweeter than sugar, so it is used in very small amounts. It leaves a bitter aftertaste. In 1977 the US Food and Drug Administration (FDA) banned its use when large amounts were found to cause cancer in rats. The US Congress issued moratoriums to allow saccharin to remain on the market but carry the warning on food labels that saccharin may be a health hazard and that it causes cancer in laboratory animals. In 2000, the government removed saccharin from the National Toxicology Program's (NTP) list of cancer-causing chemicals. Industry leaders are expected to petition for permission to stop using the warning label on products containing saccharin. Opponents charge that the best human study on saccharin, conducted by the National Cancer Institute, showed a correlation between exposure to saccharin and bladder cancer.
  - **Aspartame** is found in the tabletop sweeteners Equal, Nutrasweet, and Sweet-Mate. Because it is not heat stable, aspartame is used commercially in products that do not require cooking or baking, such as puddings, gelatins, frozen desserts, yogurt, powdered drink mixes, soft drinks, and chewing gum. It is made commercially from two amino acids, aspartic acid and phenylalanine, which do not naturally taste sweet. The amino acids in aspartame are digested and absorbed just as they are when they occur naturally in meat, milk, fruit, and vegetables. Aspartame provides 4 cal/g, like other amino acids, but because

it is used in small quantities the amount of calories provided is negligible. People with phenylketonuria (PKU), an inborn error of metabolism that causes phenylalanine to accumulate in the blood to toxic levels, must control their intake of phenylalanine, including aspartame. Aspartame is 180 to 200 times sweeter than sugar and does not leave an aftertaste.

- **Acesulfame-K,** marketed as Sunette, is approved for use in chewing gum, desserts, yogurt, alcoholic beverages, and the tabletop sweeteners Sweet One and Swiss Sweet. It is 200 times sweeter than sugar and maintains its sweet taste during heating and cooking. Acesulfame-K is often blended with other nutritive and nonnutritive sweeteners to synergize the sweetness and minimize its slight aftertaste. It is not digested and therefore is excreted in the urine unchanged.
- **Sucralose,** which is 600 times sweeter than sugar, was approved in 1998 for use as the tabletop sweetener Splenda and in numerous desserts and nonalcoholic beverages. Like acesulfame-K, it is not digested and is excreted in the urine unchanged.

At first glance nonnutritive sweeteners appear to answer Americans' passion for calorie-free sweetness. But do they really help people manage their weight? Are they appropriate for diabetics? Are they safe for everyone, including pregnant women and children?

- **Weight management.** Nonnutritive sweeteners are not a panacea for weight control. In theory, use of nonnutritive sweeteners in place of sugar can save 16 cal/teaspoon, or 160 cal in a 12-ounce can of cola. Eliminating one regularly sweetened soft drink per day for 22 days (160 cal × 22 days = 3520 cal) translates to a 1-pound loss (3500 calories equals 1 pound of body weight) without any other changes in eating or activity. This is because *all* of the calories in the regular soft drink have been eliminated. But foods whose calories come from a mixture of sugar, starch, protein, and fat still provide calories after sugar calories are reduced or eliminated. For instance, sugar-free cookies can provide as many or more calories than cookies sweetened with sugar. Many people falsely believe that low sugar means low calories and therefore overeat because they overestimate the calories saved by replacing sugar. Ironically, the prevalence of obesity has increased significantly as the intake of nonnutritive sweeteners has increased. Nonnutritive sweeteners may help manage weight, but only when they are used within the context of an otherwise varied, balanced, and moderate meal plan.
- **Diabetes mellitus.** Contrary to what was previously believed, regular sugar does not raise blood glucose levels more than complex carbohydrates do; a food's effect on blood glucose levels is influenced by several factors, not just sugar content. The focus in management of blood glucose levels has shifted from avoiding simple sugars to maintaining a relatively consistent total carbohydrate intake, with less emphasis on the source. For that reason, sweets can be included within the context of a nutritious, calorie-appropriate, diabetic diet. However, because most type 2 diabetics are overweight, substitution of calorie-free sweets for calorie-containing ones has the potential to improve blood glucose levels by promoting weight management.
- **Safety.** The FDA is responsible for approving the safety of all food additives, including nonnutritive sweeteners. An *acceptable daily intake (ADI)*, or the estimated

amount per kilogram of body weight that a person can safely consume every day over a lifetime without risk, is established as a safety limit for each sweetener. The ADI is a conservative value that usually reflects an amount 100 times less than the maximum level at which no observed adverse effects have occurred in animal studies. For instance, the ADI of aspartame is 50 mg/kg of body weight; therefore, someone weighing 132 pounds (60 kg) could safely consume 3000 mg of aspartame daily, or the equivalent of 13 cans of aspartame-sweetened soft drinks. Currently, apartame users consume an average of just 3.0 g/kg, or 6% of the safety limit.

For most adults, nonnutritive sweeteners are safe when used within approved guidelines; for pregnant women, the issue is less straightforward. Some physicians recommend that women avoid all nonnutritive sweeteners during pregnancy, but others suggest that they may be used in moderation. The position of the American Dietetic Association is that if pregnant women use saccharin they should do so cautiously, because saccharin crosses the placenta and is slowly cleared from fetal tissues. Aspartame is safe during pregnancy but should not be used by women with PKU. Acesulfame-K is safe during pregnancy.

Saccharin has not been well studied in children, so prudent use is advised. Other nonnutritive sweeteners are relatively safe for children, with the exception of aspartame for children with PKU. The qualifier *relatively* refers to the fact that any substance becomes toxic at some level, but average consumption of nonnutritive sweeteners among children is less than the ADIs set for them. But even if they are relatively safe, are they really necessary? The alternative to nonnutritive sweeteners—regular sugar—is not plagued with safety concerns and can fit within the context of a nutritious and balanced meal plan. One must look at the risk-benefit ratio to decide whether use of nonnutritive sweeteners is appropriate for children.

Questions You May Hear

Isn't the sugar in fruit better for you than the sugar in candy? No, sugar is sugar, whether it is lactose in milk, fructose in fruit, sucrose in jelly, or sucrose in sweet potatoes. When the process of digestion is completed, monosaccharides remain, regardless of the original source. The body cannot distinguish between sugars present naturally and those added through food processing. What does matter to the body is the "package" that contained the sugar. The fruit package provides various vitamins, minerals, fiber, and phytochemicals; the candy package may provide fat and little else—no difference in sugar, big difference in nutrition.

What is glycemic response? Glycemic response is the effect a food has on the blood glucose concentration: how quickly the glucose level rises, how high it goes, and how long it takes to return to normal. Traditionally it was believed that, because simple sugars are rapidly and completely absorbed, they produce a quicker and higher effect on blood glucose levels than complex carbohydrates do. Actually, the amounts of fat and fiber, the method of preparation, and the amount eaten influence a food's glycemic response. The *glycemic index* is a numeric measure of the glycemic response of 50 g of a food sample; the higher the number, the higher the glycemic response. For instance, cornflakes (low fiber, low fat) have a higher glycemic index than does ice cream (high fat). For diabetics, the glycemic index can help fine-tune optimal meal planning (see Chapter 19). Athletes can use the glycemic index to choose optimal fuels for before, during, and after exercise (see Chapter 7). Within each category in Table 2–2, foods are ranked from highest to lowest glycemic index.

Aren't starches fattening? At 4 cal/g, starches are no more fattening than sugar or protein, and less than half as fattening as fat at 9 cal/g. The misconception that starches are fattening is promoted by high-protein fad diet propaganda that claims starches stimulate insulin secretion (which hastens the conversion of excess glucose into body fat), whereas high-protein diets do not stimulate insulin secretion and effectively promote rapid weight loss. In truth, both proteins and carbohydrates stimulate insulin secretion, whether they are eaten alone or together. If high-protein diets promote weight loss, it is because they are low in calories. The key to weight management is always the balance between calories consumed and calories expended.

"Light" breads are high in fiber. Can I use them in place of whole-grain breads? So-called light breads usually have processed fiber from peas or other foods added in place of some of the starch; the result is a lower-calorie, higher-fiber bread that may help prevent constipation but lacks the "package" of vitamins, minerals, and phytochemicals found in whole grains.

TABLE 2.2 ***Glycemic Indices of Selected Foods***

High (>60)	Moderate (40–60)	Low (<40)
Glucose	Bran muffin	Apple
Gatorade	Bran Chex	Pear
Potato, baked	Orange juice	PowerBar
Cornflakes	Boiled potato	Chocolate milk
Rice cakes	Rice, white	Fruit yogurt, low-fat
Potato, microwaved	Rice, brown	Chickpeas
Jelly beans	Popcorn	P R Bar
Vanilla Wafers	Corn	Lima beans
Cheerios	Sweet potato	Split peas, yellow
Cream of Wheat, instant	Pound cake	Skim milk
Graham crackers	Banana, overripe	Apricots, dried
Honey	Peas, green	Green beans
Watermelon	Bulgur	Banana, underripe
Bagel	Baked beans	Lentils
Bread, white	Rice, white parboiled	Kidney beans
Bread, whole wheat	Lentil soup	Barley
Shredded wheat	Orange	Grapefruit
Soft drink	All-Bran cereal	Fructose
Mars Bar	Spaghetti (no sauce)	
Grape-Nuts cereal	Pumpernickel bread	
Stoned Wheat Thins	Apple juice	
Cream of Wheat, regular		
Table sugar		
Raisins		
Oatmeal		
Ice cream		

KEY CONCEPTS

- Carbohydrates, found almost exclusively in plants, provide the major source of energy in almost all human diets.
- The two major groups are simple carbohydrates (monosaccharides and disaccharides) and complex carbohydrates (polysaccharides).
- Monosaccharides and disaccharides are composed of one or two sugar molecules, respectively. They vary in sweetness.
- Polysaccharides, namely starch, glycogen, and fiber, are made up of many glucose molecules. They do not taste sweet because their molecules are too large to sit on taste buds in the mouth that perceive sweetness.
- Fiber, the part of plant cell walls that is indigestible, is commonly classified as either water-soluble or water-insoluble; each type has different physiologic effects.
- The majority of carbohydrate digestion occurs in the small intestine, where disaccharides and starches are digested to monosaccharides. Monosaccharides are absorbed through intestinal mucosal cells and transported to the liver through the portal vein. In the liver, fructose and galactose are converted to glucose. The liver releases glucose into the bloodstream.
- The major function of carbohydrates is to provide energy, which includes sparing protein and preventing ketosis. Glucose can be converted to glycogen, used to make nonessential amino acids, used for specific body compounds, or converted to fat and stored in adipose tissue.
- Carbohydrates are found in every Food Guide Pyramid group. Starches are most abundant in the Bread, Cereal, Rice, and Pasta group and the Vegetable group; natural sugars occur in the Fruit group and in the Milk, Yogurt, and Cheese group; and the apex contains sugars and other sweets such as candy, gelatin, and soft drinks.
- Because the body can make glucose from certain amino acids (protein) and glycerol (fat), an RDA for carbohydrate has not been established. Most experts recommend that 50% to 60% of total calories come from carbohydrates and that added sugars be limited to 6% to 10% of calories. Twenty to 35 g of fiber is recommended daily.
- All sources of fiber contain a mix of insoluble and soluble fibers. The most popular American foods do not represent rich sources of fiber. Whole grains, bran cereals, dried peas and beans, and unpeeled fruits and vegetables are the best sources of fiber.
- Sugar satisfies the inborn preference for sweets; it does not cause hyperactivity, diabetes, or heart disease. Sugars—as well as starches—promote dental decay by feeding bacteria in the mouth that produce an acid that damages tooth enamel. Sugar is also a source of empty calories. The higher the intake of empty calories, the greater the risk of an inadequate nutrient intake, an excessive calorie intake, or both. Americans' intake of sugar and nonnutritive sweeteners is rising.
- Sugar alcohols are considered to be low-calorie sweeteners because they are incompletely absorbed and therefore provide fewer calories per gram than regular sugar does. Because they do not promote dental decay, they are well suited for use in gum and breath mints, which stay in the mouth a long time.
- Nonnutritive sweeteners provide negligible or no calories. Their use as food additives is regulated by the FDA, which sets safety limits known as ADIs. The ADI, a level per kilogram of body weight, reflects an amount 100 times less than the maximum level at

which no observed adverse effects have occurred in animal studies. Nonnutritive sweeteners have intense sweetening power, ranging from 180 to 700 times sweeter than that of sucrose.

ANSWER KEY

1. **TRUE** Starches (including bread) promote dental decay in the same way as sugars (including candy), by feeding bacteria in the mouth that damages tooth enamel.
2. **TRUE** Nonnutritive sweeteners do not promote tooth decay.
3. **FALSE** The potential risks associated with eating too much fat are higher than those associated with eating too much sugar.
4. **FALSE** The insoluble fiber found in wheat bran and vegetables helps aid in bowel elimination, as opposed to the physiologic effect of soluble fiber, which is responsible for lowering elevated levels of blood cholesterol.
5. **TRUE** Oats and fruit are excellent sources of soluble fiber, which delays the absorption of glucose from the small intestine and lowers elevated blood cholesterol levels.
6. **TRUE** Soft drinks contribute more sugar to the average American diet than any other food or beverage.
7. **FALSE** Fruit is better than candy because it provides vitamins, some minerals, and phytochemicals—but not because its sugar is healthier than the sugar in candy. The body cannot distinguish between natural and added sugars.
8. **FALSE** Although Nutrition Facts labels do not distinguish between natural and added sugars, they do list the total sugar content per serving.
9. **TRUE** Soluble fiber slows the absorption of glucose, thus delaying and stifling the rise in serum glucose that occurs after eating.
10. **TRUE** If a very-low-calorie, low-carbohydrate diet is consumed, the body will first use dietary protein for energy. If still more energy is needed, the body will begin to break down its own protein tissue.

REFERENCES

American Dietetic Association. (1997). Position of the American Dietetic Association: Health implications of dietary fiber. *J Am Diet Assoc*, 97(10), 1157–1159.

American Dietetic Association. (1998). Position of the American Dietetic Association: Use of nutritive and nonnutritive sweeteners. *J Am Diet Assoc*, 98(5), 580–586.

Liebman, B. (1997). Sugar: The sweetening of the American diet. *Nutrition Action Health Letter*, 25(9), 1, 3–6.

Liebman, B. (1997). The whole grain guide. *Nutrition Action Health Letter*, 24(2), 1, 7–11.

Marlett, J., Cheung, T. (1997). Database and quick methods of assessing typical dietary fiber intakes using data for 228 commonly consumed foods. *J Am Diet Assoc*, 97(10), 1139–1148.

Pennington, J. (1998). *Bowes and Church's food values of portions commonly used.* (17th ed.). Philadelphia: Lippincott-Raven.

Subar, A., Krebs-Smith, S., Cook, A., Kahle, L. (1998). Dietary sources of nutrients among US adults, 1989 to 1991. *J Am Diet Assoc*, 98(5), 537–547.

CHAPTER 3

Protein

TRUE	FALSE	Check your knowledge of protein.
		1 Most Americans eat more protein than they need.
		2 Protein is the nutrient most likely to be deficient in a purely vegetarian diet.
		3 The body stores extra amino acids in muscle tissue.
		4 The quality of soy protein is comparable to or greater than that of animal proteins.
		5 Nutritionally, the limiting factor in building muscle tissue is calorie intake, not protein intake.
		6 A protein classified as "high quality" has the majority of calories provided by protein, with few fat or carbohydrate calories.
		7 Protein is found in all Food Guide Pyramid groups.
		8 Healthy adults are in a state of positive nitrogen balance.
		9 Vegetarian diets are not adequate during pregnancy.
		10 There are no risks associated with eating too much protein.

Upon completion of this chapter, you will be able to

- Explain the difference between high-quality proteins and lower-quality proteins and name sources of each.
- Explain how an adequate calorie intake "spares" protein.
- Explain why protein must be consumed daily.
- Discuss the Recommended Dietary Allowance (RDA) for protein for adults and compare the RDA with the average American intake for protein.
- Discuss the nutrients that are most likely to be deficient in a vegetarian diet and vegetarian sources of each.
- Discuss how protein is used in the body.
- Describe protein digestion and absorption.

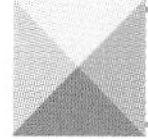

Keys to Understanding Protein

Proteins are large, complex molecules composed of individual building blocks known as amino acids. Like carbohydrates, **amino acids** are organic compounds made from carbon, hydrogen, and oxygen atoms. Unique to amino acids is their nitrogen component, which distinguishes them from the other energy nutrients. Protein is a component of every living cell.

AMINO ACIDS

All amino acids have a carbon atom core with four bonding sites: one site holds a hydrogen atom, one an amino group (NH_2), and one an acid group (COOH). Attached to the fourth bonding site is a side group (R group), which contains the atoms that give each amino acid its own distinct identity. For instance, the R group of the amino acid glycine is simply one hydrogen atom, whereas that of lysine is NH_2-CH_2-CH_2-CH_2-CH_2. Some side groups contain sulfur; some are acidic, and some are basic. The differences in these side groups account for the differences in size, shape, and electrical charge among amino acids.

There are 20 common amino acids (Box 3–1). Nine of them are classified as **essential amino acids** because they cannot be made by the body and therefore must be consumed through food. The remaining 11 are **nonessential amino acids** because they can be synthesized in the liver if nitrogen and other precursors are available. All 20 amino acids must be available for cells to synthesize the proteins they need.

PROTEINS

Proteins come in various sizes and shapes and are composed of different amino acids joined in various proportions and sequences. The complex structure of protein molecules can be considered from four different levels.

- **Primary structure** refers to a protein's unique sequence of amino acids. The number of amino acids in most proteins ranges from several dozen to several hundred. Just as the 26 letters of the alphabet can be used to form an infinite number of words, so can amino acids be joined in different amounts, proportions, and sequences to form a great variety of proteins. The body may contain as many as 100,000 different proteins.
- **Secondary structure** refers to the protein's shape along one dimension, such as whether it is straight, folded, or coiled.
- **Tertiary structure** pertains to the three-dimensional shape that forms when polypeptides fold back on themselves into spheres or globes.
- **Quaternary structure** refers to the joining of two or more three-dimensional polypeptides as they assemble into larger protein molecules.

BOX 3.1

Common Amino Acids

Essential Amino Acids	Nonessenial Amino Acids
Histidine	Alanine
Isoleucine	Arginine
Leucine	Asparagine
Lysine	Aspartic acid
Methionine	Cystine (cysteine)
Phenylalanine	Glutamic acid
Threonine	Glutamine
Tryptophan	Glycine
Valine	Proline
	Serine
	Tyrosine

The shapes of protein molecules are important because they determine the protein's function. For instance, *globular proteins* are highly water-soluble, ball-shaped proteins that circulate throughout the body's fluids. Immunoglobulins, hormones, hemoglobin, and most enzymes are examples of globular proteins. *Fibrous proteins* are long, thread-like strands of polypeptide chains that provide strength and support for tissues. Elastin and collagen are fibrous proteins located in the connective tissue of tendons, cartilage, bone, and ligaments. Tubular-shaped fibrous proteins, contained within cells, are important in cell movement and in cell shape maintenance. Actin and myosin in muscle cells are examples of tubular fibrous proteins.

HOW THE BODY HANDLES PROTEIN

Digestion

Chemical digestion of protein begins in the stomach, where hydrochloric acid denatures protein to make the peptide bonds more available to the actions of enzymes (Fig. 3–1). Hydrochloric acid also converts pepsinogen to the active enzyme pepsin, which begins the process of breaking down proteins into smaller polypeptides and some amino acids.

The majority of protein digestion occurs in the small intestine, where pancreatic proteases reduce polypeptides to shorter chains, tripeptides, dipeptides, and amino acids. The enzymes trypsin and chymotrypsin act to break peptide bonds between specific amino acids. Carboxypeptidase breaks off amino acids from the acid (carboxyl) end of polypeptides and dipeptides. Enzymes located on the surface of the cells that line the small intestine complete the digestion: aminopeptidase splits amino acids from the amino ends of short peptides, and dipeptidase reduces dipeptides to amino acids.

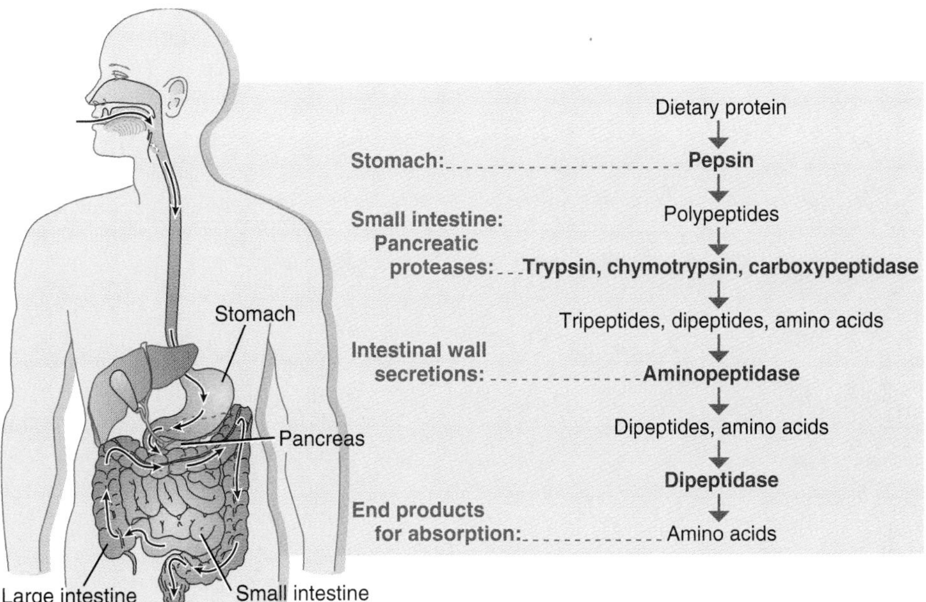

FIGURE 3-1 Protein digestion. Chemical digestion of protein begins in the stomach. Hydrochloric acid converts pepsinogen to the active enzyme pepsin, which begins the process of breaking down proteins into small polypeptides and some amino acids. The majority of protein digestion occurs in the small intestine, where pancreatic proteases reduce polypeptides into shorter chains, tripeptides, dipeptides, and amino acids. Enzymes located on the surface of the cells that line the small intestine complete the digestion: aminopeptidase splits amino acids from the amino ends of short peptides, and dipeptidase reduces dipeptides to amino acids.

Absorption

Amino acids, and sometimes a few dipeptides or larger peptides, are absorbed through the mucosa of the small intestine by active transport with the aid of vitamin B_6. Intestinal cells release amino acids into the bloodstream for transport to the liver via the portal vein.

Metabolism

The liver acts as a clearinghouse for the amino acids it receives: it uses the amino acids it needs, releases those that are needed elsewhere, and handles the extra. For instance, the liver retains amino acids to make liver cells, nonessential amino acids, and plasma proteins such as heparin, prothrombin, and albumin. The liver regulates the release of amino acids into the bloodstream and removes excess amino acids from the circulation. As enzymes are needed, the liver synthesizes specific enzymes to degrade excess amino acids. The liver removes the nitrogen from amino acids so that they can be burned for energy, and it converts amino acids to glucose or fat, as appropriate. The liver coordinates amino acid metabolism.

The pathways available to amino acids are either anabolic (building up) or catabolic (breaking down). Primarily, amino acids are used by all body cells to synthesize proteins that are either lost through normal wear and tear or are needed to build new tissue, such as during pregnancy or adolescent growth. Amino acids can also be used to make other molecules (eg, nonessential amino acids, other nitrogen-containing compounds, fat) when protein is consumed in excess of need. Catabolically, amino acids stripped of their nitrogen can be broken down for energy. Some amino acids can be converted to glucose.

Used for Protein Synthesis

Part of what makes every individual unique is the minute differences in body proteins, which are caused by variations in the sequencing of amino acids determined by genetics. Genetic material created at conception holds the instructions for making all of the body's proteins. This genetic material is contained in the deoxyribonucleic acid (DNA) located in the nucleus of every cell.

Protein synthesis is a complicated but efficient process that quickly assembles amino acids to create proteins needed by the body. The genetic codes for creating proteins are contained in the DNA. Cell function and life itself depend on the precise replication of these codes. An alteration in the structure of DNA, whether from radiation, chemicals, or other causes, impairs its ability to replicate and synthesize proteins. Unrepaired damage leads to abnormal cell function and possibly cell death. Such may be the sequence of events that leads to many types of cancer. Some important concepts related to protein synthesis are metabolic pool, nitrogen balance, and protein turnover.

METABOLIC POOL

Unlike glucose and fat, the body is not able to store excess amino acids for later use. However, a limited supply of free amino acids exists within cells in a dynamic *metabolic pool*, which accepts and donates amino acids as needed. This metabolic pool is constantly changing in response to the constant buildup and breakdown of body proteins and the influx of amino acids from food.

NITROGEN BALANCE

Body cells continuously make proteins to replace those that break down from normal wear and tear. For example, red blood cells are replaced every 60 to 90 days, gastrointestinal cells are replaced every 2 to 3 days, and enzymes used in the digestion of food are continuously replenished. When the amount of protein made is equal to the amount lost, the body is said to be in a state of neutral *nitrogen balance*. Healthy adults are in neutral nitrogen balance. When protein synthesis exceeds protein breakdown, such as during growth, pregnancy, or recovery from injury, a *positive nitrogen balance* exists. A *negative nitrogen balance* is an undesirable state that occurs when protein breakdown exceeds protein synthesis, such as during starvation or the catabolic phase after injury.

The state of nitrogen balance is determined by comparing nitrogen intake with nitrogen excretion over a 24-hour period. To calculate nitrogen intake, protein intake is measured for a 24-hour period. The total grams of protein consumed is then divided by

6.25, because protein is 16% nitrogen by weight. The result is the grams of nitrogen consumed per 24 hours. Nitrogen excretion is calculated by having a 24-hour urine sample analyzed for the amount (grams) of urinary urea nitrogen it contains. To this number a coefficient of 4 is added to account for the estimated daily nitrogen loss in feces, hair, nails, and skin. Finally, the amount of nitrogen consumed is compared with the total amount of nitrogen excreted to reveal a positive, negative, or neutral nitrogen balance (Box 3–2).

PROTEIN TURNOVER

The body's supply of amino acids comes from food (exogenous) and from its own protein tissue (endogenous). Amino acids released when body proteins break down may be recycled to build new proteins or stripped of their nitrogen and burned for energy. This constant breakdown and synthesis of endogenous protein is known as *protein turnover*. Body proteins vary in their rate of turnover. For instance, protein turnover in the liver, pancreas, and small intestine is rapid; during times of need, these tissues give up amino acids for protein synthesis or energy. The turnover of muscle proteins is slower, and the turnover in the brain and nervous system is negligible.

Used to Make Nonessential Amino Acids

Cells have the ability to remedy a shortage of nonessential amino acids by the process of *transamination*, which involves removing the amino group from one amino acid and com-

BOX 3.2

Calculating Nitrogen Balance

Mary is a 25-year-old woman who was admitted to the hospital with multiple fractures and traumatic injuries from a car accident. A nutritional intake study indicated a 24-hour protein intake of 64 g. A 24-hour urinary urea nitrogen (UUN) collection result was 19.8 g.

1. Determine nitrogen intake by dividing protein intake by 6.25:

$$64 \div 6.25 = 10.24 \text{ g of nitrogen}$$

2. Determine total nitrogen output by adding a coefficient of 4 to the UUN:

$$19.8 + 4 = 23.8 \text{ g of nitrogen}$$

3. Calculate nitrogen balance by subtracting nitrogen output from nitrogen intake:

$$10.24 - 23.8 = -13.56 \text{ g in 24 hours}$$

4. Interpret the results.

A negative number indicates that protein breakdown is exceeding protein synthesis. Mary is in a catabolic state.

bining it with carbon fragments of glucose molecules to create the particular amino acid that is needed. However, the body cannot make essential amino acids; they must be furnished through the diet or from the breakdown of body proteins.

Used to Make Nitrogen-containing Compounds

Cells use amino acids to synthesize other nitrogen-containing compounds. For instance, amino acids are needed to create the purine bases of DNA, the neurotransmitter epinephrine, and creatine, which combines with phosphate to form the high-energy compound creatine phosphate. Specific amino acids have specific functions within the body. For instance, tryptophan is a precursor of the vitamin niacin, and tyrosine is the precursor of melanin, the pigment that colors hair and skin.

Used for Glucose

Certain body tissues, such as brain and nervous tissue, rely solely on glucose for energy. When carbohydrate intake is inadequate and glycogen reserves are exhausted, the body resorts to converting amino acids into glucose. Approximately 58% of the amino acids in proteins are *glucogenic*, which means they can be used to synthesize glucose. First, these amino acids are stripped of their nitrogen-containing amino group (NH_2) by the process of *deamination*. The three–carbon atom fragment that remains is converted to pyruvate; then, two pyruvate molecules are joined together to form the six–carbon atom molecule, glucose. Although only glucogenic amino acids can be converted to glucose, whole proteins must be broken down to make them available. The remaining amino acids are not glucogenic and are used for energy by other body cells.

Ammonia (NH_3) is produced from the deamination of amino acids. In the liver, some of this ammonia is used in the synthesis of nonessential amino acids. The remaining ammonia combines with carbon dioxide to make urea, which is released into the blood, circulates to the kidneys, and is excreted in the urine.

Burned for Energy

Normally the body uses very little protein for energy, so long as intake and storage of carbohydrate and fat are adequate. If insufficient carbohydrate and fat are available for energy use, or if protein is consumed in amounts greater than those needed for protein synthesis, amino acids are broken down for energy. However, the use of protein for energy is a physiologic and economic waste, because amino acids that are used for energy are not available to be used for protein synthesis, a function unique to amino acids. Another disadvantage of using protein for energy is the burden placed on the kidneys to excrete the nitrogenous waste. Protein is also more expensive to buy than carbohydrates, and rich sources of protein are often high in fat.

There are three routes by which deaminated amino acids can be catabolized for energy in the tricarboxylic acid (TCA) cycle, depending on the number of carbon atoms they contain. Glucogenic amino acids (three carbon atoms) enter the cycle by way of pyruvate; pyruvate can form glucose or be catabolized for energy. Ketogenic amino acids (two carbon atoms) are first converted to acetyl coenzyme A (acetyl-CoA). Other amino acids (eg, those with six carbon atoms) enter the TCA cycle directly. All proteins provide 4 cal/g of energy, regardless of their amino acid composition.

Converted to Fat

At this point, protein that has not been used for specific protein functions has been deaminated, leaving a carbon fragment that is ready to be burned for energy. But if energy needs are already satisfied, the carbon fragment (initially or eventually acetyl-CoA) undergoes lipogenesis to form fatty acids, which combine with glycerol to form triglycerides, the storage form of fat in the body. Protein is converted to fat only when it is consumed in excess of need.

FUNCTIONS OF PROTEIN IN THE BODY

By now the prevalence and diversity of protein throughout the body should be apparent. All body cells are made of protein, and all body cells make protein. Protein functions are many and varied.

- **Structure and framework.** Proteins function to grow, repair, and maintain body structures. Bones, muscles, tendons, ligaments, blood vessels, skin, hair, and nails all contain protein.
- **Enzymes.** Enzymes are proteins that facilitate specific chemical reactions in the body without undergoing change themselves. Some enzymes (eg, digestive enzymes) break down larger molecules into smaller ones; others (eg, enzymes involved in protein synthesis, in which amino acids are combined) join molecules together to form larger compounds.
- **Other body secretions and fluids.** Hormones (eg, insulin, thryoxine, epinephrine), neurotransmitters (eg, serotonin, acetylcholine), and antibodies are all made from protein, as are breast milk, mucus, sperm, and histamine.
- **Fluid and electrolyte balance.** Proteins help regulate fluid balance because they attract water, thereby creating osmotic pressure. Circulating proteins, such as albumin, maintain the proper balance of fluid among the intravascular (within veins and arteries), intracellular (within the cells), and interstitial (in the fluid between the cells) compartments of the body. A symptom of low albumin is edema, which is characterized by the swelling of body tissues secondary to accumulation of fluid in the interstitial spaces.
- **Acid–base balance.** Because amino acids contain both an acid (COOH) and a base (NH_2), they can act as either acids or bases depending on the pH of the surrounding fluid. This ability to buffer or neutralize excess acids and bases enables proteins to maintain normal blood pH, which protects body proteins from being denatured (with subsequent loss of function).
- **Transport molecules.** Globular proteins transport other substances through the blood. For instance, lipoproteins transport fats, cholesterol, and fat-soluble vitamins; hemoglobin transports oxygen; and albumin transports free fatty acids, bilirubin, and many drugs.

- **Other compounds.** As previously stated, protein is included in numerous body compounds, such as opsin, the light-sensitive visual pigment in the eye, and thrombin, a protein necessary for normal blood clotting.
- **Energy.** Like carbohydrates, protein provides 4 cal/g. Although it is not the body's preferred fuel, protein is a source of energy when it is consumed in excess of need or when calorie intake from carbohydrates and fat is inadequate.

DIETARY PROTEIN: SOURCES AND QUALITY

Just as body proteins contain different quantities and proportions of amino acids, so do the proteins in food. It is these differences in amino acid profiles that determine the *quality* of a food protein (ie, its ability to support protein synthesis). For most Americans, protein quality is not important because the amounts of protein and calories consumed are more than adequate. But when protein needs are increased or protein intake is marginal, quality becomes a crucial consideration. Any discussion of protein sources must also consider protein quality, because quality influences the quantity of protein needed.

Protein Sources

Dietary proteins can be classified by their origin: plant or animal. Based on the Food Guide Pyramid (see Chapter 8), plant sources of protein are found in the Bread, Cereal, Rice, and Pasta group and in the Vegetable group; dry beans and nuts also provide plant protein. As a group, fruits provide only small amounts of protein. Animal sources of protein are found in the Milk, Yogurt, and Cheese group and in the Meat, Poultry, Fish, Dry Beans, Eggs, and Nuts group. Fats, oils, and sweets generally do not provide protein. For both plant and animal sources, protein quantity and quality vary among the items within each group (Table 3–1).

Protein Quality

The quality of a protein is determined by the balance of essential amino acids it provides.

- **Complete proteins,** which are said to have *high biologic value*, provide all nine essential amino acids in adequate amounts and proportions needed by the body for growth and tissue maintenance. With the exception of gelatin, all animal sources of protein (meat, fish, poultry, eggs, milk, and dairy products) are complete proteins. Soy protein is the only complete plant protein.
- **Incomplete proteins,** those of *low biologic value*, provide all the essential amino acids, but one or more of these amino acids is present at levels insufficient for human needs. The essential amino acid that is present in the smallest amount is known as the *limiting* amino acid because it limits protein synthesis to the extent

TABLE 3.1 *Variations in Protein Content Among Items in Each Food Guide Pyramid Food Group*

Food Group	Amount	Average Protein Content (g)
Bread, Cereal, Rice, and Pasta		
Whole-grain products	1 serving	2.3
Enriched grain products	1 serving	2.1
Vegetables		
Dark green vegetables	1 serving	1.9
Deep yellow vegetables	1 serving	0.9
Starchy vegetables	1 serving	2.5
Other vegetables	1 serving	0.8
Fruits	1 serving	0.9
Milk, Yogurt, and Cheese		
Milk	1 cup	8.0
Yogurt	1 cup	10.0
Cottage cheese	2 cups*	48.0
Hard cheese	1 oz	6.0–8.0
Meat, Poultry, Fish, Dry Beans, Eggs, and Nuts		
Meat, fish, and poultry	1 oz	7.0
Dry beans	½ cup cooked	7.0
Eggs	1 large	7.0
Peanut butter	2 tablespoons	8.0–9.0
Fats, Oils, and Sweets		
Fat	1 tsp	0
Sugar	1 tsp	0

*Serving size based on calcium equivalents, not on protein or calorie content.

of its availability. Once it is used up, protein synthesis cannot continue, and the remaining amino acids are either wasted or used for something else.

With the exception of soybeans, all plant proteins are incomplete. However, the limiting amino acids differ among plant proteins. For instance, grains are typically low in lysine, legumes are low in methionine and cysteine, and nuts are low in lysine and isoleucine. Combining two different incomplete proteins, or a small amount of any complete protein with an incomplete protein, boosts the overall quality to that of a complete protein. Proteins that can be combined to obtain sufficient quantities and proportions of all essential amino acids are called *complementary proteins*. Examples include

- Two different complementary plant proteins combined to form a complete protein:
  - Black beans and rice
  - Bean tacos
  - Pea soup with toast
  - Lentil and rice curry

  - Falafel sandwich (ground chickpea patties on pita bread)
  - Peanut butter sandwich
  - Pasta e fagioli (pasta and white bean stew)
- A plant protein complemented by a small amount of an animal protein to form a complete protein:
  - Bread pudding
  - Rice pudding
  - Corn pudding
  - Cereal and milk
  - Macaroni and cheese
  - Cheese fondue
  - Bean soup and milk
  - French toast
  - Cheese sandwich
  - Vegetable quiche

Historically, vegetarians were advised to eat complementary proteins at every meal. Experts now contend that it is not necessary to consciously complement proteins at every meal, so long as a variety of proteins is eaten and calorie intake is adequate. Over the course of a day, if calories are adequate and a variety of grains, legumes, seeds, nuts, and vegetables are consumed, adequate amounts of all the essential amino acids will be provided.

INTAKE RECOMMENDATIONS

The Recommended Dietary Allowance (RDA) for protein for a healthy adult is 0.8 g/kg, which is approximately 10% of recommended total calories. This protein allowance is derived from the absolute minimum requirement needed to maintain nitrogen balance plus an additional factor to account for individual variations and the mixed quality of proteins typically consumed. This allowance is also based on the assumption that calorie intake is adequate. The information in Box 3–3 can be used to calculate how much protein should be consumed daily.

The RDAs for protein for the "reference man" and "reference woman" (medians for the U.S. population) are 63 g and 50 g, respectively. Table 3–2 lists the protein RDAs for various age groups and conditions. Notice that the protein allowance per kilogram of body weight is highest during infancy and gradually decreases until it stabilizes sometime during middle to late adolescence, corresponding to the completion of growth. Likewise, higher protein allowances are set for pregnancy and lactation to account for tissue growth and milk production.

In addition to age, growth, and body weight, other factors influence how much protein the body needs. For instance, muscle tissue is metabolically active and requires protein to maintain itself, so protein needs are higher for people with a large muscle mass than for people with less muscle. That is why men actually need more protein than women (who typically have less muscle mass than men) and bodybuilders need more

BOX 3.3

Calculating Daily Protein Allowance

John is a 30-year-old man who weighs 184 pounds. What is his daily protein allowance?

1. Determine the weight in kilograms by dividing the weight in pounds by 2.54:

$$184 \div 2.54 = 72.44 \text{ kg}$$

2. Multiply the weight in kilograms by 0.8 g/kg (the RDA for men 19 years of age and older or women 15 years and older):

$$72.44 \times 0.8 = 57.95 \text{ g}$$

John should consume 58 g of protein per day.

TABLE 3.2 *Recommended Dietary Allowances for Protein*

Category	Age (y) or Condition	Weight (kg)	RDA (g/kg)*	RDA (g/d)
Both sexes	0–0.5	6	2.2	13
	0.5–1	9	1.6	14
	1–3	13	1.2	16
	4–6	20	1.1	24
	7–10	28	1.0	28
Men	11–14	45	1.0	45
	15–18	66	0.9	59
	19–24	72	0.8	58
	25–50	79	0.8	63
	51+	77	0.8	63
Women	11–14	46	1.0	46
	15–18	55	0.8	44
	19–24	58	0.8	46
	25–50	63	0.8	50
	51+	65	0.8	50
Pregnancy	1st trimester			+10
	2nd trimester			+10
	3rd trimester			+10
Lactation	1st 6 mo			+15
	2nd 6 mo			+12

*The amino acid score of the typical U.S. diet is 100 for all age groups except young infants. These figures take into account the quality and digestibility of the typical American amino acid intake. Values have been rounded upward to the nearest 0.1 g/kg.

+: means in addition to a person's normal RDA.

Source: National Research Council (1989).

protein than adults with a stable muscle mass. Emotional or physical stress, infection, and high environmental temperatures increase nitrogen excretion, thereby increasing protein needs. Protein needs are increased when calorie intake is inadequate, because protein that is required for energy production cannot be used for protein synthesis. Also, whenever the body needs to heal itself, whether from surgery, trauma, or burns, protein requirements increase. Protein restriction is used for people with severe liver disease and those with renal failure who are unable to excrete nitrogenous wastes. It is important to remember that the RDA is intended for healthy people only.

Protein intake, per se, is not addressed in the *Dietary Guidelines for Americans* (see Chapter 8), and among leading health agencies that make diet recommendations the issue of protein appears to be more of an afterthought than a key element. The decades-long focus on limiting fat has expanded to include eating more whole grains, fruits, and vegetables (carbohydrates). Most experts agree that fat should be limited to 30% or less of total calories and that 50% to 60% of calories should come from carbohydrates. That leaves the remaining 10% to 20% of calories to be obtained from protein.

In a 1600-cal diet, 10% to 20% of total calories would be equivalent to 160 to 320 cal from protein. Because protein provides 4 cal/g, the corresponding range of protein intake per day is 40 to 80 g (160 cal ÷ 4 cal/g = 40 g, and 320 cal ÷ 4 cal/g = 80 g protein).

Shown here is the amount of protein obtained from the minimum recommended number of servings from each of the Food Guide Pyramid groups (see Chapter 8).

Food Group	No. Servings		Protein Content per Serving (g)		Total Protein (g)
Bread, Cereal, Rice, and Pasta	6	×	3.0	=	18.0
Vegetables					
Dark green	1	×	1.9		
Deep yellow	1	×	0.9	=	5.3
Starchy	1	×	2.5		
Fruits	2	×	0.9	=	1.8
Milk, Yogurt, and Cheese	2	×	8.0	=	16.0
Meat, Poultry, Fish, Dry Beans, Eggs, and Nuts	5 oz	×	7.0 g/oz	=	35.0
Total					76.1

As this example shows, eating the minimum number of servings from each group (totaling approximately 1600 cal) provides 76.1 g of protein (19% of total calories), exceeding the reference RDA for adult men and women (76.1 g × 4 cal/g = 304.4 protein calories, and 304.4 ÷ 1600 = 19% of total calories). Yet for most Americans, this example of 5 ounces from the Meat, Poultry, Fish, Dry Beans, Eggs, and Nuts group significantly underestimates average daily intake from this group. For example, a queen-size steak at a restaurant can weigh 10 to 12 ounces—double the recommended intake for an *entire day* from this food group in the example just cited. Likewise, one fast food double cheeseburger provides 41 g of protein, more than half the total daily protein intake.

What amazes meat-loving Americans is that even *without any* selections from the Meat, Poultry, Fish, Dry Beans, Eggs, and Nuts group, the total protein intake is 40.1 g, or 10% of total calories. No one recommends eliminating this or any of the Food Guide Pyramid groups (vegetarians don't eliminate this group but choose selectively from it); this case simply shows that, for most Americans, obtaining enough protein is not a problem. In fact, average protein consumption for American women is 55 to 65 g/day (compared with an RDA of 50 g). For adult men, with an RDA of 63 g, average intakes range from 105 g/day among 19- to 29-year-olds, to 93 g for 30- to 59-year-olds and 79 g for 60- to 69-year-olds.

The National Academy of Sciences Committee on Diet and Health recommends that protein intake not exceed twice the RDA, or 1.6 g/kg of body weight for adults. High protein intakes are associated with increased urinary excretion of calcium, which may contribute to the risk of osteoporosis. High protein intake also burdens the kidneys to excrete nitrogen, which may play a role in the loss of renal function that occurs with aging. Finally, high intakes of animal proteins are linked to atherosclerosis (related to their saturated fat and cholesterol content) and to colon and prostate cancers (possibly related to animal fat or to something else in meat that promotes tumor formation).

In the average American diet, protein provides 16% to 17% of total calories consumed. According to data from the *Continuing Survey of Food Intakes by Individuals* (Subar, Krebs-Smith, Cook, et al. 1998), from 1989–1991 the top five sources of protein in the American diet were beef, poultry, milk, yeast bread, and cheese.

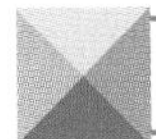

Protein in Health Promotion

VEGETARIAN DIETS

Vegetarianism, loosely defined as the abstinence from animal products, encompasses a variety of eating styles. Pure vegetarians, or **vegans,** eat only plants; they form the smallest group of vegetarians. Most vegetarians in the United States are classified as either **lacto-vegetarians,** whose diets include milk products, or **lacto-ovovegetarians,** who eat both milk products and eggs. Many Americans consider themselves vegetarians simply because they avoid red meat. Within each general category, individuals vary as to how strictly they adhere to their eating style. For instance, some vegans do not eat refried beans that contain lard because lard is an animal product, but other vegans do not avoid animal products so conscientiously. People who generally abstain from red meat may allow themselves an occasional steak or hamburger.

In addition to the political, philosophical, religious, and economic motivations for becoming vegetarian, the potential health benefits are attracting a growing number of recruits. Because they eat fewer or no animal products, vegetarians consume less saturated fat and cholesterol. Eating more plants—grains, legumes, fruits, and vegetables—translates into consuming more fiber, folate, antioxidants, and phytochemicals. Health benefits may come from eating less of certain nutrients, eating more of others, or a combination of the two. Or health benefits may be related to some other lifestyle practice vegetarians may adopt, such as participating in regular exercise, abstaining from tobacco, or using alcohol only moderately, if at all. Whatever the reasons, the end result is that vegetarians have lower incidences of obesity, coronary artery disease, hypertension, diabetes mellitus, lung cancer, and colorectal cancer, compared with nonvegetarians. Vegetarians may also be at lower risk for osteoporosis, kidney stones, gallstones, and breast cancer.

Vegetarian diets are not automatically healthier than nonvegetarian diets. Poorly planned vegetarian diets may be lacking in certain essential nutrients, endangering health. Also, vegetarian diets can be excessive in fat and cholesterol if whole milk, whole-milk cheeses, eggs, nuts, and high-fat desserts are used extensively. Whether a vegetarian diet is healthy or detrimental to health depends on the actual food choices made over time.

Nutrients of Concern

A nutrient that does not make this list, even among vegans, is protein. Vegetarian diets meet or exceed the RDA for protein, even though they contain less protein and lower-quality protein than nonvegetarian diets do. Over the course of a day, if a variety of foods are consumed and calories are adequate, sufficient amounts of all essential amino acids can be obtained from plants. In addition, the quality of soy protein is comparable to or exceeds that of animal proteins, so products such as tofu (soybean curd), tempeh (caked fermented soybeans), meat analogs (eg, soy burgers, soy hot dogs), and textured soy protein (soy flour modified to resemble ground beef when rehydrated) are excellent alternatives to meat. Furthermore, avoiding excessive protein offers the benefits of improved calcium retention and decreased renal workload.

Iron, zinc, calcium, vitamin D, and linolenic acid are nutrients of concern—not because they cannot be obtained in sufficient quantities from plants, but because they may not be adequately consumed, depending on an individual's food choices. Vitamin B_{12} is of concern because it does not occur naturally in plants.

- **Iron.** Iron in plants (nonheme iron) is not as well absorbed as the heme iron in meat. Although vegetarians have lower stores of iron than nonvegetarians, they do not have higher rates of iron deficiency anemia. This may be because vegetarians consume more vitamin C, which enhances the absorption of nonheme iron. Vegetarian sources of iron include iron-fortified bread and cereals, sea vegetables, legumes, soybeans, tofu, and greens.
- **Zinc.** Many plants provide zinc, but it is not absorbed as well as the zinc in meats. Vegetarians may eat less zinc than nonvegetarians, but they are able to maintain adequate zinc levels in hair, serum, and saliva, possibly because compensatory mechanisms enable them to adapt to lower zinc intakes. Still, vegetarians are urged to meet or exceed the RDA for zinc. Plant sources of zinc include whole grains (especially the bran and germ), legumes, soybean products, seeds, and nuts. Lacto-ovovegetarians obtain zinc from milk, yogurt, and eggs.

- **Calcium.** Calcium intake of lacto-vegetarians and lacto-ovovegetarians is comparable to or higher than that of nonvegetarians. Vegans consume less calcium, but, because their lower total protein intake promotes calcium retention, their actual calcium requirement may be lower than normal. However, all vegetarians are advised to consume at least the level of calcium recommended for their age group. For people who do not use milk or dairy products, calcium-fortified orange juice, calcium-fortified or calcium-processed soyfoods, legumes, tortillas made from lime-processed corn, and some dark green leafy vegetables can provide adequate calcium. Calcium supplements are recommended for people who do not meet their requirement from food.
- **Vitamin D.** Vitamin D is low in all diets that do not include vitamin D–fortified foods. Fortified milk is the biggest dietary source of vitamin D. The other major source of vitamin D is sunlight, which converts vitamin D precursors in the skin to vitamin D. In fact, humans have the potential to obtain adequate vitamin D from just 5 to 15 minutes of daily sun exposure on the face, hands, and arms. In practice, sunlight alone is not enough for many people, including people with dark skin, people living in northern climates, people who use sunscreens, and the elderly (because aging impairs vitamin D synthesis). Fortified ready-to-eat cereals, fortified soymilk, and other fortified nondairy milk products provide vitamin D.
- **Linolenic acid.** Diets that do not include fish or eggs lack the omega-3 fatty acid docosahexanoic acid (DHA). Some studies show that vegetarians have low levels of DHA in their blood, but the significance of this is not known. As a safety measure, vegetarians are advised to consume good sources of the essential fatty acid linolenic acid, because the body can convert linolenic acid to DHA. Flaxseed, walnuts, walnut oil, canola oil, and soybean oil are sources of linolenic acid.
- **Vitamin B_{12}.** Vitamin B_{12} is a concern for vegans, because it is naturally found only in animals. If plants contain vitamin B_{12}, it is either because they have been fortified with it or because they are contaminated with soil that contains microorganisms producing vitamin B_{12}; food handling and sanitation practices in the United States virtually eliminate the possibility of vitamin B_{12} on fruits and vegetables. Reliable sources of vitamin B_{12} are fortified foods, including ready-to-eat cereals, meat analogs, and soymilk. Supplements containing *cyanocobalamin*, the most readily absorbed form of vitamin B_{12}, are also reliable. Some brands of nutritional yeast contain vitamin B_{12}, and some do not (baking yeast does not provide vitamin B_{12}). Products that are *not* reliable for this vitamin are seaweed, algae, spirulina, tempeh, miso, beer, and other fermented foods; they contain a form of vitamin B_{12} the body cannot use.

Is Vegetarianism for Everyone?

Vegetarianism is a personal choice, subject to personal interpretation. Although some view vegetarianism as a way of life, others prefer to simply opt for occasional meatless meals. Whatever the level of restriction, properly planned lacto-vegetarian, lacto-ovovegetarian, and vegan diets are nutritionally adequate during all phases of the life cycle, including pregnancy and lactation. *Proper planning* means paying close attention to the nutrients of concern (listed earlier) and choosing wisely. A vegetarian Food Guide Pyramid appears in Figure 3–2.

Tips for Choosing a Healthy Vegetarian Diet

- **Eat a variety of foods.** Vary choices from each of the Food Guide Pyramid groups; the greater the variety, the greater the likelihood that adequate amounts of essential nutrients will be consumed. For instance, variety in the Meat, Poultry, Fish, Dry Beans, Eggs, and Nuts group can be achieved by choosing different types of legumes, different types of soyfoods, and various nuts and seeds. The only group ever actually eliminated is the Milk, Yogurt, and Cheese group by pure vegans; they need to be sure to consume enough calcium from alternative sources. Calcium-fortified orange juice ranks as a comparable alternative to milk, at least in terms of calcium content.
- **Eat enough calories.** Adequate calories are necessary to avoid using amino acids for energy, which could lead to a shortage of amino acids for protein synthesis.

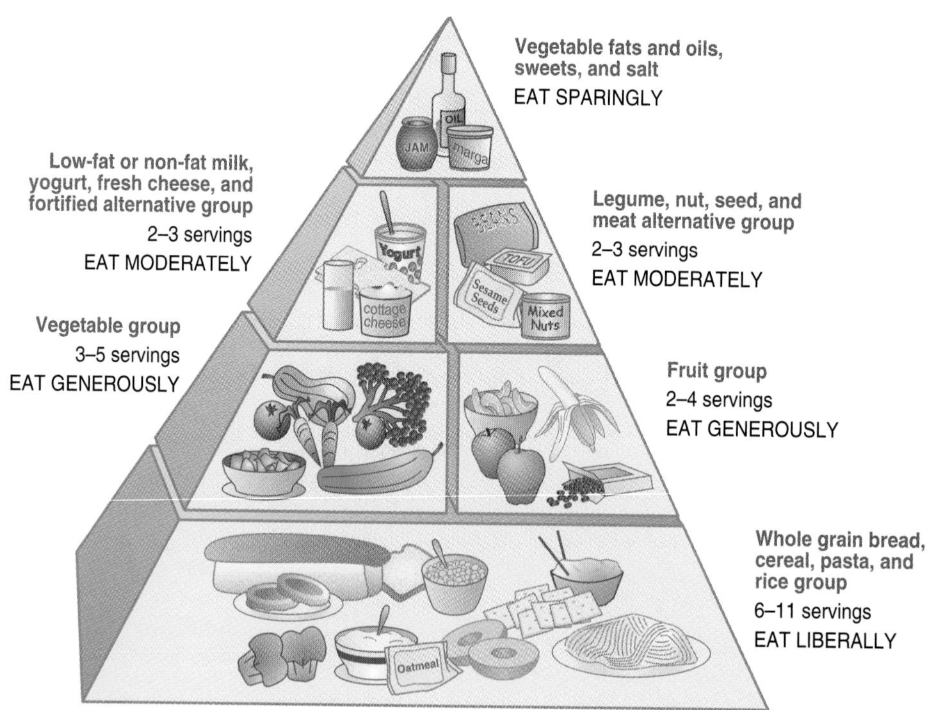

FIGURE 3-2 Lacto-vegetarian Food Guide Pyramid.

Attention to calories is especially important whenever protein requirements are high, such as during pregnancy and lactation and during childhood and adolescence, when protein requirements per kilogram of body weight are higher than those of adults. But calories should not be eaten just for the sake of calories: focus on sources of calories that also provide nutrients.

- **Choose grains wisely.** Grains are the foundation of a healthy diet for both vegetarians and meat-eaters. Whole grains provide fiber, iron, and zinc, and fortified cereals are rich sources of iron and folic acid. Experimenting with a variety of grains—barley, amaranth, buckwheat, bulgur, millet, kasha, quinoa, triticale—can turn familiar meals into exciting new feasts.
- **Consume a rich source of vitamin C at every meal.** Sources of vitamin C include citrus fruits and juices, tomatoes, broccoli, green and red peppers, guava, brussels sprouts, strawberries, and cabbage. Eating a good source of Vitamin C at every meal helps maximize nonheme iron absorption.
- **Avoid excess fat.** If milk and dairy products are in the meal plan, select low-fat varieties. Limit high-fat desserts and snacks that are calorie-rich but nutritionally bankrupt. Like nonvegetarians, vegetarians should limit egg yolks to four or fewer per week. Go easy on nuts, nut butters, and seeds.
- **Supplement nutrients that are lacking from food.** For vegans, that means vitamin B_{12} (unless reliable fortified foods are consumed) and perhaps vitamin D. The adequacy of calcium, iron, and zinc intakes is evaluated on an individual basis.

Box 3–4 lists resources available on the World Wide Web that can provide additional information on vegetarian diets.

PROTEIN FOR BODYBUILDERS

Bodybuilders easily fall prey to advertising claims that protein is the key to building muscle. They forsake starches for mounds of beef, chicken, tuna, and eggs. For extra measure, they take protein or amino acid supplements in pills, powders, and potions. They reason that more protein means more energy, more strength, and more muscles. In truth, high-protein diets—with or without amino acid supplements—are neither beneficial nor harmless.

BOX 3.4

Internet Addresses for Information on Vegetarian Diets

North American Vegetarian Society
www.cyberveg.org/navs

Vegetarian Resource Group
www.vrg.org

Building Muscles

Logic would indicate that to increase the size of a muscle, a protein tissue, one must feed it more protein. To some extent this is true; in theory, to gain 1 pound of muscle per week, an extra 14 g of protein is needed daily (the amount of protein in only 2 ounces of meat). In general, experts recommend that athletes consume 1.0 to 1.5 g of protein per kilogram of body weight, up from the RDA of 0.8 g/kg. Considering that the average American diet contains ample amounts of protein, most people already eat more than enough protein to build muscle. If muscle building were simply a matter of eating enough protein, Americans would be bulging with muscles. Although muscles do take up extra protein as they increase in size, they are not able to simply grab extra amino acids and convert them to muscle. The only way to build and strengthen muscle is through resistance exercises, such as weight lifting and pushups. Nutritionally, the limiting factor for building muscle is calorie intake, not protein. Although actual calorie requirements vary among individuals and with the frequency and intensity of athletic training, it is recommended that carbohydrates contribute 60% to 65% of total calories, up slightly from the normal recommendation of 50% to 60%. To bulk up, athletes need exercise, enough calories, and adequate protein.

More is not Better

Not only are high-protein diets not able to stimulate muscle gain, but they are potentially harmful. High-protein diets burden the kidneys to excrete excess nitrogen; some experts believe that a high-protein diet over time leads to loss of renal function with aging. High-protein diets are often high in fat; like the general public, athletes are urged to limit total fat intake to 30% or less of total calories. High-protein diets are proportionately low in carbohydrates; inadequate carbohydrate intake compromises glycogen storage in the liver and muscles, risking fatigue and poor performance that can hinder exercise and muscle building. Finally, protein consumed in excess of need is used for energy or converted to fat and stored; for everyone, health risks increase as the percentage of body fat increases.

Amino Acid Supplements

Health food stores, health clubs, and Internet outlets offer a vast selection of protein and amino acid supplements with reputed benefits ranging from muscle development to cures for obesity, depression, pain, and infections. Unlike food, which contains all 20 amino acids in proper balance, supplements may contain disproportionate amounts of one or more amino acids. Because protein synthesis in the body uses all amino acids, there is no advantage to having an excess of any of them: protein synthesis cannot continue after the supply of the limiting amino acid has been depleted. In fact, too much of one amino acid can impair the absorption and use of others, thereby inducing deficiencies. The body is not equipped to handle an excessive or unbalanced supply of amino acids.

Supplements of single amino acids have been linked with health problems. Most notably, supplements of tryptophan, an amino acid promoted as a sleep aid, have been blamed for 38 deaths and hundreds of cases of permanent neurologic damage. Although contaminants introduced in the manufacturing process are suspected, experts have not ruled out the possibility that other factors may have contributed.

Compared with getting amino acids from food, getting them from supplements is expensive. A person can obtain 1050 mg of the amino acid arginine from 27 pills of a supplement costing $2.60, or from 3 cups of skim milk costing 60 cents. Compared with protein powders, tuna, milk, and eggs are more economical, are subjectively tastier, and provide other nutrients in addition to protein.

Tips for Eating to Build Muscles

- **Stick to the Food Guide Pyramid.** Athletes need the same balance and proportion of foods as the general public, but they may need to choose the highest number of servings for each food group. Use fats and sugars sparingly.
- **Eat enough calories.** Extra nutrient-dense calories should come from high-carbohydrate, low-fat foods. Depending on calorie requirements, athletes may need more servings, larger portions, or more frequent meals.
- **Eat protein every day.** Because the body cannot store amino acids, they need to be consumed daily. It is not essential to eat meat in order to obtain adequate protein.
- **Drink plenty of fluid.** Muscle activity generates heat, which is dissipated through evaporation of water on the skin. Water must be replaced faster than it is lost, or dehydration will occur. Actual fluid requirements vary with the intensity of the exercise and environmental temperatures. Guidelines suggest that urine output be monitored to evaluate the adequacy of fluid intake: dark and scanty urine means that more fluid is needed; pale yellow urine with normal volume means that fluid intake is adequate. Body weight is another indicator of fluid adequacy: for each 1 pound of weight lost during exercise, 2 cups of fluid should be consumed.
- **Think wholesome.** The requirements for certain vitamins and minerals increase in response to the increased need for calories. A high-carbohydrate, moderate-protein, low-fat diet featuring a variety of wholesome foods is the best way to meet increased needs.
- **Be wary of potions and pills that sound too good to be true.** Researchers have failed to substantiate claims that ergogenic aids such as bee pollen, glycine, carnitine, lecithin, and gelatin improve strength or endurance.

Questions You May Hear

What is a macrobiotic diet? The Zen-macrobiotic diet, promoted as a cure for cancer, is an extreme type of vegetarian diet that progresses through ten increasingly restrictive levels. The "ultimate" diet consists mainly of brown rice and small amounts of fluid. The "higher" diets have caused dehydration, severe cases of malnutrition, and even death.

Does gelatin make fingernails stronger? There is nothing magical about gelatin that enables it to grow or fortify fingernails. Gelatin, like all other dietary proteins, is digested into its amino acids and used by the body as needed.

KEY CONCEPTS

- Protein is a component of every living cell. Except for bile and urine, every tissue and fluid in the body contains some protein.
- Amino acids, composed of carbon, hydrogen, oxygen, and nitrogen atoms, are the building blocks of protein. There are 20 common amino acids, 9 of which are considered essential because they cannot be made by the body. The remaining 11 amino acids are no less important, but they are considered nonessential because they can be made by the body.
- Amino acids are joined in different amounts, proportions, and sequences to form the thousands of different proteins in the body.
- The small intestine is the principal site of protein digestion; amino acids and some dipeptides are absorbed through the portal bloodstream.
- In the body, amino acids are used to make proteins, nonessential amino acids, and other nitrogen-containing compounds. Some amino acids can be converted to glucose. Amino acids consumed in excess of need are burned for energy or converted to fat and stored.
- Protein in the body provides structure and framework. Proteins are also components of enzymes, hormones, neurotransmitters, and antibodies. Proteins play a role in fluid balance and acid-base balance and are used to transport substances through the blood. Protein provides 4 cal/g of energy.
- Healthy adults are in nitrogen balance, which means that protein synthesis is occurring at the same rate as protein breakdown. Nitrogen balance is determined by comparing the amount of nitrogen consumed with the amount of nitrogen excreted in urine, feces, hair, nails, and skin.
- All of the Food Guide Pyramid groups provide protein; pure fats and pure sugars do not contain protein.
- The quality of proteins varies. Complete proteins, those with high biologic value, provide adequate amounts and proportions of all essential amino acids needed for protein synthesis. Animal proteins and soy protein are complete proteins. Incomplete proteins lack adequate amounts of one or more essential amino acids. Except for soy protein, all plants are sources of incomplete proteins.
- The RDA for protein for adults is 0.8 g/kg of body weight. Most experts recommend that protein contribute 10% to 20% of total calories in the diet. Most Americans consume more protein than they need.
- High protein intakes may increase the risk of osteoporosis and renal insufficiency. High intakes of animal protein are linked to atherosclerosis and to colon and prostate cancers.
- Pure vegans eat no animal products. Most American vegetarians are lacto-vegetarians or lacto-ovovegetarians, whose diets include, respectively, milk products or milk products and eggs.

- Most vegetarian diets meet or exceed the RDA for protein and are nutritionally adequate across the life cycle. Pure vegans who do not have reliable sources of vitamin B_{12} and vitamin D need supplements.
- Although body building requires more than the RDA for protein, the limiting factor in adding muscle mass is energy intake, not protein. Muscle building requires resistance exercise, adequate calories, and moderate protein.

ANSWER KEY

1. **TRUE** Most Americans consume more protein than they need.
2. **FALSE** Over the course of a day, if the food consumed is varied and contains sufficient calories, most vegetarian diets meet or exceed the RDA for protein.
3. **FALSE** Unlike glucose and fat, the body is not able to store excess amino acids for later use.
4. **TRUE** Soy protein is complete, or has high biologic value, protein, and is comparable in quality to animal protein.
5. **TRUE** The limiting factor in muscle building is energy intake (calories), not protein.
6. **FALSE** The quality of a protein is determined by the balance of essential amino acids provided.
7. **TRUE** Protein is found in almost all of the food groups in the Food Guide Pyramid; however, protein is represented only in limited amounts in the Fruit group, and fats, oils, and sweets generally do not provide protein at all.
8. **FALSE** Healthy adults are in neutral nitrogen balance: Protein synthesis is occurring at the same rate as protein breakdown.
9. **FALSE** Properly planned vegetarian diets are nutritionally adequate during all phases of pregnancy and lactation.
10. **FALSE** High protein intake may increase the risk of osteoporosis and renal insufficiency. In addition, high intake of animal protein is associated with atherosclerosis and colon and prostate cancers.

REFERENCES

American Dietetic Association. (1993). Position of the American Dietetic Association and the Canadian Dietetic Association: nutrition for physical fitness and athletic performance for adults. *J Am Diet Assoc*, 93(6), 691–696.

American Dietetic Association. (1997). Position of the American Dietetic Association: vegetarian diets. *J Am Diet Assoc*, 97(11), 1317–1321.

Clark, N. (1997). *Nancy Clark's sports nutrition guidebook*. (2nd ed.). Champaign, IL: Human Kinetics.

Liebman, B. (1996). Plants for supper? Ten reasons to eat more like a vegetarian. *Nutrition Action Health Letter 23*(8), 10–12.

National Research Council. (1989). *Recommended dietary allowances*. (10th ed.). Washington, DC: National Academy Press.

Subar, A., Krebs-Smith, S., Cook, A., Kahle, L. (1998). Dietary sources of nutrients among US adults, 1989 to 1991. *J Am Diet Assoc*, 95(5), 537–547.

CHAPTER 4

Lipids

TRUE	FALSE	Check your knowledge of lipids.
		1 Ounce for ounce, saturated fats are higher in calories than unsaturated fats.
		2 A statement on a label that a product is 98% fat free means that 2% of that product's calories are from fat.
		3 In a "healthy" diet, no foods have more than 30% of their calories from fat.
		4 Margarine is less healthy than butter.
		5 Because omega-3 fatty acids provide so many health benefits, people who do not eat fish should take omega-3 supplements.
		6 Beef is the biggest source of fat in the typical American diet.
		7 Cheese is the biggest source of saturated fat in the typical American diet.
		8 *Trans*-fatty acids raise blood levels of LDL-cholesterol (the "bad" cholesterol).
		9 The % Daily Value on the Nutrition Facts label is the same as the percentage of calories from fat.
		10 Reduced-fat foods are always low in calories.

Upon completion of this chapter, you will be able to

- Discuss the differences between saturated, monounsaturated, and polyunsaturated fats and name sources of each.
- Discuss the digestion and absorption of fat.
- List functions of fat in the body.
- Discuss recommendations regarding fat intake.
- Discuss the health problems associated with high-fat diets.
- Explain labeling regulations as they pertain to fat content.
- Describe ways to limit fat intake.

Keys to Understanding Lipids

Lipids, commonly known as **fats,** are a group of water-insoluble organic compounds that include triglycerides (fats and oils), phospholipids (eg, lecithin), and sterols (eg, cholesterol). Like carbohydrates, triglycerides are composed of carbon, hydrogen, and oxygen atoms. Because triglycerides have proportionately less oxygen, they provide more than double the amount of calories as an equivalent amount of carbohydrate.

TRIGLYCERIDES

Triglycerides account for approximately 95% of the fats in foods and are the major storage form of fat in the body. All **triglycerides** have a glycerol molecule (with its chain of three carbon atoms) as their backbone, with three fatty acids attached. **Diglycerides** consist of glyceride molecules that have only two fatty acids attached; **monoglycerides** have one fatty acid attached to a glyceride.

Fatty acids are composed of a chain of carbon atoms to which hydrogen atoms are attached. An acid group (COOH) is attached at one end and a methyl group (CH_3) at the other end. Fatty acids vary in the length of their carbon chain and in their degree of saturation.

Carbon Chain Length

Almost all fatty acids have an even number of carbon atoms in their chain, the range being 2 to 24. Short-chain fatty acids contain 2 to 4 carbon atoms, medium-chain fatty acids contain 6 to 12 carbon atoms, and long-chain fatty acids contain 14 or more carbon atoms. The length of the carbon chain determines how the fatty acid is absorbed. Most food fats contain predominately long-chain fatty acids.

Degree of Saturation

Saturated Fatty Acids

Each carbon atom has four potential bonding sites; when all four sites hold single bonds, that carbon atom is said to be *saturated* with the maximum number of hydrogen atoms. Because all of the carbon atoms in **saturated fatty acids** are bonded to as many hydrogen atoms as they can hold, no double bonds exist. All short- and medium-chain fatty acids are saturated. The most common saturated fatty acids are myristic, palmitic, and stearic acids, all of which are long-chain fatty acids.

Unsaturated Fatty Acids

Unsaturated fatty acids are not saturated with hydrogen atoms, so double bonds form between the carbon atoms to satisfy nature's law that each carbon atom must have four bonds connecting it to other atoms. Unsaturated fatty acids are unstable; the greater the number of double bonds, the less stable the molecule. **Monounsaturated** fatty acids have only one double bond between carbon atoms.

Polyunsaturated fatty acids (PUFAs) have two or more double bonds between carbon atoms. Linoleic acid is the most common PUFA found in foods. It contains 18 carbon atoms and has 2 double bonds. Because the first double bond occurs after carbon number 6 from the methyl (CH_3) end of the fatty acid, it is known as an **omega-6 fatty acid** (n-6).

Omega-3 fatty acids (n-3) are polyunsaturated fatty acids that have their first double bond three carbon atoms from the methyl carbon atom. Eicosapentaenoic acid (EPA) and docosahexaenoic acid (DHA) are n-3 fatty acids found primarily in cold-water fish and fish oils. Mackerel, albacore tuna, salmon, sardines, and lake trout are excellent sources of n-3 fatty acids. Alpha-linolenic acid, which is found in green leafy vegetables, flax oil, canola oil, soybean products, walnuts, and hazelnuts, is the n-3 fatty acid in plants. To a limited extent humans can convert alpha-linolenic acid to EPA and DHA in the body.

Omega-3 fatty acids have been shown to lower serum triglyceride levels, reduce blood pressure, and decrease factors involved in blood clotting and stroke. They also have antiinflammatory effects that may benefit people with ulcerative colitis, rheumatoid arthritis, or asthma. Animal studies indicate n-3 fatty acids may inhibit the development of certain cancers. It is not known whether the reduced risk of sudden cardiac death among people who eat one fish meal per week results from consumption of n-3 fatty acids, or of some other component in fish, or both.

Linoleic acid (n-6) and alpha-linolenic acid (n-3) are termed **essential fatty acids** because they cannot be synthesized in the body; all other fatty acids are made by the body. Essential fatty acids are important for maintaining healthy skin and promoting normal growth in children. As part of phospholipids, essential fatty acids are a component of cell membranes and are precursors of eicosanoids, a group of hormone like substances involved in inflammation and blood clotting. Prostaglandins, thromboxanes, and leukotrienes are types of eicosanoids. The actions on platelets, endothelial cells, and leukocytes of eicosanoids made from the fatty acid EPA (n-3) are more desirable than are those of eicosanoids derived from linoleic acid.

TRIGLYCERIDES IN FOOD

Just as amino acids can be arranged in limitless combinations to form different proteins, fatty acids can attach to glycerol molecules in various ratios and combinations to form a variety of triglycerides within a single food fat. Ninety-eight percent of triglycerides are classified as *mixed* because they contain more than one kind of fatty acid. For instance, a triglyceride may contain one saturated fatty acid, one monounsaturated fatty acid, and one polyunsaturated fatty acid. *Simple* triglycerides, which contain three molecules of the same fatty acid, occur rarely.

All food fats contain a mixture of saturated, monounsaturated, and polyunsaturated fatty acids. The types and amounts of fatty acids present influence the sensory and functional properties of the food fat. For instance, butter tastes and acts differently from corn oil, which tastes and acts differently from lard. When applied to sources of fat in the diet, "unsaturated" and "saturated" are not absolute terms used to describe the only types of fatty acids present; rather, they are relative descriptions that indicate which kinds of fatty acids are present in the largest proportion (Fig. 4–1).

Unsaturated Fats

Generally, unsaturated fats have the following characteristics:

- They are soft or liquid at room temperature.
- They have low melting points—the more double bonds in a fatty acid, the lower the melting point. For instance, soft margarine (high in unsaturated fatty acids) melts quicker than butter (lower in unsaturated fatty acids).

Monounsaturated fats and oils

	% Monounsaturated fatty acids
Olive oil	71%
Canola oil	53%
Peanut oil	49%
Soft margarine	47%
Chicken, turkey	42%

Polyunsaturated fats and oils

	% Polyunsaturated fatty acids
Safflower oil	75%
Sunflower oil	64%
Soybean oil	58%
Corn oil	55%

Saturated fats and oils

	% Saturated fatty acids
Coconut oil	88%
Palm kernel oil	81%
Butter	65%
Beef fat	53%

FIGURE 4-1 Predominate types of fatty acids in selected fats and oils. All food fats contain a mix of saturated, monounsaturated, and polyunsaturated fatty acids.

- They are susceptible to rancidity when exposed to light and oxygen over a prolonged period. The chemical change that occurs results in an offensive taste and smell and the loss of vitamins A and E (fat-soluble vitamins). Antioxidants added to fats, such as butylated hydroxyanisole (BHA) and butylated hydroxytoluene (BHT), help extend shelf life, as does minimizing storage time and avoiding high temperatures.
- They are predominately found in plant fats and oils, with the exceptions of coconut, palm, and palm kernel oils.

Saturated Fats

Generally, saturated fats exhibit the following characteristics:

- They are solid at room temperature. Saturated fatty acids have a straight configuration (no double bonds) and so are usually capable of being packed into a solid at room temperature. Exceptions to this generalization are coconut oil, palm kernel oil, and palm oils, the so-called "tropical oils."
- They have high melting points.
- They are more stable (less likely to become rancid) than unsaturated fats.
- They are animal in origin, except for the tropical oils.

Hydrogenated Fats

Hydrogenated fats are unsaturated vegetable oils (usually corn, soybean, cottonseed, safflower, or canola oil) in which hydrogen atoms have been added to some of the double bonds, making the fat more saturated. The purpose of hydrogenation is to improve the stability of a fat or oil, change its texture, and increase its functionality. The degree of hydrogenation varies from "light" to "partial" according to the desired outcome. For instance, lightly hydrogenated oils are more stable because they have fewer double bonds, but they are still in liquid form. A higher degree of hydrogenation ("partially hydrogenated") creates solid shortenings from liquid oils. The resulting product is more stable (eg, can be reused more times in deep frying) and produces flakier pie crusts and crispier French fries. Partially hydrogenated fats bear little resemblance to their original oil. Any health benefits from the use of unsaturated oils are eliminated when the fatty acids are changed into saturated fats.

A consequence of hydrogenation is that some of the remaining double bonds are structurally altered from the *cis* position to the *trans* position, meaning that hydrogen atoms then occur on opposite sides of the double bond. The position of the double bond may also change. *Trans*-fatty acids contribute to the stability of hydrogenated fats.

***Trans*-fats** are not common in nature. The only natural sources of *trans*-fats are beef and dairy products, which account for only 20% of total *trans*-fat intake. The remaining 80% of *trans*-fats comes from processed foods that contain or are made from partially hydrogenated oils (eg, stick margarine, commercially prepared baked goods, crackers, snack chips, microwave popcorn) and from fried foods. An estimated 2% to 4% of total calories in the typical American diet comes from *trans*-fats.

The impact of *trans*-fats on health has made headlines in recent years. Declarations that "margarine is worse than butter" stemmed from reports that show *trans*-fats act like saturated fat in the body to raise "bad" cholesterol. Yet, labeling laws have not required manufacturers to disclose the *trans*-fat content of their products, so consumers were unable to tell how much *trans*-fat they were eating.

In November 1999, the FDA proposed changes in labeling laws be enacted to require the amount of *trans*-fat per serving to be added to the amount of saturated fat per serving so that the amount and percent Daily Value (%DV) per serving on the Nutrition Facts label will reflect the sum of the two. The FDA has also proposed limits on *trans*-fat on several nutrient content claims found on food labels, such as the "low saturated fat" claim and a proposed new "*trans*-fat free" claim. In all likelihood the proposed changes will be adopted sometime in 2000 and food manufacturers will have up to 2 to 3 years to comply with the new labeling format and regulations. As this book goes to print, it is not known what the new label will actually look like or where the actual *trans*-fat content will be listed.

PHOSPHOLIPIDS AND STEROLS

The other 5% of lipids in foods (remember that triglycerides account for 95%) is made up of phospholipids and sterols.

Phospholipids

Phospholipids are a group of compound lipids that are similar to triglycerides in that they contain a glycerol molecule and two fatty acids. In place of the third fatty acid, phospholipids have a phosphate group and a molecule of choline or another nitrogen-containing compound. The fatty acids make phospholipids fat-soluble, and the phosphate group makes them water-soluble. Because of this unique feature, phospholipids are used extensively by the food industry as emulsifiers. Phospholipids occur naturally in almost all foods; excellent sources include liver, eggs, wheat germ, and peanuts.

Phospholipids perform many vital functions in the body. They work as emulsifiers to keep fats suspended in blood and other body fluids. As a component of all cell membranes, phospholipids not only provide structure but help transport fat-soluble, substances across cell membranes. Phospholipids are precursors of prostaglandins.

Lecithin is the best known phospholipid. Claims that it lowers blood cholesterol, improves memory, controls weight, and cures arthritis, hypertension, and gallbladder problems are unfounded. Studies show no benefit from taking supplements, because lecithin is digested in the gastrointestinal tract into its component parts, not absorbed intact to perform super functions. Lecithin is not even an essential nutrient, because it is synthesized in the body. Many people who take lecithin supplements do not realize that they provide 9 cal/g, just like all other fats in the diet.

Sterols

Sterols contain carbon, hydrogen, and oxygen atoms arranged in rings; each particular sterol has a unique side group attached to the ring structure. Cholesterol, bile acids, sex hormones, the adrenocortical hormones, and vitamin D are all sterols.

Cholesterol is found in all cell membranes and in myelin; brain and nerve cells are especially rich in cholesterol. Cholesterol is also used to synthesize bile acids, steroid hormones, and vitamin D.

Cholesterol is found in all animal products with the exception of egg whites. Organ meats and egg yolks are the richest sources of cholesterol; smaller amounts are found in muscle meats, shellfish, poultry, and dairy products. The cholesterol in food is just cholesterol; descriptions of "good" and "bad" cholesterol refer to the lipoprotein packages that move cholesterol through the blood (see Chapter 18). You cannot eat more "good" cholesterol, but you can make lifestyle changes that increase the amount of "good" cholesterol in the blood, such as quitting smoking, exercising, and losing weight if overweight.

Cholesterol is not an essential nutrient, because it is synthesized in the body. In fact, every day the liver makes approximately twice as much cholesterol as the typical American diet provides. When dietary cholesterol decreases, endogenous cholesterol production increases to maintain an adequate supply. The body makes cholesterol from acetyl coenzyme A (acetyl-CoA), which can originate from carbohydrates, protein, fat, or alcohol.

HOW THE BODY HANDLES FAT

Digestion

A minimal amount of chemical digestion of fat occurs in the mouth and stomach through the action of lingual lipase and gastric lipases, respectively (Fig. 4–2).

As fat enters the duodenum, it stimulates the release of the hormone cholecystokinin, which in turn stimulates the gallbladder to release bile. Bile, an emulsifier produced in the liver from bile salts, cholesterol, phospholipids, bilirubin, and electrolytes, prepares fat for digestion by suspending the hydrophobic molecules in the watery intestinal fluid. Emulsified fat particles have enlarged surface areas on which digestive enzymes can work.

Most fat digestion occurs in the small intestine. Pancreatic lipase, the most important and powerful lipase, splits off one fatty acid at a time from the triglyceride molecule, working from the outside in until two free fatty acids and a monoglyceride remain. Usually the process stops at this point, but sometimes digestion continues and the monoglyceride splits into a free fatty acid and a glyceride molecule. The end products of digestion—mostly monoglycerides with free fatty acids and little glycerol—are absorbed into intestinal cells. It is normal for a small amount of fat (4–5 g) to escape digestion and be excreted in the feces.

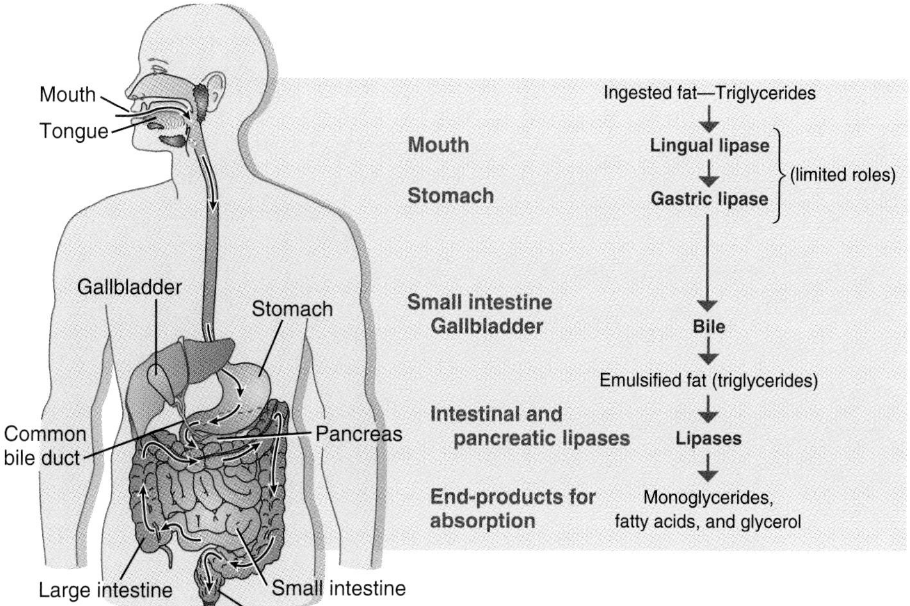

FIGURE 4-2 Fat digestion. A minimal amount of chemical digestion of fat occurs in the mouth and stomach through the action of lingual lipase and gastric lipases, respectively. As fat enters the duodenum, it stimulates the release of the hormone cholecystokinin, which in turn stimulates the gallbladder to release bile. Bile prepares fat for digestion by suspending the hydrophobic molecules in the watery intestinal fluid. Most fat digestion occurs in the small intestine. Pancreatic lipase splits off one fatty acid at a time from the triglyceride molecule, working from the outside in until two free fatty acids and a monoglyceride remain. Usually, the process stops at this point, but sometimes digestion continues and the monoglyceride spits into a free fatty acid and glyceride molecule. The end products of digestion—mostly monoglycerides with free fatty acids and little glycerol—are absorbed into intestinal cells. It is normal for a small amount of fat (4 to 5 g) to escape digestion and be excreted in the feces.

The digestion of phospholipids is similar, with the end products being two free fatty acids and a phospholipid fragment. Cholesterol does not undergo digestion; it is absorbed as is.

Absorption

About 95% of consumed fat is absorbed, mostly in the duodenum and jejunum. Small fat particles, such as short- and medium-chain fatty acids and glycerol, are absorbed directly through the mucosal cells into capillaries leading to the portal vein and liver.

The absorption of larger fat particles, namely monoglycerides and long-chain fatty acids, is more complex. Although they are insoluble in water, monoglycerides and long-chain fatty acids dissolve into micelles, compounds created by bile salts that encircle fat particles to facilitate their diffusion into intestinal cells. After achieving their goal of delivering fat to the intestinal cells, most of the released bile salts are reabsorbed in the terminal ileum, transported back to the liver, and recycled (enterohepatic circulation).

Some of the bile salts become bound to fiber in the intestine and are excreted in the feces.

Once inside the intestinal cells, the monoglycerides and long-chain fatty acids combine to form triglycerides. The reformed triglycerides, along with phospholipids and cholesterol, become encased in protein to form chylomicrons. **Chylomicrons** transport absorbed lipids from intestinal cells through the lymph and eventually into the bloodstream for distribution throughout the body.

Metabolism

In the bloodstream, triglycerides in the chylomicrons are broken down into glycerol and fatty acids by lipoprotein lipase, a fat-digesting enzyme located on the surface of adipose cells and other body cells. These fatty acids and glycerol enter cells, where they can be catabolized for energy or rebuilt into triglycerides for storage. Fat metabolism is regulated by hormones: adrenocorticotropin (ACTH), epinephrine, glucagon, glucocorticoids, and thyroxine promote fat mobilization (catabolism); insulin stimulates fat synthesis (anabolism).

Fat Catabolism

Fatty acids and glycerol for use by cells come from the most recent meal (triglycerides in chylomicrons) or from stored triglycerides. Most cells are able to store only minute amounts of fat; the exception is adipose cells, which have a virtually boundless capacity to store fat. Adipose cells give up stored fat when an enzyme within the adipose cell (hormone-sensitive lipase) reacts to the need for energy by splitting triglycerides into glycerol and fatty acids, which are released into the bloodstream and picked up by cells as needed.

Within cells, the process of fat catabolism is the same whether the fatty acids and glycerol originate from chylomicrons or from storage. Both components—fatty acids and glycerol—enter the tricarboxylic acid (TCA) cycle as acetyl-CoA to produce energy, but they do so by different routes and yield different amounts of energy. Fatty acids undergo the process of beta-oxidation, a complex series of reactions that split off two carbon atoms at a time into molecules of acetyl-CoA. This process continues until the entire fatty acid chain is separated into fragments containing two carbon atoms. For instance, linoleic acid (18 carbon atoms) is broken down into 9 molecules of acetyl-CoA. Fatty acids provide the majority of energy derived from triglycerides.

Glycerol is easily converted to pyruvate, which continues on through the metabolic pathway of glucose to become acetyl-CoA. Pyruvate can be converted to glucose, whereas acetyl-CoA cannot (see Chapter 7). That is why only a small portion of a triglyceride molecule (the glycerol backbone, which is 5% of the molecule by weight) can be converted to glucose.

As part of normal fatty acid catabolism in the liver, beta-oxidation stops at the last four carbon atoms and yields the ketone bodies beta-hydroxybutyric acid and acetone.

Ketones leave the liver, travel through the bloodstream, and diffuse into other body cells, where they are catabolized into acetyl-CoA and enter the TCA cycle.

During starvation or uncontrolled diabetes, when carbohydrate intake is inadequate or unavailable, the body meets its energy needs by increasing the catabolism of fatty acids. However, in the absence of adequate glucose, fatty acids are incompletely broken down and ketone formation increases. Ketosis and acidosis may result.

Fat Anabolism

The body makes triglycerides for storage from any excess calories, but the ease and efficiency of doing so varies among nutrients. The steps to convert carbohydrates and protein to fat are complex and numerous; the pathway for dietary fat is quick and easy. For instance, excess glucose (six carbon atoms) must first be split into pyruvate molecules (three carbon atoms) and then into acetyl-CoA (two carbon atoms). Molecules of acetyl-CoA are then put together to form fatty acids, which combine with glycerol to make triglycerides. Each step of this lengthy process requires energy; approximately 23% of the original carbohydrate calories are used to convert glucose to fat. The process with protein differs for glycogenic and ketogenic amino acids. Most excess amino acids can only enter the pathway of fat anabolism as pyruvate to be converted to glycerol; a few are able to enter by way of acetyl-CoA to become fatty acids. Either way, amino acids must first go through the step of being deaminated. By comparison, the pathway for turning excess dietary fat into body fat is much more direct and efficient: the body simply puts the glycerol and fatty acids back together into triglycerides. The body uses little energy, only about 3% of the original calories, to make fat from fat. That is why an excess of dietary fat is more likely to become body fat than an excess of either carbohydrate or protein.

Lipid Carriers

Lipoproteins are a group of compounds that are made by the body to move water-insoluble lipids through the (watery) bloodstream. The four major types of lipoproteins all contain lipids (triglycerides, phospholipids, and cholesterol) and protein, but in different ratios. The density of lipoproteins varies depending on their proportion of fat to protein. As the protein concentration increases, the density of the molecule increases. Each type of lipoprotein has a distinct function.

CHYLOMICRONS

Chylomicrons are lipoproteins that:

- Are composed mostly of triglycerides absorbed from food, with smaller amounts of phospholipid and cholesterol and little protein
- Function to transport dietary lipids from the intestine to the liver and other body cells
- Are the least dense and largest of the lipoproteins. Chylomicrons get increasingly smaller as they come in contact with lipoprotein lipase, causing the release of triglycerides for use by body cells. When virtually all the lipids have been removed, the liver breaks down the protein remnant.

VERY-LOW-DENSITY LIPOPROTEINS

Very-low-density lipoproteins (VLDLs):

- Are synthesized and secreted mostly by liver cells. They contain approximately 50% triglycerides, with some cholesterol, phospholipids, and protein.
- Transport lipids made in the liver (eg, triglycerides, cholesterol) to body tissues
- Lose triglycerides to body cells and gain cholesterol from other lipoproteins. The resulting triglyceride-depleted, cholesterol-enriched molecule is called an intermediate-density lipoprotein (IDL).
- When present in large concentrations in the blood may increase the risk of atherosclerosis.

LOW-DENSITY LIPOPROTEINS

Low-density lipoproteins (LDLs):

- Are the major source of cholesterol in blood. They are approximately 50% cholesterol, with lesser amounts of phospholipid and protein and small amounts of triglycerides. About half of all IDLs become LDLs.
- Function to transport cholesterol from the liver to the tissues.
- Are commonly referred to as the "bad" cholesterol. High levels of LDL are atherogenic.

HIGH-DENSITY LIPOPROTEINS

High-density lipoproteins (HDLs):

- Are made by liver and intestinal cells. They are made up of approximately 50% protein, with lesser amounts of cholesterol, phospholipid, and triglycerides.
- Function to carry cholesterol from the tissues to the liver, where it can be recycled or degraded.
- Are commonly referred to as the "good" cholesterol. High levels of HDL decrease the risk of atherosclerosis.

FUNCTIONS OF FAT IN THE BODY

As already mentioned, specific lipids have specific functions in the body. Phospholipids and cholesterol are vital components of cell membranes, and cholesterol is a precursor of vitamin D, steroid hormones, and bile acids. Essential fatty acids, as a component of phospholipids, help maintain cell membrane integrity; they also regulate cholesterol metabolism and are precursors of eicosanoids. Omega-3 fatty acids affect triglyceride metabolism, blood pressure regulation, and blood clotting. General functions of fat in the body are to provide energy, protect vital organs, insulate against cold environmental temperatures, and facilitate the absorption of fat-soluble vitamins.

- **Energy contribution.** At 9 cal/g, fat provides more than double the amount of calories as an equivalent amount of either carbohydrate or protein. Still, fat is not the body's preferred fuel, because its metabolism is more complex than that of

glucose and it requires some glucose in order to be completely oxidized. Although certain cells, such as red blood cells, brain cells, and cells of the central nervous system, rely solely on glucose for energy, muscles at rest use mostly fatty acids. The body's normal mix of fuels at rest is approximately 55% fat and 45% carbohydrate. Stored fat in adipose cells represents the body's largest and most efficient energy reserve. Unlike glycogen, which can be stored only in limited amounts and is accompanied by water, adipose cells have a virtually limitless capacity to store fat and carry very little additional weight as intracellular water. Each pound of body fat provides 3500 calories. Although normal glycogen reserves may last for half a day of normal activity, fat reserves can last up to 2 months during a complete fast in people of normal weight. Although cholesterol is made from acetyl-CoA, it is an irreversible reaction. The body cannot break down cholesterol into CoA molecules to generate energy (calories) through the TCA cycle.
- **Support and protection for internal organs.** Fat deposits insulate and cushion internal organs to protect them from mechanical injury.
- **Temperature regulation.** Fat under the skin provides a layer of insulation against the cold.
- **Absorption of fat-soluble vitamins.** Dietary fat facilitates the absorption of vitamins A, D, E, and K, the fat-soluble vitamins.

FUNCTIONS OF FAT IN FOODS

Anyone who has tried to eliminate or reduce fat in a recipe knows that fat does more than simply provide calories. Fat contributes to the sensory appeal of foods by:

- Absorbing flavors and aromas of ingredients to improve overall taste
- Providing flavor of its own, depending on the source. Peanut oil and olive oil have distinct tastes; canola oil and corn oil have mild tastes.
- Providing a creamy and smooth "mouth feel"
- Tenderizing and adding moisture, as in baked goods such as cookies, pies, and cakes

SOURCES OF FAT

According to the Food Guide Pyramid (see Chapter 8), which depicts naturally occurring and added fats as gold dots in the background of the graphic illustration, fat is found in all food groups except the Fruit group. The type and amounts of fat vary considerably within each group. Some fat is visible: for example, butter, salad dressings, and the fat surrounding a piece of steak are easily identified as fat. More often, fat is invisible; examples are the fats in cheese, milk, nuts, cookies, and pancakes and the fat marbled through meat.

Animal sources account for approximately 57% of total fat intake, and plant fats account for 43%. The top five sources of fat (in descending order) among American adults are beef, margarine, salad dressings/mayonnaise, cheese, and milk. The top five sources of saturated fat are cheese, beef, milk, cakes/cookies/quick breads/doughnuts, and margarine.

Bread, Cereal, Rice, and Pasta Group

Grains naturally contain very little fat. It is the prepared items within this group that provide significant added fat, such as granola cereals, crackers, pancakes, croissants, doughnuts, cakes, cookies, and pies.

Low Fat (< 1 g fat/serv)		Higher Fat	
Serving Size	Fat (g)	Serving Size	Fat (g)
Bread, 1 slice	<1.0	French toast, 1 slice	7.0
Rice, ½ cup	<1.0	Rice with herbs and butter, ½ cup	4.5
Pasta, ½ cup	<1.0	Chow mein noodles, ½ cup	7.0
Oatmeal, ½ cup	<1.0	Muffin, 1	6.0
Ready-to-eat cereals (most types)	<1.0	Granola, ⅓ cup	10.0
Bagel, ½	<1.0	Croissant, 1 medium	12.0
Pita bread, ½	<1.0	Danish pastry, ½	6.5

Vegetable Group

Unadulterated vegetables contain little or no fat. Vegetables that are fried, creamed, served with cheese, or mixed with mayonnaise provide significantly more fat.

Serving Size	Fat (g)
Boiled potato, ½ cup	trace
Mashed potatoes, ½ cup	4.4
Scalloped potatoes, ½ cup	4.5
French fries, 10	8
Potato salad, ½ cup	10.3
Homemade hash browns, ½ cup	10.8

Fruit Group

With the exception of the three fruits listed here, fruits do not contain appreciable amounts of fat. Note the saturated fat content of coconut.

Serving Size	Fat (g)	Saturated Fat (g)
Avocado, 1 medium	15	2.3
Coconut, 2 tbsp shredded	4.0	4.0
Coconut milk, 1 cup	48.2	42.7
Olives (green or ripe), 5 large	3.0	0.5

Milk, Yogurt, and Cheese Group

Items within this group come in fat-free, reduced-fat, and whole-fat varieties. Label reading is a must to make accurate comparisons between varieties. Because dairy foods originate from animals, they contain cholesterol.

Serving Size	Fat (g)	Cholesterol (mg)
Milk, 1 cup		
Skim	trace	4
1%	3.0	10
2%	5.0	18
Whole	8	33
Yogurt, 1 cup		
Nonfat	trace	5
Low-fat	2.5	15
Custard-style	4.0	20
Cheddar cheese, 1 oz		
Nonfat	0	5
Low-fat	2.0	6
Reduced-fat	5.0	20
Natural	9.4	30
Ice cream (vanilla), 1/2 cup		
Nonfat	0	12
Ice milk	2.8	9
Regular	7.3	29
Premium	12.0	45

Meat, Poultry, Fish, Dry Beans, Eggs, and Nuts Group

Generalizations about this group include:

- Three ounces of meat is about the same size as a deck of cards.
- Untrimmed meats are higher in fat than lean-only portions.
- White poultry meat is lower in fat than dark meat.
- Cooking methods can add fat (eg, frying, basting with fat).
- Crab, lobster, and shrimp are high in cholesterol but very low in fat and saturated fat.
- Plant items (beans, nuts) are cholesterol free and contain little or no saturated fat.

Serving Size	Fat (g)	Saturated Fat (g)	Cholesterol (g)
Beef, 3-oz portion, lean part only			
Lean eye of round	4	2	59
Chuck blade	11	4	90
Ground beef, cooked 3 oz patty			
Extra lean	14	5	71
Lean	16	6	73
Regular	17	7	76
Beef liver, 3 oz	4	2	331
Beef kidney, 3 oz	3	1	332
Pork, 3 oz roasted lean only			
Arm picnic	11	4	81
Loin blade	13	5	80
Chicken, 3 oz, light and dark meat			
Without skin	6	2	75
With skin	12	3	74
Fish, 3 oz cooked			
Cod	0.7	0.1	47
Salmon	5	0.8	47
Shrimp	0.9	0.2	166
Turn in water (light, drained)	0.7	0.2	26
Tuna in oil (light, drained)	7	1.3	15
Dry beans, 1/2 cup	trace	trace	0
Egg, 1 large			
White only	0	0	0
Yolk	5	2	213
Nuts, 1 oz dry roasted			
Almonds	15	1.4	0
Cashews	13	2.6	0
Macadamia	21	2.5	0
Peanuts	14	2.0	0
Pecans	18	1.5	0

Fats, Oils, and Sweets

Notice the small serving sizes. A little bit goes a long way.

Serving Size	Fat (g)	Saturated Fat (g)	Cholesterol (g)
Butter, 1 tsp	4.0	2.0	10
Margarine, 1 tsp			
Diet	1.5	0.3	0
Liquid (squeezable)	4.0	0.7	0
Tub	4.0	0.7	0
Stick	4.0	0.7	0

(continued)

Serving Size	Fat (g)	Saturated Fat (g)	Cholesterol (g)
Mayonnaise, 1 tbsp	12	2	7
Salad dressing, 1 tbsp	7	1	4
Sour cream, 2 tbsp	6	4	12
Cream cheese, 1 oz	10	6	32
Chocolate bar, 1 oz	9	6	6

INTAKE RECOMMENDATIONS

Recommended Allowance

The need for fat is actually very small, because the body can make saturated fatty acids, monounsaturated fatty acids, and cholesterol from acetyl-CoA molecules. Cells cannot make n-6 or n-3 fatty acids or convert fatty acids from one omega family to the other, so dietary sources of these essential fatty acids are needed. Adequate intakes of essential fatty acids are estimated to range between 5% and 10% of total calorie intake, but as little as 1% to 2% of calories from n-6 fatty acids and 1% of calories from n-3 fatty acids prevents deficiency symptoms. This level of n-6 fatty acids is easily achieved within the context of an oral diet, but most Americans consume only small amounts of n-3 fatty acids.

Essential fatty acid deficiencies are extremely rare in people eating a mixed diet. Those at risk for deficiency include infants and children consuming low-fat diets (their need for essential fatty acids is proportionately higher than that of adults), clients with anorexia nervosa, and people receiving lipid-free parenteral nutrition for long periods. People with fat malabsorption syndromes are also at risk. Symptoms of essential fatty acid deficiency include growth failure, reproductive failure, skin lesions, and kidney and liver disorders.

Fat Intake Guidelines

A recommendation of the *Dietary Guidelines for Americans* (see Chapter 8), consistent with advice from the American Heart Association, the National Cholesterol Education Program, the U.S. Surgeon General, the American Cancer Society, and the American Diabetes Association, suggests that consumers "Choose a diet low in fat, saturated fat, and cholesterol and moderate in total fat." Specifically, this means to:

- Limit fat to 30% or less of total calories.
- Limit saturated fat to less than 10% of total calories.
- Limit cholesterol to 300 mg or less daily.

For someone consuming 1600 calories a day, these guidelines translate into:

- A total of 53 g or less of fat daily:

$$1600 \text{ cal} \times 0.3 = 480 \text{ cal}$$
$$480 \text{ cal} \div 9 \text{ cal/g} = 53.3 \text{ g total fat}$$

- Less than 18 g of saturated fat daily:

$$1600 \text{ cal} \times 0.1 = 160 \text{ cal}$$
$$160 \text{ cal} \div 9 \text{ cal/g} = 18 \text{ g saturated fat}$$

Considering that one fast food ¼-pound hamburger with cheese (30 g fat, 13 g saturated fat) and one large order of French fries (22 g fat, 4 g saturated fat) supplies a total of 52 g fat and 17 g saturated fat, it is obvious that the effort is to "limit" not "get to" the guideline values. Findings from the *Third Report on Nutrition Monitoring in the United States* revealed that only 20.9% of men and 25.2% of women age 20 years and older consume 30% or less of their total calories from fat. The average American adult consumes 33% of calories from fat and 11% of calories from saturated fat. Although 33% fat appears to be an improvement from earlier surveys, the total fat grams consumed have actually remained stable as total calorie intake has increased. Currently, daily cholesterol intake averages 217 mg for adult women and 337 mg for adult men.

The following guidelines are designed to limit fat, saturated fat, and cholesterol intake.

- Use fats and oils sparingly in cooking and at the table.
- Use small amounts of salad dressings and spreads such as butter, margarine, and mayonnaise. Consider using low-fat or fat-free dressing for salads.
- Choose vegetable oils and soft margarines most often, because they are lower in saturated fat than solid shortenings and animal fats even though their caloric content is the same.
- Check the Nutrition Facts label to see how much fat and saturated fat are in a serving; choose foods that are lower in fat and saturated fat.
- Choose low-fat sauces with pasta, rice, and potatoes.
- Use as little fat as possible to cook vegetables and grain products.
- Season with herbs, spices, lemon juice, and fat-free or low-fat salad dressings.
- Choose two to three servings of lean fish, poultry, meats, or other protein-rich foods such as beans each day.
- Use meats labeled "lean" or "extra lean." Trim fat from meat; take skin off poultry. (Three ounces of cooked lean beef or chicken without skin provides about 6 g of fat; 3 ounces of chicken with skin or untrimmed meat may have as much as 12 g of fat.) Most beans and bean products are almost fat free and are a good source of protein and fiber.
- Limit intake of high-fat processed meats such as sausages, salami, and other cold cuts; choose lower-fat varieties by reading the Nutrition Facts label.
- Limit intake of organ meats (3 ounces of cooked chicken livers provides about 540 mg of cholesterol); use egg yolks in moderation. Egg whites contain no cholesterol and can be used freely.
- Choose skim or low-fat milk, fat-free or low-fat yogurt, and low-fat cheese.
- Choose two to three servings of low-fat milk and milk products daily. Add extra calcium without added fat by choosing fat-free yogurt and low-fat milk more often. If you do not consume foods from the Milk, Yogurt, and Cheese group, eat other calcium-rich foods.

To eat more "heart-healthy" fats, such as monounsaturated fats and omega-3 fatty acids, Americans should do the following:

- Make olive oil or canola oil your oil of choice, but use sparingly.
- Eat nuts that are rich in monounsaturated fats and n-3 fats (in moderation): walnuts, almond, hazelnuts, pecans, cashews, and macadamia nuts.
- Eat fish once a week.

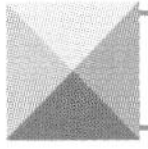

Fat in Health Promotion

DISEASE PREVENTION

Today, health promotion has more to do with avoiding chronic disease than with avoiding nutrient deficiencies. And fat, more than any other nutrient, is singled out as a public health enemy based on the overwhelming evidence that high-fat diets increase the risk of certain chronic diseases, namely, cardiovascular disease, certain cancers, obesity, hypertension, insulin resistance, and gallbladder disease. Independently, obesity increases the risk of type 2 diabetes, several types of cancer, and heart disease. It is no wonder that dietary fat has a notorious reputation. A brief summary on the role of fat in chronic diseases follows.

Cardiovascular Disease

Atherosclerotic coronary heart disease (CHD) is the leading cause of death among Americans. Atherosclerosis starts early in life with the formation of fatty streaks related to apparent chronic microscopic injury to the arterial endothelium. Plaque develops as the result of a complex series of chemical and physical events that appears to be triggered by increased amounts of oxidized LDL-cholesterol. Adding to the problem of narrowed arteries is the increased propensity to form blood clots on the plaque. Eventually a clot may grow until it fully blocks the narrowed artery (causing a heart attack), or it may break off and travel until it gets stuck in an artery (causing a stroke if it gets stuck in a brain artery). Many risk factors have been identified in the development of CHD, including high blood LDL-cholesterol and a high–saturated fat, high-cholesterol diet (Fig. 4–3).

By far the strongest connection between diet and heart disease lies with saturated fats, which raise LDL-cholesterol in the blood more than any other dietary component. It is well known that eating less saturated fat lowers LDL-cholesterol levels, which in turn reduces the risk of CHD. Yet research has shown that not all saturated fats are equally atherogenic; in particular, stearic acid is unique in that it has a neutral effect on blood cholesterol levels. What this means in terms of practical application has yet to be determined, because sources of stearic acid—namely beef, cocoa butter, and fully hydrogenated vegetable oils—are also sources of other saturated fats that definitely raise the LDL-cholesterol.

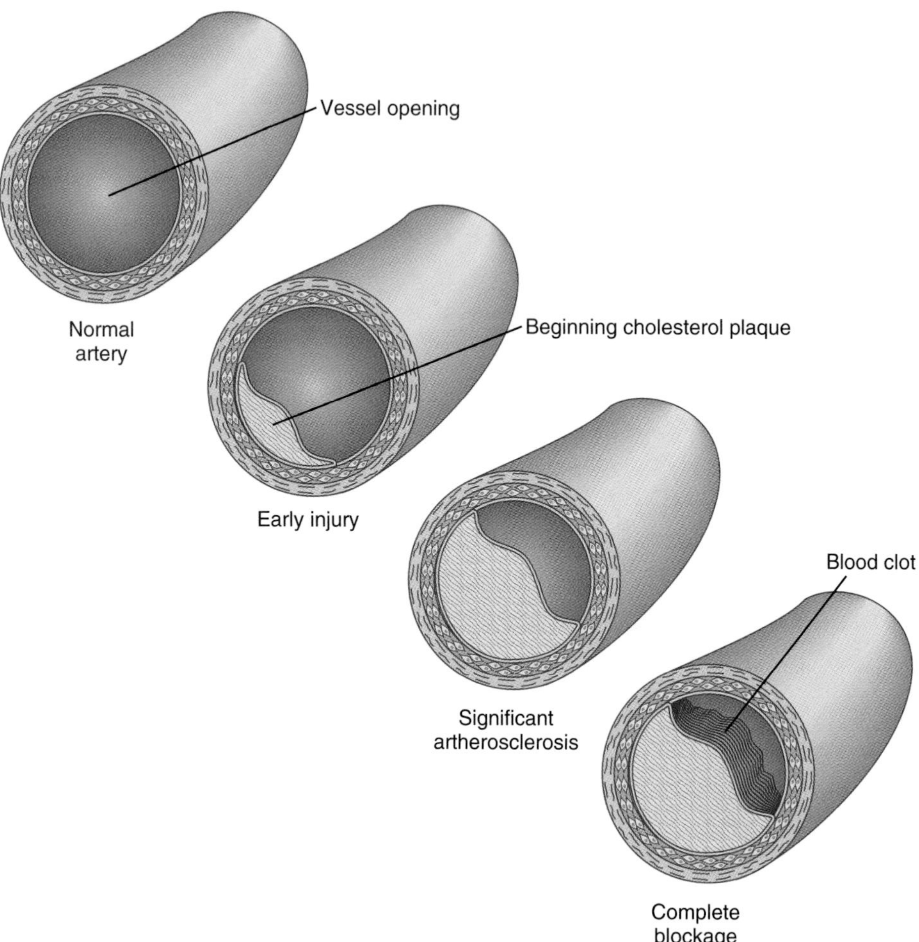

FIGURE 4-3 Schematic of formation of atheromatous plaque. The plaque develops by a series of events that apparently are triggered by increased amounts of oxidized LDL cholesterol. The arteries narrow, and the condition is exacerbated by the propensity of blood clots to form on the plaque.

Dietary cholesterol increases total and LDL-cholesterol, but the effect is lessened when saturated fat intake is low. Dietary cholesterol may have an independent effect on heart disease risk beyond its effect on serum cholesterol.

Although polyunsaturated fats lower levels of total and LDL-cholesterol (a positive effect), they appear to make it more susceptible to oxidation (a negative effect). A growing body of evidence suggests that oxidized LDL triggers the sequence of events leading to CHD. At high levels, polyunsaturated fats decrease HDL-cholesterol and may increase platelet aggregation, increasing the risk of clot formation, stroke, and heart attack.

Studies on the effects of other types of fats on cardiovascular disease are inconclusive and controversial:

- Monounsaturated fats are beneficial in that they lower LDL-cholesterol and appear to make it less susceptible to oxidation. Low-fat diets with half of their fat content provided by monounsaturated fats decrease HDL-cholesterol or leave it unchanged.
- *Trans*-fatty acids raise LDL-cholesterol. Not all studies agree that *trans*-fats lower HDL-cholesterol.
- The effect of n-3 fatty acids on LDL-cholesterol is variable. They may have no effect on either LDL- or HDL-cholesterol in people with normal blood lipid levels, but they may increase LDLs in people with high blood lipid levels. However, n-3 fatty acids are considered heart-healthy because they decrease platelet aggregation, increase resistance to cardiac arrhythmias, and lower blood pressure.

Cancers

Dietary fat may promote, not cause, certain cancers, but the relationship between fat and cancer is much more cloudy than that between fat and atherosclerosis. According to the 1996 *American Cancer Society Dietary Guidelines*, high-fat diets are associated with an increased risk of cancers of the colon, rectum, prostate, and endometrium. However, it is not known whether the increased risk is related to the amount of fat, the type of fat, the total energy intake, or some other food-related factor.

Obesity

Obesity results from a chronic imbalance between energy intake and energy expenditure, and it appears that excessive fat intake may be more to blame for that imbalance than either carbohydrates or protein. First, fat is denser in calories than either carbohydrate or protein. Second, the body is able to increase oxidation (burning) of carbohydrates and proteins to balance high intakes of these nutrients, but it does not immediately do so for fat. Excess fat intake does not stimulate its own oxidation until after 3 to 7 days of consistent high-fat eating; shorter periods of high-fat eating result in increased fat storage. Finally, the body appears to prioritize maintaining both carbohydrate balance and protein balance over limiting fat storage. When energy intake is excessive, the body burns the excess carbohydrate and protein to maintain balance; as the oxidation of these nutrients increases, fat oxidation decreases and, consequently, fat storage increases. Although increased fat storage is the common response to increased fat intake, individuals vary in their resistance or susceptibility to obesity, probably as a result of genetic differences.

Clients who need or want to eat less fat should be advised to:

- **Think small.** Small changes can add up to big results. For instance, someone who drinks 3 cups of whole milk daily can save 9 g of fat per day by switching to 2% milk, 15 g of fat by using 1% milk, or 24 g of fat with skim milk.
- **Make changes gradually.** Gradual changes in food choices are more likely to result in long-lasting lifestyle modifications than are drastic "quick fixes" that are difficult to maintain over the long haul. People who are accustomed to whole

milk are much more likely to accept 2% milk than skim milk. After they have become accustomed to 2% milk, they should try 1% and then skim milk. Each change makes subsequent changes easier.

- **Be positive.** Focus on all the things the client can eat, not on what should not be eaten. Natural and wholesome plant foods are naturally low in fat and are loaded with essentials for good health, such as vitamins, minerals, fiber, and phytochemicals.
- **Rethink the importance of meat.** Meats are a mainstay in the typical American diet, but many are high in fat and saturated fat. Encourage the client to experiment with meatless entrees. Clients who absolutely must have meat should think of it as a condiment or side dish and focus on fruits, vegetables, and grains.
- **Use the plate method.** Divide the dinner plate into two parts: three quarters for grains and vegetables and one quarter for the entree. This arrangement turns out to be approximately equivalent to 50% to 60% complex carbohydrates, 20% to 30% protein, and 20% to 30% fat—right on target.
- **Be mindful of portion sizes.** Three ounces of meat is the size of a deck of cards; 1 teaspoon is about the size of a thumbnail; a tennis ball is approximately 1 cup.
- **Opt for color.** Color most certainly comes from fruits and vegetables.
- **Season with spices, not fat.** Picante, salsa, ginger, flavored vinegars, and Italian spice blends are rich in fat-free flavor.
- **Choose low-fat varieties over full-fat foods.** Encourage the client to comparison shop, because there are big differences in taste and texture among different brands of the same item.
- **Be careful when eating out.** Restaurant portion sizes tend to be much bigger than the recommended serving sizes. Encourage clients to order a regular burger instead of a super-sized or specialty burger. Other ideas are to ask for a "doggie bag" and take home part of the meal, to split dessert with a companion, to ask that dressings be served on the side, to forgo gravies and sauces, and to select baked or broiled foods over fried foods.

WITH FAT, THE LOWER THE INTAKE THE BETTER . . . OR IS IT?

"Eat less fat" has long been a nutritional mantra. But decades of study have shown that the relationship between fat and chronic disease is far more complex than that simple advice implies. Is low fat consumption appropriate for everyone? Is the type of fat as important as the amount of fat eaten? How low is too low?

Is a Low-fat Diet Appropriate for Everyone?

The suggestions in the *Dietary Guidelines for Americans*—including the recommendation to choose a diet low in saturated fat and cholesterol, and moderate in total fat—are intended for healthy Americans age 2 years and over for the purpose of promoting health and preventing disease. Key words in that sentence are "healthy" and "age 2."

- **Healthy.** Originally, lowering and modifying fat intake was a recommendation aimed at *treating* people with existing heart disease. But, as more and more evidence revealed that dietary interventions could actually help *prevent* heart disease (and perhaps reduce the risk of obesity and certain cancers), dietary recommendations were simplified and generalized to the "well" population. Conversely, low-fat diets are not appropriate for certain "ill" clients, such as a person with high nonprotein calorie needs related to chronic renal failure or a frail elderly person whose need for calorie density takes precedence over restricting the amount and type of fat consumed.
- **Age 2.** Because of the relationship between diet and chronic disease risk in children, more than ten scientific groups have issued dietary recommendations for children 2 years of age and older. The American Academy of Pediatrics Committee on Nutrition recommends that children older than 2 years of age gradually change their eating styles so that, by the age of 5 years, total fat intake ranges between 20% to 30% of total calories, saturated fat intake is less than 10% of calories, and cholesterol intake is less than 300 mg/day. Although opponents argue that children may experience growth failure because they cannot obtain adequate calories and nutrients when fat intake is limited, studies have shown the opposite to be true: despite a decrease in fat intake among American children, the prevalence of obesity has increased. Likewise, other studies have shown that decreasing the fat intake actually increases the vitamin and mineral density of the diet. So long as calories are adequate and there is variety and moderation in the diet, children who limit fat to 30% of total energy do not experience any adverse health effects. Low-fat diets are not recommended for children younger than 2 years of age because their need for fat is high.

Is the Type of Fat as Important as the Amount?

Absolutely, but all of the answers are not yet known, and fat is not the only consideration in eating healthy. It is known that:

- Saturated fats raise LDL-cholesterol.
- Low-fat diets containing high levels of polyunsaturated fats lower both LDL- and HDL-cholesterol.
- Low-fat diets containing high levels of monounsaturated fats lower LDL-cholesterol; they may decrease HDL-cholesterol or leave it unchanged.
- High-fat diets that are high in monounsaturated fats and low in saturated fats may produce the most favorable change in LDL- and HDL-cholesterol levels. But high-fat diets increase the risk of weight gain, which can increase the risk of heart disease. High-fat diets may also promote the formation of blood clots.

Of recent interest is the so-called Mediterranean diet, the traditional eating style of people living in Greece, parts of Italy, Lebanon, Morocco, Portugal, Spain, Syria, Tunisia, and Turkey. Although it is high in fat (approximately 40% of calories), it is associated with a long life expectancy and low rates of heart disease, certain cancers, and other diet-related chronic diseases. Granted, its high monounsaturated fat content and very low saturated fat content impart definite health benefits, but they are probably only one piece of the healthy diet and lifestyle puzzle. The minimally processed plant-based diet with added nuts and olive oil contains very little meat, eggs, or dairy products. Daily fruit and vegetable intake is approximately 1 pound, and moderate amounts of red wine are consumed with meals. High levels of physical activity, a less stressful lifestyle, and lean body weights play a role in disease prevention. The bottom line is that although the Mediterranean diet and lifestyle may be optimal for health and longevity, it cannot be achieved simply by adding olive oil and red wine to the typical American diet. It is not as easy as drizzling olive oil on a cheeseburger. See Chapter 18 for more on the Mediterranean diet.

How Low is Too Low?

According to the Food and Agriculture Organization of the United Nations and the World Health Organization, fat should supply at least 15% of total calories for adults. Too little fat causes HDL-cholesterol levels to decrease, but that may not be harmful as long as fat intake is low, because the ratio of LDL to HDL actually improves when fat is restricted. Also, very-low-fat diets can worsen glucose tolerance in non–insulin-dependent diabetics. At the current American intake of 33% of calories from fat, most people have a long way to go before they need to worry about getting too little fat. In a culture and environment where high-fat foods are abundant, cutting fat can be a challenge.

Consider Dean Ornish's Reversal Diet, which is part of a lifestyle program that includes exercise, meditation, and yoga. This program has been proven to not only reduce LDL-cholesterol and body weight but to actually cause clearing in clogged arteries. Although the potential benefits are tremendous, long-term compliance with the diet is difficult. This vegetarian eating plan, which eliminates meat, cheese, and butter and restricts nuts and oils, provides only 10% of calories from fat. Compliance requires a high level of motivation, frequent and ongoing follow-up, and major lifestyle changes.

Avid dieters dedicated to counting fat grams can take the concept of restricting fat too far. Although low-fat diets may be among the best options for promoting weight loss, simply counting fat grams does not guarantee a low-calorie eating plan nor a healthy intake. For instance, many "low-fat" and "fat-free" foods are loaded with sugar and calories and are devoid of vitamins, minerals, phytochemicals, and fiber. Extreme fat phobia, a common characteristic of clients with anorexia nervosa, can have devastating physical and psychological consequences. Variety, balance, and moderation remain the cornerstones of healthy eating.

DECODING FOOD LABELS

Dietary advice on how much fat to eat is always given as a percentage of total calories, from a minimum of 15% to the almost universal guideline of 30% or less. However, Nutrition Facts labels do not list the percentage of calories from fat (see Chapter 8). Instead, they indicate the number of calories from fat, the total fat grams, and the Percent Daily Value (%DV) contained in one serving of the product. But is all that information really useful? And if so, how should it be used? What about claims that a product is, for instance, "97% fat free"? And are terms like "light" and "low fat" valid and reliable?

Calories From Fat

On the Nutrition Facts label, "Calories from fat" is found on the same line as "Calories." Alone, this figure is meaningless because it is not needed for either of the popular methods used to track fat intake: counting total fat grams or concentrating on foods that provide 30% or fewer calories from fat. But this number, divided by the total calories and then multiplied by 100, can be used to determine the percentage of calories from fat. For example, 2 tablespoons of reduced-fat peanut butter provides 180 cal, 90 of which come from fat:

$$90 \text{ cal} \div 180 \text{ cal} \times 100 = 50\% \text{ of calories from fat}$$

It's not a difficult calculation, but without a calculator some people may not find it worth the trouble. A short cut approach for *most* foods is to use the guideline of 3 g of fat for every 100 cal provided (3 g of fat, at 9 cal/g, equals 27 cal from fat, or 27% of the 100 cal). For instance:

If the total calories are . . .	Fat grams should not exceed . . .
50	1.5
100	3
200	6
300	9

This method ensures that the food has less than 30% of its calories from fat. But remember that the guideline of 30% calories from fat pertains to the total diet, not to individual foods. Higher-fat foods such as peanut butter need not be excluded from the diet, because, when they are averaged over an entire day with foods that provide little or no fat (vegetables, fruits, skim milk, and grains), the percentage of total calories from fat is lessened.

Fat Grams

It's possible, but not practical, to keep track of fat intake by counting fat grams. To use this method as a reliable means of monitoring fat intake, an individual must know his or her daily fat gram budget as well as the fat content of all foods eaten.

The problem in counting fat grams is that not all foods are labeled. The fact that fresh fruits and vegetables are not labeled is inconsequential because they generally provide insignificant amounts of fat. But foods eaten away from home account for an estimated 25% of fat consumed—a significant unknown amount. Comparing labels for fat grams does allow consumers to make informed choices. However, information on grams of polyunsaturated fat and monounsaturated fat is not required on food labels, so tracking the type of fat consumed is almost impossible.

To determine the fat gram budget:

1. Multiply the number of calories needed daily by 30% for the maximum daily intake. (The same calculation may be made using 25% to provide a daily range.)
2. Divide the maximum daily intake by 9 cal/g to find total fat grams per day.

The following table eliminates the need to do the math.

	Fat Grams	
Total daily calories	30% of Calories From Fat	25% of Calories From Fat
1600	53	44
1800	60	50
2000	65	56
2200	73	61
2500	80	69

Percentage of Daily Value From Fat

As a reflection of the significance of monitoring fat intake, information on fat grams and %DV for fat is located directly under the line for calories on the Nutrition Facts label. What many people do not know is that %DV is not the same thing as percentage of calories from fat. For all food labels except infant foods, the Daily Value (DV) is how much of each nutrient should be consumed by an individual who needs 2000 calories daily; the %DV indicates what percentage of the day's total for that nutrient is contained in one serving of the food. In a diet of 2000 cal/day, up to 65 g/day should come from fat:

$$2000 \text{ cal} \times 30\% \div 9 \text{ cal/g} = 65 \text{ g/day from fat}$$

According to the Nutrition Facts label, 2 tablespoons of reduced-fat peanut butter contains 11 g of fat, and the %DV is listed as 17%:

$$11 \text{ g fat} \div 65 \text{ g/day} \times 100 = 16.4\% \text{ (rounded to 17\%)}$$

People who mistakenly think that 17% refers to total calories instead of DV grams of fat are greatly underestimating the percentage of calories from fat, which is really 50% in this reduced-fat peanut butter.

Moreover, although all noninfant food labels use 2000 cal as the basis for the DV, a 2000-cal diet is not appropriate for everyone. For people who need less than 2000 cal (including most women), the %DV listed on the label underestimates the contribution to the total day's allowance. The %DV overestimates the contribution when calorie needs exceed 2000 per day. Also, for anyone who wants to limit fat to less than 30% of total calories, the %DV on food labels underestimates the actual contribution.

Fat Content Claims

Can you believe whole milk is 97% fat free? It's true, but it is 97% fat free *by weight*, not by calories. And our concern is calorie content, not weight. The 3% fat by weight of whole milk (which contains a lot of heavy, but calorie-free, water) actually translates to 48% calories from fat. Follow the math found on the label:

1 cup of whole milk contains 8 g of fat and 150 cal
$8 \text{ g} \times 9 \text{ cal/g} = 72$ cal from fat per cup
$72 \text{ cal} \div 150 \text{ cal/cup} \times 100 = 48\%$ calories from fat

Fat content claims, which frequently appear on packaged meat labels, can be used to compare one brand to another but not to determine the percentage of calories from fat. For instance, packaged ham labeled "94% fat free" is lower in fat than ham labeled "92% fat free," but it cannot be assumed that it falls within the guideline of 30% or fewer calories from fat.

Defined Terms

Thanks to nutrition labeling laws, terms such as "light" and "low fat" have a legal meaning. You can trust that:

If the label says . . .	One serving contains . . .
Fat-free	<0.5 g fat
*Saturated fat–free	<0.5 g of fat, and the level of *trans*-fatty acids does not exceed 1% of total fat
Low fat	3 g fat or less
*Low saturated fat	1 g or less, and not more than 15% of calories are from saturated fatty acids
Reduced or less fat	At least 25% less fat than the reference food (but not necessarily "low fat")
*Reduced or less saturated fat	At least 25% less fat than the reference food (but not necessarily "low fat")
Light	One-third fewer calories or 50% less fat than the reference food
*Low cholesterol	20 mg or less cholesterol, and 2 g or less saturated fat
Reduced or less cholesterol	At least 25% less cholesterol than the reference food, and <2 g saturated fat

*The definition of these may change slightly due to proposed labeling changes regarding *trans*-fat.

FAT REPLACERS

The proliferation of low-fat foods in the marketplace is a result of increased consumer demand and recommendations by the American Heart Association and the National Institutes of Health. Although some foods can be made low fat by simply reducing the fat content (eg, milk), others use fat replacers to simulate the functional properties of fat while reducing total fat, saturated fat, and calories. Depending on how well they are digested, replacers made from carbohydrates or protein supply 4 cal/g or less, compared with 9 cal/g in the fat they replace; the calorie content of replacers made from fats varies from 0 to 5 cal/kg. Each type has its own advantages, disadvantages, and most practical food uses.

Carbohydrate-Based Replacers

These fat replacers are made from modified food starch, gels, gums, and grain- or fruit-based fibers. Examples include Lighter Bake (made from prune puree) and Litesse (made from polydextrose). Carbohydrate-based fat replacers are used most often in dairy products, sauces, frozen desserts, salad dressings, baked goods, candy, chewing gum, and dry cake and cookie mixes. They offer the advantage of retaining moisture in foods and adding texture, but they cannot be used for frying. Some can have a laxative effect when consumed in large amounts.

Protein-Based Replacers

A special cooking and blending process can be used to convert protein in whey, milk, egg, or corn into fat replacers. Protein-based fat replacers, such as Simplesse, are found most often in dairy products (cheese, ice cream, sour cream, yogurt); baked goods; and mayonnaise, butter, salad dressings, and spreads. Although they can be used in a variety of foods, most are not suitable at high temperatures because the protein coagulates and loses its function.

Fat-Based Replacers

Olestra (brand name, Olean) combines fatty acids from vegetable oils with a sugar backbone. Enzymes in the gastrointestinal tract are not able to split the fatty acids from the sugar molecule, so olestra passes through the body unabsorbed. Because it is not absorbed, it provides no calories, may cause gastrointestinal upset (abdominal cramping, flatulence, diarrhea), and impairs the absorption of fat-soluble vitamins when eaten at the same time as those nutrients. Manufacturers are required to add specified amounts of vitamins A, D, E, and K to products containing olestra to compensate for the potential loss of these nutrients, and they must disclose on the product label that vitamins have been added and that potential gastrointestinal side effects may occur. The mouth feel and flavor of olestra are similar to those of fat, and olestra is used as a replacement for up to 100% of the fat in salty snack foods (eg, potato chips, corn chips, cheese puffs) and crackers.

Salatrim, a fat replacer made from selected short- and long-chain fatty acids that are only partially absorbed, contributes 5 cal/g. It is used in baked goods, dairy products, and candy.

Safety

The U.S. Food and Drug Administration (FDA) is responsible for ensuring the safety of the nation's food supply. Most fat replacers have been approved for use under the heading "Generally Recognized as Safe" (GRAS) because they are made from components already found in the food supply. Examples of GRAS fat replacers include those made from gums, gels, and starches. The other fat replacers are considered food additives because they are substances not previously found in foods. The FDA approves their use only after the manufacturer submits extensive data on the ingredient's safety and intended use. After an item is approved, the FDA sets recommended limits of consumption and may require ongoing monitoring of use and safety. Despite its approval as a food additive, many people are concerned about the safety of olestra. One consumer watchdog agency, the Center for Science in the Public Interest, has placed olestra on its list of food additives to avoid (Jacobson, 1999).

Efficacy

According to the American Dietetic Association, "Fat replacers may offer a safe, feasible, and effective means to maintain the palatability of diets with controlled amounts of fat and/or energy." Whether they actually help Americans eat less fat and fewer calories depends on whether they are used in addition to foods normally eaten or take the place of regular fat foods that would otherwise be eaten. Furthermore, diets low in fat are not guaranteed to be low in calories. People who choose to use fat replacers should do so with the understanding that they are only one component of a total diet, and as such they, by themselves, cannot transform an "unhealthy" diet into a healthy one. Fat replacers should be consumed only at levels that are well tolerated. Only time will tell whether fat replacers will help Americans eat less fat, maintain healthy body weight, and reduce the risk of chronic diseases.

Questions You May Hear

Is there such a thing as a "fat tooth"? Yes, it appears that some people have a preference for fats, a "fat tooth" (similar to a "sweet tooth"). Experts are not sure whether this results from our high-fat environment and culture, from the sensory qualities of fat itself, or as a side effect of intermittent dieting. Whatever the cause, it is more common in overweight people than in those who are thin. Indulging a fat tooth (in small portion sizes) and using foods containing fat replacers may help control high-fat cravings.

Is it okay to use fish oil supplements if you don't like to eat fish? Fish oil supplements are not recommended for several reasons. Foremost, the safety, effectiveness, and proper dosages for fish oil supplements have not been determined. Tests on supplements have shown that often they contain less active ingredients than those stated on the label, and some fish oil supplements may contain pesticides. Adding supplements to a poor diet does not make up for mediocre food choices. Potential side effects include gastrointestinal upset, increased bleeding time (which may cause nosebleeds and easy bruising), and, with some preparations, vitamin A and D toxicity. Because they contain oil, they provide calories and can contribute to weight gain. They are more expensive than eating fish. At high doses, supplements act more like drugs than nutrients; although it is almost impossible to overdose on nutrients in food, the same is not true for supplements. Rather than discount all seafood as unpalatable, try different varieties and different seafood dishes—you may find something you like.

KEY CONCEPTS

- Ninety-five percent of lipids consumed in the diet are triglycerides, which are composed of one glyceride molecule and three fatty acids. Most fatty acids in foods are long-chain fatty acids. Phospholipids and sterols are the other two types of dietary lipids.
- Saturation refers to the hydrogen atoms attached to the carbon atoms in the fatty acid chain. Saturated fatty acids do not have any double bonds between carbon atoms; each carbon is "saturated" with as much hydrogen as it can hold. Unsaturated fats have one (monounsaturated) or more than one (polyunsaturated) double bond between carbon atoms. When used to describe food fats, these terms are relative descriptions of the type of fatty acid present in the largest amount. All foods contain a mixture of saturated, monounsaturated, and polyunsaturated fats.
- Omega-3 fatty acids help lower serum triglyceride levels, may lower blood pressure, and decrease platelet aggregation. They may also have antiinflammatory effects. The best sources of n-3 fatty acids are marine oils; walnuts, soybeans, flaxseed, and canola oil are plant sources.
- *Trans*-fatty acids are produced through the process of hydrogenation. They are chemically unsaturated fats but function like saturated fat in the body.
- Linoleic acid (n-6) and linolenic acid (n-3) are essential fatty acids because they cannot be made by the body. They are important constituents of cell membranes, and they function to maintain healthy skin and promote normal growth. Deficiencies of essential fatty acids are rare.
- Phospholipids are structural components of cell membranes that facilitate the transport of fat-soluble substances across cell membranes. They are widespread in the diet.
- Cholesterol, a sterol, is a constituent of all cell membranes and is used to make bile acids, steroid hormones, and vitamin D. Cholesterol is found in all foods of animal origin except egg whites. Most Americans eat about half as much cholesterol as the body makes each day.
- Fat digestion occurs mostly in the small intestine. Short-chain and medium-chain fatty acids and glycerol are absorbed through mucosal cells into capillaries leading to the portal vein. Larger fat molecules—namely cholesterol, phospholipids, and reformed triglycerides made from monoglycerides and long-chain fatty acids—are absorbed in chylomicrons and transported through the lymph system.
- Lipids are transported through the blood in vehicles known as lipoproteins. The four major classes of lipoproteins vary in their density and function. Chylomicrons transport exogenous lipids to the liver. VLDLs are made mostly in the liver for the purpose of transporting endogenous lipids. LDLs are highly atherogenic and are commonly referred to as "bad" cholesterol; their function is to transport cholesterol to cells. HDLs

are the "good" cholesterol; HDLs pick up cholesterol from the cells and take it back to the liver.

- The major function of fat is to provide energy; 1 g of fat supplies 9 cal of energy. Fat also provides insulation, protects internal organs from mechanical damage, and promotes the absorption of the fat-soluble vitamins. The essential fatty acids are important for cell membrane integrity and eicosanoid synthesis.
- Fat in foods contributes sensory qualities. It absorbs flavors and aromas, imparts flavor, aerates batters, and has a creamy "mouth feel."
- All Food Guide Pyramid food groups provide fat except the Fruit group. The type and quantity of fat varies considerably among items within each group. In the typical American diet, beef is the biggest source of fat, and cheese is the biggest source of saturated fat.
- Most leading health authorities recommend that Americans limit total fat intake to 30% of total calories or less, saturated fat intake to less than 10% of total calories, and cholesterol intake to 300 mg/day. The majority of Americans fail to meet the guidelines for fat and saturated fat.
- High-fat diets are linked to several chronic diseases, namely heart disease, certain cancers, obesity, hypertension, insulin resistance, and gallbladder disease. Obesity is an independent risk factor for diabetes, certain cancers, and heart disease.
- Generally, saturated fats raise LDL-cholesterol; polyunsaturated fats lower both LDL- and HDL-cholesterol; and monounsaturated fats lower LDL-cholesterol and may or may not lower HDL.
- A diet containing 30% or fewer calories from fat is recommended for all healthy Americans older than 2 years of age. However, population studies show that the higher-fat Mediterranean diet (approximately 40% of calories from fat, with most from monounsaturated fats) may actually be optimal for disease prevention. Other lifestyle differences (exercise, normal body weight, less stress) contribute to the diet's positive effect on health. Diets that are very low in fat decrease LDL- and HDL-cholesterol, increase blood triglycerides, and are difficult to comply with on a long-term basis. Extreme low-fat diets, as seen in people with anorexia nervosa, can cause physical and psychological damage.
- Label reading helps consumers make informed food choices. The %DV for fat on the Nutrition Facts label is appropriate only for people who need 2000 cal/day in their diet; it underestimates or overestimates the contribution of fat to overall intake in people who need less or more, respectively, than 2000 cal/day.
- Fat replacers are safe and may help Americans reduce their fat and calorie intake if they are used to replace high-fat foods normally eaten. Their use does not guarantee a low-calorie or healthy diet. Because olestra is not absorbed, it may cause abdominal cramping, flatulence, and diarrhea.

ANSWER KEY

1. **FALSE** All fats, whether saturated or unsaturated, provide 9 cal/g.
2. **FALSE** A label that states a product is 98% fat free is indicating that it is 98% fat free by weight, not by calories.

3. **FALSE** The 30% calories from fat guideline pertains to the entire diet, not individual foods.
4. **FALSE** The total *trans*-fats and saturated fat in margarine is always less than the saturated fat content of butter.
5. **FALSE** The safety, effectiveness, and proper dosage for fish oil supplements have not been determined; therefore, the supplement is not recommended.
6. **TRUE** Beef is the top source of fat in American diets.
7. **TRUE** Cheese is the biggest source of saturated fat in the typical American diet.
8. **TRUE** *Trans*-fatty acids act like saturated fatty acids to raise blood levels of LDL-cholesterol (the "bad" cholesterol).
9. **FALSE** Nutrition Facts labels do not list the percent of calories from fat; however, they do indicate the amount of calories from fat, total fat grams, and the Percent Daily Value of fat in a serving of a product.
10. **FALSE** Reduced-fat foods are at least 25% less fat than the reference food, but not necessarily low fat and not necessarily lower in calories.

REFERENCES

Albert, C., Hennekens, C., O'Donnell, C., Ajani, U., Carey, V., & Willett, W. (1998). Fish consumption and risk of sudden cardiac death. *Journal of the American Medical Association*, 279, 23–28.

American Dietetic Association. (1999). Position of the American Dietetic Association: Dietary guidance for healthy children aged 2 to 11 years. *Journal of the American Dietetic Association*, 99, 93–101.

American Dietetic Association. (1998). Position of the American Dietetic Association: Fat replacers. *Journal of the American Dietetic Association*, 98, 463–468.

Harrison, G. (1997). Reducing dietary fat: Putting theory into practice. Conference summary. *Journal of the American Dietetic Association*, 98(Suppl.), S93–S96.

International Food Information Council. (1998). *Sorting out the facts about fat*. Washington, DC: International Food Information Council Foundation.

Jacobson, M. (Ed.). (1999). A guide to food additives. *Nutrition Action Health Letter*, 26(2), 1, 4–9.

Kris-Etherton, P., & Burns, J. (Eds.). (1998). *Cardiovascular nutrition: Strategies and tools for disease management and prevention*. Chicago: The American Dietetic Association.

Kuller, L. (1997). Dietary fat and chronic diseases: Epidemiologic overview. *Journal of the American Dietetic Association*, 98(Suppl.), S9–S15.

Masley, S. (1998). Dietary therapy for preventing and treating coronary artery disease. *American Family Physician*, 57, 1299–1313.

Prince, D., & Welschenbach, M. (1998). Olestra: A new food additive. *Journal of the American Dietetic Association*, 98, 565–569.

Ravussin, R., & Tataranni, P. (1997). Dietary fat and human obesity. *Journal of the American Dietetic Association*, 97(Suppl.), S42–S46.

Subar, A., Krebs-Smith, S., Cook, A., & Kahle, L. (1998). Dietary sources of nutrients among US adults, 1989 to 1991. *Journal of the American Dietetic Association*, 98, 537–547.

Wootan, M., Liebman, B., & Rosofsky, W. (1996). Trans: The phantom fat. *Nutrition Action Health Letter*, 23(7), 1, 10–13.

CHAPTER 5

Vitamins

TRUE	FALSE	Check your knowledge of vitamins.
⬭	⬭	1 Most people need a daily multivitamin supplement.
⬭	⬭	2 Cooking vegetables in the microwave destroys more vitamins than does cooking them on the stove.
⬭	⬭	3 Taking large doses of water-soluble vitamins is harmless.
⬭	⬭	4 Vitamin pills give people energy.
⬭	⬭	5 With vitamin pills, the higher the price, the better the quality.
⬭	⬭	6 "Natural" vitamins are superior to "synthetic" ones.
⬭	⬭	7 Even though the final verdict on antioxidants and disease has not been decided, it is prudent to take antioxidant supplements.
⬭	⬭	8 Natural folate in foods is better absorbed than synthetic folic acid added to foods.
⬭	⬭	9 All people who do not adequately absorb vitamin B_{12} require parenteral injections of B_{12}.
⬭	⬭	10 People under emotional stress need "stress" vitamins.

Upon completion of this chapter, you will be able to

- Compare and contrast fat- and water-soluble vitamins.
- Describe general functions and uses of vitamins.
- Identify the major vitamins provided in each Food Guide Pyramid food group.
- Name vitamins most likely to be deficient in the typical American diet.
- Discuss criteria for choosing a vitamin supplement.
- Discuss why some people need supplements of folic acid, vitamin B_{12}, and vitamin D.
- Discuss why the adage "If a little is good, a lot is better" does not apply to vitamins.

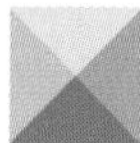

Keys to Understanding Vitamins

Vitamins are organic compounds made of carbon, hydrogen, oxygen, and sometimes nitrogen or other elements. Vitamins promote biochemical reactions within cells to help regulate body processes such as growth and metabolism. They are essential to life.

Unlike the organic compounds covered previously in this section (carbohydrates, protein, and fat), vitamins:

- Are individual molecules, not long chains of molecules linked together
- Do not provide energy but are needed for the metabolism of energy
- Are needed in microgram or milligram quantities, not gram quantities. Because they are needed in such small amounts, they are referred to as **micronutrients.**

Vitamins were discovered a mere 100 years ago as scientists searched to identify what components in food prevented the development of deficiency diseases such as scurvy. As knowledge of vitamin functions and requirements grew, fortification and enrichment policies were put in place and have virtually eliminated vitamin deficiency diseases in the general American population. Today the focus of vitamin research has evolved from preventing deficiencies to reducing the risk of chronic diseases such as heart disease and cancer. Somewhere between the brink of deficiency and the point of toxicity lies the optimal dosage for optimal health.

GENERAL CHEMISTRY

Vitamins are extremely complex chemical substances that differ widely in their structure. One of the most complex vitamin structures is vitamin B_{12}. See the figure on page 101.

Because vitamins are defined chemically (eg, any molecule labeled as vitamin B_{12} must look exactly like the structure shown), the body cannot distinguish between natural vitamins extracted from food and synthetic vitamins produced in a laboratory. However, the absorption rates of natural and synthetic vitamins sometimes differ because of different chemical forms of the same vitamin (eg, synthetic folic acid is better absorbed than natural folate in foods) or because the synthetic vitamins are "free," not "bound" to other components in food (eg, synthetic vitamin B_{12} is not bound to small peptides, as natural vitamin B_{12} is).

As organic substances, vitamins in food are susceptible to destruction and subsequent loss of function. For instance, thiamine is heat sensitive and is easily destroyed by high temperatures and long cooking times. Riboflavin is resistant to heat, acid, and oxidation but is quickly destroyed by light. That is why riboflavin-rich milk is sold in opaque containers, not transparent ones. Baking soda added during cooking, a practice used by some cooks to retain the color of beets and red cabbage, destroys thiamine. Fifty percent to 90% of folate in foods may be lost during preparation, processing, and storage. Vitamin C is destroyed by heat, air, and alkalis.

Many vitamins exist in more than one active form. Different forms perform different functions in the body. For instance, vitamin A exists as retinol (important for reproduction), retinal (needed for vision), and retinoic acid (which acts as a hormone to regulate

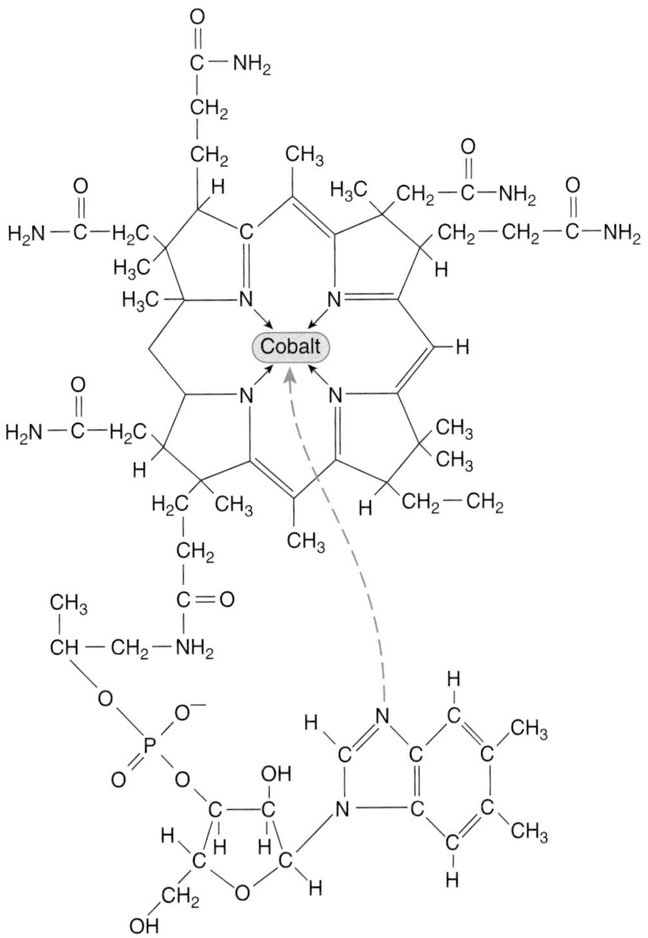

Vitamin B_{12} (cyanocobalamin). The arrows indicated that the spare electron pairs on the nitrogens attract them to the cobalt.

growth). The form of vitamin C that is added to foods as an antioxidant lacks the ability to prevent scurvy, the vitamin C deficiency disease. Recommended allowances take into account the biologic activity of vitamins as they exist in different forms.

Vitamins are essential in the diet because, with few exceptions, the body cannot make vitamins. The body can make vitamin A, vitamin D, and niacin if the appropriate precursors are available. Microorganisms in the gastrointestinal tract synthesize vitamin K and vitamin B_{12}, but not in amounts sufficient to meet the body's needs.

SOLUBILITY

The 13 known vitamins are classified according to their solubility. Vitamins A, D, E, and K are fat-soluble vitamins. Vitamin C and the B vitamins (thiamine, riboflavin, niacin, folate, B_6, B_{12}, biotin, and pantothenic acid) are water soluble.

Fat-soluble Vitamins

Fat-soluble vitamins:

- Are absorbed with fat in chylomicrons, which enter the lymphatic system before circulating in the bloodstream. Whenever fat absorption is impaired, such as in the case of cystic fibrosis or pancreatic insufficiency, secondary deficiencies of the fat-soluble vitamins can develop.
- Attach to protein carriers to be transported through the blood, because fat is not soluble in watery blood. For instance, most circulating vitamin E is found in low-density lipoprotein (LDL)–cholesterol.
- Are stored, not excreted, when consumed in excess of need. The liver and adipose tissue are the primary storage sites. Because these vitamins are stored, deficiency symptoms can take months or years to develop when intake is less than adequate.
- Can be toxic when consumed in large doses over a prolonged period. This applies primarily to vitamins A and D; large doses of vitamins E and K are considered relatively nontoxic. Vitamin toxicities are not likely to be caused by food; inappropriate use of supplements is usually to blame.
- Do not have to be eaten every day, because the body can retrieve them from storage as needed.
- Are found in the fat and oil portion of foods.

Water-soluble Vitamins

Water-soluble vitamins:

- Are absorbed directly into the bloodstream
- Move freely through the watery environment of blood and within cells
- Are excreted in the urine when consumed in excess amounts. Some tissues may hold limited amounts of certain water-soluble vitamins. For instance, adult men can store up to 3000 mg of vitamin C (most of which is contained within cells) at daily intakes of about 200 mg. (The Dietary Reference Intake [DRI] for adult men is 90 mg/d.)
- Were historically believed to be nontoxic because the body can protect itself from large doses by increasing excretion. This belief has come under scrutiny since the discovery of neurologic abnormalities caused by high-dose vitamin B_6 supplements used for a prolonged period.
- Must be consumed daily because there is no reserve in storage.
- Are found in the watery portion of foods.

GENERAL FUNCTIONS AND USES

Vitamins work as coenzymes. Some vitamins are antioxidants and therefore have important roles in the body and in food preservation. Some vitamins are used as drugs in pharmacologic doses. Although their roles in the body may be similar and interdependent, vitamins cannot replace each other.

Coenzymes

Enzymes are proteins produced by cells that catalyze chemical reactions within the body without themselves undergoing change. Many enzymes are not active without a **coenzyme,** which is an organic molecule that makes up the nonprotein portion of the enzyme. Vitamins function as coenzymes; without vitamins, thousands of chemical reactions could not take place. For instance, as a coenzyme, folacin facilitates both amino acid metabolism and nucleic acid synthesis by transferring carbon fragments from one compound to another. Without adequate folacin, protein synthesis and cell division are impaired.

Antioxidants

Free radicals are highly unstable, highly reactive molecular fragments with one or more unpaired electrons that are produced continuously in cells as they burn oxygen during normal metabolism. Ultraviolet radiation, air pollution, ozone, and smoking can also generate free radicals in the body. The problem with free radicals is that, in their quest to gain an electron and become stable, they oxidize body cells and DNA. These structurally and functionally damaged cells are believed to contribute to aging and various health problems such as cancer, heart disease, and cataracts. Polyunsaturated fatty acids in cell membranes are particularly vulnerable to damage by free radicals.

Antioxidants are substances that donate electrons to free radicals. In doing so, the antioxidants are oxidized (destroyed), the free radicals are stabilized and rendered harmless, and body cells are protected from damage. In the body, vitamin C, vitamin E, and beta-carotene (a precursor of vitamin A) are major antioxidants. Each has a slightly different role, so one cannot completely substitute for another. For instance, water-soluble vitamin C works within cells to disable free radicals, and fat-soluble vitamin E functions within fat tissue. Because antioxidants complement each other, an excess or deficiency of one may impair the action of other antioxidants.

Headlines and advertisements often tout antioxidants as "magic bullets" to prevent aging and chronic disease. Although population studies show that diets rich in fruits and vegetables appear to be protective against heart disease and cancer, it is not known whether this effect is caused by antioxidants, other vitamins, phytochemicals, or (most likely) a combination of substances in those foods. A study in which large doses of beta-carotene supplements were given to smokers to reduce their risk of lung cancer was aborted when it became apparent that the supplements actually increased the risk of lung cancer in the study subjects. Fruits and vegetables are safe and protective; research has yet to prove whether the same is true for antioxidant supplements.

Food Additives

Some foods have vitamins added to them simply to boost their nutritional content; examples include vitamin C–enriched fruit drinks, fortified ready-to-eat cereals, and enriched flour and breads. Other foods have certain vitamins added to them to help preserve quality. For instance, added vitamin C helps prevent rancidity in frozen fish and stabilizes the red color of luncheon meats and other cured foods. Small amounts of vitamin E added to vegetable oils help prevent rancidity. Beta-carotene adds color to margarine.

Drugs

In megadoses (amounts at least ten times greater than the RDA), vitamins function like drugs, not nutrients. Large doses of niacin are used to lower cholesterol, LDL-cholesterol, and triglycerides in people with hyperlipidemia who do not respond to diet and exercise. Tretinoin (retinoic acid, a form of vitamin A) is used as an antineoplastic drug to induce remission in patients with acute promyelocytic leukemia and as a topical treatment for acne vulgaris. Acitretin (Soriatane) is a retinoid, another form of vitamin A; large oral doses are used to treat severe psoriasis. Gram quantities of vitamin C promote wound healing in patients with thermal injuries.

VITAMIN REQUIREMENTS

Until recently, two standards were used for vitamin intake recommendations. The RDAs, introduced in 1941 and periodically updated, represented average daily dietary intake amounts sufficient to meet the nutrient requirements of almost all healthy people in a group. RDAs were established as goals for healthy individuals. All vitamins except biotin and pantothenic acid had RDAs. Because there were insufficient data to determine allowances for biotin and pantothenic acid, they had Estimated Safe and Adequate Daily Dietary Intakes ranges instead of RDAs.

A new set of standards called **Dietary Reference Intakes** (DRIs) are gradually replacing the RDAs. The DRIs are actually a set of four reference values of estimates of nutrient intake to be used for planning and assessing diets for healthy people. They include updated RDAs and three other types of reference values: the Estimated Average Requirement (EAR), the Adequate Intake (AI), and the Tolerable Upper Intake Level (UL).

DRIs have already been released for calcium and related nutrients and for the B vitamins, vitamin C, vitamin E, and selenium. At least three more reports on groups of nutrients and related compounds are scheduled to be released over the next 3 to 4 years. Until the new DRI system is fully implemented, reference standards will be a mixture of old and new. Definitions of the new standards are as follows.

Recommended Dietary Allowance

The **RDA** continues to represent the average daily dietary intake level that is sufficient to meet the nutrient requirement of 97% to 98% of all healthy people in a life stage and gender group. This definition is similar to past descriptions of the RDA, but in the DRI framework, this is the only use of the RDA—as a goal for individuals.

Estimated Average Requirement

The **EAR** is the amount of a nutrient that is estimated to meet the requirement of 50% of healthy people in a life stage or gender group. It is necessary to establish EAR values for nutrients in order to determine RDA values.

Adequate Intake

An **AI** is set when an RDA cannot be determined owing to lack of sufficient data on requirements. It is a recommended daily intake level based on observed or experimentally determined estimates of nutrient intake by a group of healthy people. Its primary use is as a goal for the nutrient intake of individuals.

Tolerable Upper Intake Level

The **UL** is the highest level of daily nutrient intake that is likely to pose no risk of adverse health effects to almost all individuals in the general population. The term *Tolerable Upper Intake Level* does not imply a possible beneficial effect in consuming that amount, but rather indicates the level that can be physiologically tolerated. It is not intended to be a recommended level of intake. There is no benefit in consuming amounts greater than the RDA or AI.

VITAMIN SOURCES

Because micronutrient deficiencies are unusual in the general population and excessive fat is widespread, the focus of the Food Guide Pyramid is to avoid fat, not to obtain adequate amounts of vitamins. Still, the Food Guide Pyramid can help Americans choose a nutritionally adequate diet, especially if the concepts of variety and balance are followed.

The vitamin content of items within each food group varies considerably. Figure 5–1 illustrates major vitamins within each food group. The following are generalizations.

Bread, Cereal, Rice, and Pasta Group

Items within this group provide thiamine, riboflavin, and niacin and are fortified with folic acid. Whole-grain items also contain vitamin E. Fortified breakfast cereals provide varying amounts of most vitamins.

Vegetable Group

Vegetables are among the best choices for beta-carotene, vitamin C, folate, and vitamin K. Generally, with vegetables it is best to:

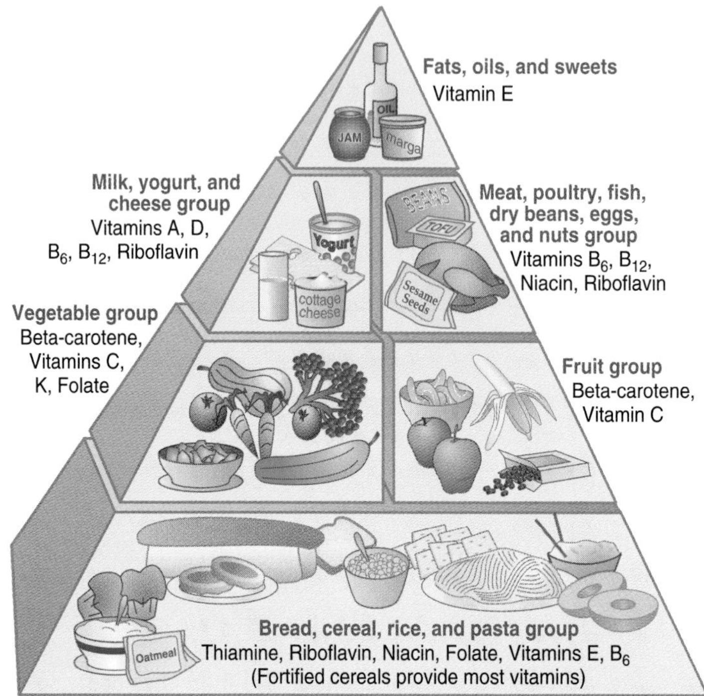

FIGURE 5-1 Major vitamins provided in the Food Guide Pyramid Groups. Actual vitamin content varies by selection within each group.

- Use minimal preparation techniques. Cooking and soaking can destroy vitamins.
- Eat a wide variety, because each one contains a unique package of vitamins, minerals, fiber, and phytochemicals.
- Go beyond the recommendation of three to five servings daily. It is impossible to overdose on nutrients from vegetables.

Fruit Group

As a group, fruits and fruit juices are also known for their beta-carotene and vitamin C content. Orange and grapefruit juice are the biggest sources of vitamin C among American adults, and they also provide significant folate. Although some fruit drinks and ades are enriched to provide 100% of the RDA for vitamin C in a single serving, they are basically sugar-water solutions with no other nutritional value except calories. Stick to 100% fruit juice.

Milk, Yogurt, and Cheese Group

Milk is fortified with vitamins A and D, is the leading source of riboflavin, and contains smaller amounts of other B vitamins. Cheese supplies vitamin A and riboflavin.

Meat, Poultry, Fish, Dry Beans, Eggs, and Nuts Group

Animal proteins provide vitamin B_{12}, niacin, vitamin B_6, and some riboflavin. Pork is rich in thiamine, dry beans are rich in folate, eggs have vitamin A, and nuts and seeds provide vitamin E.

Fats, Oils, and Sweets Group

Margarine supplies vitamins A, E, and D; vegetable oils and salad dressings are rich in vitamin E.

INDIVIDUAL FAT-SOLUBLE VITAMINS

Salient features for each fat-soluble vitamin are presented in the following paragraphs. Table 5–1 highlights each vitamin's requirements, sources, functions, deficiency symptoms, and toxicity symptoms.

TABLE 5.1 ***Summary of Fat-Soluble Vitamins***

Vitamin and Sources	Functions	Deficiency/Toxicity Signs and Symptoms
Vitamin A ***Adult RDA*** Men: 1000 μg RE* Women: 800 μg RE • Retinol: Liver, milk, butter, cheese, cream, egg yolk, fortified milk, margarine, and ready-to-eat cereals • Carotenoids: Spinach, collards, kale, mustard greens, broccoli, carrots, peaches, pumpkin, red peppers, sweet potatoes, winter squash *RE = retinol equivalents 1 RE = 1 μg retinol or 6 μg β carotene	The formation of visual purple, which enables the eye to adapt to dim light Normal growth and development of bones and teeth The formation and maintenance of mucosal epithelium to maintain healthy functioning of skin and membranes, hair, gums, and various glands Important role in immune function	*Deficiency* Night blindness, or the slow recovery of vision after flashes of bright light at night Bone growth ceases; bone shape changes; enamel-forming cells in the teeth malfunction; teeth crack and tend to decay. Skin becomes dry, scaly, rough, and cracked; keratinization or hyperkeratosis develops; mucous membrane cells flatten and harden: Eyes become dry (xerosis); irreversible drying and hardening of the cornea can result in blindness Decreased saliva secretion → difficulty chewing, swallowing → anorexia Decreased mucous secretion of the stomach and intestines → impaired digestion and absorption → diarrhea, increased excretion of nutrients

(continued)

TABLE 5.1 *Summary of Fat-Soluble Vitamins (continued)*

Vitamin and Sources	Functions	Deficiency/Toxicity Signs and Symptoms
		Susceptibility to respiratory, urinary tract, and vaginal infections increases. *Toxicity* Headaches, vomiting, double vision, hair loss, bone abnormalities, liver damage Can cause birth defects during pregnancy
Vitamin D ***Adult AI**** Men and Women: 5 μg/d to age 50 10 μg/d ages 51–70 15 μg/d over age 70 ***Adult UL:*** 50 μg/d • Sunlight on the skin • Liver, fatty fish, egg yolks, fortified milk, ready-to-eat cereals, and margarine *In the absence of sunlight and as cholecalciferol. 1 μg cholecalciferol = 40 IU Vit D	Maintains serum calcium concentrations by: Stimulating GI absorption Stimulating the release of calcium from the bones Stimulating calcium reabsorption from the kidneys	*Deficiency* Rickets (in infants and children) Retarded bone growth Bone malformations (bowed legs) Enlargement of ends of long bones (knock-knees) Deformities of the ribs (bowed, with beads or knobs) Delayed closing of the fontanel → rapid enlargement of the head Decreased serum calcium and/or phosphorus Malformed teeth; decayed teeth Protrusion of the abdomen related to relaxation of the abdominal muscles Increased secretion of parathyroid hormone Osteomalacia (in adults) Softening of the bones → deformities, pain, and easy fracture Decreased serum calcium and/or phosphorus, increased alkaline phosphatase Involuntary muscle twitching and spasms *Toxicity* Kidney stones, irreversible kidney damage, muscle and bone weakness, excessive bleeding, loss of appetite, headache, excessive thirst, calcification of soft tissues (blood vessels, kidneys, heart, lungs), death
Vitamin E ***Adult RDA*** Men and Women: 15 mg*/d	Acts as an antioxidant to protect vitamin A and PUFA from being destroyed Protects cell membranes	*Deficiency* Increased RBC hemolysis In infants, anemia, edema, and skin lesions

(continued)

TABLE 5.1 *Summary of Fat-Soluble Vitamins (continued)*

Vitamin and Sources	Functions	Deficiency/Toxicity Signs and Symptoms
Vitamin E continued ***Adult UL:*** 1000 mg/d • Vegetable oils, margarine, salad dressing, other foods made with vegetable oil, nuts, seeds, wheat germ *As α tocopherol		*Toxicity* Relatively nontoxic High doses enhance action of anticoagulant medications
Vitamin K ***Adult RDA*** Men: 80 μg Women: 65 μg • Bacterial synthesis green leafy vegetables, liver, milk, vegetables of the cabbage family	Synthesis of blood clotting proteins and a bone protein that regulates blood calcium	*Deficiency* Hemorrhaging *Toxicity* No symptoms have been observed from excessive vitamin K

Vitamin A

Vitamin A exists as a group of compounds known as **retinoids**; they include retinol, retinaldehyde, and retinoic acid. Preformed vitamin A, which is converted to retinol in the intestine, is found in animal fats such as liver, milk, butter, cheese, cream, and egg yolk. Low-fat milk, skim milk, margarine, and ready-to-eat cereals are fortified with vitamin A.

Carotenoids are the red and yellow pigments in plants. Approximately 10% of the 600 carotenoids in foods can be converted to vitamin A in the body. Beta-carotene, lutein, and lycopene are among the most common carotenoids in plasma. Deep yellow and orange fruits and vegetables and most dark-green leafy vegetables are rich in beta-carotene. Beta-carotene accounts for about half of the usual intake of vitamin A.

Vitamin A is best known for its roles in night vision, normal growth of bones and teeth, and the formation and maintenance of mucosal epithelium for the normal function of skin, hair, gums, various glands, and mucous membranes. The role of vitamin A is less well understood in reproduction, cell-membrane stability, the synthesis of corticosterone (a hormone produced by the adrenal glands), the output of thyroxine (the hormone secreted by the thyroid gland), the development of the nervous system, red blood cell production, and immune system functioning. Because carotenes are important antioxidants in the body (by comparison, vitamin A is a relatively poor antioxidant), there is much interest in their possible role in the prevention of heart disease and cancer. To date, results of studies are conflicting, and widespread supplementation is not recommended.

The body can store large amounts of vitamin A. Because deficiency symptoms do not develop until body stores are exhausted, it may take years for vitamin A deficiency to become apparent. Severe vitamin A deficiency is rare in the United States. Mild deficiency symptoms may be seen in low socioeconomic groups. Vitamin A deficiency is a major health problem worldwide, and it is the major cause of blindness.

Only preformed vitamin A is toxic in high doses. Toxicity is not likely to occur from food alone, but rather from megadoses of supplements. Children are more susceptible to vitamin A toxicity than adults are. Because large doses are teratogenic, vitamin A supplementation is not recommended during the first trimester of pregnancy unless there is specific evidence of vitamin A deficiency. In adults, toxicity symptoms can be reversed if they are detected early and vitamin supplementation is stopped, although complete recovery may take several weeks. Damage can be permanent if prompt action is not taken.

Beta-carotene is not converted to vitamin A quickly enough to cause toxicity. Instead, carotene is stored primarily in adipose tissue and may accumulate under the skin to the extent that it causes the skin color to turn yellowish-orange, a harmless condition known as hypercarotenemia.

Vitamin D

Vitamin D is unique in that the body can synthesize it from cholesterol and ultraviolet light absorbed through the skin (Fig. 5–2). In theory, with regular exposure to sunlight under optimal conditions (10–15 minutes of exposure on the hands, face, and arms between 8 a.m. and 4 p.m., two to three times per week), a dietary source of vitamin D is not necessary. In reality, a dietary source is considered essential because few people meet those conditions. For instance, only people living in southern states make vitamin D in the winter. Dense clouds, heavy smog, sunscreen, clothing, window glass, and dark-colored skin block vitamin D synthesis. Also, the ability to produce vitamin D decreases with aging.

Vitamin D occurs naturally in only a few foods: liver, fatty fish, and egg yolks. Fortified foods (milk, margarine, and some ready-to-eat breakfast cereals) are important sources. Vitamin D–fortified milk is credited with eliminating vitamin D deficiency in American children.

Another unique feature of vitamin D is that it acts more like a hormone than a vitamin. It is synthesized in one part of the body and stimulates functional activity elsewhere. Vitamin D promotes bone formation and maintenance by optimizing blood levels of calcium and phosphorus, which it achieves by stimulating:

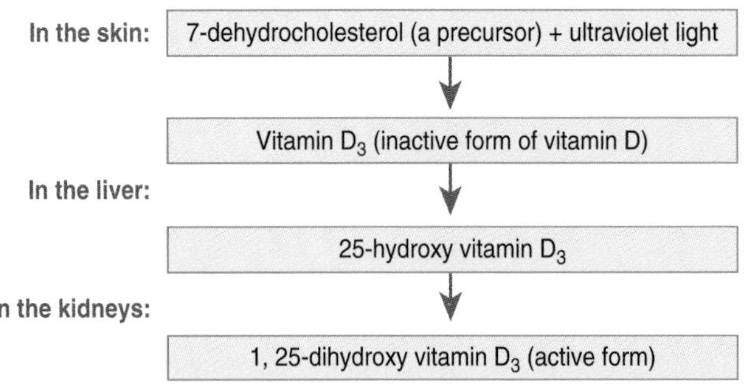

FIGURE 5-2 Vitamin D synthesis.

- The gastrointestinal tract to absorb more calcium and phosphorus
- The bones to release calcium and phosphorus
- The kidneys to retain calcium and phosphorus

Without vitamin D, calcium is not absorbed regardless of the amount consumed; as a result, blood calcium levels fall and bones lose minerals. Elderly persons are particularly at risk for vitamin D deficiency because their kidneys produce less, their exposure to the sun may be limited, and many have a low intake of vitamin D because they do not drink milk. Older adults with borderline or overt vitamin D deficiency may appear asymptomatic.

Conversely, too much vitamin D heightens calcium absorption and raises blood calcium levels. Hypercalcemia can damage the kidneys and other soft tissues. Because vitamin D has the narrowest range of safe intake among all the vitamins, it is the one most likely to produce toxic symptoms when consistently consumed at levels a few times higher than recommended. Neither excessive sun exposure nor eating a normal mixed diet causes vitamin D toxicity. Toxicity occurs in people who take vitamin D supplements despite consuming an adequate diet and getting ample exposure to sunlight.

Vitamin E

Vitamin E is a generic term that describes a group of at least eight compounds that have the biologic activity of alpha-tocopherol, which is the most active and most abundant form of vitamin E. Because different tocopherols have different potencies, the standard used to measure vitamin E activity is alpha-tocopherol equivalents.

As the primary antioxidant in the body, vitamin E protects polyunsaturated fatty acids (PUFAs) and other lipid molecules from oxidative damage, thereby helping to maintain the integrity of PUFA-rich cell membranes; protects red blood cells against hemolysis; and protects vitamin A from oxidation. Vitamin E is also important for immune system functioning.

Vitamin E is being studied for its role in preventing the oxidation of LDL-cholesterol and subsequent development of coronary artery disease, but the doses used in clinical trials (100 to 400 IU) cannot be achieved through food alone. Other studies are investigating the role of vitamin E in wound healing, Parkinson's disease, and treatment of Alzheimer's disease. Doctors often recommend large doses of vitamin E to help relieve the pain of fibrocystic disease.

Although vitamin E is vital for maintaining health, it is not a miracle nutrient. There is no evidence to support claims that vitamin E cures infertility, diabetes, ulcers, skin disorders, shortness of breath, and muscular dystrophy. Nor does vitamin E increase physical performance and sexual potency, protect against air pollution, reverse gray hair and wrinkles, or slow the aging process.

Because vitamin E is so abundant in plant fats, deficiencies are rare except among very-low-birthweight infants. People with chronic fat malabsorption syndromes are at risk for vitamin E deficiency, but symptoms may take 5 to 10 years to develop. The need for vitamin E increases as the intake of PUFA increases. Fortunately, vitamin E and

PUFA have the same food sources: vegetable oils, margarine, salad dressings, other foods made with vegetable oils, nuts, seeds, and wheat germ.

Large amounts of vitamin E are relatively nontoxic but can interfere with vitamin K action (blood clotting) by decreasing platelet aggregation. Large doses may also potentiate the effects of blood-thinning drugs, increasing the risk of hemorrhage.

Vitamin K

Vitamin K occurs naturally in two forms: phylloquinone, which is found in plants such as green leafy vegetables, and menaquinones, which are synthesized in the intestinal tract by bacteria. Animal sources, such as liver and milk, provide both forms of vitamin K. Approximately half of vitamin K requirements are met through food sources, the other half through bacterial synthesis. Unlike other fat-soluble vitamins, stores of vitamin K are quickly depleted when requirements are not obtained.

Vitamin K is essential for the synthesis of prothrombin and at least four other proteins required for normal blood clotting. Without adequate vitamin K, life is threatened: even a small wound can cause someone deficient in vitamin K to bleed to death. Vitamin K is also involved in the synthesis of other proteins needed by blood, bones, and the kidneys.

Newborns are prone to vitamin K deficiency because their sterile gastrointestinal tracts cannot synthesize vitamin K and it may take weeks for bacteria to establish themselves in the newborn's intestines. To prevent hemorrhagic disease, a single oral or parenteral dose of vitamin K is given prophylactically at birth.

A secondary deficiency of vitamin K occurs from fat malabsorption syndromes and the use of vitamin K antagonists, such as coumarin and indanedione, anticoagulants that interfere with hepatic synthesis of vitamin K–dependent clotting factors. People who take anticoagulants do not need to avoid vitamin K, but they should try to maintain a consistent intake. Vitamin K deficiency may also occur secondary to prolonged use of antibiotics or sulfa drugs, which kill the intestinal bacteria that synthesize vitamin K.

INDIVIDUAL WATER-SOLUBLE VITAMINS

Salient features for each water-soluble vitamin are presented in the following paragraphs. Requirements, sources, functions, deficiency symptoms, and toxicity symptoms are highlighted in Table 5–2.

Thiamine

Thiamine (vitamin B_1) is a vital component of the coenzyme thiamine pyrophosphate, which is involved in the conversion of pyruvate to acetyl coenzyme A (acetyl-CoA) and in the tricarboxylic acid (TCA) cycle. In addition to its role in energy metabolism, thiamine is important in nervous system functioning.

Actual thiamine requirements are stated in milligrams of thiamine per 1000 cal consumed, because the thiamine requirement increases as calorie intake increases. Usually, a

TABLE 5.2 *Summary of Water-Soluble Vitamins*

Vitamin and Sources	Functions	Deficiency/Toxicity Signs and Symptoms
Thiamine (Vitamin B_1) ***Adult RDA*** Men: 1.2 mg/d Women: 1.1 mg/d • Whole grain and enriched breads and cereals, liver, legumes, nuts	Coenzyme in energy metabolism Promotes normal appetite and nervous system functioning	*Deficiency* Beriberi Mental confusion Fatigue Peripheral paralysis Muscle weakness and wasting Painful calf muscles Anorexia Edema Enlarged heart Sudden death from heart failure *Toxicity* No toxicity symptoms reported
Riboflavin (Vitamin B_2) ***Adult RDA*** Men: 1.3 mg/d Women: 1.1 mg/d • Milk and other dairy products; whole grain and enriched breads and cereals; eggs, meat, green leafy vegetables	Coenzyme in energy metabolism Aids in the conversion of tryptophan into niacin	*Deficiency* Ariboflavinosis Dermatitis Cheilosis Glossitis Photophobia Reddening of the cornea *Toxicity* No toxicity symptoms reported
Niacin (Vitamin B_3) ***Adult RDA**** Men: 16 mg/d Women: 14 mg/d ***Adult UL:*** 35 mg/d • All protein foods, whole grain and enriched breads and cereals *As niacin equivaents (NE) 1 mg niacin = 60 mg tryptophan	Coenzyme in energy metabolism Promotes normal nervous system functioning	*Deficiency* Pellagra: 4 (Ds) Dermatitis (bilateral and symmetrical) and glossitis Diarrhea Dementia, irritability, mental confusion → psychosis Death, if untreated *Toxicity* (from supplements/drugs) Flushing, liver damage, gastric ulcers, low blood pressure, diarrhea, nausea, vomiting
Vitamin B_6 ***Adult RDA*** Men: 1.3 mg/d to age 50 1.7 mg/d after 50	Coenzyme in amino acid and fatty acid metabolism Helps convert tryptophan to niacin Helps produce insulin, hemoglobin, myelin sheaths and antibodies	*Deficiency* Dermatitis, cheilosis, glossitis, abnormal brain wave pattern, convulsions, and anemia

(continued)

TABLE 5.2 *Summary of Water-Soluble Vitamins (continued)*

Vitamin and Sources	Functions	Deficiency/Toxicity Signs and Symptoms
Vitamin B_6 continued Women: 1.3 mg/d to age 50 1.5 mg/d after 50 ***Adult UL:*** 100 mg/d • Meats, fish, poultry, legumes, fruits, green leafy vegetables, whole grains, nuts		*Toxicity* Depression, fatigue, irritability, headaches; sensory neuropathy characteristic
Folate ***Adult RDA**** Men and women: 400 µg/d ***Adult UL:*** 1,000 µg/d (applies to forms obtained from food, supplements, or combination) • Leafy vegetables, legumes, seeds, liver, orange juice, some fruits; breads, cereals and other grains are fortified with folic acid	Coenzymes in DNA synthesis therefore vital for new cell synthesis and the transmission of inherited characteristics	*Deficiency* Glossitis, diarrhea, macrocytic anemia, depression, mental confusion, fainting, fatigue *Toxicity* Too much can mask B_{12} deficiency
*As dietary folate equivalent (DFE) 1 DFE = 1 µg food folate = 0.6 µg folic acid (from fortified food or supplement) consumed with food = 0.5 µg synthetic (supplemental) folic acid taken on an empty stomach		
Vitamin B_{12} ***Adult RDA*** Men & women: 2.4 µg/d (people over 50 should meet their RDA mainly by consuming foods fortified with vitamin B_{12} or a supplement containing vitamin B_{12}) • Animal products: meat, fish, poultry, shellfish, milk, dairy products, eggs • Some fortified foods	Coenzyme in the synthesis of new cells Activates folate Maintains nerve cells Helps metabolize some fatty acids and amino acids	*Deficiency* GI changes: glossitis, anorexia, indigestion, recurring diarrhea or constipation, and weight loss Macrocytic anemia: pallor, dyspnea, weakness, fatigue, and palpitations Neurologic changes: paresthesia of the hands and feet, decreased sense of position, poor muscle coordination, poor memory, irritability, depression, paranoia, delirium, and hallucinations *Toxicity* No toxicity symptoms reported

(continued)

TABLE 5.2 *Summary of Water-Soluble Vitamins (continued)*

Vitamin and Sources	Functions	Deficiency/Toxicity Signs and Symptoms
Pantothenic Acid ***Adult AI*** Men and women: 5 mg/d • Widespread in foods • Meat, poultry, fish, whole grain cereals, and legumes are among best sources.	Part of coenzyme A used in energy metabolism	*Deficiency* Rare; general failure of all body systems *Toxicity* No toxicity symptoms reported, although large doses may cause diarrhea
Biotin ***Adult AI*** Men and women: 30 μg/d • Widespread in foods • Eggs, liver, yeast breads, and cereals are among best choices • Synthesized by GI flora	Coenzyme in energy metabolism, fatty acid synthesis, amino acid metabolism, and glycogen formation	*Deficiency* Rare; anorexia, fatigue, depression, dry skin, heart abnormalities *Toxicity* No toxicity symptoms reported
Vitamin C ***Adult RDA*** Men: 90 mg/d Women: 75 mg/d ***Adult UL:*** 2 g/d • Citrus fruits and juices, peppers, broccoli, cauliflower, Brussels sprouts, cantaloupe, kiwifruit, mustard greens, strawberries, tomatoes	Collagen synthesis Antioxidant Promotes iron absorption Involved in the metabolism of certain amino acids Thyroxin synthesis Immune system functioning	*Deficiency* Bleeding gums, pinpoint hemorrhages under the skin Scurvy, characterized by Hemorrhaging Muscle degeneration Skin changes Delayed wound healing: reopening of old wounds Softening of the bones → malformations, pain, easy fractures Soft, loose teeth Anemia Increased susceptibililty to infection Hysteria and depression *Toxicity* Diarrhea, abdominal cramps, nausea, headache, insomnia, fatigue, hot flashes, aggravation of gout symptoms

person who consumes adequate calories obtains adequate thiamine. Sources of thiamine include whole-grain and enriched breads and cereals, liver, dried peas and beans, and nuts.

In the United States and other countries, the use of enriched and fortified grains has virtually eliminated the thiamine deficiency disease known as beriberi. Today, thiamine deficiency is usually seen only in alcoholics, because chronic alcohol abuse impairs thiamine intake, absorption, and metabolism.

Riboflavin

Riboflavin (vitamin B_2) is part of the coenzymes flavin adenine dinucleotide (FAD) and flavin mononucleotide (FMN), which function to release energy from nutrients in all body cells. As with thiamine, riboflavin requirements are based on the amount of calories consumed. Riboflavin is found in milk and other dairy products; whole-grain and enriched breads and cereals; eggs; milk; and green leafy vegetables.

Riboflavin deficiency is rare in the United States, and symptoms may take several months to appear. Groups most likely to consume inadequate riboflavin are those with marginal calorie intakes, such as fad dieters, alcoholics, and the elderly.

Niacin

Niacin (vitamin B_3) exists as nicotinic acid and nicotinamide. The body converts nicotinic acid to nicotinamide, which is the major form of niacin in the blood. All protein foods provide niacin, as do whole-grain and enriched breads and cereals.

A unique feature of niacin is that the body can make it from the amino acid tryptophan: approximately 60 mg of tryptophan is used to synthesize 1 mg of niacin. Because of this additional source of niacin, niacin requirements are stated in niacin equivalents (NEs). As with thiamine and riboflavin, niacin requirements are based on the calorie content of the diet.

Niacin is part of the coenzymes nicotinamide adenine dinucleotide (NAD) and nicotinamide adenine dinucleotide phosphate (NADP), which are involved in energy transfer reactions in the metabolism of glucose, fat, and alcohol. Reduced NADP is used in the synthesis of fatty acids, cholesterol, and steroid hormones.

Pellagra, the disorder caused by severe niacin deficiency, is rare in the United States and usually is seen only in alcoholics. However, pellagra is widespread in areas that rely on corn as a staple, such as parts of Africa and Asia, and it occurred frequently in the southern United States before grain products were enriched with niacin. Niacin deficiency may be treated with niacin, or tryptophan, or both. Because a deficiency of niacin rarely occurs alone, treatment is most effective when other B-complex vitamins are also given, especially thiamine and riboflavin.

Large doses of niacin in the form of nicotinic acid (1 g to 6 g/d) are used therapeutically to lower total cholesterol and LDL-cholesterol and raise high-density lipoprotein (HDL)–cholesterol. Flushing is a common side effect that is caused by vasodilation. Large doses may also cause liver damage and gout. Large doses of niacin should be used only with a doctor's supervision.

Vitamin B_6

Vitamin B_6 and pyridoxine are group names for a class of related chemicals that include pyridoxine, pyridoxal, and pyridoxamine. All three forms can be converted to the coenzyme pyridoxal phosphate, which participates in more than 60 biochemical reactions, especially those involving amino acid and fatty acid metabolism. Vitamin B_6 is also important for the conversion of tryptophan to niacin, the formation of heme for hemoglobin, the synthesis of myelin sheaths, and the maintenance of cellular immunity. Unlike other B vitamins, vitamin B_6 is stored extensively in muscle tissue.

Dietary sources of vitamin B_6 are meats, fish, poultry, dried peas and beans, fruits, green leafy vegetables, whole grains, and nuts. Deficiencies of vitamin B_6 are uncommon but are usually accompanied by deficiencies of other B vitamins. Secondary deficiencies are related to alcohol abuse (the metabolism of alcohol promotes the destruction and excretion of vitamin B_6) and to other drug therapies such as isoniazid, the antituberculosis drug that acts as a vitamin B_6 antagonist.

Vitamin B_6 has been used experimentally to relieve malaise and depression in women who use oral contraceptives and in doses of 50 g to 100 mg to alleviate symptoms of premenstrual syndrome, even though its efficacy has not been proven in controlled, double-blind studies. Vitamin B_6 has been used with some success to relieve nausea and vomiting during pregnancy and after radiation therapy.

Acute toxicity occurs infrequently. Intakes greater than the UL (100 mg) may cause sensory neuropathy, a nerve disorder characterized by pain, numbness, and weakness in the limbs. Damage is not permanent, and symptoms improve gradually when the vitamin is discontinued.

Folate

Folate is the group name for this B vitamin, and folic acid is the form used in vitamin supplements and fortified foods. Natural folate in foods—found in green leafy vegetables, dried peas and beans, seeds, liver, and orange juice—is only half as available to the body as manmade folic acid is.

As part of the coenzymes tetrahydrofolate (THF) and dihydrofolate (DHF), folate's major function is in the synthesis of DNA. Thus folate, with the aid of vitamin B_{12}, is vital for synthesis of new cells and transmission of inherited characteristics.

Because folate is recycled through the intestinal tract (much like the enterohepatic circulation of bile), a healthy gastrointestinal tract is essential to maintain folate balance. When gastrointestinal integrity is impaired, as in malabsorption syndromes, failure to reabsorb folate quickly leads to folate deficiency. Gastrointestinal cells are particularly susceptible to folate deficiency because, as rapidly dividing cells, they depend on folate for new cell synthesis. Without the formation of new cells, gastrointestinal function declines and widespread malabsorption of nutrients occurs.

Folate deficiency is prevalent in all parts of the world. In developing countries, folate deficiency commonly is caused by parasitic infections that alter gastrointestinal integrity. In the United States, alcoholics are at highest risk of folate deficiency because of alcohol's toxic effect on the gastrointestinal tract. Groups at risk because of poor intake include the elderly, fad dieters, and people of low socioeconomic status. Because the growth of new tissue increases folate requirements, infants, adolescents, and pregnant women may have difficulty consuming adequate amounts.

Studies show that adequate intake of folate before conception and during the first trimester of pregnancy can reduce the incidence of neural tube defects (eg, spina bifida) by as much as 50%. This discovery has prompted the U.S. Public Health Service to recommend that all women of childbearing age who are capable of becoming pregnant consume 400 μg of synthetic folic acid from food and/or supplements in addition to folate from a varied diet. To increase folate intake, mandatory folic acid fortification of enriched bread and grain products began on January 1, 1998. However, this policy alone does not ensure adequate folate intake among women of childbearing age; supplements and wise food choices continue to be important.

The UL for folic acid is 1000 μg/day. Consistently high intakes of folate can mask vitamin B_{12} deficiency, which can cause permanent neurologic damage if left untreated. Large doses may interfere with anticonvulsant therapy and precipitate convulsions in patients with epilepsy controlled by phenytoin.

Vitamin B_{12}

Vitamin B_{12} (cobalamin) has several interesting features. First, vitamin B_{12} has an interdependent relationship with folate: each vitamin must have the other to be activated. Because it activates folate, vitamin B_{12} is involved in DNA synthesis and maturation of red blood cells. Unlike folate, vitamin B_{12} has important roles in maintaining the myelin sheath around nerves. For this reason, large doses of folate can alleviate the anemia caused by vitamin B_{12} deficiency (a function of both vitamins), but folate cannot halt the progressive neurologic impairments that only vitamin B_{12} can treat. Nervous system damage may be irreversible without early treatment with vitamin B_{12}.

Vitamin B_{12} also holds the distinction of being the only water-soluble vitamin that does not occur naturally in plants. Fermented soy products and algae may be enriched with vitamin B_{12}, but it is in an inactive form. Some ready-to-eat cereals are fortified with vitamin B_{12}. All animal foods contain vitamin B_{12}.

Another unique feature of vitamin B_{12} is that it requires an intrinsic factor, a glycoprotein secreted in the stomach, in order to be absorbed from the terminal ileum. But before it can bind with the intrinsic factor, vitamin B_{12} must first be separated from the small peptides to which it is bound in food sources. This is accomplished by pepsin and gastric acid.

Vitamin B_{12} deficiency symptoms may take 5 to 10 years or longer to develop, because the liver can store relatively large amounts of B_{12} and the body recycles B_{12} by reabsorbing it.

Dietary deficiencies of vitamin B_{12} are rare and are likely to occur only in strict vegans who consume no animal products and do not adequately supplement their diet. A more frequent cause of deficiency is the lack of intrinsic factor, which prevents absorption of vitamin B_{12} regardless of intake; this condition is known as pernicious anemia. People with pernicious anemia, which can occur secondary to gastric surgery or gastric cancer, require parenteral injections of vitamin B_{12}. Most commonly, B_{12} deficiency arises from inadequate gastric acid secretion, which prevents protein-bound vitamin B_{12} in foods from being freed. As many as 10% to 30% of adults older than 51 years of age may have this type of vitamin B_{12} deficiency as a result of gastric resection, atrophic gastritis, use of medications that suppress gastric acid secretion, or gastric infection with *Helicobacter pylori*. Because people with protein-bound vitamin B_{12} deficiency are able to absorb synthetic (free) vitamin B_{12}, the National Academy of Sciences Institute of Medicine recommends that people in this age group obtain most of their requirement from fortified foods or supplements.

Pantothenic Acid

Pantothenic acid is part of CoA, the coenzyme involved in the formation of acetyl-CoA and in the TCA cycle. Pantothenic acid participates in more than 100 different metabolic reactions. It is widespread in the diet. The best sources of pantothenic acid are meat, fish, poultry, whole-grain cereals, and dried peas and beans.

Pantothenic acid has an established AI of 5 mg for nonpregnant adults. The estimated usual adult daily intake of pantothenic acid is 5 to 10 mg. No cases of pantothenic acid deficiency from natural causes have been reported.

Biotin

As a coenzyme, biotin is involved in the TCA cycle, gluconeogenesis, fatty acid synthesis, and chemical reactions that add or remove carbon dioxide from other compounds.

Biotin is widely distributed in nature and is most abundant in eggs, liver, yeast breads, and cereals. Gastrointestinal flora synthesize significant amounts of biotin, but it is not known how much is available for absorption.

Biotin has an AI of 30 μg/day for nonpregnant adults. It is assumed that the average American diet provides adequate amounts of biotin to meet the needs of most healthy adults.

Biotin deficiency symptoms have been induced in humans only by adding the equivalent of 24 raw egg whites to a biotin-deficient diet. Avidin, a chemical in raw egg white, prevents the absorption of biotin from the intestinal tract and leads to a dry, scaly dermatitis and other deficiency symptoms.

Vitamin C

Vitamin C (ascorbic acid), which is found in citrus fruits and juices, peppers, broccoli, kiwifruit, greens, strawberries, and tomatoes, may be the most famous vitamin. Its long history dates back to more than 250 years ago, when it was determined that something in citrus fruits prevents scurvy, a disease that killed as many as two thirds of sailors on long journeys. Years later, British sailors acquired the nickname "Limeys" because of Great Britain's policy to prevent scurvy by providing limes to all navy men. It wasn't until 1928 that the antiscurvy agent was identified as vitamin C. Since then, vitamin C has been touted as a cure for a variety of ills, including cancer, colds, and infertility.

Vitamin C prevents scurvy by promoting the formation of collagen, the most abundant protein in fibrous tissues such as connective tissue, cartilage, bone matrix, tooth dentin, skin, and tendon. Without adequate vitamin C, the integrity of collagen is compromised; muscles degenerate, weakened bones break, wounds fail to heal, teeth are lost, and infection occurs. Hemorrhaging begins as pinpoints under the skin and progresses to massive internal bleeding and death. Even though scurvy is deadly, it can be cured within a matter of days with moderate doses of vitamin C.

Vitamin C also acts as an antioxidant to protect vitamin A, vitamin E, PUFA, and iron from destruction. As an antioxidant, vitamin C is being studied for its ability to prevent heart disease, certain cancers, and cataracts. It is involved in many metabolic reactions, including the promotion of iron absorption, the formation of some neurotransmitters, the synthesis of thyroxine, the metabolism of some amino acids, and normal immune system functioning.

There is a lack of consensus on how much vitamin C is needed for optimal health. RDAs for vitamin C differ widely among nations, ranging from 20 mg for women in Canada to 100 mg in Japan. The need for vitamin C increases in response to fever, chronic illness, infection, wound healing, and smoking. The new RDA for vitamin C represents an increase from the previous recommendation. The new RDA is set at 90 mg/d for adult men and 75 mg/d for adult women. Cigarette smokers should increase their intake by 35 mg/d. An upper limit (UL) is set at 2 g/d. Intakes higher than this may cause osmotic diarrhea and gastrointestinal disturbances.

There is no clear and convincing evidence that large doses of vitamin C prevent colds, although some studies suggest that it may lessen the severity of cold symptoms because vitamin C reduces blood histamine levels. Its role in normal immune system functioning may also be involved. Epidemiologic studies have shown an association between increased dietary or tissue levels of vitamin C and a reduced incidence of cancer, but most of those studies looked at vitamin C intake from food, not supplements.

Vitamins in Health Promotion: Vitamin Supplements

Headlines and research findings fuel strong consumer interest in supplements. Intrigued by the prospect of defying aging and avoiding disease without the effort of changing their eating and exercise behaviors, Americans swallow supplements with abandon. They rationalize that supplements make up for "bad" food choices. They are spurred on by the misplaced philosophy that "if a little is good, a lot is better." It is no wonder that the dietary supplement industry is a $6 billion a year business. But can vitamin supplements prevent chronic disease? Do they provide insurance against bad food choices? Who really needs them? What should one look for when buying supplements?

CAN VITAMIN SUPPLEMENTS PREVENT CHRONIC DISEASE?

Without doubt, vitamin supplements can prevent *deficiency* diseases (eg, scurvy, beriberi) that occur when vitamin intake is inadequate. But can certain vitamins in amounts greater than the RDA help prevent *chronic* diseases? That is the area of current of vitamin research.

Researchers continue to find a strong association between increased fruit and vegetable intake and decreased risk of chronic diseases such as cancer, heart disease, and stroke.

Convincing evidence is emerging about the protective role of fruits and vegetables in reducing the incidence of cataracts, diverticulosis, hypertension, and chronic obstructive pulmonary disease. Fruits and vegetables are also shown to be important in weight management and diabetes control. But that does not specifically mean that the credit goes to vitamins. Nor does it mean that vitamin supplements can potentiate or even duplicate the benefits from eating fruits and vegetables. The most important point to note is that in most cases health benefits are seen from whole foods, not from supplements.

Clients who are tempted to use vitamin supplements to prevent chronic disease should be advised that:

- **Proof is hard to come by.** Observational studies, such as those that detect an association between lower cancer rates and diets rich in fruits and vegetables, do not *prove* anything. To prove cause-and-effect (eg, that vitamin C prevents cancer), all types of research must be considered—clinical, pathologic, animal, experimental, epidemiologic, and, when available, randomized, double-blind, placebo-controlled clinical intervention trials. As of yet there is not conclusive evidence to prove that supplements prevent chronic disease. In fact, several well-designed clinical trials have shown that the beneficial effects associated with high intakes of fruits and vegetables may not be replicated by the use of supplements of individual nutrients such as vitamin E, C, or beta-carotene.
- **The responsible substances are not even known.** Perhaps the antioxidant vitamins do help prevent cancer, but maybe that is only true when they are consumed with other food components. But which ones? And how much of each substance is optimal? People eat food, not nutrients, and food provides a variety of nutrients and compounds, not single active ingredients.
- **Abnormally high intakes of one or more vitamins may adversely affect other vitamins.** For instance, high doses of vitamin E interfere with the function of vitamin K, and excess folic acid can mask vitamin B_{12} deficiency. In contrast, it is almost impossible to overdose on vitamins from foods.
- **Potential long-term risks are unknown.** Controlled studies testing supplement use in humans have been of relatively short duration. They have not lasted long enough (eg, years) to indicate whether there are any risks from high doses of multiple or single vitamins taken for a prolonged period.

CAN VITAMIN SUPPLEMENTS PROVIDE INSURANCE AGAINST LESS-THAN-OPTIMAL FOOD CHOICES?

The answer to that question is both yes and no. For instance, someone who cannot tolerate citrus juices because of gastric reflux may not consistently obtain adequate vitamin C without the use of a vitamin supplement. But vitamin C supplements or multivitamins are not nutritionally equivalent to citrus juices.

Leading health and nutrition authorities agree that the best way to get nutrients is through food, not supplements. Although vitamin supplements may provide a sense of security against bad food choices, they are extremely limited in what they offer: vitamins, maybe some minerals, perhaps some non-nutrients such as lecithin, and probably other incidental ingredients such as starch, sugar, and coloring. They hardly compare to the array of vitamins, minerals, and fibers found in foods. And perhaps the biggest shortcoming of vitamin supplements used in place of fruits and vegetables is that they lack the hundreds to thousands of phytochemicals, naturally occurring chemicals produced by plants to protect themselves against viruses, bacteria, and fungi. For instance, it is estimated that tomatoes have 10,000 phytochemicals, but vitamin pills have none.

At this time, researchers are not able to create a perfect pill to substitute for a varied diet rich in plants. We simply do not know what all of the components in plant foods are, how they function, which ones are beneficial, which ones are potentially harmful, and the ideal combination and concentration of these chemicals. More than likely it is the total package of nutrients, fiber, and phytochemicals that makes fruits and vegetables so healthy. Until science catches up to nature, the best advice is to eat a diet rich in plants. And variety is important, because different plants supply different types and amounts of nutrients and phytochemicals.

WHEN ARE SUPPLEMENTS A GOOD IDEA?

Supplement use is most common among people with higher personal incomes, people with more education, nonsmokers, and people who are not heavy alcohol users. Studies show that supplement users eat more fruits and vegetables than do people who do not take supplements. In other words, the people who take supplements may not be the people who need them.

In theory, almost all healthy people should be able to obtain all the nutrients they need through food alone. In reality, not everyone eats according to the Food Guide Pyramid. Encourage clients to:

- Eat at least five servings of fruits and vegetables every day. More is even better.
- Choose wholesome, nutrient-dense foods over refined or processed foods. For instance, fortified whole-grain cereal (eg, Total) is more nutritious than refined cereal (eg, puffed wheat), and orange juice is more nutritious than carbonated beverages.
- Concentrate on variety. For instance, people who habitually limit their fruit intake to apples and bananas may not be getting adequate vitamin C.
- Make an effort to preserve the vitamin content of foods during storage and preparation; avoid overcooking vegetables and to microwave them instead of boiling.

In reality, food choices are often less than optimal, especially concerning fruits and vegetables. Only 27% of women and 19% of men report eating 5 or more servings of fruits and vegetables every day. On average, American adults eat 1.5 servings of fruit and 3.5 vegetables daily. The intake of dark green and deep yellow vegetables continues to be low despite recommendations to eat more. These figures suggest that the majority of Americans may be cheating themselves out of important nutrients and benefits. In fact, adult women tend to eat less than the RDA for vitamins E and B_6; men tend to consume inadequate vitamin E.

Although it cannot substitute for a healthy diet, a balanced multivitamin and mineral supplement that provides no more than 100% of the Daily Value (DV) for each vitamin is harmless and provides a basic safeguard. Because vitamins work best together and when they are in balanced proportions, a multivitamin is usually better than single vitamin supplements, which tend to provide doses much greater than the RDA. Remember that pills are not a substitute for healthy food: "supplement" means "add to," not "replace."

In addition to people whose food choices fall short of the ideal, the following groups of clients may benefit from vitamin supplements:

- **The elderly.** Food (and vitamin) intake may be inadequate among the elderly because of income restraints, impaired chewing and swallowing, social isolation, physical limitations that make shopping or cooking difficult, or a decreased sense of taste leading to poor appetite. Their vitamin requirements may be elevated as a result of chronic disease or as a side effect of certain medications. The ability to synthesize vitamin D decreases with aging, as does the ability to absorb vitamin B_{12}. Studies show that multivitamin and mineral supplements may improve immune function in the elderly.
- **People on very-low-calorie diets and finicky eaters.** It is difficult to meet vitamin requirements when calorie intake is below 1200 per day. Also, people who eliminate one or more food groups from their diets, such as strict vegans and people with food intolerances or allergies, may not obtain adequate levels of vitamins.
- **Smokers.** Smokers need more vitamin C than nonsmokers, but they can easily meet their requirement by choosing foods high in vitamin C. The need for supplements depends on their actual food choices.
- **People with certain clinical conditions and those who use certain medications.** Therapeutic vitamin supplements are used to treat or prevent deficiencies related to clinical conditions that increase vitamin requirements (eg, vitamin C for thermal injuries), impair vitamin intake (eg, anorexia secondary to cancer treatment), impair vitamin absorption (eg, vitamin B_{12} malabsorption related to pernicious anemia secondary to gastric resection), or increase vitamin excretion (eg, fat malabsorption syndromes). Medications may alter vitamin absorption, metabolism, or excretion.
- **Alcoholics.** Alcohol alters vitamin intake, absorption, metabolism, and excretion. The nutrients most profoundly affected are thiamine, riboflavin, niacin, folic acid, and pantothenic acid.
- **Pregnant and lactating women.** Most notably, folic acid supplements taken before conception and in the early weeks of pregnancy help prevent neural tube defects. All women of childbearing age who can become pregnant are advised to consume synthetic folic acid through fortified foods or supplements. During pregnancy, prenatal vitamins are routinely prescribed as a safeguard against a less-than-optimal diet.

SUPPLEMENTS: BUYING BASICS

Seventy percent of Americans use vitamin and mineral supplements at least occasionally. The FDA now requires a standardized **Supplement Facts label** on all supplements manufactured after March 23, 1999. Like the Nutrition Facts label, the new supplement label is intended to provide consumers with better information. Labels must divulge serving sizes, calories per serving (if any), and a complete ingredient list. Vitamins with established DVs must appear at the top of the panel. Ingredients that have not been proven to be important in health (eg, inositol, garlic, bioflavonoids) must appear at the bottom of the panel and must be separated from the established nutrients by a solid line. The amount of each ingredient and the Percent Daily Value (%DV) must be listed. For ingredients that do not have a DV, an asterisk must be used to indicate that there is no official government recommendation for that substance.

Clients who need or want a vitamin supplement should be advised about the following points.

Composition

For most people, the best bet for an all-purpose, safeguard-type supplement is one that provides no more than 100% of the DV for the 12 vitamins and 8 minerals for which there are established DVs. Clients who opt for megavitamins should be aware that, with few exceptions, manufacturers are free to add or leave out whatever nutrients they choose. What they put in is often based on economics, not health. For instance, because biotin is expensive, only small amounts, if any, are found in supplements. Conversely, most of the other B vitamins are cheap, so they are often used abundantly. The buyer should be aware that:

- The nutrient content on some brands is listed as a "serving," but two or three "servings" may be needed daily.
- Taking more than 100% of the DV for vitamins such as thiamine, riboflavin, and niacin is usually not harmful, but it does not offer any advantage.
- Taking more than 100% of the DV for vitamins A, D, and B_6 is potentially harmful.
- Most people get more than the RDA for vitamin C from foods.
- Deficiencies of biotin and pantothenic acid almost never occur.
- Studies on vitamin E and its role in reducing the risk of heart disease have used doses of 100 to 400 IU or more daily—more than the amount in any diet or multivitamin. To get that much, separate supplements are needed.
- Because studies on beta-carotene supplements have failed to show health benefits, and some have shown increased health risks, it is best to get beta-carotene from fruits and vegetables, not supplements.
- Ingredients such as bee pollen, silica, and yarrow flowers add to the price but not the nutritional value.

Natural is Not Naturally Better

Marketing tactics that promote vitamins as "natural" and "organic" are open to interpretation. In this situation, "natural" often means synthetic mixed with plant extracts. Sometimes synthetic is even better than natural. For instance, synthetic folic acid is much better absorbed than natural folate in foods.

Cost is Not Necessarily an Indication of Quality

Vitamin supplements do not necessarily follow the dictum, "You get what you pay for." Because large retail chains are high-volume customers, they can demand and get their own top-quality private-label brand supplements from vitamin manufacturers. The cost of these supplements is usually significantly less than that of brand-name varieties, yet the quality and content are similar.

Quality Indicators

The United States Pharmacopeia (USP) has established strict quality standards for vitamins and minerals to enable consumers to identify products whose quality can be trusted. The designation *USP* on the label means that the product passes tests for several parameters:

- **Disintegration.** If a tablet does not break down into small pieces, it may not be able to dissolve. Such tablets may pass through the body without any of their ingredients being absorbed.
- **Dissolution.** This is the next step after disintegration. Ingredients in tablets that do not dissolve are not digested.
- **Strength.** To get the USP stamp, the amount of ingredients present must be within a limited range of the amount declared on the label.
- **Purity.** USP standards set a range for acceptable impurities resulting from contamination or degradation of the product due to processing or storage.
- **Expiration date.** Beyond this date, the ingredients may no longer meet USP standards of purity, strength, and/or quality.

Questions You May Hear

What is the difference between the terms "enriched" and "fortified"? *Enriched* foods have nutrients added back that were lost during processing. For instance, white flour is enriched with B vitamins that are lost when the bran and germ layers are removed from the endosperm portion of wheat. The term *fortified* means that nutrients have been added that are not naturally found in the food. For instance, milk is fortified with vitamin D, and some breakfast cereals are fortified with vitamin B_{12}.

How can I eat more fruits and vegetables? Make gradual changes in the way you eat. Strategies that may help are to:

- Start at least one meal each day with a fresh salad.
- Eat raw vegetables or fresh fruits for snacks.
- Add vegetables to other foods, such as zucchini to spaghetti sauce, grated carrots to meat loaf, or spinach to lasagna.
- Double your normal portion size.
- Buy a new fruit or vegetable when you go grocery shopping.
- Eat occasional meatless entrees, such as pasta primavera, vegetable stir fry, or black beans and rice.
- Order a vegetable when you eat out.
- Choose 100% fruit juice instead of drinks, cocktails, ades, and/or carbonated beverages.
- Eat fruit for dessert.
- Make fruits and vegetables more visible. Leave a bowl of fruit on the center of your table. Keep fresh vegetables on the top shelf of the refrigerator in plain view.

What food preparation techniques can I use to minimize the loss of vitamins from food? When you prepare vegetables:

- Use fresh or frozen vegetables instead of canned ones. Canned vegetables have lower levels of vitamins and added sodium.
- Cook in a small amount of water (or no water) and for the shortest period possible. Steamed or microwaved vegetables retain more vitamins than boiled ones do.
- Do not add baking soda during cooking.
- Save the cooking water and use it as a base for soups, gravies, or sauces.

Is it better to take vitamin supplements with meals or between meals? In general it is better to take supplements with meals, because the absorption of some vitamins is enhanced by food.

Should I choose vitamin-fortified foods over those that are not fortified? For the most part, fortified foods are a good bet. Fortified milk and fortified cereals provide nutrients (vitamin D and iron, respectively) that otherwise may not be consumed in adequate amounts by some people. On the other hand, a vitamin-fortified candy bar is still a candy bar. Be aware of slick marketing techniques that might lead you to believe that junk food with vitamins is healthy.

I am under a lot of emotional stress. Should I take stress vitamins? Although significant physical stress (eg, thermal injury, trauma) increases the requirements for certain vitamins, mental stress does not. Misleading advertising is to blame for this widespread misconception.

Are claims on food packages regarding vitamin content valid and reliable? Yes. Guidelines for nutrient claims are clearly defined. Compared with a standard serving size of the traditional food:

- A food claimed to be *High in*, *Rich in*, or an *Excellent source of* a nutrient must supply at least 20% of the DV for that particular nutrient in each serving.

- A food whose label indicates that it is a *Good source of*, *Contains*, or *Provides* a nutrient must supply 10% to 19% of the DV per serving.
- A food labeled as having *More*, being *Enriched with* or *Fortified with*, or containing an *Added* nutrient must provide 10% or more of the DV for that nutrient per serving.

KEY CONCEPTS

- Vitamins are organic compounds that are soluble in either water or fat; their solubility determines how they are absorbed, transported through the blood, stored, and excreted.
- Vitamins do not provide energy (calories) but are needed for the metabolism of energy. Most vitamins function as coenzymes to activate enzymes.
- Vitamins are needed by the body in small amounts (microgram or milligram quantities). They are essential in the diet because they cannot be made by the body or are synthesized in inadequate amounts.
- Fortification and enrichment have virtually eliminated vitamin deficiencies in healthy Americans. It is assumed that if a variety of foods and the recommended number of servings from each of the Food Guide Pyramid food groups are chosen, the vitamin content of the diet will be adequate.
- Vitamins A, D, E, and K are the fat-soluble vitamins. Because they are stored in liver and adipose tissue, they do not need to be consumed daily. Vitamins A and D are toxic when consumed in large quantities over a long period.
- The B-complex vitamins and vitamin C are water-soluble vitamins. Although some tissues are able to hold limited amounts of certain water-soluble vitamins, they are not generally stored in the body, so a daily intake is necessary. Because they are not stored, they are considered nontoxic; however, adverse side effects can occur from taking megadoses of certain water-soluble vitamins over a prolonged period.
- Although diets rich in fruits and vegetables appear to be protective against chronic diseases such as heart disease, cancer, and hypertension, it is not known what components in them are responsible for the health benefits. Antioxidant vitamins in foods are suspected of being beneficial, but high-dose supplements have not been proven to prevent disease and may disrupt nutrient balances. Long-term safety has not been established; some reports indicate that single-nutrient supplements may actually increase, not decrease, health risks.
- In theory, most healthy people can obtain all the vitamins they need through food. Vitamin intake is maximized by eating at least five servings of fruits and vegetables daily; choosing wholesome, nutrient-dense foods; focusing on variety; and using preparation techniques that minimize vitamin loss.
- Multivitamin supplements provide a limited safeguard when food choices are less than optimal. Other groups who may benefit from taking a daily multivitamin are the elderly, fad dieters, finicky eaters, smokers, alcoholics, and pregnant and lactating women.
- People who choose to take an all-purpose multivitamin should select one that provides 100% of the DV for vitamins with an established DV. The USP stamp ensures the quality of vitamin supplements. High-cost supplements are not necessarily superior to lower-cost ones.

ANSWER KEY

1. **FALSE** In theory, healthy people should be able to obtain all the nutrients they need from food alone.
2. **FALSE** Steamed or microwaved vegetables retain more nutrients than boiled vegetables.
3. **FALSE** Adverse side effects can occur from taking large doses of certain water-soluble vitamins over a long period of time.
4. **FALSE** Vitamins do not provide energy (calories); they are necessary for the metabolism of energy.
5. **FALSE** Cost and quality are not necessarily related.
6. **FALSE** "Natural" vitamins are not naturally better.
7. **FALSE** Long-term safety has not been determined, and it is possible that antioxidant supplements may actually increase health risks.
8. **FALSE** Natural folate in foods is only half as available to the body as man-made folic acid.
9. **FALSE** People with inadequate absorption of vitamin B_{12} due to inadequate gastric acid secretion, are able to absorb synthetic (free) Vitamin B_{12} from fortified food and supplements. Only people with pernicious anemia (lack of intrinsic factor) require Vitamin B_{12} parenterally.
10. **FALSE** Physiologic stress increases the requirement of certain vitamins; however, emotional stress does not.

REFERENCES

American Dietetic Association. (1996). Position of the American Dietetic Association: Vitamin and mineral supplementation. *Journal of the American Dietetic Association*, 96, 73–77.

Gershoff, S. (Ed.). (1999). Making a case for more vitamin C. *Tufts University Health and Nutrition Letter*, *17*(4), 3.

Ho, C., Kauwell, G., & Bailey, L. (1999). Practioners' guide to meeting the vitamin B_{12} Recommended Dietary Allowance for people aged 51 years and older. *Journal of the American Dietetic Association*, 99, 725–727.

Hundall, M. (1999). *Vitamins, minerals, and dietary supplements*. Written for the American Dietetic Association. Minneapolis: Chronimed Publishing.

Kloeblen, A. (1999). Folate knowledge, intake from fortified grain products, and periconceptional supplementation patterns of a sample of low-income pregnant women according to the Health Belief Model. *Journal of the American Dietetic Association*, 99, 33–38.

National Academy of Sciences, Institute of Medicine, Produce for a Better Health Foundation. (1999). *Year 2000 dietary guidelines: The case for fruits and vegetables first. A scientific overview for the health professional*. Wilmington, DE: Produce of Better Health Foundation.

Rock, C. (1998). Dietary Reference Intakes, antioxidants, and beta carotene. *Journal of the American Dietetic Association*, 98, 1410–1411.

Rock, C., Jacob, R., & Bowen, P. (1996). Update on the biological characteristics of the antioxidant micronutrients: Vitamin C, vitamin E, and the carotenoids. *Journal of the American Dietetic Association*, 96, 693–702.

Yates, A., Schlicker, S., & Suitor, C. (1998). Dietary Reference Intakes: The new basis for recommendations for calcium and related nutrients, B vitamins, and choline. *Journal of the American Dietetic Association*, 98, 699–706.

National Academy of Sciences, Institute of Medicine. (1997). *Dietary Reference Intakes for calcium, phosphorus, magnesium, vitamin D, and fluoride*. Washington DC: National Academy Press.

CHAPTER 6

Fluids and Minerals

TRUE	FALSE	Check your knowledge of fluids and minerals.
		1 Calcium in supplements is better absorbed when taken with food rather than between meals.
		2 All minerals consumed in excess of need are excreted in the urine.
		3 Sodium is the most plentiful mineral in the body.
		4 High temperatures and prolonged cooking times reduce the mineral content of foods.
		5 Bottled water lacks fluoride, a mineral important for dental health.
		6 The biggest source of sodium in the typical American diet is processed foods.
		7 Macrominerals are more important for health than microminerals.
		8 For most people, thirst is a reliable indicator of fluid needs.
		9 All Americans are urged to limit their sodium intake to the amount contained in about 1 tablespoon of salt.
		10 A chronically low intake of calcium leads to hypocalcemia.

Upon completion of this chapter, you will be able to

- Name sources of fluids.
- Discuss fluid requirements.
- Explain mechanisms by which the body maintains mineral homeostasis.
- Describe general functions of minerals.
- Identify minerals provided in each Food Guide Pyramid food group.
- Discuss why some people need supplements of calcium and iron.

Keys to Understanding Fluid

Life as we know it does not exist without water. It is the most abundant compound in the body, accounting for one half to four fifths of total body weight. It is the medium in which all biochemical reactions take place. Although most people can survive 6 weeks or longer without food, death occurs in approximately 1 week without water.

FUNCTIONS OF WATER

Water occupies essentially every space within and between body cells and is involved in virtually every body function. It:

- **Provides shape and structure to cells.** Approximately two thirds of the body's 10 to 12 gallons of water is located within cells (intracellular fluid). Muscle cells have a higher concentration of water (73%) than fat, which is only about 25% water. Men generally have more muscle mass than women and therefore have a higher percentage of body water.
- **Regulates body temperature.** Because water absorbs heat slowly, the large amount of water contained in the body helps maintain body temperature homeostasis despite fluctuations in environmental temperatures. Evaporation of water (sweat) from the skin cools the body.
- **Aids in the digestion and absorption of nutrients.** Approximately 7 to 9 L of water is secreted in the gastrointestinal tract daily to aid in digestion and absorption. Except for the approximately 100 mL of water excreted through the feces, all of the water contained in the gastrointestinal secretions (saliva, gastric secretions, bile, pancreatic secretions, and intestinal mucosal secretions) is reabsorbed in the ileum and colon.
- **Transports nutrients and oxygen to cells.** By moistening the air sacs in the lungs, water allows oxygen to dissolve and move into blood for distribution throughout the body. Approximately 92% of blood plasma is water.
- **Serves as a solvent for vitamins, minerals, glucose, and amino acids.** The solvating property of water is vital for health and survival.
- **Participates in chemical reactions.** For instance, water is used in the synthesis of hormones and enzymes.
- **Eliminates waste products.** Water helps excrete body wastes through urine, feces, and expirations.
- **Is a major component of mucus and other lubricating fluids.** As such, it reduces friction in joints, where bones, ligaments, and tendons come in contact with each other, and it cushions contacts between internal organs that slide over one another.

WATER REQUIREMENT

Water is an essential nutrient because the body cannot produce as much water as it needs. To maintain water balance, intake should approximate output. On average, adults lose approximately 1450 to 2800 mL of water daily from *insensible* (unmeasurable) and *sensible* (measurable) means. Insensible water losses from the skin and expirations account for approximately half of the total water lost daily. Sensible water losses from urine and feces make up the remaining water loss.

Source of Water Loss	Average Amount Lost (mL/d)
Perspiration	450 to 900
Exhalations	350
Urine	500 to 1400
Feces	150
Total	1450 to 2800

Another way to calculate the water requirement is to allow 1 to 1.5 mL of water per calorie consumed. For instance, someone consuming 2000 calories daily needs 2000 to 3000 mL of fluid.

Actual water requirement is highly variable. Extreme environmental temperatures (very hot or very cold), high altitude, low humidity, and strenuous exercise increase insensible losses. Water evaporation from the skin is also increased by prolonged exposure to heated or recirculated air, such as during long airplane flights. Vomiting, diarrhea, and fever increase water losses. Water requirements increase during pregnancy and lactation. People who eat a high-fiber diet need to consume more water because fiber works by absorbing water in the gastrointestinal tract. Certain other clinical conditions are characterized by high water losses, including thermal injuries, fistulas, uncontrolled diabetes, hemorrhage, and certain renal disorders. The use of drainage tubes contributes to increased water losses.

Among healthy adults, thirst is usually a reliable indicator of water need. However, thirst is blunted in the elderly, in children, and during hot weather or strenuous exercise. For these people and conditions, drinking fluids should not be delayed until the sensation of thirst occurs, because by then fluid loss is significant. Because the body cannot store water, it should be consumed throughout the day.

Dehydration

Dehydration may be acute, such as from a strenuous workout, or chronic, as occurs when daily water intake is below requirements for a prolonged period. Both types of dehydration are defined as a loss of 1% or more of body weight due to water loss. For a 150-pound person, 1% of weight translates to a mere 1.5 pounds. Because 480 mL (2 cups) of fluid weighs 1 pound, a 1.5-pound water loss means a water deficit of 720 mL (3 cups).

Early signs of dehydration include headache, fatigue, loss of appetite, flushed skin, heat intolerance, lightheadedness, dry mouth and eyes, and dark, scanty urine. The effects are progressive and cumulative over time. Dehydration leads to delirium and death when water loss exceeds 10% of body weight.

Fluid Overload

Normally, fluid consumed in excess of need is excreted through the urine. Fluid overload from excessive fluid intake is rarely seen in healthy adults. Fluid overload is most likely to occur as a result of impaired fluid output or abnormal sodium retention, such as in renal failure, congestive heart failure, corticosteroid therapy, and cirrhosis.

SOURCES OF WATER

Drinking water is obviously the best source of water, but it is not Americans' favorite drink. Other liquids, such as milk, juice, carbonated beverages, coffee, and tea, provide more fluid in the typical American diet than plain water does. Only liquids are considered as sources of water available to meet the body's need, although solid foods and metabolic water also contribute to total fluid intake. The water provided by solid foods and metabolic processes usually is not factored in when water intake is calculated, because it is difficult to accurately estimate the amounts they provide.

Solid foods range from 0% water by weight in vegetable oil to 95% in lettuce. Although few people would be surprised to learn that watermelon is 92% water by weight, many may be amazed by the percentages in other foods: broccoli, 91%; carrot, 87%; chicken, 65%; and whole wheat bread, 38%. It is estimated that solid foods supply 700 to 1000 mL of water daily in an average diet.

Metabolism is the other, less obvious source of water. Approximately 240 mL of water is produced daily as an end product of carbohydrate, protein, and fat metabolism.

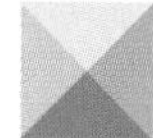

Fluid in Health Promotion

PROMOTING ADEQUATE FLUID INTAKE

Little information is available on how much fluid adults usually consume, and the adequacy of fluid intake may be overlooked in routine health assessments. Some experts believe that intake typically is less than required, placing a significant portion of the population at risk for chronic mild dehydration. Possible adverse effects associated with chronic mild dehydration and inadequate fluid intake include reduced physical performance, increased risk of kidney stones in susceptible people, and increased risk of cancers of the urinary tract, colon, and breast. Total fluid and water intake should always be part of the diet record.

Water is the best fluid for several reasons. It is as close as the nearest tap and relatively inexpensive or free. It quenches thirst better than all other liquids and contains no caffeine, calories, fat, or cholesterol. Honorable mention goes to low-fat milk and 100% juice, which supply essential nutrients. Carbonated beverages provide fluid, but their concentrated sugar content delivers empty calories. Caffeinated beverages and alcohol promote fluid loss through increased urination and are not good choices for satisfying fluid requirements.

Tips to encourage adequate fluid intake are listed in Box 6–1.

BOX 6.1

Tips to Encourage Adequate Fluid Intake

Drink before you become thirsty. People who are thirsty need to drink to satisfy thirst plus a little extra.

Choose liquids with appealing taste. Clients who dislike their tap water should be urged to consider buying a water filter or bottled water. Refrigeration usually improves the taste of tap water.

Keep a water bottle at your desk. Iced water in a sports bottle enables "sippers" to drink at their leisure.

Make water part of your meals. Served with a meal, water does not seem like a troublesome extra that requires thought and planning.

Drink a glass of water before each meal, especially if weight control is a concern. Water can blunt appetite and help people eat less. Weight management programs often urge participants to drink adequate water as a means to control appetite.

Buy bottled water in place of carbonated beverages. It is better on the teeth, better at quenching thirst, and doesn't provide empty calories.

Pack bottled water in your lunch. This tactic eliminates the need to patronize the soda machine.

Drink enough low-fat milk. Fluid, calcium, vitamin D, and protein are provided in one package.

Try sparkling water with a wedge of lemon or lime, for a little variety. Seltzer is pure, calorie free, and loaded with bubbles.

Eat enough fruits and vegetables. Fruits and vegetables are generally high in water, even though the water they provide is usually not counted when fluid intake is calculated. Six ounces of 100% fruit juice counts as a serving from the Fruit group.

Drink extra fluids before, during, and after exercise, especially in hot weather. General guidelines are to drink:

- A least 16 oz of beverages up to 2 h before a competitive event
- 4–8 oz or more of waer or sports drink 5–10 min before your workout or competition
- 8–10 oz every 15–20 minutes during strenuous exercise

Try using herbal tea, decaffeinated tea, or decaffeinated coffee in place of some or all caffeinated beverages.

THE BOTTLED WATER BOOM

Bottled water is the fastest-growing segment of the beverage industry. It offers an alternative to people who are tired of carbonated beverages or dislike the taste of tap water. It is encroaching on places once reserved only for carbonated beverages, such as fast food restaurants, street vendors, and vending machines. About 700 brand labels of bottled water are currently sold in the United States.

The U.S. Food and Drug Administration regulates bottled water to ensure its safety, quality, and accurate labeling. The following terms are legally defined:

- **Artesian water** is water that comes from a confined aquifer (rock formation containing water) in which the water level stands above the natural water table.
- **Mineral water** contains no less than 250 ppm of total dissolved, naturally occurring (not added) solids, or minerals. Mineral water is required to be labeled "low mineral content" if the content is less than 500 ppm or "high mineral content" if it is more than 1500 ppm.
- **Purified water** has been processed to remove minerals (demineralized). Minerals may be removed by deionization, reverse osmosis, or other processes. *Distilled water* is a type of purified water in which water is evaporated to steam and then recondensed to remove minerals.
- **Sparkling water** is water that contains carbon dioxide gas either naturally ("natural sparkling water") or added at levels not to exceed those of natural sparkling water. Soda water, tonic water, and club soda are carbonated soft drinks, not sparkling water.
- **Spring water** is water from a natural spring in the ground; it may or may not be carbonated.

But is bottled water better than tap water? Both are safe, and both have advantages. Bottled water:

- Is usually chlorine free, so the taste is more appealing to some people
- Is lead-free, unlike tap water in some areas. Lead can accumulate in the body, damaging the brain, nervous system, kidneys, and red blood cells. Unborn babies, infants, and children are especially vulnerable to lead poisoning.
- Is fashionable to drink, an "in" thing to do
- Is easily packed and carried in lunches, cars, picnics, and family outings

In contrast, tap water:

- Is conveniently available in an unlimited supply right in your home; there is no need to go out to buy it
- Is treated with chlorine to keep away the threat of cholera, hepatitis, and other diseases
- May be a source of minerals, such as fluoride, calcium, sodium, iron, and magnesium. The actual mineral content varies with the water source and how it is processed. The American Dental Association recommends that water that is low in fluoride be fluoridated to 1 ppm because adding fluoride to water is safe, economical, and practical and offers effective protection against dental caries.

In the end, the decision to use bottled water instead of tap water is a personal choice that is usually based on taste. If nonfluoridated bottled water is used by children, a fluoride supplement may be prescribed by the dentist to help strengthen and protect teeth from decay.

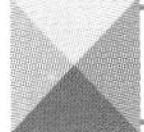

Keys to Understanding Minerals

Although minerals account for only about 4% of the body's total weight, they are found in all body fluids and tissues. **Macrominerals,** also known as *major minerals*, are present in the body in amounts greater than 5 g (the equivalent of 1 teaspoon) and are needed in relatively large quantities (>100 g). Calcium, phosphorus, and magnesium are macrominerals. **Microminerals,** also known as *trace minerals* or *trace elements*, are present in the body in amounts less than 5 g and are needed in very small amounts (≤15 mg/day). Microminerals include iron, iodine, zinc, selenium, copper, manganese, fluoride, chromium, and molybdenum. Both groups are essential for life. As many as 30 other, potentially harmful minerals are present in the body, such as lead, gold, and mercury. Their presence appears to be related to environmental contamination.

GENERAL CHEMISTRY

Unlike the energy nutrients and vitamins, minerals are *inorganic elements* that originate from the earth's crust, not from plants or animals. Minerals do not undergo digestion, nor are they broken down or rearranged during metabolism. Although they combine with other elements to form salts (eg, sodium chloride) or with organic compounds (eg, iron in hemoglobin), they always retain their chemical identity.

Unlike vitamins, minerals are not destroyed by light, air, heat, or acids during food preparation. In fact, when food is completely burned, minerals are the ash that remains. Minerals are lost only when foods are soaked in water.

GENERAL FUNCTIONS

Minerals function to provide structure to body tissues and to regulate body processes, such as fluid balance, acid-base balance, nerve cell transmission, muscle contraction, and vitamin, enzyme, and hormonal activity:

- **Structure.** Calcium, phosphorus, magnesium, and fluorine provide structure to bones and teeth. Soft tissues gain structural support from phosphorus, potassium, iron, and sulfur. Sulfur is also a fundamental constituent of skin, hair, and nails.
- **Fluid balance.** The volume of water in the body and how it is distributed among body compartments are determined largely by the concentrations of solutes in solution. Fluid balance is influenced by sodium, potassium, chloride, and all the major minerals (calcium, phosphorus, magnesium).
- **Acid-base balance.** This term refers to the maintenance of the body's concentration of hydrogen ions. Sodium hydroxide and sodium bicarbonate are part of the carbonic acid–bicarbonate system that regulates the pH of blood. Phosphorus is involved in buffer systems that regulate the pH of red blood cells and the kidney tubular fluids.

- **Nerve cell transmission and muscle contraction.** The exchange of sodium and potassium across nerve cell membranes causes the transmission of nerve impulses. Calcium stimulates muscles to contract. Sodium, potassium, and magnesium are involved in muscle relaxation. Mineral imbalances interfere with normal muscle functioning.
- **Vitamin, enzyme, and hormone activity.** Minerals help regulate body processes through their role in activation of vitamins, enzymes, and hormones. For instance, cobalt's sole function is as an essential component of vitamin B_{12}. Zinc is a constituent of many enzymes used in energy and nucleic acid metabolism, and manganese is part of an enzyme involved in fat synthesis. Iodine is needed for synthesis of the hormone thyroxine, and chromium is involved in insulin production.

MINERAL BALANCE

The body has several mechanisms by which it maintains mineral balance, depending on the mineral involved. Some minerals can be released from storage and redistributed as needed, which is what happens when calcium is released from bones to restore normal serum calcium levels. The body can also compensate for low or high levels of some minerals by increasing or decreasing the rate of absorption. For example, normally only about 10% of the iron consumed is absorbed, but the rate increases up to 50% when the body is deficient in iron. Another way the body maintains homeostasis is to alter the excretion rate of some minerals. Virtually all of the sodium consumed in the diet is absorbed; the only way the body can rid itself of excess sodium is to increase urinary sodium excretion. For most people, the higher the intake of sodium, the greater the amount of sodium excreted in the urine.

Mineral Toxicities

Minerals that are easily excreted, such as sodium and potassium, do not accumulate to toxic levels in the body under normal circumstances. Minerals that are stored can produce toxicity symptoms when intake is excessive, but excessive intake is not likely to occur from eating a balanced diet. Instead, mineral toxicity is related to excessive use of mineral supplements, environmental or industrial exposure, human errors in commercial food processing, or alterations in metabolism. For instance, more than a dozen Americans developed selenium toxicity after taking an improperly manufactured dietary supplement than contained 27.3 mg of selenium per tablet (500 times the Recommended Dietary Allowance [RDA] of 55 μg/day).

Mineral Interactions

Mineral balance is significantly influenced by hundreds of interactions that occur among minerals and between minerals and other dietary components. For instance, a high intake of zinc impairs copper absorption. Nonheme iron absorption is enhanced by vitamin C and animal protein and inhibited by tannins in tea and phytates in vegetables. Caffeine promotes calcium excretion, whereas vitamin D promotes its absorption. Therefore, mineral status should be viewed as a function of the total diet, not simply from the standpoint of the quantity consumed.

MINERAL REQUIREMENTS

Like the references for vitamin requirements, those for mineral requirements are under revision. Four reference standards are currently being used for minerals:

1. Dietary Reference Intakes (DRIs), in the new system that includes four sets of reference values, have been established for calcium, phosphorus, magnesium, and selenium. DRIs for trace elements will be released over the next few years.
2. The 1989 RDAs are still being used for iron, zinc, and iodine.
3. Estimated Safe and Adequate Daily Intakes, which are intake ranges assumed to be appropriate for healthy people, are set for the remaining trace minerals. Because scientists do not know enough about the roles, interactions, and regulation of these minerals, actual requirements have not been determined.
4. Estimated Minimum Requirements of Healthy Persons have been established for sodium, chloride, and potassium.

SOURCES OF MINERALS

Generally, unrefined or unprocessed foods have more minerals than refined foods. Trace mineral content varies with the content of soil from which the food originates. Within all food groups, processed foods are high in sodium and chloride. Drinking water contains varying amounts of calcium, magnesium, and other minerals; sodium is added to soften water. Fluoride may be a natural or added component of drinking water. Figure 6–1 illustrates minerals within the Food Guide Pyramid food groups.

Bread, Cereal, Rice, and Pasta Group

Enriched and whole-grain breads and cereals provide magnesium and several trace minerals, such as iron, chromium, and manganese. Bran contains potassium. Depending on where they are grown, grains may also be a source of selenium.

Vegetable Group

Vegetables provide iron, potassium, and magnesium. Green leafy vegetables provide calcium, although it is not well absorbed owing to naturally present compounds that bind with calcium, such as oxalic acid.

Fruit Group

Fruits are generally not considered good sources of minerals, except for potassium.

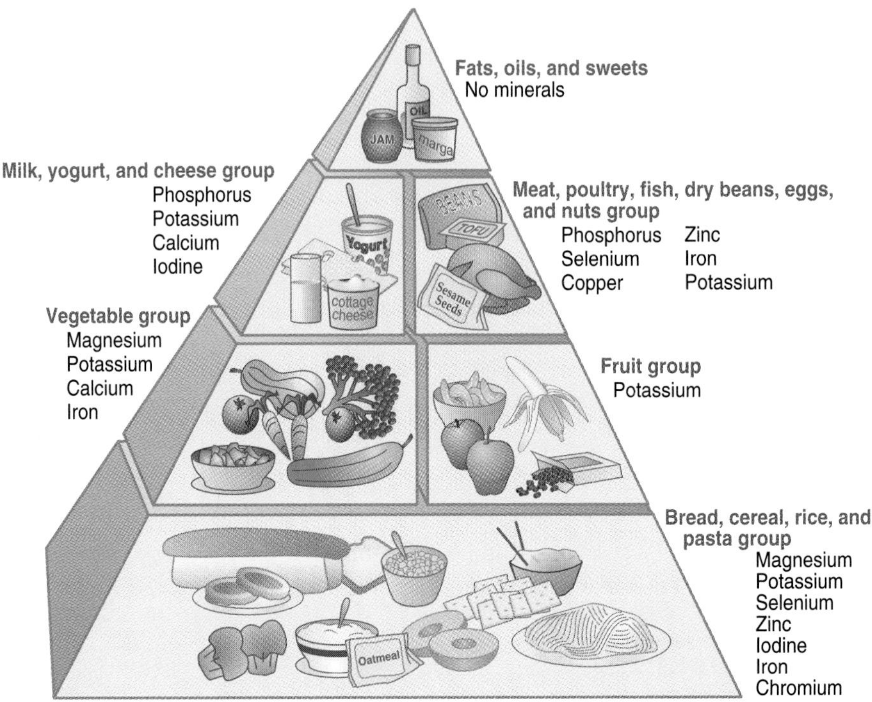

FIGURE 6-1 Minerals within the Food Guide Pyramid groups. Processed foods within every food group provide sodium chloride (salt). The actual mineral content varies by selection within each group.

Milk, Yogurt, and Cheese Group

This group provides potassium and phosphorus and is the richest source of calcium in the diet. People who do not consume milk or yogurt are not likely to obtain adequate calcium from foods alone.

Meat, Poultry, Fish, Dry Beans, Eggs, and Nuts Group

Generally, animal proteins are sources of phosphorus, potassium, sulfur, zinc, and iron. Dried peas and beans provide iron, potassium, and calcium.

Fats, Oils, and Sweets Group

Fats, oils, and sugars contain almost no minerals.

THE ELECTROLYTES

Sodium, chloride, and potassium are major minerals that are also major electrolytes in the body. Their sources, functions, and recommended intakes are summarized in Table 6–1.

TABLE 6.1 *Summary of Major Electrolytes*

Electrolyte and Sources	Functions	Deficiency/Toxicity Signs and Symptoms
Sodium (Na) ***Adult Estimated Minimum Requirement:*** 500 mg • ¼ tsp salt = 500 mg Na • 75% of Na intake is from processed foods: canned soups, meats, vegetables; convenience and restaurant foods; pizza; processed meats	Fluid and electrolyte balance, acid–base balance, maintains muscle irritability, regulates cell membrane permeability and nerve impulse transmission	*Deficiency* Rare except with chronic diarrhea or vomiting and renal disorders; nausea, dizziness, muscle cramps *Toxicity* Excess is normally excreted. Impaired excretion (eg, secondary to renal disorders) causes edema and acute hypertension
Potassium (K) ***Adult Estimated Minimum Requirement:*** 2000 mg • Fruits and vegetables, legumes, whole grains, milk, meats, coffee	Fluid and electrolyte balance, acid–base balance, nerve impulse transmission, catalyst for many metabolic reactions, involved in skeletal and cardiac muscle activity	*Deficiency* Muscular weakness, paralysis, anorexia, confusion (occurs with dehydration) *Toxicity* (from supplements/drugs) Muscular weakness, vomiting
Chloride (Cl) ***Adult Estimated Minimum Requirement:*** 750 mg • ¼ tsp salt = 750 mg Cl • Same sources as sodium	Fluid and electrolyte balance, component of hydrochloric acid in stomach	*Deficiency* Rare; may occur secondary to chronic diarrhea or vomiting and certain renal disorders *Toxicity* Vomiting, hypertension in chloride-sensitive people.

Sodium

As the major extracellular cation, sodium is largely responsible for regulating fluid balance. It also regulates cell permeability and the movement of fluid, electrolytes, glucose, insulin, and amino acids. Sodium is pivotal in acid-base balance, nerve transmission, and muscular irritability.

By weight, 39% of salt (sodium chloride) is sodium. Approximately 75% of the sodium consumed in the typical American diet comes from processed food. Only 10% of total sodium intake is from sodium that occurs naturally in foods, such as sodium from milk and certain vegetables. Salt added during cooking or at the table accounts for the remaining sodium intake.

Almost all of the sodium that is consumed is absorbed. Sodium balance is achieved by eliminating excesses in the urine. For instance, a salty meal causes a transitory increase in serum sodium, which triggers thirst. Drinking fluids dilutes the sodium in the blood to normal concentration, even though the volume of both sodium and fluid are increased. The increased volume stimulates the kidneys to excrete more sodium and fluid together to restore normal blood volume. Conversely, low blood volume or low extracellular sodium stimulates the hormone aldosterone to increase sodium reabsorption by the kidneys. Normally, the amount of sodium consumed equals the amount of sodium excreted.

There is no RDA for sodium. The minimum amount of sodium that is needed by a healthy adult to replace obligatory losses is probably only 115 mg/day. To compensate for wide variations in physical activity and climate, 500 mg/day has been set as the estimated minimum requirement of healthy adults. This amount is roughly the equivalent of ¼ teaspoon of salt. The Daily Value (DV) for sodium used on food labels is 2400 mg. Average sodium intakes from food alone in the United States are more than 4000 mg for men and at most, 3000 mg for women. Wide variations in intake exist, largely related to the amount of processed foods consumed. Sodium deficiencies occur only as a result of prolonged vomiting or diarrhea or from certain renal disorders.

Potassium

Most of the body's potassium is located in the cells as the major cation of the intracellular fluid. The remainder is in the extracellular fluid, where it works to maintain fluid balance, maintain acid-base balance, transmit nerve impulses, catalyze metabolic reactions, aid in carbohydrate metabolism and protein synthesis, and control skeletal muscle contractility.

As with sodium, an excessive intake of potassium does not lead to an increase in serum concentration because of the action of hormones. Aldosterone increases urinary excretion of potassium when serum levels rise. However, the kidneys cannot conserve potassium as efficiently as sodium, and urinary losses may be 200 to 400 mg/day, even when the body is depleted in potassium.

The estimated minimum requirement for potassium for healthy adults is 2000 mg/day. However, some experts recommend intakes of 3500 mg/day because of potassium's protective role against hypertension. Potassium deficiency in healthy people does not occur from inadequate intake but rather from conditions that increase potassium excretion, such as vomiting, diarrhea, certain renal impairments, and certain medications.

Potassium intake varies widely, depending on actual food choices. Diets high in fruits and vegetables may provide as much as 11 g/day. Generally, sodium and potassium content are inversely related: processed foods are low in potassium and high in sodium; fresh, wholesome foods are high in potassium and lower in sodium.

Chloride

Chloride is the major anion in the extracellular fluid, where it helps maintain fluid and electrolyte balance in conjunction with sodium. Chloride is an essential component of hydrochloric acid in the stomach and therefore plays a role in digestion and acid-base balance. Its concentration in most cells is low.

Almost all of the chloride in the diet comes from salt (sodium chloride). One-quarter teaspoon of salt provides 750 mg of chloride, the minimum daily amount recommended for healthy adults. Sodium and chloride share dietary sources, conditions that cause them to become depleted in the body, and signs and symptoms of deficiency.

MAJOR MINERALS

Calcium, phosphorus, magnesium, and sulfur are major minerals. Their sources, functions, and recommended intakes are summarized in Table 6–2.

Calcium

Calcium is the most plentiful mineral in the body; it makes up about half of the body's total mineral content. Almost all of the body's calcium (99%) is found in bones and teeth, where it combines with phosphorus, magnesium, and other minerals to provide rigidity and structure. Bones serve as a large, dynamic reservoir of calcium that readily releases calcium when serum levels drop; this helps maintain blood calcium levels within normal limits when calcium intake is inadequate.

The remaining 1% of calcium in the body is found in plasma and other body fluids, where it has important roles in blood clotting, nerve transmission, muscle contraction and relaxation, cell membrane permeability, and the activation of certain enzymes. Studies suggest that calcium plays a role in the prevention and treatment of hypertension, and a possible protective effect of calcium on the development of colon cancer has also been shown.

Calcium balance—or, more accurately, calcium balance in the blood—is achieved through the action of vitamin D and hormones. When blood calcium levels fall, the parathyroid gland secretes parathormone (PTH), which promotes calcium reabsorption in the kidneys and stimulates the release of calcium from bones. Vitamin D has the same effects on the kidneys and bones, and in addition, it increases the absorption of calcium from the gastrointestinal tract. Together the actions of PTH and vitamin D restore low blood calcium levels to normal, even though bone calcium content may fall. A chronically low calcium intake compromises bone integrity without affecting blood calcium levels. When blood calcium levels are too high, the thyroid gland secretes calcitonin, which promotes the formation of new bone by taking excess calcium from the blood. A high calcium intake does not lead to hypercalcemia but rather maximizes bone density.

Abnormal blood concentrations of calcium occur from alterations in the secretion of PTH. Inadequate PTH secretion (hypoparathyroidism) causes a decrease in calcium mobilization from the bone, an increase in serum phosphorus, decreased urinary excretion of both calcium and phosphorus, and hypocalcemia. Hypocalcemia increases neuromuscular irritability and can lead to tetany (painful, involuntary muscle spasms); tingling, numbness, and cramping in the extremities; bronchospasms; laryngeal spasms; Trousseau's sign (carpopedal spasm that occurs when circulation is occluded in the arm with a blood pressure cuff); and Chvostek's sign (facial muscle spasms that occur when muscles or branches of facial nerves are tapped). Excessive PTH (hyperparathyroidism) causes calcium to leave the bones and enter the bloodstream. The rise in serum calcium causes a corresponding drop in serum phosphorus and a decrease in neuromuscular irritability, which may be evidenced by

TABLE 6.2 ***Summary of Major Minerals***

Mineral and Sources	Functions	Deficiency/Toxicity Signs and Symptoms
Calcium (Ca) ***Adult AI*** 19–50 yr: 1000 mg 51+ yr: 1200 mg ***Adult UL:*** 2.5 g/d • Milk and milk products, fortified orange juice, green leafy vegetables, small fish with bones, legumes	Bone and teeth formation and maintenance, blood clotting, nerve transmission, muscle contraction & relaxation, cell membrane permeability, blood pressure	*Deficiency* Children: impaired growth Adults: osteoporosis *Toxicity* Constipation, increased risk of renal stone formation, impaired absorption of iron and other minerals
Phosphorus (P) ***Adult RDA*** Men and women: 700 mg ***Adult UL:*** To age 70: 4 g/d 70+ yr: 3 g/d • All animal products (meat, poultry, eggs, milk), bread, ready-to-eat cereal	Bone and teeth formation and maintenance, acid–base balance, energy metabolism, cell membrane structure, regulation of hormone and coenzyme activity	*Deficiency* Rare; weakness and bone pain *Toxicity* Low blood calcium
Magnesium (Mg) ***Adult RDA*** Men: 19–30 yr: 400 mg 31+ yr: 420 mg Women: 19–30 yr: 310 mg 31+ yr: 320 mg ***Adult UL:*** 350 mg/d from supplements only (does not include intake from food and water) • Green leafy vegetables, nuts, legumes, whole grains, seafood, chocolate, cocoa	Bone formation, nerve transmission, smooth muscle relaxation, protein synthesis, CHO metabolism, enzyme activity	*Deficiency* Weakness, confusion. Growth failure in children. Severe deficiency: convulsions, hallucinations, tetany *Toxicity* Rare; nausea, vomiting, low blood pressure
Sulfur (S) No recommended intake • All protein foods (meat, poultry, fish, eggs, milk, legumes, nuts)	Component of disulfide bridges in proteins; component of biotin, thiamine, and insulin	*Deficiency* Unknown *Toxicity* In animals, excessive intake of sulfur-containing amino acids impairs growth

apathy, fatigue, depression, paranoia, muscular weakness, nausea, vomiting, constipation, and anorexia. Renal and gastrointestinal complications may develop. The loss of calcium from the bone may cause back and joint pain, pain on weight bearing, pathologic fractures, skeletal deformities, and loss of height.

Many factors influence calcium absorption, which averages about 30% of the total calcium consumed. The percentage of calcium absorbed increases in response to body need, such as during pregnancy, lactation, growth, and recovery from bone fractures. Lactose, the carbohydrate in milk and yogurt, and vitamin D promote calcium absorption. Calcium absorption is impaired by vitamin D deficiency, phytates, and oxalates. Fat malabsorption syndromes cause calcium to precipitate into insoluble calcium soaps, which are excreted in the feces.

An adequate calcium intake early in life helps maximize bone density and strength and therefore offers protection against the inevitable net bone loss that occurs in all people after the age of about 35 years. Daily Adequate Intake (AI) recommendations are set at 1300 mg for adolescents up to 18 years of age, 1000 mg between the ages of 19 and 50 years, and 1200 mg thereafter. Three daily servings of milk, yogurt, or cheese, in addition to nondairy sources of calcium, are needed to ensure an adequate calcium intake. Women older than 12 years of age in almost all racial and ethnic groups consistently fail to consume adequate calcium, often because they forsake milk in an attempt to control calorie intake, even though skim milk provides approximately 300 mg of calcium in a mere 80 cal.

Phosphorus

Phosphorus is the second most abundant mineral (after calcium) in the body. Approximately 85% of the body's phosphorus is combined with calcium in bones and teeth. The rest is distributed in every body cell, where it performs various functions, such as regulating acid-base balance (phosphoric acid and its salts), metabolizing energy (adenosine triphosphate), and providing structure to cell membranes (phospholipids). Phosphorus is an important component of RNA and DNA and is responsible for activating many enzymes and the B vitamins.

Normally about 55% of phosphorus in the adult diet is absorbed. As with calcium, phosphorus absorption is enhanced by vitamin D and regulated by PTH. The major route of phosphorus excretion is in the urine.

Because phosphorus is pervasive in the food supply, dietary deficiencies of phosphorus do not occur. Animal proteins, soft drinks, and food additives are major sources of phosphorus.

Magnesium

There is approximately 1 ounce of magnesium in an adult body. More than half is deposited in bone with calcium and phosphorus; the rest is distributed in various soft tissues, muscles, and body fluids. Magnesium is a cofactor for more than 300 enzymes in the body, including those involved in energy metabolism, protein synthesis, and cell membrane transport.

Median magnesium intake among American adult men is the same as the Estimated Average Requirement (EAR), 330 mg; women consume less than the EAR. Magnesium intake has declined over the past few decades, possibly from the replacement of whole grains with refined grains. Yet, despite chronically low intakes, deficiency symptoms appear only in conjunction with certain diseases, such as alcohol abuse, protein malnutrition, renal impairments, endocrine disorders, and prolonged vomiting or diarrhea.

Net magnesium absorption in a typical diet is approximately 50%. Phytates, oxalates, and fat inhibit magnesium absorption.

Sulfur

Sulfur does not function independently as a nutrient, but it is a component of biotin, thiamine, and the amino acids methionine and cysteine. The proteins in skin, hair, and nails are made more rigid by the presence of sulfur. There is no recommended intake for sulfur, and no deficiency symptoms are known. A sulfur deficiency is likely only when protein deficiency is severe.

TRACE MINERALS

Dietary Sources

The trace mineral content of foods varies with several factors. First, the mineral content of the soil from where the food originates largely influences trace mineral content. For instance, grains, vegetables, and meat raised in South Dakota, Wyoming, New Mexico, and Utah are high in selenium, whereas the selenium content is much lower in foods from the southern states and from both coasts of the United States. The quality of the water supply also influences the trace mineral content of foods, as does food processing. For instance, the amount of manganese, zinc, and copper in refined white flour is less than half of that found in 100% whole wheat flour. Because trace mineral content varies with soil content, water quality, and food processing, the trace mineral content listed in food composition tables may not represent the actual amount in a given sample.

Food composition tables generally include data on iron, zinc, manganese, and copper; data on other trace elements may appear in supplemental lists. Data are not available for all trace minerals.

Bioavailability

Even when trace element intake can be estimated, the amount available to the body may be significantly less because the absorption and metabolism of individual trace elements is strongly influenced by mineral interactions and other dietary factors. An excess of one trace mineral may induce a deficiency of another. For instance, an excess of iron impairs zinc absorption, and calcium impairs iron absorption. A deficiency of one trace mineral may potentiate toxic effects of another, as when iron deficiency increases vulnerability to lead poisoning.

Trace Mineral Assessment

Reliable and valid indicators of trace element status (eg, measured serum levels, results of balance studies, enzyme activity determinations) are not available for all microminerals, so assessment of trace element status is not always possible.

Each trace mineral has its own range of Estimated Safe and Adequate Daily Intake over which the body can maintain homeostasis. The margin of safety is narrow, with toxicity occurring at intakes not much higher than the recommended intake. People who consume an adequate diet derive no further benefit from supplementing their intake with minerals and may induce a deficiency by upsetting the delicate balance that exists between minerals. Routine supplementation is not recommended.

RDAs have been established for the trace minerals iron, zinc, iodine, and selenium. Table 6–3 summarizes the sources, functions, recommended intakes, and signs and symptoms of deficiency and toxicity of these trace minerals. Copper, manganese, fluoride, chromium, and molybdenum have Estimated Safe and Adequate Daily Intake recommendations.

Iron

Approximately two thirds of the body's 3 to 5 g of iron is contained in the heme portion of hemoglobin. Iron is also found in transferrin, the transport carrier of iron, and in enzyme systems that are active in energy metabolism. Ferritin, the storage form of iron, is located in the liver, bone marrow, and spleen.

Iron in foods exists in two forms: *heme iron*, which is the major type of iron found in animal sources (meat, fish, and poultry), and *nonheme iron*, the major form of iron in plants (grains, vegetables, legumes, and nuts). The majority of iron in the diet is nonheme iron.

On average, only about 10% of total iron consumed is absorbed, but the rate is influenced by several factors. For both types of iron, absorption becomes more efficient when the body needs more iron, such as during growth, pregnancy, or iron deficiency. The overall absorption rate may increase to as high as 50% during periods of increased need.

The rate of absorption also differs between the two types of iron. Under normal conditions, 15% to 35% of heme iron is absorbed. This rate is influenced only by body need. Nonheme iron is absorbed at a rate of only 3% to 8% and is greatly influenced by the presence of absorption enhancers and inhibitors. Vitamin C consumed at the same meal, certain animal proteins, alcohol, and gastric acidity make nonheme iron more soluble and thus enhance its absorption. Nonheme iron absorption is inhibited by tea, coffee, bran, phosphates, oxalates, phytates, and alkalinity (eg, antacids).

Because the body maintains iron balance primarily by adjusting the rate of absorption, little or no iron is excreted in the urine. Iron contained in hemoglobin and other body substances is recycled as the cells are replaced. However, a small amount of iron is lost daily through the skin, hair, feces, nails, sweat, and gastrointestinal cells. Additional iron is lost through menstrual bleeding.

To compensate for an average absorption rate of 10% and daily (and monthly) iron losses, the RDA for iron is set at 10 mg for men and postmenopausal women and 15 mg

TABLE 6.3 *Summary of Trace Minerals*

Mineral and Sources	Functions	Deficiency/Toxicity Signs and Symptoms
Iron (Fe) ***Adult RDA*** Men: 10 mg Women (19–50 yr): 15 mg (51+ yr): 10 mg • Beef liver, red meats, clams, tofu, legumes, fortified cereals, bread	Oxygen transport via hemoglobin and myoglobin; constituent of enzyme systems	*Deficiency* Lower immunity, decreased work capacity, weakness, fatigue, itchy skin, pale nailbeds and eye membranes, impaired wound healing, intolerance to cold temperatures *Toxicity* Increased risk of infections, lethargy, joint disease, hair loss, organ damage, enlarged liver, amenorrhea, impotence. Accidental poisoning in children causes death
Zinc (Zn) ***Adult RDA*** Men: 15 mg Women: 12 mg • Meat, poultry, fish, egg yolks, legumes, whole grains, milk	Tissue growth and wound healing, sexual maturation and reproduction; constituent of many enzymes in energy and nucleic acid metabolism; immune function; vitamin A transport, taste perception, associated with insulin	*Deficiency* Abnormal glucose tolerance, growth retardation, impaired wound healing, impaired sense of smell, weight loss, diarrhea, nausea, night blindness, delayed onset of puberty, anorexia, irritability, low sperm count *Toxicity* Anemia, elevated LDL, lowered HDL, diarrhea, vomiting, impaired calcium absorption, fever, renal failure, muscle pain, dizziness, reproductive failure
Iodine ***Adult RDA*** 150 μg • Iodized salt, seafood, bread, dairy products	Component of thyroid hormones that regulate growth, development, and metabolic rate	*Deficiency* Goiter, weight gain, lethargy During pregnancy may cause severe and irreversible mental & physical retardation (cretinism) *Toxicity* Enlarged thyroid gland
Selenium (Se) ***Adult RDA*** Men and women: 55 μg ***Adult UL:*** 400 μg/d • Seafood, liver, kidney, other meats. • Grains grown in selenium-rich soil	Works as an antioxidant with vitamin E	*Deficiency* Heart disease *Toxicity* Nausea, vomiting, abdominal pain, diarrhea, hair and nail changes, nerve damage, fatigue

(continued)

TABLE 6.3 ***Summary of Trace Minerals (continued)***

Mineral and Sources	Functions	Deficiency/Toxicity Signs and Symptoms
Copper (Cu) ***Adult Estimated Safe and Adequate Intake:*** 1.5–3.0 mg • Organ meats, seafood, nuts, seeds	Used in the production of hemoglobin; component of several enzymes; used in energy metabolism	*Deficiency* Rare; anemia, bone abnormalities *Toxicity* Vomiting, diarrhea
Manganese (Mn) ***Adult Estimated Safe and Adequate Intake:*** 2.0–5.0 mg • Widely distributed in foods. Best sources are whole grains, tea, pineapple, kale, strawberries	Component of enzymes involved in fat synthesis, growth, reproduction, and blood clotting	*Deficiency* Rare *Toxicity* Rare; nervous system disorders
Fluoride (Fl) ***Adult AI:*** Men: 3.8 mg Women: 3.1 mg • Fluoridated water, water that naturally contains fluoride, tea	Formation and maintenance of tooth enamel, promotes resistance to dental decay, role in bone formation and integrity	*Deficiency* Susceptibility to dental decay, may increase risk of osteoporosis *Toxicity* Fluorosis (mottling of teeth), nausea, vomiting, diarrhea, chest pain, itching
Chromium (Cr) ***Adult Estimated Safe and Adequate Intake:*** 50–200 µg • Meat, whole grains, nuts, cheese	Cofactor for insulin	*Deficiency* Insulin resistance, impaired glucose tolerance *Toxicity* Dietary toxicity unknown Occupational exposure to chromium dust damages skin and kidneys
Molybdenum (Mo) ***Adult Estimated Safe and Adequate Intake:*** 75–250 µg • Milk, legumes, bread, grains	Component of many enzymes; works with riboflavin to incorporate iron into hemoglobin	*Deficiency* Unknown *Toxicity* Occupational exposure to molybdenum dust causes gout-like symptoms

for women of childbearing age. Iron requirements increase during growth and in response to heavy or chronic blood loss related to menstruation, surgery, injury, gastrointestinal bleeding, or aspirin abuse. Adult men typically consume more than their RDA for iron; adult women usually consume less than their RDA.

Zinc

The small amount of zinc contained in the body (about 2 g) is found in almost all cells and is especially concentrated in the eyes, bones, muscles, and prostate gland. Zinc in tissues is not available to maintain serum levels when intake is inadequate, so a regular and sufficient intake is necessary.

Zinc is a component of DNA and RNA and is part of more than 70 enzymes involved in growth, metabolism, sexual maturation and reproduction, and the senses of taste and smell.

On average, only 15% to 35% of ingested zinc is absorbed, but absorption is more efficient during times of need. Fiber and phytates reduce the bioavailability of zinc. For instance, the proportion of zinc available from red meat is much greater than that from whole-grain products, wheat germ, and black-eyed peas.

Zinc homeostasis is strongly regulated, and its excretion, primarily through the feces, is directly proportional to zinc status. Fecal excretion includes unabsorbed dietary zinc and zinc from enteropancreatic circulation. Small amounts of zinc are excreted in bile. Normally zinc is not excreted in the urine.

It is estimated that men consume 90% or more of the RDA for zinc and that women consume less than 81% of the RDA. This difference appears to be related to calorie intake, not to the zinc density of foods consumed: zinc intake increases as calorie intake increases. Although average zinc intake among Americans may be marginal, deficiency symptoms are not observed.

Iodine

Iodine is found in muscles, the thyroid gland, skin, the skeleton, endocrine tissues, and the bloodstream. It is an essential component of thyroxine (T_4) and triiodothyronine (T_3), the thyroid hormones responsible for regulating basal metabolic rate.

Even though half of the salt sold in the United States is not iodized, iodized salt is the biggest source of iodine in the American diet. One-half teaspoon of iodized salt provides more than the RDA for iodine. Seafood is naturally high in iodine derived from ocean water. Food processing techniques incidentally add iodine to the food supply. For instance, milk is naturally low in iodine, but it has become a significant source of iodine because of the iodized salt licks given to cows and the use of iodine chemicals to sanitize and disinfect udders, milking machines, and milk tanks. Iodate dough conditioners increase the iodine content of bread.

The RDA for iodine includes a built-in measure of safety for the unquantified effect of goitrogens (thyroid antagonists found in members of the cabbage family) on iodine requirements. The average American adult consumes more than the RDA for iodine, and it is recommended that no new sources of iodine be added to the U.S. food supply.

Selenium

Selenium is a component of enzymes that work to protect cells from oxidative damage. As such, its role as an antioxidant in the prevention of heart disease and cancer are being investigated.

Although areas of the country with selenium-poor soil produce selenium-poor foods, mass transportation mitigates the effect on total selenium intake. Also, because selenium is associated with protein, meats and other animal products are high in selenium. The average American adult intake exceeds the RDA for selenium.

Copper

Copper is distributed in muscles, liver, brain, bones, kidneys, and blood. Copper is a component of several enzymes, aids in the synthesis of hemoglobin, and is used in energy metabolism.

A dietary deficiency of copper is not likely, but excess zinc intake has the potential to induce copper deficiency by impairing its absorption. Supplements, not food, may cause copper toxicity.

Manganese

Manganese is found in the liver, kidneys, pancreas, and bones. It works as part of enzymes involved in fat synthesis, growth, reproduction, and blood clotting.

Because manganese is widespread in the diet, a deficiency is not likely. Toxicities from food alone are rare. The average American adult consumes amounts within the Estimated Safe and Adequate Daily Intake range.

Fluoride

Only minute amounts of fluoride occur in the body. After being absorbed into the bloodstream, fluoride is either deposited into forming teeth or combines with calcium and phosphorus in bones to add strength. Even after teeth eruption is complete, fluoride excreted through the saliva offers lifetime protection against dental decay.

Fluoride is naturally present in varying concentrations in all drinking water and soil, and most foods contain some fluoride. Major sources of fluoride are supplements and fluoridated water; fluoridation of municipal water is considered to be the most effective dental public health intervention in existence. However, not all municipal water supplies are fluoridated, and most bottled waters are not. Approximately half of the American population has access to water with an optimal fluoride concentration that delivers about 1 mg of fluoride per liter.

Chromium

Chromium functions with the hormone insulin to help regulate blood glucose levels. In fact, a deficiency of chromium is characterized by high blood glucose and impaired insulin response.

Even though chromium is widespread in foods, an estimated 90% of American adults consume less than the minimum daily recommendation of chromium. Unrefined foods are higher in chromium than processed foods.

Molybdenum

Molybdenum plays a role in red blood cell synthesis and is a component of several enzymes. Average American intake falls within the recommended range, and neither dietary deficiencies nor toxicities occur.

Other Trace Elements

Although definitive evidence is lacking, future research may reveal that other trace elements are essential for human nutrition. However, evidence is difficult to obtain, and quantifying human need is even more formidable. In addition, as with all trace minerals, the potential for toxicity exists. Consider that:

- Nickel, silicon, and boron are recognized as essential nutrients for animals and may someday be classified as essential for humans.
- Cobalt is an essential component of vitamin B_{12}, but it is not an essential nutrient and does not have an RDA.
- It is possible that minute amounts of cadmium, lithium, tin, and vanadium are also essential to human life.

Minerals in Health Promotion

Arguably, sodium, calcium, and iron are the minerals with which nutritionists are most concerned. Most Americans consume much more sodium than they need, increasing their risk of hypertension. Conversely, most American adults consume less than optimal amounts of calcium, placing them at risk of osteoporosis and perhaps hypertension, colon cancer, and premenstrual syndrome. Iron deficiency anemia is the most common nutritional deficiency disorder in the United States.

CUTTING BACK ON SODIUM

The *Dietary Guidelines for Americans* suggests that Americans "Choose and prepare foods with less salt" because studies show that a high sodium intake is linked to higher blood pressure (see Chapter 8). Even though only a small percentage of the population is truly sodium-sensitive, all Americans are advised to limit their intake of sodium to approximately 2400 mg/day, a little more than is contained in 1 level teaspoon of salt. Likewise, the American Heart Association recommends that salt intake not exceed 6 g of sodium chloride, which is the equivalent of 2400 mg of sodium. The average intakes from foods alone (not counting salt added at the table) are more than 4000 mg for men and almost 3000 mg for women. Only 25% of American adults think they eat too much sodium.

Clients who need or want to limit sodium should be advised to:

- **Reduce sodium intake gradually.** People are born with a preference for sweets but acquire a taste for salt. In other words, the more salt and salty foods a person eats, the more salt the person likes or wants. Fortunately, the converse is also true: reducing salt intake gradually reduces the desire for salt.
- **Read the Nutrition Facts label.** The DV for sodium on the Nutrition Facts label is 2400 mg; the Percent Daily Value (%DV) of sodium in a serving of food is based on this reference. For instance, the %DV of sodium in a serving of canned pasta is 41%, or 990 mg ($990 \text{ mg} \div 2400 \text{ mg} \times 100 = 41.25\%$). As a general guideline, limit foods that provide 20% of the DV (480 mg) to 1 serving per day.
- **Compare labels among different brands of the same items.** For instance, the sodium content in a cup of spaghetti sauce ranges from about 500 mg to more than 1200 mg. Know what the terms used to describe sodium content mean (Box 6–2).
- **Concentrate on freshness and remember that "natural" is usually best.** Approximately 75% of the sodium in a typical American diet comes from restaurant and processed foods such as canned vegetables and meats; convenience foods such as hamburger mixes and prepared spaghetti sauces; frozen dinners and entrees; canned and dried soups; pizza; and lunch meats, hot dogs, and ham. The following examples illustrate the difference in sodium content between natural foods and their processed counterparts. Whenever possible, choose fresh over processed foods.

Food	Serving Size	Sodium Content (mg)
Fresh tomato	1 medium	11
Diced canned tomatoes	½ cup	477
Baked potato	1 medium	16
Frozen potato puffs	½ cup	463
Shredded wheat	1 oz	0
Raisin Bran	1.3 oz	330
Swiss cheese	1 oz	74
Swiss cheese food	1 oz	440
Homemade chicken potpie	1 serving	594
Frozen chicken potpie	1 serving	1023

- **Be aware that high-sodium foods do not necessarily taste salty.** Sometimes "salty" foods actually have the same or less sodium than foods that don't taste salty. For instance, fast food French fries have less sodium than fast food sandwiches, even though the fries taste saltier. A serving of potato chips has approximately the same amount of sodium as a serving of many breakfast cereals.

BOX 6.2

Descriptors of Sodium Content

If the label says . . .	One serving contains . . .
Sodium free	<5 mg
Very low sodium	<35 mg
Low sodium	<140 mg
Reduced or less sodium	At least 25% less sodium compared with a standard serving size of the traditional food
Light in sodium	50% less sodium than the traditional food (restricted to >40 cal/serving or >3 g fat/serving)
Salt free	<5 mg
Unsalted or no added salt	No salt added during processing (this does not necessarily mean the food is sodium free)

- **Balance high-sodium foods with lower-sodium foods.** What matters is sodium intake over several days, not necessarily the sodium content of individual foods. For instance, if the client has canned soup for lunch, other food choices for the rest of the day should not be high in sodium.
- **Taste food before adding salt.** Some salt users do so out of habit, even before tasting their food. Salt should be used judiciously, not automatically.
- **Experiment with herbs, spices, and vinegars as alternatives to salt.** Some suggestions to use in place of salt are:
  - Beef: dry mustard, pepper, marjoram, red wine, or sherry
  - Chicken: parsley, thyme, sage, tarragon, curry, or white wine
  - Seafood: bay leaf, cayenne pepper, dill, curry, onions, or garlic
  - Eggs: oregano, curry, chives, pepper, tomatoes, or a pinch of sugar
- **Focus on the positive.** When it comes to reducing the risk of hypertension, consuming adequate potassium and calcium may be as important as limiting sodium. Encourage the client to eat ample amounts of a variety of fruits and vegetables (not canned), whole grains, and low-fat milk and yogurt.

GETTING ENOUGH CALCIUM

Most of the body's 3 pounds or so of calcium is located within bones, providing strength and density as part of the mineral matrix. Bones actually serve as a dynamic reservoir of calcium to help maintain blood calcium levels despite variations in calcium intake. When calcium intake is low, bones donate calcium to prevent blood levels from dropping; when intake is high, bones take up the excess to keep blood levels from rising. A chronically low calcium intake compromises the density and strength of bones; adequate calcium helps maximize bone density.

Dietary Calcium

An adequate calcium intake is important throughout the life cycle. During the first few decades of life, attaining maximum bone density is a safeguard against the inevitable net bone loss that occurs with aging: the greater the peak bone mass, the less likely it is that subsequent bone loss will cause problems. After age 30 to 35 years, adequate calcium alone cannot stop net bone loss, but it can slow the rate. Adequate calcium may also play a role in preventing hypertension and colon cancer in susceptible people. Some studies show that calcium helps reduce symptoms of premenstrual syndrome. The latest recommendations for calcium intake, higher than the previous RDAs, are set at levels associated with maximum retention of body calcium.

Many Americans do not consume the recommended quantity of calcium: although they may be getting enough to meet their *requirement*, they fall short of the *recommendation*, which is set higher to reduce the risk of osteoporosis. At least three 8-ounce glasses of milk or yogurt are needed within the context of a varied, balanced diet to ensure that total calcium intake will be adequate. According to 1994–1996 survey data, the average number of daily servings consumed from the dairy group was 1.5. Selecting more calcium-fortified foods, such as calcium-fortified orange juice, boosts calcium intake. Calcium supplements are appropriate for people who cannot or will not consume adequate calcium from foods alone.

Calcium Supplements

Although it is possible to get adequate calcium through foods, many people do not. Women interested in weight loss often forsake dairy products, rationalizing that they cannot "afford" the calories in milk. Many adults perceive milk as a children's beverage and replace it with more "adult" drinks such as carbonated beverages, coffee, and tea. People with lactose intolerance avoid milk because they are unable to digest the sugar in milk. They experience gas, bloating, cramping, and diarrhea that varies with individual tolerance and lactose load. For many, calcium supplements are necessary to ensure adequate intake.

Clients who use calcium supplements should be advised to:

- **Determine how much calcium is needed from supplements based on the requirement and the usual calcium intake.** A Tolerable Upper Intake Level (UL) for calcium is set at 2500 mg/day. Intakes higher than this offer no benefit and may pose potential harm. An estimate of the number of daily servings of milk and yogurt consumed provides an approximation of the usual calcium intake, which can be used to calculate the amount of calcium needed through supplements.
- **Keep the doses small.** Calcium from supplements is absorbed best in doses of 500 mg or less. If two or three doses are needed, they should be spread throughout the day.
- **Know whether the supplement should be taken with or between meals.** The most common type of calcium supplement, calcium carbonate, is better absorbed

with food, especially with acidic foods such as citrus juice or fruit. Calcium citrate is better absorbed on an empty stomach, because it does not require gastric acid for absorption. For this reason, calcium citrate is the preferred calcium supplement for people with low stomach acid and those taking medications that block gastric acid secretion.

- **Read the label.** Supplements differ greatly in their calcium content. For instance, calcium carbonate (eg, Tums) is the most concentrated calcium source at 40% calcium, so it provides more per tablet.
- **Do not take calcium and iron supplements at the same time.** Calcium interferes with iron absorption.
- **Drink plenty of fluids.** Extra fluid helps prevent constipation, a common side effect of calcium supplements.
- **Stay away from supplements that include dolomite or bonemeal.** These sources of calcium may contain small amounts of lead and other heavy metals.
- **Remember that "supplement" means "add to" not "replace."** Calcium supplements provide an important source of calcium, but that is all. Milk and yogurt, on the other hand, provide calcium, protein, vitamin D, phosphorus, and other essential nutrients that are important for general health as well as bone health. Calcium-fortified orange juice is also an excellent source of vitamin C and potassium. Supplements should not be relied on to provide total calcium requirements.

PREVENTING IRON DEFICIENCY ANEMIA

Iron deficiency anemia occurs when total iron stores become depleted, leading to a decrease in hemoglobin. This type of anemia is classified as microcytic (small blood cells) and hypochromic (pale red blood cells, related to the decrease in hemoglobin pigment). People with mild anemia may not even know that they are deficient in iron. People with symptomatic anemia may complain of fatigue, weakness, pallor, sensitivity to cold, anorexia, dizziness and headaches, stomatitis, and glossitis. Fingernails may be thin and spoon shaped. Some people with iron deficiency anemia practice pica (ingestion of nonfood substances such as dirt, clay, or laundry starch), which impairs iron absorption.

Iron deficiency anemia is the most common nutritional deficiency disorder in the United States. The incidence rate among high-risk populations may be as high as 10% to 50%. Groups who are most vulnerable include infants younger than 2 years of age, menstruating women, elderly persons, and members of minority and/or low-income groups.

There are several reasons why inadequate intake is a frequent cause of iron deficiency anemia. First, the typical American diet provides 10 to 20 mg/day. Men, who typically consume more food than women, can easily meet their requirement for iron (10 mg). Women tend to eat less iron—the mean intake for women 12 to 49 years of age is 12.4 mg/day—but they require more iron (RDA, 15 mg). Also, on the average, only 10% of the iron that is consumed is absorbed. To reduce the risk of iron deficiency anemia, rich sources of iron should be consumed regularly and steps should be taken to maximize iron absorption.

Clients who have or are at risk for iron deficiency anemia should be advised to:

- **Eat more iron from all sources.** Sources of heme iron include beef, poultry (especially the dark meat), egg yolk, lamb, oysters, pork, shellfish, shrimp, tuna, and veal. Sources of nonheme iron include bran flakes, brown rice, enriched and whole grains, fortified cereals, dried peas and beans, soybeans, dried fruit, greens, nuts, oatmeal, and sweet potatoes.

- **Eat a source of heme iron at every meal.** Add a little meat, poultry, or fish to plant foods to boost the absorption of nonheme iron. For instance, use ground beef in chili or tuna fish in pasta salad.
- **Include a rich source of vitamin C at every meal to maximize absorption.** These sources include citrus fruits and their juices, brussels sprouts, strawberries, broccoli, greens, cabbage, cantaloupe, and tomatoes.
- **Drink coffee and tea between meals, not with meals.** Coffee and tea interfere with nonheme iron absorption.
- **Choose iron-fortified cereals and whole-grain products.** Check the label to find breakfast cereals fortified with 100% DV of iron. Crush the cereal and use it as a breading for meat, fish, poultry, and vegetables; mix it with butter or margarine for a casserole topping; use it as a meat extender in meat loaf, meatballs, and meat burgers; sprinkle it on ice cream; or add it to yogurt and pudding for extra crunch.
- **Cook in iron pots whenever possible, especially when cooking acidic foods such as dishes made with tomatoes.** Acid enhances leaching of some of the iron from the pot into the food.

Questions You May Hear

Is tea good for you? Like most nutritional issues, the answer to whether tea is "good" or "bad" is not absolute. On the down side, tea contains tannins, which significantly impair iron absorption when they are consumed at the same time as the iron. Brewed black tea also contains caffeine (about half as much as an equivalent amount of brewed coffee), which in high amounts can cause a jittery feeling, insomnia, and a transitory increase in heart rate. On the other hand, studies have failed to link caffeine consumption to any health problems, including cancer, heart disease, or birth defects. Also, tea contains phytochemicals that may help protect against cancer and heart disease. If you like tea, drink it in moderation, and try to avoid having it 1 hour before or after a meal to minimize its impact on iron absorption. But if you don't like tea, it is not necessary to drink it for optimal health.

Are diet soft drinks bad for you? Diet soft drinks have an advantage over regular soft drinks in that they contain no sugar and are essentially calorie free. The sugar alternatives used in soft drinks are safe at normal doses for most people. (The exception—people with the genetic disorder phenylketonuria, who should not use products sweetened with aspartame.) In moderation, diet soft drinks provide a sweet-tasting alternative to water, but they do not provide any nutrients and should not displace the use of milk or 100% fruit juice.

Does chlorine in drinking water cause cancer? When organic matter is present in water, chlorine reacts with it to form a byproduct called trihalomethane (THM). If THM does forms, it is in such small quantities that it is not a cancer risk. The benefits of chlorine in preventing outbreaks of cholera, hepatitis, and other diseases far outweigh the negligible effects of THM.

Do zinc lozenges help relieve cold symptoms? To date, approximately half of the studies done on zinc gluconate lozenges showed that they shorten the duration of colds, and half found no effect. Until more studies are done, it's not unreasonable or unsafe to try the lozenges when you have a cold. However, long-term use to prevent colds is not recommended; regular consumption of too much zinc can impair the immune system and lower the concentration of high-density lipoprotein ("good") cholesterol.

KEY CONCEPTS

- Because it is involved in almost every body function, is not stored, and is excreted daily, water is more vital to life than food.
- Under normal conditions, water intake equals water output to maintain water balance. In most healthy people, thirst is a reliable indicator of need.
- The body's need for water is influenced by many variables. General guidelines suggest 1.0 to 1.5 mL of fluid per calorie consumed.
- Minerals are inorganic substances that cannot be broken down and rearranged in the body.
- Mineral toxicities are not likely to occur from diet alone. They are most often related to excessive use of mineral supplements, environmental exposure, or alterations in metabolism.
- Depending on the mineral involved, the body can maintain mineral balance by altering the rate of absorption, altering the rate of excretion, or releasing minerals from storage when needed.
- The absorption of many minerals is influenced by mineral-mineral interactions. Too much of one mineral may promote a deficiency of another mineral.
- Sodium, potassium, and chloride are electrolytes because they carry electrical charges when they are dissolved in solution.
- Macrominerals are needed in relatively large amounts (>100 mg/day) and are found in the body in quantities greater than 5 g. Trace minerals are needed in very small amounts (<15 mg/day) and are found in the body in amounts less than 5 g.
- As much as 75% of sodium consumed in the average American diet is from processed food. Americans are urged to reduce their intake of sodium because of its potential role in the development of hypertension.
- Many American adults consume less than optimal amounts of calcium, placing them at risk of osteoporosis and possibly hypertension and colon cancer. Milk and yogurt are the richest sources of calcium, and their vitamin D and lactose content promote its absorption. Calcium-fortified orange juice is also an excellent source of well-absorbed calcium. Calcium supplements should be used to boost calcium intake in people who are unable or unwilling to consume adequate calcium through foods.

ANSWER KEY

1. **FALSE** It depends on the type of calcium supplement. Calcium carbonate, the most common calcium supplement, is better absorbed with food. Calcium citrate is better absorbed on an empty stomach.

2. **FALSE** Increased urinary excretion helps rid the body of an excess of some minerals (eg, sodium and potassium), but not all minerals are excreted in the urine when consumed in excess of need. Some minerals, such as iron and selenium, can accumulate in the body to toxic levels.
3. **FALSE** Calcium is the most plentiful mineral in the body.
4. **FALSE** Minerals are lost only when foods are soaked in water.
5. **TRUE** Bottled water lacks fluoride. If children drink non-fluoridated bottled water, a fluoride supplement may be necessary to help prevent dental cavities.
6. **TRUE** Americans get approximately 75% of dietary sodium from processed foods.
7. **FALSE** Both macro- and microminerals are essential to health. Neither is more important than the other.
8. **TRUE** Among healthy adults, thirst is generally a reliable indicator of fluid need.
9. **TRUE** The Nutrition Facts label lists a Daily Value of 2400 mg of sodium per day, a little more than the amount contained in 1 level teaspoon of salt.
10. **FALSE** A chronically low intake of calcium compromises the density and strength of bones.

REFERENCES

American Dietetic Association. (1994). Position of The American Dietetic Association: The impact of fluoride on dental health. *Journal of the American Dietetic Association, 94*(12), 1428–1431.

Hudnall, M. (1999). *Vitamins, minerals, and dietary supplements*. Written for the American Dietetic Association. Minneapolis: Chronimed Publishing.

Jacobson, M. (Ed.). (1998). No cold comfort. *Nutrition Action Healthletter, 25*(8), 13.

Kleiner, S. (1999). Water: An essential but overlooked nutrient. *Journal of the American Dietetic Association*, 99(2), 200–206.

National Academy of Sciences Institute of Medicine. (1997). *Dietary Reference Intakes for calcium, phosphorus, magnesium, vitamin D, and fluoride*. Washington, DC: National Academy Press.

Shardt, D. (1998). Zinc or swim. *Nutrition Action Healthletter, 25*(3), 9.

Subar, A., Krebs-Smith, S., Cook, A., & Kahle, L. (1998). Dietary sources of nutrients among US adults, 1989 to 1991. *Journal of the American Dietetic Association*, 98(5), 537–547.

Whitney, E., Cataldo, C., & Rolfes, S. (1998). *Understanding normal and clinical nutrition* (5th ed.). Belmont, CA: Wadsworth Publishing Company.

CHAPTER 7

Eating, Energy, and Exercise

TRUE	FALSE	Check your knowledge of eating, energy, and exercise.
		1 A food that is high in "energy" is high in calories.
		2 No matter how much body fat you have, the limiting factor in how long and how well you exercise is the amount of glycogen in storage.
		3 The most effective way to increase your metabolism is to build muscle tissue.
		4 Exercise promotes hunger and a higher calorie intake.
		5 To lose 2 pounds a week, you must incur a daily deficit of 1000 calories.
		6 You may burn more body fat with a low-calorie diet than by fasting.
		7 To lose fat, you have to do low-intensity, fat-burning exercise.
		8 After 35 years of age, loss of muscle tissue is an unavoidable consequence of aging.
		9 To reap health benefits, you must participate in continuous activity for at least 30 minutes.
		10 Fasting and starvation lower the metabolic rate.

Upon completion of this chapter, you will be able to

- Describe how carbohydrates, proteins, and fats are digested and absorbed.
- Discuss the role of each of the three energy nutrients in supplying energy to the body.
- Explain changes in metabolism that occur as a result of fasting.
- Explain the factors that affect basal energy requirements.
- Discuss the benefits of aerobic and resistance exercises.
- Describe the nutritional implications of (1) increasing activity for health benefits, (2) exercising for optimal fitness, and (3) exercising for weight management.

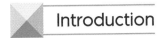

Introduction

Energy is relatively abstract in that it cannot be defined by its size, shape, or mass. According to basic principles of thermodynamics, energy is neither created nor destroyed but changes from one form to another without being used up. In the body, energy is extracted from nutrients. Tiny amounts of energy are stored within cells as a source of immediate fuel. Much larger amounts of energy are available in glycogen and fat tissue to fuel activity of longer duration. The metabolism of energy is a dynamic process that constantly changes with the influx of nutrients, the availability of stored energy, and the demands of fueling activity.

This chapter discusses how the body extracts energy from food, the body's use of energy under various conditions, and total energy requirements. The Health Promotion section focuses on physical activity and various nutritional supplements promoted as fat burners.

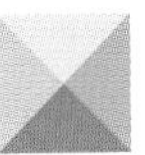

Keys to Understanding How the Body Extracts Energy From Food

Food provides energy (calories) in carbohydrates, proteins, and fats (and alcohol). The processes of digestion and absorption precede the actual release of energy from food.

DIGESTION

Digestion mechanically (physically) and chemically transforms food into nutrients the body can absorb.

Mechanical Digestion

Mechanical digestion breaks down food into smaller particles, thereby increasing the surface area on which digestive enzymes can work. It begins in the mouth as the teeth and tongue transform food into a soft, pliable mass and continues as muscles of the gastrointestinal tract contract and relax to push and mix the gastrointestinal contents.

The gastrointestinal tract has longitudinal (long) muscles on the outside surface and circular muscles that surround the tube (Fig. 7-1). Contraction of these muscles propels matter forward by a rhythmic, wavelike movement known as **peristalsis.** Peristaltic contractions occur continuously, regardless of whether food is present. Peristalsis is strongest in the esophagus and weakest in the small intestine.

A layer of circular muscles surrounds the gastrointestinal tract, under the long outer muscles. These circular muscles control the diameter of the tube by contracting and relaxing. **Segmentation** is a localized contraction in the small intestine that occurs as circu-

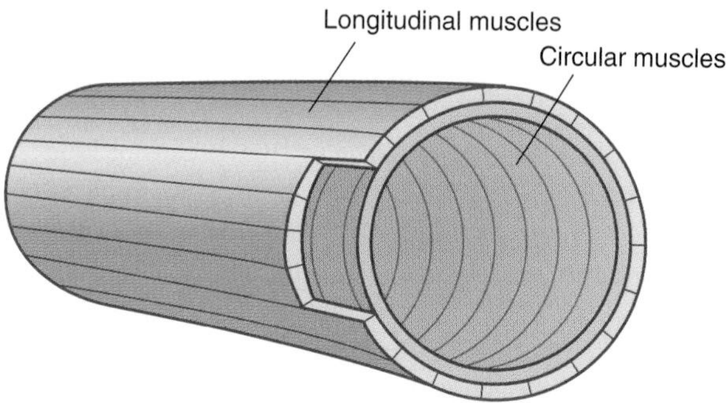

FIGURE 7-1 Muscles of the gastrointestinal wall.

lar muscles periodically squeeze to constrict the diameter of the tube, giving the gastrointestinal tract the appearance of "sausage links" (Fig. 7-2). This action forces the gastrointestinal contents backward a few inches, thereby prolonging the time they are in contact with digestive juices and the absorptive surface.

Chemical Digestion

Most chemical digestion occurs as food mixes with digestive enzymes secreted by the pancreas and small intestine (Fig. 7-3). Digestive enzymes are complex protein molecules that hasten the rate of reaction without being consumed. They are very specific; that is, they work on only one substrate. Because they are reused, only small quantities of enzymes are needed. About 90% of digestion occurs in the first half of the small intestine.

The large amount of fluid that is pumped into the gastrointestinal tract facilitates digestion. Normal adults secrete about 6 to 10 L of fluid into the gastrointestinal tract daily, in addition to the 1 to 2 L that is normally consumed. Most of the fluid is reabsorbed in the small intestine.

ABSORPTION

Absorption is the actual movement of substances across the mucosal membrane. Most nutrients are absorbed in the jejunum and ileum. Some nutrients are absorbed through *passive diffusion*, in which a substance moves freely and continuously from an area of high concentration to one of lower concentration until it becomes evenly dispersed. Other

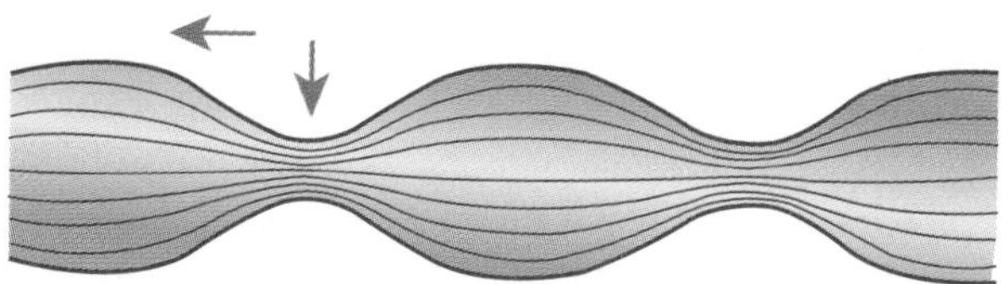

FIGURE 7-2 Segmentation.

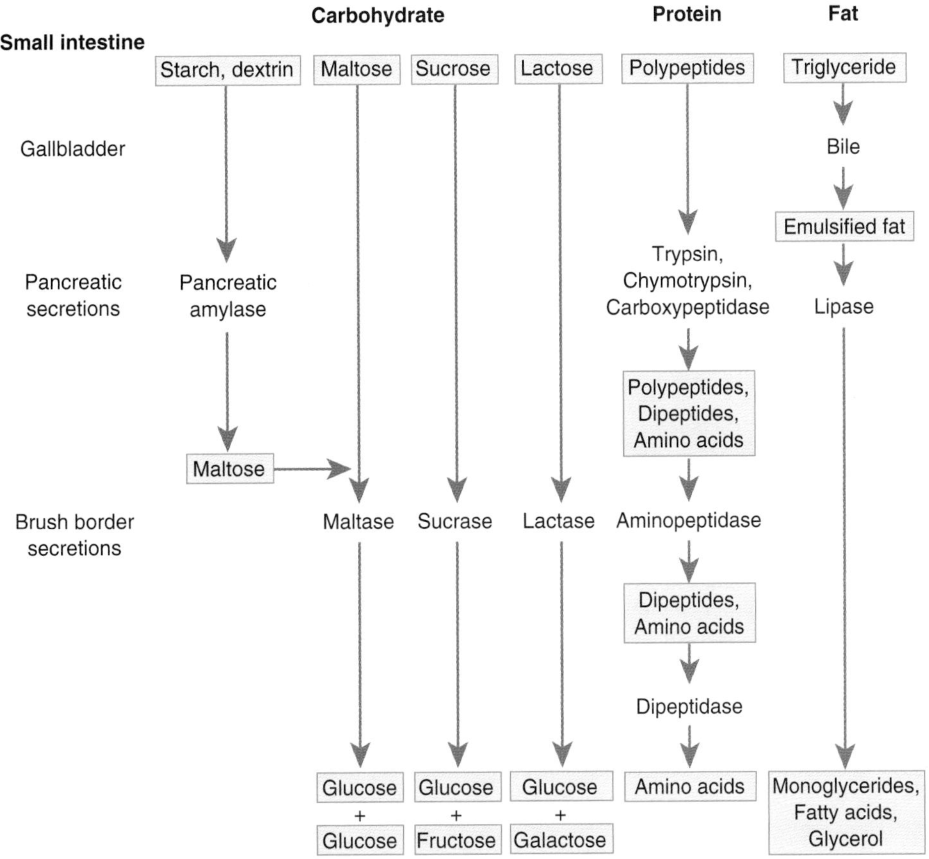

FIGURE 7-3 Chemical digestion within the small intestine.

nutrients are absorbed by *active transport*, which requires energy to move the nutrient from an area of low concentration to one of higher concentration. Water is absorbed by the process of *osmosis*; it passes through a selectively permeable membrane to equalize the concentration of water molecules on both sides of the membrane.

OVERVIEW OF DIGESTION AND ABSORPTION

The entire process of digestion, absorption, and elimination usually takes 1 to 3 days after eating. Although motility is affected by numerous variables, including actual food and fluid intake, activity and muscle tone, emotional factors, certain drug therapies, and gastrointestinal integrity, it is controlled primarily by the actions of nerves and hormones.

Digestion and absorption details are presented in each of the energy nutrient chapters. Figure 7-4 summarizes the functions of the digestive system organs. A quick overview follows.

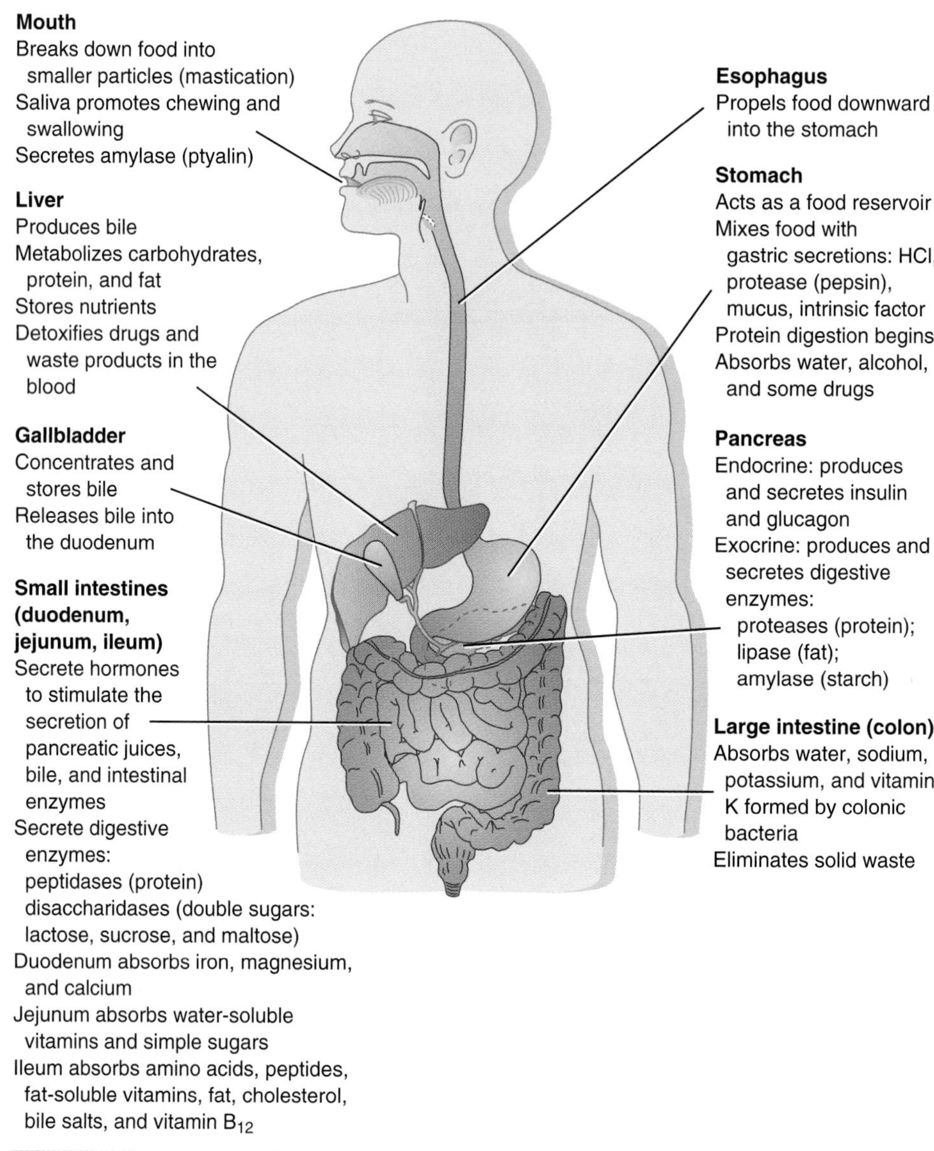
Mouth
Breaks down food into smaller particles (mastication)
Saliva promotes chewing and swallowing
Secretes amylase (ptyalin)
Liver
Produces bile
Metabolizes carbohydrates, protein, and fat
Stores nutrients
Detoxifies drugs and waste products in the blood
Gallbladder
Concentrates and stores bile
Releases bile into the duodenum
Small intestines (duodenum, jejunum, ileum)
Secrete hormones to stimulate the secretion of pancreatic juices, bile, and intestinal enzymes
Secrete digestive enzymes:
peptidases (protein)
disaccharidases (double sugars: lactose, sucrose, and maltose)
Duodenum absorbs iron, magnesium, and calcium
Jejunum absorbs water-soluble vitamins and simple sugars
Ileum absorbs amino acids, peptides, fat-soluble vitamins, fat, cholesterol, bile salts, and vitamin B_{12}
Esophagus
Propels food downward into the stomach
Stomach
Acts as a food reservoir
Mixes food with gastric secretions: HCl, protease (pepsin), mucus, intrinsic factor
Protein digestion begins
Absorbs water, alcohol, and some drugs
Pancreas
Endocrine: produces and secretes insulin and glucagon
Exocrine: produces and secretes digestive enzymes:
proteases (protein);
lipase (fat);
amylase (starch)
Large intestine (colon)
Absorbs water, sodium, potassium, and vitamin K formed by colonic bacteria
Eliminates solid waste

FIGURE 7-4 Functions of the digestive system organs.

The Mouth

Saliva moistens mucous membranes and food to promote chewing and swallowing. Saliva also enhances the sense of taste and facilitates chemical digestion. Salivary amylase *(ptyalin)* begins the process of breaking down starch into maltose, but because food is usually held in the mouth only briefly, limited starch digestion occurs there. However, swallowed amylase may continue to work for another 15 to 30 minutes in the stomach, until it is inactivated by gastric acids.

The Esophagus

Swallowed food, called **bolus,** is directed into the esophagus (and away from the trachea) by closure of the epiglottis. Food is moved downward through the esophagus by peristalsis and gravity. Very soft foods and liquids may reach the stomach in about 1 second; solid or semisolid foods may take 4 to 8 seconds. No chemical digestion or absorption occurs in the esophagus.

At both ends of the esophagus, circular muscles called **sphincters** control the passage of food. The upper esophageal sphincter relaxes (opens) during swallowing to allow food to pass from the laryngopharynx into the esophagus. The lower esophageal sphincter relaxes to allow food to pass from the esophagus into the stomach. Both sphincters contract (close) to prevent the backflow of food.

The Stomach

As food enters the upper portion of the stomach (cardia), gentle churning and mixing with gastric secretions transforms it into a semiliquid paste called **chyme.** Chyme may remain in the fundus for 1 hour or longer, during which time muscular activity is slight but salivary amylase can continue digesting starch. Vigorous churning occurs when chyme enters the body of the stomach. Chyme must pass through the pyloric sphincter to enter the duodenum, and it does so in very small amounts so as not to overwhelm the small intestine. As "gatekeeper" for the duodenum, the pyloric sphincter normally remains almost, but not quite, completely closed. Wavelike forward and backward "splashing" of gastrointestinal contents helps force chyme through the sphincter, but some backflow does occur. This continued churning accounts for most of the mixing of the gastrointestinal contents.

The pH of the stomach is about 2 because of the presence of hydrochloric acid (HCl). The acid environment has many advantages, including activating gastric enzymes, killing most food bacteria, and promoting the absorption of calcium and iron.

Chemically, the primary function of the stomach is to begin breaking down protein into smaller peptide molecules through the action of the enzyme *pepsin*. Pepsin is first secreted in its inactive form, pepsinogen; it is converted to pepsin in the presence of HCl. To help protect the stomach lining from being digested, activated pepsin stimulates the secretion of mucus, which coats and protects the mucosa.

The position and size of the stomach change continuously: The stomach seemingly "shrinks" when empty but stretches to accommodate a large meal. The stomach's volume averages about 1.5 L. The rate at which the stomach empties is influenced by many factors, including the volume and composition of the food that is consumed. Liquids leave the stomach faster than solids do; carbohydrates empty more quickly than protein, and fat is the slowest mover. Gastric emptying usually takes 1 to 4 hours, but it may take as long as 6 hours after a high-fat meal.

Because the stomach wall is impermeable to most substances, its absorptive capacity is limited to some water, certain drugs, and alcohol.

The Small Intestine

Chyme then proceeds through the three portions of the small intestine: the duodenum, jejunum, and ileum. In the duodenum, digestion continues as chyme mixes with bile and pancreatic enzymes. Pancreatic secretions, which contain enzymes, bicarbonate, and electrolytes, are delivered into the duodenum through a duct. Pancreatic enzymes (amylases, proteases, and lipases) are responsible for the digestion of carbohydrates, proteins, and fats, respectively. Sodium bicarbonate and fluid transform the acidic chyme into a neutral or slightly alkaline semiliquid.

Bile, which is made in the liver and concentrated and stored in the gallbladder, passes through the common bile duct to reach the duodenum. Its secretion is stimulated by fat in the duodenum; bile is not an enzyme but an emulsifier that promotes fat digestion by suspending fat particles in solution, thereby increasing the surface area on which lipases can work.

The small intestine is the primary site of absorption for the end products of carbohydrate, protein, and fat digestion and for most vitamins, minerals, water, and drugs (Fig. 7-5). The lining of the small intestine has hundreds of folds covered with *villi*, which are fingerlike projections into the intestinal lumen (Fig. 7-6). Each villus is covered with a layer of epithelial cells that are coated with projections called *microvilli;* these microvilli greatly increase the surface area of the small intestine. The microvilli collectively form what is known as the **brush border,** which contains both digestive enzymes that complete the process of digestion and cells that absorb nutrients.

The manner in which nutrients proceed out of the villi depends on whether they are water (blood) soluble or fat soluble. Although all nutrients eventually end up in the bloodstream, only water-soluble nutrients can pass from the villi into capillaries (Fig. 7-5) and then enter portal circulation. This is the route taken by monosaccharides, amino acids, glycerol, water-soluble vitamins, minerals, short-chain fatty acids, and medium-chain fatty acids. Long-chain fatty acids, once inside the villi, are further digested into glycerol and fatty acids; then, they are recombined to form triglycerides. The reformed triglycerides, along with cholesterol and the fat-soluble vitamins A, D, E, and K, leave the villi as chylomicrons by way of the lymphatic system, traveling into the thoracic duct, through the subclavian veins, and then to the liver.

The Colon

Unabsorbed material exits the small intestine through the ileocecal valve and enters the large intestine, which is composed of the cecum, colon, rectum, and anal canal. Here bacteria ferment the remaining undigested food residue and synthesize significant

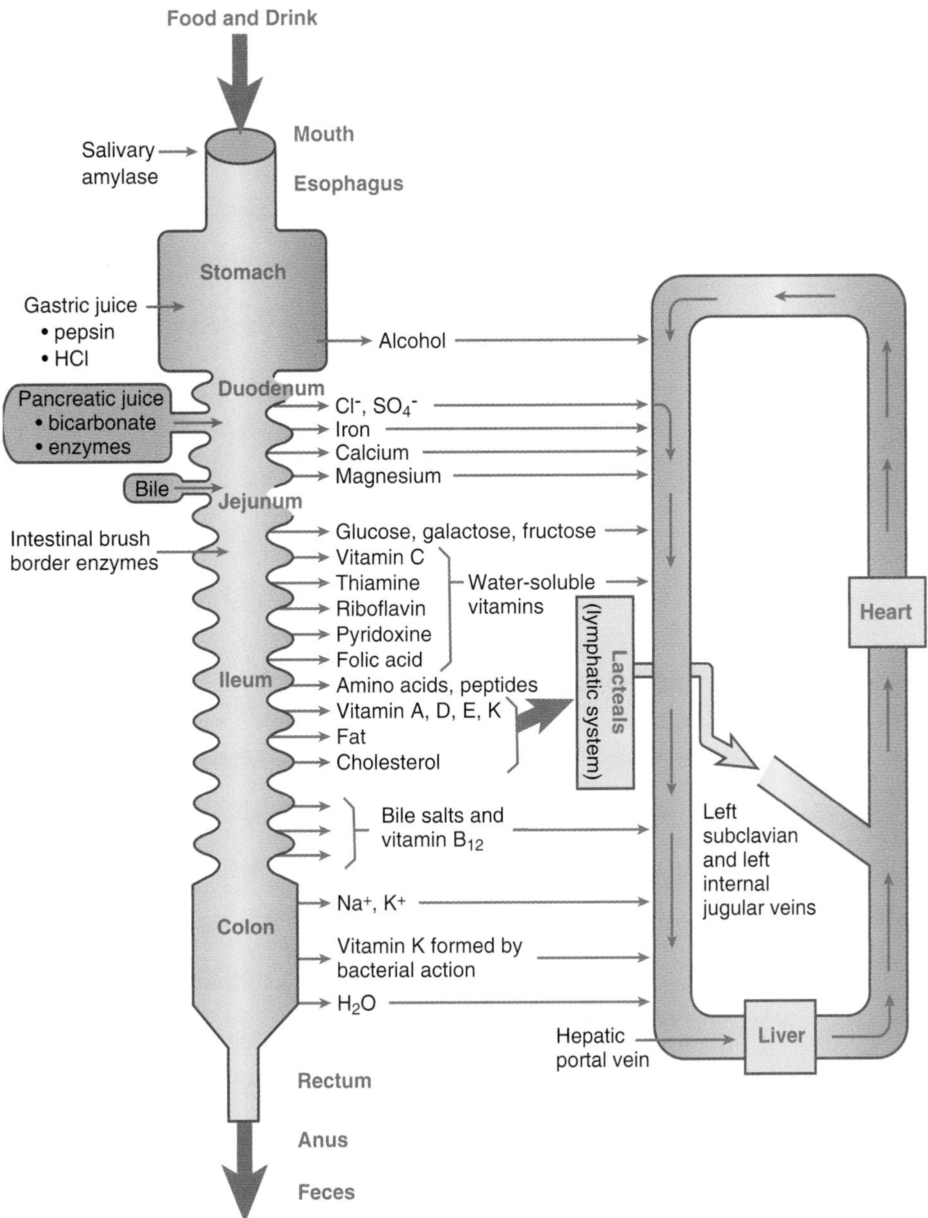

FIGURE 7-5 Sites of secretion and absorption in the gastrointestinal tract.

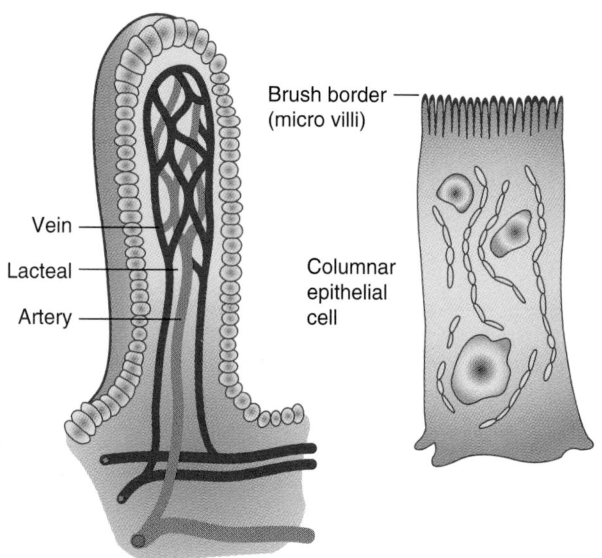

FIGURE 7-6 Villi and microvilli.

amounts of vitamin K and smaller amounts of vitamin B_{12} and biotin. Sodium, potassium, and water are absorbed in the colon. The semisolid waste that remains after absorption is completed is made of water, food residues, microorganisms, digestive secretions, and mucus. Feces is held in the rectum by muscular action until the anal sphincter opens to allow voluntary evacuation.

ENERGY METABOLISM

Metabolism is a broad term that is defined as the sum total of all chemical reactions that occur in living cells. *Energy metabolism* refers to how the body obtains and uses energy from the energy-yielding nutrients after they are absorbed—glucose from carbohydrate digestion, glycerol and fatty acids from fat digestion, and amino acids from protein digestion. It is a continuous process that includes energy-using reactions that build (*anabolism*) and energy-producing reactions that break down (*catabolism*). In a healthy adult, the rate of catabolism equals the rate of anabolism.

Anabolism occurs continuously in all people as cells or substances are replaced after normal wear and tear, and as excess nutrients are reassembled and stored for later use. Examples of anabolic reactions include glycogen synthesis from glucose, triglyceride synthesis from glycerol and fatty acids, and protein synthesis from amino acids. Accelerated anabolism occurs whenever the demand for new tissue is increased, such as during growth periods, pregnancy, and the anabolic phase that occurs after injury or illness.

Catabolism is the breakdown of large molecules into smaller ones for the purpose of releasing energy. *Oxidation* is an example of catabolism in which an electron is removed from a molecule, usually in the presence of oxygen, and usually resulting in energy release. Glucose is the body's preferred fuel for oxidation, but amino acids, glycerol, and fatty acids are also oxidized. Accelerated catabolism is an undesirable state that is marked by excessive breakdown; it may occur during starvation or during the acute period after injury or illness.

Energy for Cells

In order for cells to "work" (eg, transport ions, generate heat, synthesize chemical compounds, contract muscles), they need energy. All cells have an instant supply of energy stored in the form of **adenosine triphosphate (ATP)**. Chemically, ATP contains a purine (adenine), a sugar (ribose), and three phosphate molecules. The bonds between the phosphate molecules are considered to be high-energy bonds; they store a significant amount of the potential energy available in ATP. When energy is needed, a phosphate group splits from the ATP molecule, energy is released, and a new, lower-energy compound (adenosine diphosphate, or ADP) remains. Of the energy that is released by this reaction, half or more is lost through heat; this is why metabolism raises temperature. If necessary (eg, to maintain body temperature), ATP can release all of its energy as heat. In muscle cells, creatine phosphate also provides a limited supply of immediate energy to resynthesize ATP from ADP.

The **tricarboxylic acid (TCA) cycle** and the electron transport chain are the body's primary method of extracting energy from nutrients for storage in ATP molecules. The TCA or *Krebs' cycle* is a complex series of reactions during which acetyl coenzyme A (acetyl-CoA), a two-carbon compound, is broken down to carbon dioxide and hydrogen atoms. Reduced coenzymes (carrier molecules) transfer hydrogen to the **electron transport chain** (also known as *oxidative phosphorylation*), the final pathway in the release of energy. Through a complex series of reactions, hydrogen atoms oxidize, electrons are transferred to oxygen, and chemical energy is released. This chemical energy becomes trapped in the high-energy phosphate bonds of ATP: energy + a phosphate ion + ADP = ATP.

Of the three energy nutrients, fat generates the most calories (energy) when catabolized because it has the most hydrogen atoms and its bond are readily oxidized. For instance, 1 glucose molecule produces 36 molecules of ATP when fully oxidized. By comparison, one 18-carbon fatty acid molecule generates 147 ATP molecules when fully oxidized. Because triglycerides contain three fatty acids, 441 ATP molecules (147×3) are produced from the catabolism of the fatty acids in 1 triglyceride molecule. Add to that the 19 ATP molecules generated when the glycerol portion is catabolized, and the total amount of ATP generated through the breakdown of a single triglyceride molecule is 460 ($441 + 19 = 460$). Fats yield 9 cal/g, compared with 4 cal/g for carbohydrates and proteins. Vitamins and minerals do not provide energy, but they are constituents of many enzymes and cofactors involved in energy metabolism (Fig. 7-7).

The following illustrations highlight the details of catabolism presented in the energy nutrient chapters. Notice that all three energy nutrients enter the TCA cycle, albeit by different routes.

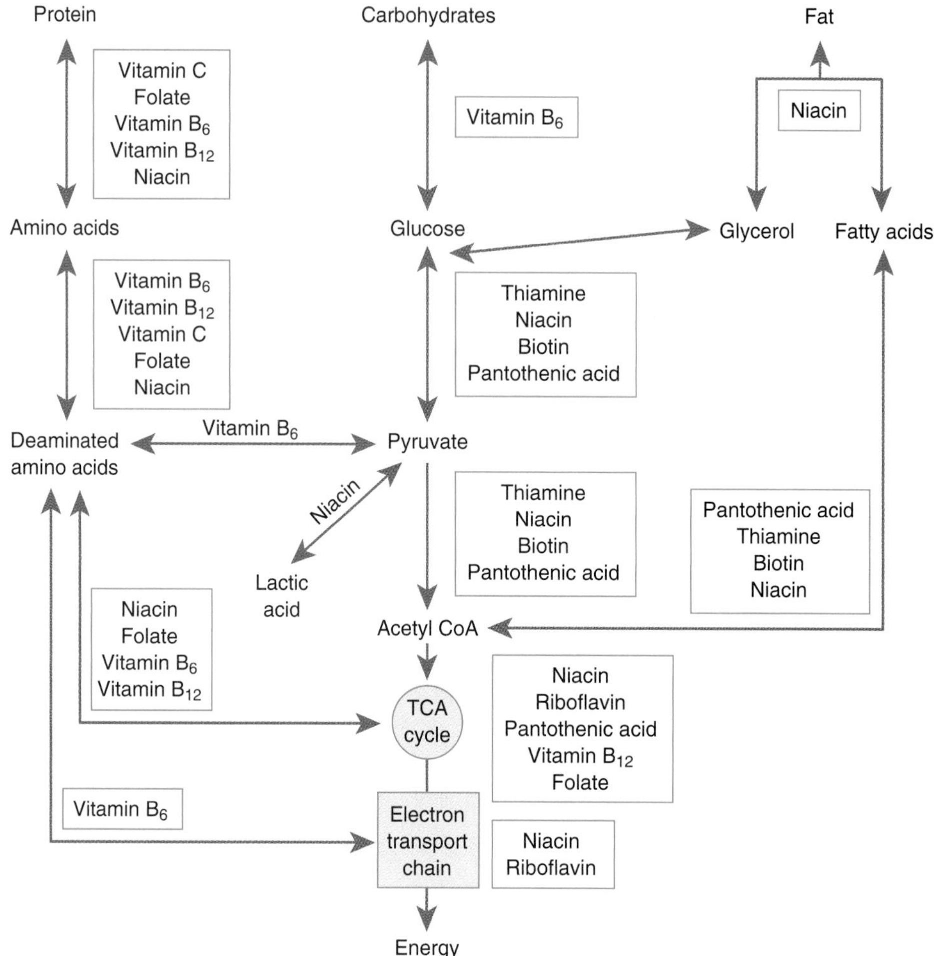

FIGURE 7-7 Vitamins involved in energy metabolism.

Energy From Glucose

Energy From Glucose

Step 1: Glucose catabolism begins with the anaerobic process of *glycolysis* (glucose splitting), in which the six-carbon molecule of glucose is broken down into two three-carbon molecules of pyruvate. Glycolysis produces only about 10% of the total energy available from glucose. Note that two pyruvate molecules (regardless of their original source) can be put back together to remake a gucose molecule, although the process isn't exactly reversible (other enzymes are needed). Glycolysis can provide the sole source of energy only briefly, because the supply of glucose is limited and because accumulated pyruvate is converted to lactate (lactic acid), which is ultimately deleterious.

(continued)

Energy From Glucose (continued)

Step 2: If the cell needs more energy and oxygen is available, aerobic catabolism continues as a carbon splits off from pyruvate. The two-carbon compound that remains combines with CoA, an enzyme, to form acetyl-CoA. (Notice the reaction from a three-carbon molecule to a two-carbon compound is irreversible: Two-carbon compounds cannot be made into glucose.) The carbon that split off joins with oxygen to form carbon dioxide, which is released into the blood and eventually exhaled through the lungs.

Step 3: Acetyl-CoA enters the TCA cycle, where it is degraded to carbon dioxide and hydrogen.

Step 4: The final step in oxidation, and the one that produces most of the energy, is the electron transport chain. Through a complex series of reactions, hydrogen atoms oxidize, electrons are transferred, and energy is captured and stored in ATP molecules.

Energy From Protein

Normally, the body uses little protein for energy as long as intake and storage of carbohydrate and fat are adequate. However, if insufficient carbohydrate and fat are available for energy use, or if protein is consumed in excessive amounts, amino acids are broken down for energy.

Energy From Protein*

Step 1: First the nitrogen-containing amino group is removed (deamination).

Step 2: Different amino acids are broken down differently: Some are converted to pyruvate, some to acetyl-CoA, and still others enter the TCA cycle directly. (Amino acids that can be converted to pyruvate can be used to synthesize glucose; therefore, a percentage of protein can be a source of glucose when carbohydrate is not available.)

*Ammonia is produced when amino nitrogen is removed from amino acids. In the liver, some of this ammonia is used in the synthesis of nonessential amino acids. The remaining ammonia combines with carbon dioxide to make urea, which is released into the blood. The body must excrete this waste product through the urine, losing water to do so. That is why high-portein, low-calorie diets cause rapid weight loss: The weight loss comes from fluid loss, not a decrease in fat tissue.

Energy From Fat

By weight, 95% of a typical fat molecule is fatty acids. Most fatty acids are composed of an even number of carbon atoms (4 to 24). The remaining 5% of fat is glycerol. Fatty acids and glycerol are catabolized differently in the body.

Energy From Fatty Acids*

Step 1: Through the process of *beta-oxidation,* fatty acids are split, two carbon atoms at a time, into two-carbon molecules that combine with CoA to form acetyl-CoA. For instance, the 18-carbon chain in the fatty acid linoleic acid is broken down into nine two-carbon molecules of

(continued)

Energy From Fatty Acids (continued)

acetyl-CoA. (It is important to note that because fatty acids are broken down into compounds containing two-carbon, not three-carbon atoms, they cannot be reformed into glucose.)

Step 2: Those acetyl-CoA molecules can then enter the TCA cycle and the electron transport chain.

*Under normal conditions, the liver produces small quantities of *ketone bodies* (acetoacetic acid and acetone) through fatty acid metabolism by condensing two molecules of CoA (*ketogenesis*). Ketones leave the liver, travel through the bloodstream, and diffuse into other body cells, where they are catabolized into CoA, which enters the TCA cycle. A higher than normal level of ketones in the blood (ketosis) occurs during starvation and periods of extremely low carbohydrate intake as the body uses fatty acids instead of glucose for energy. Beause ketones are mostly acidic, ketosis can lead to acidosis, an undesirable condition of abnormally low blood pH.

Energy From Glycerol

Glycerol (a three-carbon compound) is easily converted to pyruvate. From there, it can be oxidized through the TCA cycle and the electron transport chain. (By way of pyruvate, glycerol can be synthesized into glucose during times of need. But because it represents such a small portion of the total fat molecule, converting fat to glucose is extremely inefficient.)

Keys to Understanding the Body's Choice of Fuels

The previous section detailed how the body gets energy from carbohydrates, protein, and fat. The proportion of fuels actually used at any time depends on several variables, including energy intake (eg, the amount of time that has elapsed since the last meal) and energy output (eg, duration and intensity of physical activity).

FUEL AVAILABILITY: EATING AND FASTING

The body alternates between two metabolic states: absorptive (after eating) and postabsorptive (fasting). The absorptive phase, which occurs for about 4 hours after each meal, is the period during which nutrients that have been absorbed into the bloodstream and lymphatic system are used for energy. The postabsorptive phase is characterized by the breakdown of stored nutrients. For people who eat three meals per day, the amount of time spent in each state is about the same. Figure 7-8 depicts the anabolic and catabolic reactions summarized in the following paragraphs.

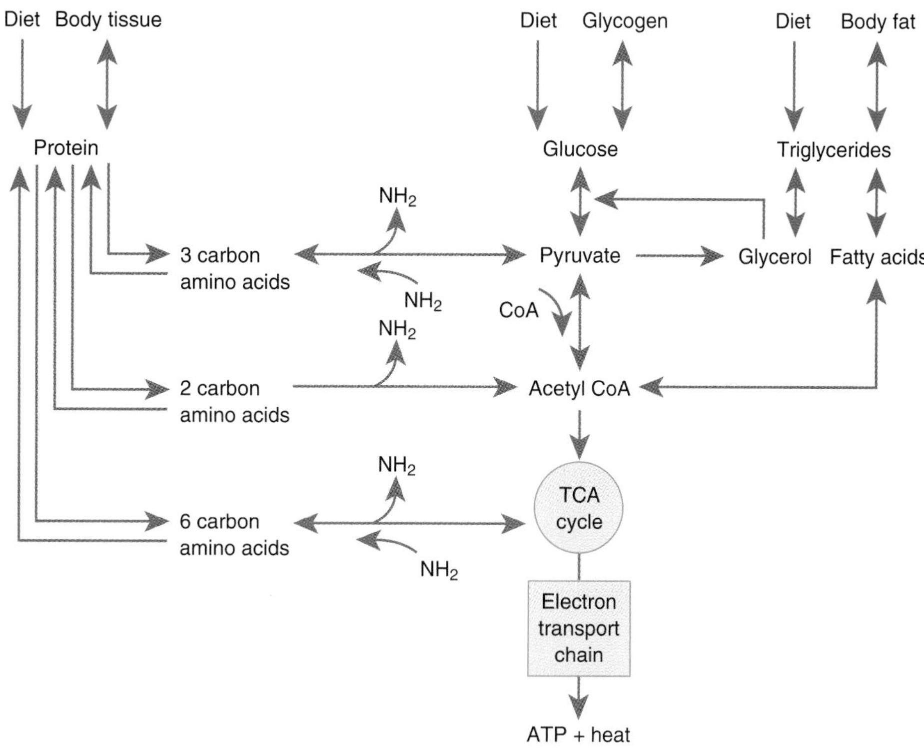

FIGURE 7-8 Summary of catabolic and anabolic reactions.

After Eating

Most of the glucose is catabolized in body cells to produce energy (ATP). Glucose that remains after energy needs are met is converted to glycogen and stored in the liver and muscle cells. Glycogen storage is limited, however, so any glucose that is left, in the form of acetyl-CoA molecules, is converted to fatty acids and stored as body fat.

The priority use for amino acids is to synthesize body proteins. If excess amino acids are eaten, or if not enough carbohydrates and fats have been consumed to meet energy needs, amino acids (stripped of their nitrogen) are catabolized to energy through several different pathways. If energy needs have been met, deaminated amino acids are converted, through the intermediates pyruvate and acetyl-CoA, to fatty acids for storage as body fat.

The glycerol portion of fat is broken down into pyruvate, which can enter the TCA cycle to produce energy, be synthesized into glucose, or be used to synthesize triglycerides for fat storage. The fatty acids are broken down into acetyl-CoA molecules, which enter the TCA cycle to produce energy. Any acetyl molecules not needed for energy are converted back to fatty acids, which combine with glycerol to form fat for storage.

The fate of each of the energy nutrients is the same when they are eaten in excess of need: regardless of which path they take to become acetyl-CoA molecules, they are ultimately converted to fatty acids, reformed into triglycerides, and stored as body fat. Over time an excessive calorie intake from any source causes an increase in body fat and consequent weight gain.

Fasting

The fasting state usually occurs during late morning, late afternoon, and most of the evening. During this time the body's energy needs are met by the breakdown of stored nutrients. Liver glycogen and fatty acids from fat storage are released into the bloodstream, where body cells catabolize them to produce energy. Triglycerides mobilized from storage account for the increase in the proportion of energy derived from fat. When glycogen stores are exhausted, usually within 4 hours or so, low blood glucose signals hunger; eating returns the body to the absorptive state.

If eating does not occur, because of either voluntary or involuntary fasting, fat breakdown continues. Most body cells can catabolize fatty acids for energy. The exceptions are cells of the brain and nerves, which normally rely exclusively on glucose for energy. During the first few days of a fast, brain and nerve cells obtain about 10% of the glucose they need from glycerol and the remaining 90% from the catabolism of body proteins, such as muscle and lean tissue. Although only certain amino acids can be converted to pyruvate and ultimately glucose, whole proteins must be broken down to make them available. The amino acids remaining from tissue breakdown that cannot be converted to glucose (ie, two-carbon molecules) are used for energy by other body cells. Breaking down body protein for energy is expensive; yet, compared to the small amount of glucose that is available from glycerol in stored triglycerides, it is more efficient. If protein catabolism were to continue at this rate, death would occur within 3 weeks, regardless of the amount of stored fat a person might have.

Fortunately, the body adapts to starvation in an attempt to conserve body protein. Some brain cells are able to use ketone bodies, derived from fatty acid catabolism, for energy. Ketone production increases to meet demand, and after several weeks of fasting about two thirds or more of the nervous system's energy requirements are supplied by ketones. However, many brain cells are unable to convert to ketone use, so some body protein catabolism continues.

Another adaptive mechanism that occurs during prolonged fasting is a reduction in energy requirement. The loss of muscle and lean tissue lowers the metabolic rate (the amount of calories used for involuntary activities, including maintenance of muscle mass). The loss of muscle also means that work capacity is lessened, so energy expenditure from physical activity declines. Hormonal changes that occur with fasting slow metabolism in an attempt to preserve life by conserving lean body mass. The ultimate result of lowered metabolism is that *fat tissue* is conserved, even though *weight loss* (due to protein loss) may be significant. In fact, because of the lowered metabolic rate, less body fat is lost during fasting than during a low-calorie diet.

In long-term fasting, fatty acids supply about 90% of total energy requirements. If adequate fluids are consumed, a normal-weight person can survive up to 60 days before fat stores are exhausted. After that, protein catabolism quickly accelerates, and death follows.

FUEL FOR ACTIVITY: AEROBIC AND ANAEROBIC METABOLISM

The body's energy needs are always met with a mixture of fuels. At rest that mixture is about 35% carbohydrate, about 60% fat, and about 2% to 5% amino acids. During activity, the mix of fuels used is constantly changing in response to the duration and intensity of the exercise. Other factors, such as the individual's fitness level and usual diet, also influence the proportion of nutrients used.

Exercise Fuel

The immediate fuel of muscle cells when activity begins is the energy trapped in ATP, of which every cell has a small supply. Because half or more of the energy released is lost as heat, exercise has an immediate warming effect. Muscle cells also use creatine phosphate, a high-energy compound, to augment the supply of ATP. Neither ATP nor creatine phosphate is dependent on the availability of oxygen. However, the supply of creatine phosphate is small, and if the activity lasts longer than 10 to 20 seconds, another source of fuel is needed.

During the first few minutes of exercise, when oxygen has not yet arrived at the muscles, stored muscle glycogen is the primary fuel; it generates energy through anaerobic glycolysis. As exercise continues, glucose from liver glycogen is released and picked up by muscle cells for their use. After several minutes, the body shifts to aerobic metabolism as increased breathing increases the supply of oxygen. The body can quickly alternate between aerobic and anaerobic metabolism as the supply of oxygen changes.

For activities lasting longer than a few minutes, the mixture of fuels used depends on the intensity and duration of the exercise (Table 7-1). In general:

- **As the intensity of activity increases, the proportion of glucose used increases,** because glucose is the only fuel that can be burned anaerobically (without oxygen).
- **As the duration of activity increases, the proportion of fat used increases.** At the onset of moderate exercise fueled aerobically, muscle glycogen serves as the primary source of energy. After 20 minutes, the proportion of fat used increases to 50% to 60% of the total in an attempt to conserve glycogen. (However, glycogen

TABLE 7.1 *Fuels Used in Various Activities*

Intensity Level	Types of Activity	Predominate Fuel
Low	Leisurely walking, ballroom dancing	Mostly fat
Moderate	Hiking	Mostly fat, some carbohydrate (after first 20 minutes)
High	Running, cycling	Mostly carbohydrate, some fat
Very high	Sprinting	Carbohydrate (anaerobic)

use continues, and if the activity is intense enough and lasts long enough, glycogen stores become depleted.) Likewise, the fuel source used in high-intensity endurance events such as marathons is a mixture of fat and glucose, whereas that used in high-intensity short-duration activities is almost exclusively glucose.

- **Physically fit people have a higher aerobic capacity, allowing them to use more fat and spare more glycogen.** Fat can be used for energy only when adequate oxygen is available. Regular aerobic exercise for at least 20 to 30 minutes, three times per week, improves heart and lung capacity, which increases oxygen delivery to muscle cells, allowing for more aerobic metabolism. It also stimulates muscle cells to produce more structures within the cell in which aerobic metabolism takes place (mitochondria), thereby increasing the rate of energy synthesis. Furthermore, trained muscles are able to store more glycogen and are better at conserving glycogen because they are able to rely more on fat for energy.

Anaerobic Metabolism

To extract all the available energy, nutrients must undergo complete oxidation by way of the TCA cycle and the electron transport chain. Both pathways are aerobic, meaning that oxygen—obtained through deep, regular breathing—is required. However, sometimes oxygen is not available, at least not quickly enough or in large enough supply, as in the case of intense bursts of activity or prolonged exercise. What happens then is anaerobic metabolism (glycolysis), the body's attempt to keep things moving when you can't "catch your breath."

During moderate aerobic exercise, a trained heart and circulatory system can adequately meet the muscles' demand for oxygen. However, when conditioning is less than optimal, or when activity is intense or prolonged, the heart and lungs cannot supply adequate oxygen quickly enough to maintain aerobic metabolism. When this occurs, muscles switch from using a glucose/fat mix to using only glucose, because it is the only fuel that can be metabolized anaerobically, albeit incompletely. Fat can be broken down for energy only when oxygen is present; in fact, more oxygen is needed to catabolize fat than glucose.

In anaerobic metabolism, glucose is broken down into pyruvate, but pyruvate catabolism cannot continue without oxygen. Instead, pyruvate accumulates, which stimulates the heart and lungs to work harder. If there is a break in the action, the increase in breathing (and therefore oxygen) allows the body to switch back to aerobic metabolism and catabolize pyruvate through the TCA cycle (aerobically). Without adequate oxygen, the accumulated pyruvate is transformed into lactic acid, which accumulates until adequate oxygen becomes available.

The accumulation of lactic acid is deleterious: It is responsible for the burning-type pain in muscles and can quickly lead to muscle exhaustion if it is not carried away by the blood. To avoid problems with lactic acid accumulation, it is necessary to rest periodically, to breathe deeply, and, most importantly, to increase the level of fitness.

Glycogen Depletion

The average lean, 150-pound man has 60,000 to 100,000 calories stored as fat. However, muscles cannot rely exclusively on fat for fuel; they need a certain amount of carbohydrate to function at any intensity. Even when muscles receive adequate oxygen and, therefore, have the ability to tap into the immense energy reserve available in fat, the depletion of muscle glycogen causes fatigue and threatens activity. So, regardless of how much fat a person has stored, the amount of carbohydrate in storage (glycogen) is the limiting factor in intense and endurance activities.

The average 150-pound man has approximately 1800 carbohydrate calories available, as follows:

Stored Carbohydrate	Calories
Muscle glycogen	1400
Liver glycogen	320
Blood glucose	80
Total	1800

Glycogen stored in muscles is not released into the bloodstream for the benefit of all cells but instead is used as a private stockpile of fuel by muscles. When exertion causes muscle glycogen depletion, athletes experience "hitting the wall," the overwhelming feeling of fatigue, muscle pain, and the inability to continue due to the exhaustion of muscle glycogen.

Liver glycogen breaks down to glucose and is released into the blood to maintain blood levels and to provide additional fuel for muscles. The proportion of glucose used by muscles from liver glycogen becomes increasingly larger as muscle glycogen becomes depleted. Eventually, the supply of blood glucose is unable to keep up with the demand for glucose by muscles, causing blood glucose levels to fall. When this occurs, athletes are said to "bonk" or "crash." The lack of adequate brain fuel impairs both physical and mental abilities, causing decreased muscle coordination, lightheadedness, inability to concentrate, and decreased exercise intensity.

Eating for Energy

Diet has a significant impact on physical performance during endurance events. Well-trained muscles regularly fed a high-carbohydrate diet can adequately replenish glycogen stores and improve overall athletic performance. The appropriate mix of fuels and fluid consumed before during competition and long-distance events maintains blood glucose levels to prevent fatigue. Adequate carbohydrate calories eaten after competition hastens glycogen replenishment. Therefore what is eaten in the long term and in the short term influences physical performance.

- **To have enough energy, you must eat enough energy (calories).** Actual calorie requirements depend on body weight, the level of fitness, and the intensity, duration, and frequency of activity. A 90-pound gymnast may require 2000 cal daily; a 350-pound football player may need more than 5000 cal daily. Too few calories means not enough energy and impaired performance. In addition, calorie needs change as training progresses, owing to changes in body composition: An increase in muscle mass raises metabolism and increases calorie needs.
- **Concentrate on carbohydrates.** Athletes are encouraged to eat 60% to 70% of total calories from carbohydrates to ensure that glycogen stores are replenished and to maximize overall athletic performance. A threshold of 500 to 800 g of carbohydrate (2000–3200 cal), regardless of total calorie intake, may be necessary to maintain maximum glycogen stores in athletes.
- **Know the difference between "quick" and "slow" carbohydrates.** A food's **glycemic index** is a measure of how quickly blood glucose levels rise after the food is eaten. High-glycemic foods—such as Gatorade, baked potatoes, cornflakes, rice cakes, jelly beans, Cheerios, and graham crackers—are best eaten during or after exercise, because they quickly release energy into the bloodstream. Low- and moderate-glycemic foods—such as bananas, yogurt, oranges, apples, pears, milk, and legumes—release energy more slowly and are desirable before exercise because they provide sustained energy.
- **Consume glucose periodically during exercise that lasts 1 hour or longer.** Drinking diluted fruit juice or other sweetened beverages helps maintain blood glucose levels and allows exercise to continue even as glycogen stores are becoming depleted.
- **Eat carbohydrate-rich foods and beverages within 15 minutes after a long workout or competition.** Enzymes responsible for making glycogen are most active immediately after exercise, and they most rapidly replenish the depleted glycogen stores when they are fed carbohydrates. A goal is to eat at least 200 to 400 carbohydrate calories as soon as tolerable after exercise, and then again 2 hours later. Eating larger amounts of carbohydrates does not hasten the recovery process. Because appetite may be suppressed after a vigorous workout, beverages may be preferred. Options include:

2 pieces of fruit (eg, banana, orange, apple)
12 oz of fruit juice (eg, orange, apple) or fruit juice cocktail (eg, cranberry)
1 cup of grapes and 1 bagel
1 cup nonfat frozen yogurt topped with 1 cup fresh fruit

- **Keep it low in fat.** Fat calories should contribute 30% of total calories or less. Most people—even lean, trained athletes—have abundant energy reserves stored in fat tissue. Because they leave the stomach slowly and can cause stomach upset, high-fat foods should be avoided before athletic events.

- **Moderate protein is adequate.** Athletes need 1.0 to 1.5 g protein per kilogram of body weight, higher than the Recommended Dietary Allowance of 0.8 g/kg. The need is increased because athletes retain more protein in exercising muscles and because some types of athletes use more amino acids for fuel. However, this amount of protein can easily be obtained from a balanced, varied diet. Eating adequate protein is secondary to consuming adequate carbohydrates.
- **Extra fluid is essential.** Fluid helps cool the body when it evaporates from the skin as sweat. Without adequate fluid, dehydration develops and impairs athletic performance and endurance. Because athletes need fluid before they actually experience thirst, they are urged to drink fluids before, during, and after exercise. The following guidelines are for endurance exercise:

Time	Action
2 h before activity	Drink at least 2 cups of fluid
15–20 min before activity	Drink 2 more cups of fluid every 15 min
During activity (in hot and humid environments)	Drink ½ to ¾ cup of fluid
After activity	Drink 2 cups of fluid for every pound of weight lost

- **Vitamin and mineral supplements are generally not needed.** Vitamins and minerals play important roles in energy metabolism and muscle function. Although physical activity increases the need for some vitamins and minerals, a varied diet that is high in carbohydrate, moderate in protein, and low in fat typically provides adequate amounts. People who have marginal intakes of vitamins and minerals from foods may benefit from supplements. Supplements do not improve athletic performance in people who obtain adequate amounts of nutrients through food.
- **Limit pregame meals to foods that are easily digested.** Meals should be eaten no closer than 3 to 5 hours before a competition, to allow time for gastric emptying. Liquids empty faster than solids, and carbohydrates faster than proteins or fats. Between 300 and 800 calories of familiar foods or liquids should be consumed. High-fiber foods, such as bran cereals, legumes, and raw vegetables, may cause discomfort and should be avoided.

Carbohydrate Loading

Endurance athletes—those who exercise for 90 minutes or longer—can maximize muscle glycogen storage and improve endurance capacity through a technique known as carbohydrate loading. By coordinating food intake with training and rest, athletes are able to increase muscle glycogen storage from 1.7 to between 4 and 5 g per 100 g of muscle.

The original format for carbohydrate loading began with exhausting exercise to deplete muscle glycogen stores, followed by a low-carbohydrate diet for 3 days, then 3 days of a high-carbohydrate diet to supersaturate the muscles with glycogen. Because research has since shown that the depletion phase offers no benefits, a modified routine has evolved that eliminates that step. The newer approach, which is said to be just as effective as the old method in maximizing glycogen storage, is to:

- Regularly consume a high-carbohydrate diet.
- Train moderately hard for approximately 90 minutes on the sixth day before a long-distance event, then gradually reduce the amount of time spent exercising each day thereafter.
- During the first 3 days of this 6-day period, eat approximately 50% of total calories from carbohydrates, then increase carbohydrate intake to 70% of total calories for the last 3 days before a competition.

Note that this method is potentially useful only for intense, long-distance events, not for activities lasting less than 90 minutes.

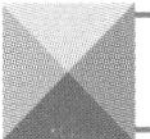

Keys to Understanding the Body's Energy Requirements

The National Research Council has set average energy intake allowances based on the assumption of light to moderate activity (Table 7-2). As averages, they may not accurately reflect *an individual's* actual calorie requirements. A more precise estimate of total energy requirements in a specific individual can be determined by calculating and adding the amount of the amount of energy spent on (1) basal metabolism, (2) the thermic effect of food, and (3) physical activity.

BASAL METABOLISM

The basal (baseline) metabolism is the amount of calories required to fuel the involuntary activities of the body at rest after a 12-hour fast. These involuntary activities include maintaining body temperature and muscle tone, producing and releasing secretions, propelling the gastrointestinal tract, inflating the lungs, and beating the heart. **Basal metabolic rate (BMR) or basal energy expendiure (BEE)** is the rate at which the body burns calories to sustain itself. It differs only slightly from **resting energy expenditure (REE)** in that REE does not adhere to the criterion of a 12-hour fast and therefore includes the energy spent on digesting, absorbing, and metabolizing food. In practice, BMR and REE are often used interchangeably. Table 7-3 gives equations for predicting REE from body weight.

A rule-of-thumb guideline for calculating BMR is to multiply healthy weight (in pounds) by 10 for women and 11 for men. For example, a 130-pound woman expends approximately 1300 cal/day on BMR:

$$130 \text{ lb} \times 10 \text{ cal/lb} = 1300 \text{ cal}$$

TABLE 7.2 ***Median Heights and Weights and Recommended Energy Intake***

Category	Age (y) or Condition	Weight (kg)	Weight (lb)	Height (cm)	Height (in)	REE* (kcal/day)	Average Energy Allowance (kcal)†		
							Multiples of Ree	*per kg*	*per day*‡
Infants	0.0–0.5	6	13	60	24	320		108	650
	0.5–1.0	9	20	71	28	500		98	850
Children	1–3	13	29	90	35	740		102	1300
	4–6	20	44	112	44	950		90	1800
	7–10	28	62	132	52	1130		70	2000
Men	11–14	45	99	157	62	1440	1.70	55	2500
	15–18	66	145	176	69	1760	1.67	45	3000
	19–24	72	160	177	70	1780	1.67	40	2900
	25–50	79	174	176	70	1800	1.60	37	2900
	51+	77	170	173	68	1530	1.50	30	2300
Women	11–14	46	101	157	62	1310	1.67	47	2200
	15–18	55	120	163	64	1370	1.60	40	2200
	19–24	58	128	164	65	1350	1.60	38	2200
	25–50	63	138	163	64	1380	1.55	36	2200
	51+	65	143	160	63	1280	1.50	30	1900
Pregnant	1st trimester								+0
	2nd trimester								+300
	3rd trimester								+300
Lactating	1st 6 months								+500
	2nd 6 months								+500

*Calculation of REE (resting energy expenditure) based on Food and Agriculture Organization equations, then rounded.

†In the range of light to moderate activity, the coefficient of variation is ±20%.

‡Figure is rounded.

From National Research Council. (1989). *Recommended Dietary Allowances* (10th ed.). Washington, DC: National Academy of Sciences.

Unless physical activity is unusually high, BMR accounts for 60% to 70% of total energy requirements in most people. The less active a person is, the greater the proportion of calories used for BMR.

BMR is influenced by numerous factors, especially body composition. Lean tissue (muscle mass) requires more calories for maintenance (ie, contributes to a higher metabolic rate) than does fat tissue. Therefore, people with more lean body compositions have higher metabolic rates than do people with proportionately more fat tissue. This explains why men (who have a greater proportion of muscle) have higher metabolic rates than women (who have a greater proportion of fat) and why metabolism is relatively high among growing children, physically active people, and pregnant women. Conversely, the loss of lean tissue that usually occurs progressively after the age of 35 years is one reason why energy requirements decrease as people get older. However, the loss of lean tissue is

TABLE 7.3 ***Equations for Predicting Resting Energy Expenditure From Body Weight****

Sex and Age Range (y)	Equation to Derive REE in kcal/day	Sex and Age Range (y)	Equation to Derive REE in kcal/day
Men		**Women**	
0–3	(60.9 × wt) – 54	0–3	(61.0 × wt) – 51
3–10	(22.7 × wt) + 495	3–10	(22.5 × wt) + 499
10–18	(17.5 × wt) + 651	10–18	(12.2 × wt) + 746
18–30	(15.3 × wt) + 679	18–30	(14.7 × wt) + 496
30–60	(11.6 × wt) + 879	30–60	(8.7 × wt) + 829
>60	(13.5 × wt) + 487	>60	(10.5 × wt) + 596

*According to the World Health Organization (1985). These equations are derived from data on basal metabolism rate (wt = weight in kilograms).

From National Research Council. (1989). *Recommended Dietary Allowances* (10th ed). Washington, DC: National Academy of Sciences.

not an inevitable consequence of aging; strength training exercises can maintain or restore muscle mass at any age.

Other factors that affect BMR include:

- **Hormones.** The thyroid gland secretes two active hormones that regulate BMR: **tetraiodothyronine (thyroxine,** or T_4) and **triiodothyronine** (T_3).

  When the body oversecretes thyroid hormones (hyperthyroidism), metabolism speeds up, often causing dramatic weight loss even though appetite is ravenous and food intake is high. BMR may increase by 15% to 25% in mild cases and up to 50% to 75% in severe cases. A rapid metabolic rate causes nervousness; decreased attention span; increased pulse rate, palpitations, and increased systolic blood pressure; intolerance to heat and profuse perspiration; and diarrhea or constipation. Drug therapy, radiation, or surgical removal of part or all of the thyroid gland is needed to treat hyperthyroidism.

  When the body's production of thyroid hormones is inadequate (hypothyroidism), the rate of metabolism slows, often by 15% to 30% or more. Significant weight gain occurs despite calorie restriction. Other symptoms of a slowed metabolism include fatigue, decreased body temperature, and pulse rate; physical and mental slowness; constipation; and an intolerance to cold. Hypothyroidism is responsible for only a small percentage of obesity.
- **Fever.** Metabolism increases 7% for each degree Fahrenheit above 98.6.
- **Body size.** When considering two people of the same gender who weigh the same, the taller one has a higher metabolic rate than the shorter one because of a larger surface area.
- **Environmental temperature.** Very hot and very cold environmental temperatures increase the metabolic rate because the body expends more energy to regulate its own temperature.

- **Starvation, fasting, and malnutrition.** Part of the decline in BMR that occurs with these conditions is attributed to the loss of lean body tissue. Hormonal changes may contribute to the decrease in metabolic rate.
- **Stress.** Stress hormones raise the metabolic rate.
- **Certain drugs,** such as barbiturates, narcotics, and muscle relaxants, decrease the metabolic rate, as does sleep and paralysis.

THERMIC EFFECT OF FOOD

The **thermic effect of food** is an estimation of the amount of energy required to digest, absorb, transport, metabolize, and store nutrients. In a normal mixed diet, the "cost" of processing food is estimated to be about 10% of the total calorie intake. For instance, people who consume 1800 cal/day use about 180 cal to process their food. The actual thermic effect of food varies with the composition of food eaten, the frequency of eating, and the size of meals consumed. Although it represents an actual and legitimate use of calories, the thermic effect of food in practice is usually disregarded when calorie requirements are estimated because it constitutes such a small amount of energy and is imprecisely estimated.

PHYSICAL ACTIVITY

Physical activity, or voluntary muscular activity, represents the second largest contributor to total energy expenditure, usually accounting for 25% to 30% of total calories used. Compared with the other components of energy expenditure (metabolic rate and the thermic effect of food), physical activity is the biggest variable on total calorie expenditure. Since the turn of the century, calorie expenditure on physical activity has declined for most Americans as a result of the increase in mechanization and the proliferation of labor-saving devices. Today Americans use less energy at work and also at leisure. The actual amount of energy that is expended on physical activity depends on the intensity and duration of the activity and the weight of the person performing the activity. The more intense and longer the activity, the greater the amount of calories burned. Heavier people, who have more weight to move, use more energy than lighter people to perform the same activity.

A rule-of-thumb guideline for estimating daily calories expended on physical activity is to calculate the percent increase above BMR based on the intensity of usual activity. Multiply calories used for BMR by:

- 20% if you are sedentary (mainly sitting, driving, lying down, standing, reading, typing, or other low-intensity activities)
- 30% for light activity, such as walking no more than 2 hours daily
- 40% for moderate activity, such as heavy housework, gardening, dancing, and very little sitting

- 50% for high activity, such as active physical sports or labor-intensive occupations (eg, construction work, ditch digging)

For example, a 130-pound woman who is lightly active expends 390 cal on physical activity:

1300 cal for BMR × 0.30 for light activity = 390 cal for physical activity

Box 7-1 describes the steps to estimating your own calorie requirements.

BOX 7.1

Estimating Total Calorie Expenditure

1. **Estimate basal metabolic rate**
   Multiply your healthy weight (in pounds) by 10 for women or 11 for men. If you are overweight, multiply by the average weight within your healthy weight range (see Chapter 14).
   _____ (weight in pounds) × _____ = __________ calories for BMR
2. **Estimate calories expended on physical activity**
   Choose the category that describes your usual activities.

Multiply BMR by	For this type of usual activity
0.20	Sedentary: mostly sitting, driving, sleeping, standing, reading, typing, other low-intensity activities
0.30	Light activity: light exercise, such as walking not more than 2 h/d
0.40	Moderate activity: moderate exercise, such as heavy housework, gardening, and very little sitting
0.50	High activity: active in physical sports or a labor-intensive occupation, such as construction work

   ____ (calories for BMR) × ____ (calories for activity level)
   = _____ total calories expended on physical activity
3. **Estimate the thermic effect of food**
   This figure is approximately 10% of calories consumed, which in people who are maintaining their weight is approximately equivalent to 10% of calories expended.
   [____ (BMR calories) + ____ (calories for activity)] × .10
   = _____ calories for thermic effect of food
4. **Calculate total calories expended**
   ____ (calories for BMR) + ____ (calories for activity)
   + ____ (calories for thermic effect) = ____ total calories expended daily

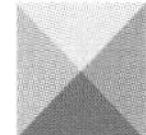

Energy in Health Promotion

The terms *activity, exercise, and fitness* are frequently used interchangeably, but they have very different meanings. **Physical activity** is voluntary muscular activity that results in energy expenditure. Washing your face is a physical activity, but it is not exercise. **Exercise** is a structured and repetitive physical activity done to improve or maintain one or more aspects of physical fitness. Running is both a physical activity and exercise. **Physical fitness** refers to a person's ability to perform physical activity. A person who is physically fit has a high level of capacity in each of three areas: cardiorespiratory endurance, muscular endurance and strength, and flexibility.

For most Americans, the topic of energy focuses on becoming more active. According to the 1996 Surgeon General's report *Physical Activity and Health*, approximately 54% of American adults are intermittently active but do not receive the recommended amount of physical activity. Twenty-four percent are classified as completely sedentary; at the other end of the spectrum are exercise enthusiasts whose focus is optimal fitness; and in the middle are people who look to exercise as a means to lose or maintain weight. This section discusses these three approaches to activity and exercise. The use of "fat-burning" supplements, promoted to both "dieters" and athletes, is addressed.

THE HEALTH BENEFITS APPROACH: INCREASE ACTIVITY

At one time, exercise recommendations were inflexible and focused exclusively on promoting optimal fitness. Mathematical calculations, a stopwatch, and a high level of dedication were part of the "go for the burn" and "no pain, no gain" philosophy of exercise. That approach eliminated options for the many sedentary people who were intimidated or overwhelmed by the thought of adopting a rigid and rigorous exercise program. Health experts have softened their approach to exercise in view of evidence that significant health benefits can be gained when sedentary people simply become more active on a regular basis and that increasing activity may be the vital first step in becoming physically fit. Today, activity and exercise recommendations are tailored to the individual client's objective—whether to reap health benefits, to manage weight, or to increase physical fitness.

The Benefits

Crossing the threshold from being sedentary to being moderately active on a regular basis improves health and well-being. The benefits of activity occur along a continuum: a modest amount of activity is enough to reduce the risk of several chronic diseases, and further exercise improves overall physical fitness. In short, doing something is better than doing nothing, and doing more is even better.

Subjectively, regular activity performed on most days of the week provides pleasure, improves productivity, instills a sense of accomplishment, increases creativity, relieves stress, and makes people feel more energetic. Objectively, activity increases bone strength, improves serum cholesterol, lowers blood pressure, relieves stiffness related to osteoarthritis, and stimulates metabolism. Improved sleep quality, improved immune system functioning, and reduced levels of body fat occur. These benefits translate to lowered risk of (or improvements in) cardiovascular disease, hypertension, type 2 diabetes, obesity, osteoporosis, depression, infection, and colon cancer. Both quality and length of life are enhanced by increasing activity.

Target Population for the Health Benefits Approach to Activity

The vast majority of American adults are classified as either "inactive" or "not regularly active." It is these people for whom the health benefits approach to activity is most suited. Other target groups include the elderly and seriously obese people, because the risks of injury and soreness with this approach are less than those of more aggressive programs. Also, as a less structured and less vigorous approach than one aimed at physical fitness, it is less likely to overwhelm people who are not accustomed to exercising. Simply stated, it is "doable." To reiterate, any activity is better than no activity.

Recommendations for Increasing Activity

To obtain health benefits that reduce the risk of chronic disease, it is recommended that the client:

- **Find some enjoyable activity.** The best chance of success comes from choosing activities that are enjoyable to the individual. The best activity or exercise is one that is done, not just contemplated.
- **Participate in at least 30 minutes of low- to moderate-intensity physical activity on most or all days of the week.** "Moderate" activity is defined as activity that uses approximately 150 cal/day or 1000 cal/week. Moderate athletic activities include walking (at 3–4 mph), swimming (with moderate effort), light calisthenics, hiking or backpacking, canoeing leisurely, horseback riding, and ice skating. Moderate activities of daily living include mopping floors, ironing, raking leaves, washing the car by hand, cleaning windows, and grocery shopping.
- **Spread activity over the entire day if desired.** This recommendation is particularly important for people who "don't have time to exercise." Many people find it easier to fit three 10-minute activity periods into a busy lifestyle than to find 30 uninterrupted minutes to dedicate to activity.
- **Start slowly and gradually increase activity.** A modest pace decreases the risks of soreness, injury, and failure. People with existing health problems such as diabetes, heart disease, and hypertension should consult a physician before beginning a physical activity program, as should all men older than 40 and all women older than 50 years of age.
- **Move more.** Just moving more can make a cumulative difference in activity. Take the stairs instead of the elevator, park at the far end of the parking lot, walk

around while talking on the portable phone, walk instead of driving short distances, play golf without a golf cart or caddy.

- **Up the ante.** After establishing a consistent activity routine, gradually increase the duration, intensity, and frequency. Adding more vigorous activities or exercises, such as brisk walking, cycling, or active recreational sports, moves people from the health benefits approach toward the direction of achieving physical fitness. See Table 7-4 for calories expended on select activities.

Nutritional Considerations for Increasing Activity

Sound nutrition and regular physical activity are synergistic components of a healthy lifestyle: practiced together, their overall impact on health and well-being is greater than when either is practiced alone. Both components rely on the same basic principles:

- **Variety.** Variety in food choices maximizes the likelihood of obtaining enough of all the good things available in food while minimizing the likelihood of nutrient toxicity or accidental contamination.

  Variety in activity reduces the risk of boredom and increases the likelihood that a greater variety of muscles will be used. For instance, the workload on muscles is different for walking compared with golfing or swimming.
- **Moderation.** Moderate food choices enable people to enjoy occasional food "indulgences" within the context of a healthy eating plan.

  Moderate activity provides health benefits without the need for more intense exercise. Moderation also implies a regular pattern, rather than alternating periods of inactivity and overactivity.
- **Balance.** Balanced food choices means that high-fat foods are balanced with low-fat selections and that serving sizes are in balance with those recommended in the Food Guide Pyramid (see Chapter 8).

  Balance in activity means that activities that promote cardiovascular fitness are balanced with activities that promote flexibility and those that increase muscular strength.

THE OPTIMAL FITNESS APPROACH

Although increasing activity provides health benefits, optimal fitness is needed to achieve maximum disease prevention benefits. Optimal fitness, as evidenced by a high level of cardiorespiratory endurance, muscular strength/endurance, and flexibility, is achieved by regularly participating in diverse exercises. Different exercises target different areas of fitness, so a variety of exercises is required for optimal overall fitness. Those people who are most interested in achieving optimal fitness exercise regularly and are highly motivated.

Cardiorespiratory Endurance: Aerobic Exercise

Cardiorespiratory endurance, or aerobic fitness, is the foundation of physical fitness that refers to the body's ability to pump oxygen-rich blood to the muscles. Aerobic fitness is achieved through aerobic or endurance exercises that (1) use large muscles of the body,

TABLE 7.4 *The Amount of Calories Expended per Minute Based on Activity and Weight*

Activity	Cal/Min	
	70-kg Men	*58-kg Women*
Sleeping, reclining	1.0–1.2	0.9–1.1
Very light activity: seated and standing activities, painting, auto and truck driving, laboratory work, typing, playing musical instruments, sewing, ironing, walking slowly	Up to 2.5	Up to 2.0
Light activity: level walking at 2.5 mph to 3 mph, tailoring, pressing, garage work, electrical trades, carpentry, restaurant trades, cannery workers, washing clothes, shopping with light load, golfing, sailing, table tennis, volleyball	2.5–4.9	2.0–3.9
Moderate activity: walking 3.5 mph to 4 mph, plastering, gardening, loading and stacking bales, scrubbing floors, shopping with heavy load, cycling, skiing, tennis, dancing	5.0–7.4	4.0–5.9
Heavy activity: walking with load uphill, tree felling, working with pick and shovel, basketball, swimming, climbing, football, jogging, chopping wood	7.5–12.0	6.0–10.0

From: Previte J. J.: Human Physiology. New York: McGraw-Hill, 1983.

especially the leg muscles, (2) are performed relatively continuously over a period of time, (3) are rhythmic in nature, and (4) elevate the heart rate. Aerobic exercises require endurance, not power.

To condition the heart and lungs, the American College of Sports Medicine recommends 20 to 60 minutes of continuous movement performed 3 to 5 days per week at a target heart rate zone equal to 60% to 90% of the maximum heart rate (for people who are accustomed to exercising and are striving for optimal fitness) or a target heart rate zone equal to 50% to 75% of the maximum heart rate (for unconditioned or sedentary people). The **maximum heart rate** is approximately 220 minus the person's age. The **target heart rate zone** is found by multiplying the target percentages by the maximum heart rate. For example, a 30-year-old client wishes to exercise at a target rate of 50% to 75%:

Step 1: Calculate maximum heart rate (beats/min)

$$220 - 30 = 190$$

Step 2: Calculate 75% of maximum heart rate as the target

$$190 \times 0.75 = 142.5$$

Step 3: From the beats per minute calculate the number of beats in 10 sec

$$143 \div 6 = \text{approximately } 24$$

This provides the upper limit of the target heart rate zone. A similar calculation is made to identify the 50% target rate. The number of pulse beats in 10 seconds can then be used by the client during exercise to determine whether the heart rate is within the target zone.

Examples of aerobic exercises (when done for more than 20 minutes) are bicycling (stationary or touring), jogging at a brisk pace, jumping rope at a brisk pace, ice skating or roller skating, cross-country skiing, steady-paced swimming, and brisk walking.

Muscular Strength and Endurance: Strength Training

Muscular strength refers to the ability to exert force, as in lifting baskets of laundry, pushing furniture, or carrying heavy backpacks. Muscular endurance is judged by how long any given muscle activity can be sustained. People who have muscular endurance can sit, stand, or walk for relatively long periods without becoming fatigued. Both muscular strength and endurance are improved with moderate-intensity strength training exercises.

Strength training exercises are short, intense exercises that require power and coordination but less endurance than aerobic exercises. Strength training involves contracting muscles a few times against a heavy load (eg, lifting free weights, using a machine, moving one's own body). Exposing the muscle to heavier loads than those to which it is normally accustomed provides a stimulus for muscle growth.

As discussed earlier, the less muscle a person has, the fewer calories are burned at rest; conversely, building muscle helps manage weight because it raises the metabolic rate. Also, all people lose muscle with age if they do not build muscle. Even aerobically fit marathon runners lose muscle mass as they age if they do not do strength training exercises. Over time, the loss of muscle lessens strength and impairs a person's ability to perform activities of daily living. All people can benefit from strength training exercises regardless of age or level of aerobic fitness.

The American College of Sports Medicine recommends the following:

- Do strength training exercises two times a week.
- Do 8–10 exercises working the major muscle groups.
- Do 8–12 continuous repetitions of the same exercise for at least 1 set.
- Use proper form and perform each exercise done through the full range of motion.
- Begin with light weights and increase gradually; select a weight that makes it hard to do more than two or three sets.
- Maintain normal breathing; lift and lower at a slow, controlled pace.

Flexibility: Stretching

Stretching improves flexibility, or the ease and extent of the range of motion through which your body is able to move. Choose stretching exercises that help maintain good posture. Other common problem areas to focus on include the shoulders, chest, lower back, front of hips, thighs, and calves. Stretch to the point of mild tension, hold for 10 to 30 seconds (no bouncing), and repeat each stretch 3 to 5 times. Stretching should not cause pain. It is ideal to stretch every day; three times per week is the minimum.

Nutritional Considerations for Optimal Fitness

The eating plan for fueling fitness is basically the same as it is for the general population: high carbohydrate, low fat, and moderate protein with an emphasis on variety, balance, and moderation. Calorie needs may increase in response to exercise, depending on body size and the duration, intensity, and frequency of exercise. Adequate fluids are needed to replace losses. Actual nutrient requirements vary with the level of fitness and the types of exercises performed. (See Eating for Energy for more details.)

THE WEIGHT MANAGEMENT APPROACH

Many people use activity and exercise to manage their weight. Understanding the basic principle of weight management—that weight changes as the balance between calorie intake and calorie output changes—enables people to tailor their activities and exercises according to their calorie intake and weight goals. The Expert Panel on the Identification, Evaluation, and Treatment of Overweight and Obesity in Adults (NHLBI, 1996) recommends that physical activity be made a component of comprehensive weight loss and weight control programs because it (1) modestly contributes to weight loss in overweight and obese adults, (2) may reduce abdominal fat, (3) improves cardiorespiratory fitness, and (4) may help with maintenance of weight loss. In practice, exercise may have limited value in stimulating weight loss *independent* of nutritional interventions.

- **Combine increased activity and exercise to maximize calorie expenditure.** Combining a variety of activities and exercises is the best approach to achieve not only weight management but also improved health and better fitness. For instance, substituting activity for nonactivity is a subtle first step in increasing calorie expenditure that sets the stage for adding more activities of greater intensity.
  - Aerobic exercise burns more calories than simply increasing activity. It is also needed to improve cardiorespiratory fitness and provides numerous health benefits.
  - Strength training builds muscle, raising the metabolic rate and increasing the likelihood of weight loss and body fat loss. Changes in body composition—more muscle, less fat—are positive outcomes of strength training that are not reflected on the scale.
  - Stretching uses few calories but increases range of motion, enabling the body to move more.
- **Start slowly; build to at least 45 minutes of moderate-intensity exercise performed at least 5 days/week.** The National Heart, Lung, and Blood Institute Obesity Education Initiative recommends the following progression of activity:
  - Begin with very light activity and progress as tolerated through each of the next sequential steps: light, moderate, high.
  - Begin with walking or swimming at a slow pace; do this for 30 minutes, 3 days a week.

- Gradually work up to 45 minutes of more intense activity done at least 5 days a week, preferably daily. Most experts recommend first increasing the duration and frequency of the activity and then the intensity. Aim to increase energy expenditure by 1000 to 2000 cal/week.
- In addition, increase every-day activities, such as standing instead of sitting, walking instead of driving, taking the stairs instead of the elevator.
- Progress to more strenuous activities, such as aerobic exercise routines, competitive sports, or bicycling.
- Incorporate stretching and strength training to round out the activity/exercise program.

- **Don't expect pounds to melt away.** Note that the goal of increasing activity is to burn an extra 1000 to 2000 cal/week. Because 1 pound of body fat is the equivalent of 3500 cal, you need to incur a daily calorie deficit of 500 calories to lose 1 pound of weight in 1 week (3500 cal ÷ 7 days/week = 500 cal/day). A 2-pound weight loss occurs when the daily deficit is 1000 cal/day. Without a reduction of food intake to contribute to this needed calorie deficit, the 1000 to 2000 extra calories burned each week would amount to a weight loss of only about ⅓ to ½ pound, an amount too low to be reflected on the bathroom scale.

  Many people overestimate the effect that activity and exercise will have on their weight. They expect rapid and sustained weight loss and become discouraged when the scale fails to reflect their hard work. It is important to remember that, even before weight changes are evident, exercise produces positive health benefits, such as improvements in blood pressure and blood cholesterol levels and lowered risks of heart disease, diabetes, and colon cancer. People who undertake activity and exercise programs with realistic expectations are more likely to remain in the program.
- **Remember that what is important is burning calories, not the actual type of fuel used.** Low- and moderate-intensity exercises performed for longer than 20 minutes are fueled primarily by fat, and when people say they want to lose weight, what they really mean is that they want to lose fat. Therefore low- and moderate-intensity exercises are desirable, particularly because they are easier on unconditioned or overweight bodies and can be performed for longer periods. But high-intensity exercise, even though fueled mostly by glucose, burns more calories per unit of time. The downside is that they usually require higher motivation to sustain, and the risk of injury is greater. Ultimately what is important is the amount of fuel used, not the type.

Nutritional Considerations for Weight Management

The efficacy of increased activity alone as a means to lose weight is controversial; increased activity appears to be more effective at maintaining weight loss than promoting it. Calorie restriction is a powerful tool for promoting weight loss, but when used alone it usually fails to maintain weight loss for 2 years or longer. Together, increased activity and calorie restriction produce the biggest impact on weight loss and on maintaining weight loss in the long term.

Traditional Low-Calorie Diets

For people who are overweight to mildly obese, low-calorie "diets" have been the cornerstone of weight loss programs. Sometimes an individual's total daily calorie needs were estimated and then 500 to 1000 cal was subtracted to achieve, theoretically, a weight loss of 1 to 2 pounds/week. For instance, someone requiring 2000 cal/day to maintain their weight would be given a 1500-calorie diet, or sometimes a 1000-calorie diet, to achieve their weekly weight loss goal. Sometimes an arbitrary calorie level was subjectively prescribed, such as 1800 cal/day for men or 1500 cal/day for women.

After total calories were determined, the "diet" would take the form of a master meal plan that specified the number and size of portions allowed from each food group for each meal and snack. Although this approach may seem appropriate, it has many drawbacks. For example:

- It does not easily allow for individual or daily variations. What if you want more for breakfast and less for lunch? What if you're more hungry on weekends, less hungry on weekdays? What if you eat at ethnic restaurants and order food that does not appear on any of the food exchange lists?
- It tends to be short-lived because of its limitations and rigidity. Some experts believe that restrictive diets actually contribute to overeating and sometimes to binge eating by promoting a "bad food/good food" dichotomy. For instance, telling someone that he or she cannot have ice cream fuels an interest in ice cream that becomes an obsession and leads to an ice cream binge. The ice cream is a "bad food," the client is "bad" for eating it, and the client views himself or herself as a failure. The result: "I've blown the diet with the ice cream so I may as well eat this cheesecake."
- It fails to teach decision-making skills that enable people to eat healthy and wise as a way of life—skills such as:
  - Identifying hunger and satiety signals to control unnecessary eating and overeating
  - Learning new ways of responding to cues to eat—for instance, taking a walk instead of eating when angry or bored
  - Self-monitoring eating behaviors to identify triggers to overeating and areas in need of improvement
  - Realistic goal setting and positive self-talk
  - Application of the principles of basic nutrition, particularly the Food Guide Pyramid and the concepts of variety, balance, and moderation

With traditional low-calorie diets, "diet" takes on the connotation of deprivation and punishment and is viewed as a short-term hurdle to be overcome in order to resume "normal" eating. Prescribed low-calorie diets are effective in some instances for some people, but they generally fail to become a way of life.

Nondiet Approach to Weight Control

A relatively new approach to "dieting" is the "nondiet" approach, which does away with counting calories, restrictive foods, and set meal patterns. It is not a single approach but rather a philosophy that promotes fitness and eating without restrictive or compulsory regimens. It can be implemented in a variety of ways. For instance, many people informally and unknowingly use a nondiet approach to weight control when they make realistic changes in their eating habits. Eliminating second helpings, substituting low-fat varieties for high-fat foods, and reducing snacking are considered lifestyle changes that, over time, help manage weight. For obese clients with long, frustrating histories of restrictive dieting, the nondiet approach offers self-regulated eating without rules and the potential to form healthier eating attitudes and behaviors (see Chapter 14).

Tips for Reducing Calories

For people who just want to eat healthier and manage their weight (maintain or lose weight gradually), subtle changes in eating can help.

- **Calories count, but counting calories is not the answer.** A calorie deficit is needed to lose weight, but counting calories does not ensure a healthy intake and is not something that can be done indefinitely.
- **Stick to the low-end range of servings from the Food Guide Pyramid, except for the Vegetable group and Fruit group.** On average, the low-end number of servings totals about 1600 cal. Eating more from the Vegetable and Fruit groups results in more nutrients and fiber with few extra calories; these are the groups to indulge in. It is difficult to get adequate amounts of all required nutrients when servings dip below the recommended minimums.
- **Choose low-fat or nonfat foods over full-fat varieties.** Because fat has more than twice the calories as equivalent amounts of protein or carbohydrate, cutting fat grams makes the biggest impact on cutting calories. Read the Nutrition Facts label to compare brands.
- **Try to divide food evenly throughout the day.** This strategy helps avoid fasting and feasting, providing a constant flow of fuel for activity.
- **Watch portion sizes.** Portion sizes are important whether the goal is getting enough nutrients or avoiding excess fat and calories.
- **Keep track of what you eat.** Periodic self-monitoring of what, when, and how much is eaten helps identify eating patterns in need of improvement.
- **Eat your favorite foods regularly.** "All foods can fit"—it's just a matter of how often and how much. When you decide to eat your favorite food, eat it slowly, enjoy every bite, and then put it behind you. This avoids feelings of "cheating" or of "blowing" the diet, which can spiral into an even bigger binge.
- **Concentrate on wholesome foods.** Wholesome foods, such as a whole apple instead of applesauce, take more time to eat, provide more nutrients and fiber, and tend to leave you feeling fuller longer.
- **Focus on the big picture.** Maintain perspective on the effect of an occasional indulgence on weight status. Eating a single piece of chocolate cake, even at 235 cal per slice, will not cause weight gain that day. But several pieces of cake topped with ice cream eaten for a few days will cause weight gain.

"FAT-BURNING" SUPPLEMENTS

People who want to lose weight actually want to burn more fat to reduce their fat stores. Athletes want to burn fat to preserve their glycogen reserves. Manufacturers of commercial supplements are eager to help consumers meet their goals with "natural" ingredients. But are they safe? And do they work?

Fat-Burning Supplements Promoted to "Dieters"

Hydroxycitric Acid

Hydroxycitric acid (HCA) is added to weight-loss supplements such as Ultra Burn and CitraLean. It is a modified form of citric acid, which is a component of the TCA cycle. Supposedly, HCA works by inhibiting the enzymes that normally help convert citric acid to fat, thereby preventing calories from being stored as fat.

Studies of HCA in animals were halted after problems with toxicities became apparent. The only two good published studies on whether HCA helps people lose weight yielded opposite conclusions. At this time, neither the effectiveness nor the safety of this product has been established.

Chitosan

The supplement Fat Trapper contains plant fiber plus chitosan, a fiber-like substance made from chitin, the material that forms the hard shells of lobsters, crabs, and other shellfish. According to one of its manufacturers, chitosan binds to fat and fat-soluble substances in the gastrointestinal tract, rendering them incapable of being absorbed and so they are excreted.

The small number of studies done to determine whether chitosan actually promotes weight loss have yielded inconsistent results. In terms of safety, the potential loss of fat-soluble nutrients and fat-soluble phytochemicals means that chitosan should not be used in the long term, even though it is marketed as a lifelong aid. Chitosan also has the potential to impair absorption of fat-soluble drugs, such as estrogen and oral contraceptives.

Conjugated Linoleic Acid

Conjugated linoleic acid (CLA) is a mixture of polyunsaturated fats that forms in the gut of cattle. Meat and milk are dietary sources. Pigs, cattle, and laboratory rats and mice given CLA acquire more muscle and less fat as they grow and develop. However, this does not appear to be the case for humans. The one study conducted with CLA was halted after it became obvious CLA was no more effective in promoting weight loss than a placebo.

Ephedrine

Ephedrine is an amphetamine-like substance derived from the Chinese herb Ephedra (ma huang). It is found in weight-loss supplements such as Diet Fuel and Metabolife. The U.S. Food and Drug Administration has received more than 800 reports of adverse side effects from ephedrine, including dizziness, headaches, chest pain, psychosis, seizures, and strokes. Ephedrine has been blamed for more than 35 deaths.

Pyruvate

Pyruvate, the substance formed during the breakdown of glucose into energy, is the major ingredient in Exercise in a Bottle and Pyruvate Punch. A company selling pyruvate supplements claims that they "contribute to a 48% greater rate of fat loss and a 37% greater rate of weight loss over non-pyruvate users in clinical studies." The actual weight loss experienced by the pyruvate users was 3.5 pounds more that that of the placebo takers; both groups consumed 1800 cal/day. The amount of pyruvate taken during the study, one-half bottle per day, costs $300/month. It is not known whether pyruvate works without a low-calorie diet or in lower amounts.

Fat-Burning Supplements Promoted to Athletes

Caffeine

Caffeine, found in strong black coffee and over-the-counter antidrowsiness preparations, has long been used by athletes to improve endurance performance. As a stimulant, it increases alertness, reduces perceived effort during exercise, and decreases reaction time. Studies show that it improves exercise capacity (probably because it increases the concentration of circulating free fatty acids), increases fatty acid oxidation, and reduces the amount of carbohydrate used during exercise. Caffeine has no effect on maximal anaerobic (sprint) exercise lasting less than 30 seconds. At high doses (>15 mg/kg body weight), caffeine can cause bradycardia, hypertension, nervousness, irritability, insomnia, and gastrointestinal upset. The Medical Commission of the International Olympics Committee classifies caffeine as a restricted drug; it is illegal at amounts greater than 12 mg/L in urine.

L-Carnitine

Carnitine is found in meats and dairy products and is synthesized in the human liver and kidneys from two essential amino acids. It transports fatty acids across the mitochondrial membrane for beta-oxidation. In fact, in all tissues, long-chain fatty acid oxidation is dependent on carnitine. Because of its central role in fatty acid metabolism, carnitine supplementation has been promoted as a means to increase fatty acid oxidation. It is especially marketed to athletes who need to meet weight specifications or to maintain low body weight, such as wrestlers, gymnasts, and bodybuilders. However, studies have failed to show that carnitine supplements enhance fatty acid oxidation, help reduce body fat, or help athletes make weight. Training does not appear to reduce carnitine levels in healthy athletes eating a normal diet, so supplementation is unnecessary. Also, some supplements contain D-carnitine, a substance that is physiologically inactive and may cause muscle weakness by depleting L-carnitine.

Questions You May Hear

Does exercise make you hungrier? During and immediately after exercise, blood flow is drawn away from the gastrointestinal tract to the muscles to deliver fuel and oxygen. Because of this, the process of digestion slows and the sensation of hunger is absent. Long, strenuous exercise can cause low blood glucose, but that is not the same as hunger. Hunger does occur when calories burned create a calorie deficit, but the increased energy expenditure allows for greater food intake without causing an increase in weight.

Do protein powders and amino acid supplements help build muscle? Expensive protein powders and amino acid pills, such as arginine, ornithine, and free amino acids, are touted as growing muscles and increasing strength. In reality, bulking up requires extra carbohydrates and extra exercise, with very little additional protein. In theory, a gain of 1 pound of muscle per week requires an extra 14 g of protein per day, the amount found in 1¾ cups of milk. By comparison, supplements provide less protein at a much higher price. Protein needs are easily met by a varied, balanced diet.

Are sports drinks a good idea? Water is the best source of fluid for most recreational athletes who exercise less than 60 to 90 minutes. It adequately replenishes fluid losses, is inexpensive, and is readily available. For endurance-type activities lasting longer than 60 to 90 minutes, such as long-distance running, long-distance cross-country skiing, and ice hockey, sugared beverages that provide 40 to 80 cal per 8 ounces (4%–8% solution) are recommended to be consumed *during* competitive exercise as a fuel boost and to enhance the rate at which water is absorbed. Consumed *before* exercise, they may stimulate insulin secretion and actually cause blood glucose levels to fall. *After* exercise they are too weak to provide the necessary carbohydrates for glycogen replacement.

What is creatine and does it help increase muscle strength? Creatine is an amino acid that is synthesized by the body; it is found in small amounts in fish and meat. It is stored in muscle primarily as free creatine and phosphocreatine. During brief, intense periods of exercise, phosphocreatine breaks down to supply the energy needed to regenerate ATP from ADP.

Because the availability of phosphocreatine stored in muscles may significantly influence the amount of energy generated during brief periods of high-intensity exercise, many athletes use creatine supplements to boost the amount of creatine in muscle and consequently improve muscle strength and endurance. Studies show that short-term creatine supplementation does increase phosphocreatine stores and improves maximal strength and muscular performance in athletes during such exercise. Supplementation also significantly increases body mass, possibly by enhancing protein synthesis or reducing protein breakdown. Increased body mass is advantageous for athletes such as bodybuilders, weight lifters, and football linemen. Although not all studies are consistent, most show that creatine supplements safely and effectively increase strength, power, sprint performance, and/or work performed during multiple sets of intense-effort muscle contractions.

KEY CONCEPTS

- Mechanical and chemical digestion break down complex molecules of carbohydrates, proteins, and fats into smaller molecules that the body can absorb. The first half of the small intestine is the primary site of nutrient digestion and absorption.
- Energy metabolism refers to how energy from carbohydrates, proteins, and fats is extracted and used. Vitamins and minerals do not provide energy (calories), but they are needed for the metabolism of energy.
- Cells' immediate source of fuel is stored in ATP, which is supplemented with a small supply of creatine phosphate, neither of which requires oxygen to be burned. Glucose is the only fuel that can be burned without oxygen through the process of glycolysis, but glycolysis extracts only a small amount of the total available energy from glucose. Aerobic metabolism includes the TCA cycle and the electron transport chain; it yields the maximum amount of available energy. Although they enter the cycle by different routes, carbohydrates, proteins, and fats are all metabolized through the TCA cycle and the electron transport chain.
- During prolonged fasting, the brain and nervous system adapt to the shortage of glucose by using ketones that are produced by fat catabolism. However, body protein catabolism does continue (although at a slower rate), because not all cells are able to adapt to ketone use.
- The body uses a mixture of fuels at rest and at work. In general, as the duration of activity increases, the amount of fat burned increases in an attempt to conserve the body's supply of glycogen. As the intensity of activity increases, the amount of glucose burned increases, because glucose is the only fuel that can be metabolized anaerobically.
- Glycogen is the limiting fuel in how long and how well physical activity can be performed. Glycogen loading is a technique that manipulates training and diet to maximize glycogen storage and thereby increase performance during endurance activities.
- Carbohydrates should supply 60% to 70% of calories in an athlete's diet. Protein needs increase above normal but are easily met from a balanced, varied diet. Fat should provide less than 30% of total calories. Athletes need fluid before they become thirsty. Calorie requirements are highly individualized.
- Total calories expended equals the amount of calories spent on voluntary activities (physical activity) and on involuntary activities (basal metabolism). For most Americans, basal metabolism represents 60% to 70% of total calories burned. The thermic effect of food is the cost of digesting, absorbing, and metabolizing food. At about 10% of total calories consumed, it is a small part of total energy requirements.
- Most Americans do not get the recommended amount of physical activity. Significant health benefits can be gained from simply increasing activity, even though optimal physical fitness is not attained. Regular physical activity can improve or lower the risks of heart disease, hypertension, type 2 diabetes, depression, and colon cancer.
- Physical activity and exercise may not be effective at promoting weight loss independent of nutritional interventions. Eating fewer calories does promote weight loss but may not be effective at independently maintaining weight loss. Together, exercise and fewer calories (plus behavior modification) provide the best strategy for promoting and maintaining weight loss.

- Traditional weight-loss diets restrict the types and amounts of food consumed. Although they may be appropriate for some people, such "diets" tend to be short term and may increase the risk of binge eating. The "nondieting" approach to weight control encourages self-regulation, skill building, and individualized lifestyle modifications.
- Fat-burning supplements capitalize on dieters' desire to reduce fat stores and athletes' desire to preserve glycogen stores. Neither safety nor efficacy has been firmly established for any fat-burning supplement.

ANSWER KEY

1. **TRUE** Food provides energy (calories) in carbohydrates, fats, and proteins (and alcohol).
2. **TRUE** Carbohydrate (glygogen) storage is the limiting factor in intense and endurance activities.
3. **TRUE** People with higher muscle mass (more lean tissue) have higher metabolic rates than people with proportionately more fat tissue.
4. **FALSE** Calorie needs may increase in response to exercise, depending on the individual's body size and the duration, intensity, and frequency of exercise.
5. **TRUE** A 2-pound weight loss in a week occurs when the daily deficit is 1000 cal/day.
6. **TRUE** Fasting leads to a lowering of metabolic rate. Fat tissue is conserved, but weight loss owing to protein loss may be significant.
7. **FALSE** As the duration of an activity increases, the proportion of fat used increases; however, strength training builds muscle, raising the metabolic rate and increasing the likelihood of body fat loss.
8. **FALSE** Strength training exercises can maintain or restore muscle mass at any age.
9. **FALSE** Significant health benefits can be obtained when sedentary people simply become more active on a regular basis. Health benefits are obtained even if the activity is spread over the course of the day.
10. **TRUE** The body adapts to fasting by lowering its energy requirement.

REFERENCES

American Dietetic Association. (1993). Position of the American Dietetic Association and the Canadian Dietetic Association: Nutrition for physical fitness and athletic performance for adults. *Journal of the American Dietetic Association*, *93*, 691–695.

American Dietetic Association Foundation. (1995). Athletes fuel up for fitness. [On-line]. Available: www.eatright.org/nfs/nfso.html. Accessed August 19, 1999.

Armsey, T., & Green, G. (June 1997). Nutrition supplements: Science vs hype. *The Physician and Sportsmedicine*, *25*. Available from McGraw-Hill, Minneapolis, MN. Accessed May 18, 2000.

Clark, N. (1997). *Nancy Clark's sports nutrition guidebook* (2nd ed.). Champaign, IL: Human Kinetics.

Hawley, J. (September 1998). Fat burning during exercise: Can ergogenics change the balance? *The Physician and Sportsmedicine*, *26*.

Kleiner, S. (October 1997). Eating for peak performance. *The Physician and Sportsmedicine, 25*. Available from McGraw-Hill, Minneapolis, MN. Accessed May 18, 2000.

Kratina, K., King, N., & Hayes, D. (1996). *Moving away from diets*. Lake Dallas, TX: Helm Seminars, Publishing.

Kreider, R. (April 1998). Creatine supplementations: Analysis of ergogenic value, medical safety, and concerns. [On-line serial]. *Journal of Exercise Physiology Online, 1*. Available from Dr. Tommy Boone, Department of Exercise Physiology, College of St. Scholastica, Duluth, MN 55811.

Leibman, B. (1999). Take a hike. *Nutrition Action Healthletter, 26*(1), 1, 3–7.

McArdle, W., Katch, F., & Katch, V. (1999). *Sports and exercise nutrition*. Philadelphia: Lippincott Williams & Wilkins.

Nash, J. (1997). *The new maximize your body potential: Lifetime skills for successful weight management*. Palo Alto, CA: Bull Publishing Company.

National Heart, Lung, and Blood Institute. (1998). *The Clinical Guidelines on the identification, evaluation, and treatment of overweight and obesity in adults*. (NIH Publication No. 98-4083). National Institutes of Health, U.S. Department of Health and Human Services, Centers for Disease Control and Prevention, and National Center for Chronic Disease Prevention and Health Promotion.

Rippe, J., & Hess, S. (1998). The role of physical activity in the prevention and management of obesity. *Journal of the American Dietetic Association*, 98(Suppl.), S31–S38.

Shardt, D. (1999). Fat burners. *Nutrition Action Healthletter, 26*, 9–11.

Volek, J., Karaemer, W., Bush, J., Boetes, M., Incledon, T., & Clark, K., (1997). Creatine supplementation enhances muscular performance during high-intensity resistance exercise. *Journal of the American Dietetic Association, 97*, 765–770.

U.S. Department of Health and Human Services. (1996). *Physical activity and health: A report of the surgeon general*. Atlanta, GA: U.S. Department of Health and Human Services, Centers for Disease Control and Prevention, and National Center for Chronic Disease Prevention and Health Promotion.

Whitney, E., Cataldo, C., Rolfes, S. (1998). *Understanding normal and clinical nutrition* (5th ed.). Belmont, CA: Wadsworth Publishing Company.

Zelasko, C. (1995). Exercise for weight loss: What are the facts? *Journal of the American Dietetic Association*, 95, 1414–1417.

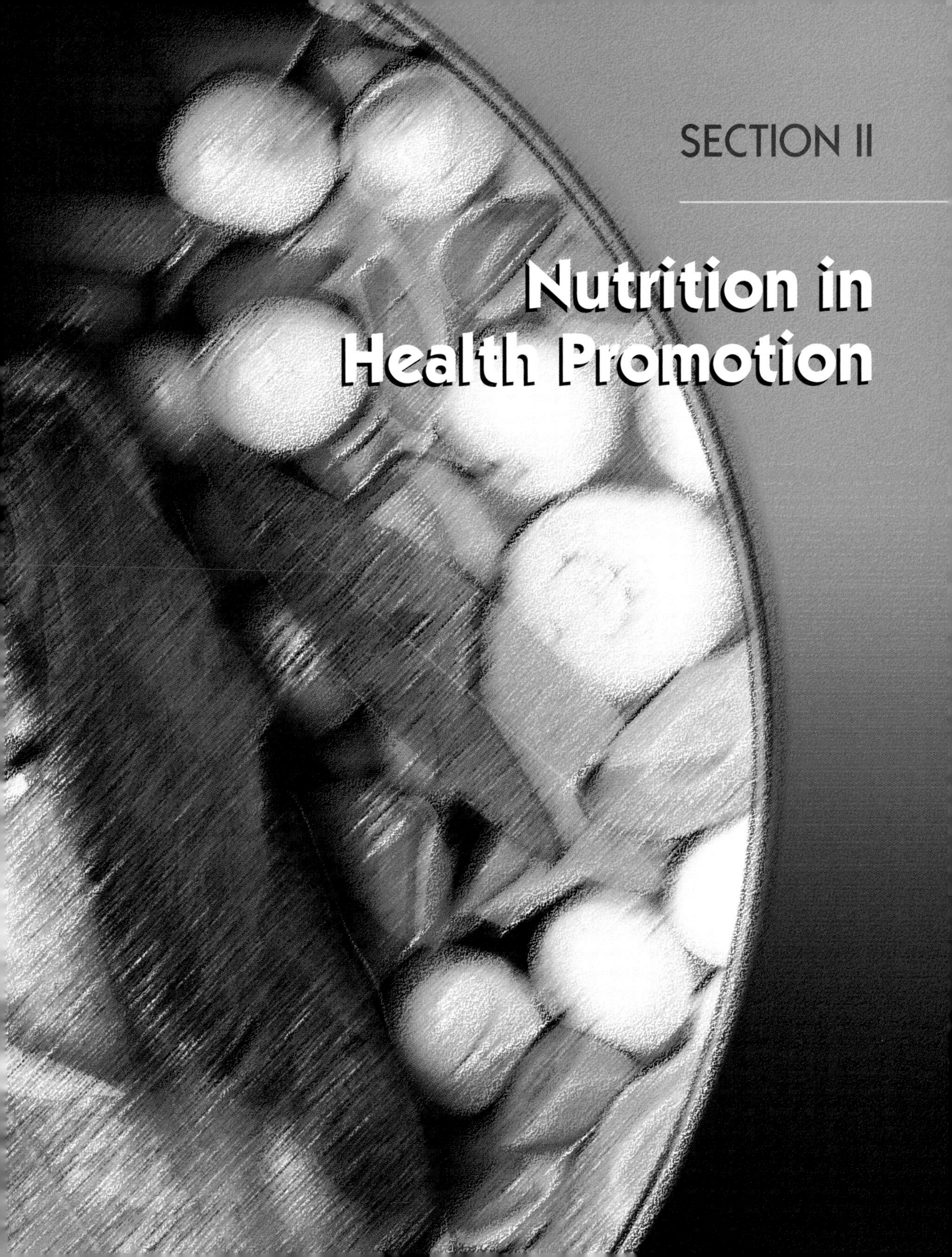

SECTION II

Nutrition in Health Promotion

CHAPTER 8

Guidelines for Healthy Eating

TRUE	FALSE	Check your knowledge of guidelines for healthy eating.
⬭	⬭	1 The Recommended Dietary Allowances (RDAs) are intended for healthy people only.
⬭	⬭	2 The old RDAs are being revised for the purpose of promoting optimal health, not just avoiding deficiency diseases.
⬭	⬭	3 The Tolerable Upper Intake Level is the optimal level of nutrients that people should try to consume.
⬭	⬭	4 The majority of nutritional problems in the United States today are related to nutrient excesses, not deficiencies.
⬭	⬭	5 The food group at the bottom of the Food Guide Pyramid is more important than all other groups.
⬭	⬭	6 Portion sizes are consistent on the Food Guide Pyramid and Nutrition Facts label.
⬭	⬭	7 It is appropriate to eat any number of servings within the specified range for each Food Guide Pyramid group.
⬭	⬭	8 Water-soluble vitamins, minerals, and fiber are most susceptible to the effects of food processing.
⬭	⬭	9 Bacteria cause the majority of foodborne illnesses.
⬭	⬭	10 Animal products are the most common vehicle for transmission of foodborne illnesses.

Upon completion of this chapter, you will be able to

- Describe how the old RDAs differ from the new Dietary Reference Intakes.
- List the three basic messages of the *Dietary Guidelines for Americans*.
- Explain the concepts of variety, balance, and moderation in relation to the Food Guide Pyramid.
- Discuss the use of the Food Guide Pyramid as a teaching tool.
- Explain the % of the Daily Value (DV) that appears on the Nutrition Facts label.

- Discuss the use of the Nutrition Facts label as a teaching tool.
- List six ways to minimize nutrient losses from food.
- List 10 rules to keep food safe.

Choosing an Adequate Diet

A healthy diet provides enough of all essential nutrients to avoid deficiencies and promote optimal health. It also is not excessive in any nutrients that may increase the risk of chronic diseases. In addition, a healthy diet is safe, that is, it is free of microorganisms and contaminants that cause foodborne illnesses.

For more than 50 years, periodic updates and revisions of the Recommended Dietary Allowances (RDAs) have served as the reference standards for nutrient intakes. The RDA represent the average daily dietary intake amounts sufficient to meet the nutrient needs of almost all healthy people. As "allowances" they differ from "requirements" in that they are requirements (the amount needed to prevent a deficiency) with a safety factor added in to account for individual variations. RDAs are established for protein, the fat-soluble vitamins (vitamins A, D, E, K), vitamin C, the B vitamins, calcium, phosphorus, magnesium, iron, zinc, iodine, and selenium. Subsets of the RDAs were established for nutrients for which definite allowances could not be determined due to the lack of sufficient data. Estimated Safe and Adequate Daily Dietary Intakes ranges were set for five trace minerals (copper, manganese, fluoride, chromium, and molybdenum). Estimated Minimum Requirements for Healthy Persons were set for sodium, chloride, and potassium.

The RDAs have been criticized for being too limited in scope. Many health experts have argued that the RDAs should be set at levels to promote optimal health, not at levels that merely prevent deficiencies. For instance, the previous RDA for folic acid for adult women was set at 180 micrograms, which was enough prevent folic acid deficiency but not enough optimize protection against neural tube defects in a developing fetus should the woman become pregnant.

DIETARY REFERENCE INTAKES

Responding to a growing knowledge base of nutrient requirements and food components, as well as an increasing awareness that the RDAs had limitations and were often misinterpreted and misused, the Food and Nutrition Board has undertaken a comprehensive, multiyear project to replace and expand the RDAs. The new references, the Daily Reference Intakes (DRIs), are not limited to preventing deficiency diseases. The DRIs incorporate current concepts about the role of nutrients and food components in reducing the risk of chronic disease, developmental disorders, and other related problems. The DRIs are intended to be used for planning and assessing diets for healthy people.

Four sets of reference values make up the DRIs. They include updated RDAs and three other sets of reference values: the Estimated Average Requirement (EAR), Adequate Intake (AI), and the Tolerable Upper Intake Level (UL). DRIs have already been released for calcium and related nutrients and the B vitamins, vitamin C, vitamin E, and selenium. At least three more reports on groups of nutrients and related compounds are scheduled to be released over the next 3 to 4 years. Until the new DRI system is fully implemented, reference standards will be a mix of old and new.

DEFINITIONS OF THE NEW STANDARDS

Recommended Dietary Allowances

The RDAs continue to represent the average daily dietary intake level sufficient to meet the nutrient requirement of 97% to 98% of all healthy people in a life stage and gender group. This definition is similar to past descriptions of the RDAs, but in the DRI framework this is the only use of the RDA—as a goal for individuals. When estimating the nutritional needs of people with health disorders, health professionals use the RDAs as a starting point and adjust them according to the individual's need.

Estimated Average Requirement (EAR)

The EAR is the amount of a nutrient that is estimated to meet the requirement of half of healthy people in a lifestyle or gender group. Rather than being based solely on the prevention of nutrient deficiencies, the EAR also considers current concepts of reducing the risk of disease and takes into account the bioavailability of the nutrient, that is, how its absorption is impacted by other food components. It is necessary to establish EAR values for nutrients in order to determine RDA values.

Adequate Intake (AI)

An AI is set when an RDA cannot be determined due to lack of sufficient data on requirements. It is a recommended daily intake level based on observed or experimentally determined estimates of nutrient intake by a group of healthy people. For instance, the AI for young infants, for whom breast milk is recommended as the sole source of nutrition, is based on the estimated daily nutrient intake provided by human milk for healthy, full-term infants who are exclusively breast-fed. The primary purpose of the AI is as a goal for the nutrient intake of individuals. This is similar to the use of the RDA except that the RDA is expected to meet the needs of almost all healthy people while in the case of an AI, it is not known what percentage of people are covered. The extent to which AI meets the needs of individuals is likely to vary among nutrients and population groups.

TOLERABLE UPPER INTAKE LEVEL (UL)

The UL is the highest level of daily nutrient intake that is likely to pose no risk of adverse health effects to almost all individuals in the general population. The term "Tolerable Upper Intake Level" does not imply a possible beneficial effect in consuming that amount, but rather indicates the level that can be physiologically tolerated with chronic daily use. It is not intended to be a recommended level of intake. There is no benefit in consuming amounts greater than the RDA or AI.

Avoiding Nutrient Excesses

Current public health concerns relating to nutrition are with overnutrition, not undernutrition. Nutrient deficiency diseases in the United States are rare, except among the poor, the elderly, alcoholics, fad dieters, and ironically, hospitalized patients. Conversely, five of the 10 leading causes of death in the US are associated with dietary excesses, namely heart disease, cancer, strokes, type 2 diabetes, and atherosclerosis. Alcohol plays a role in another three (chronic liver disease and cirrhosis, unintentional injuries, and suicide). Dietary advice issued by governmental and health agencies is intended to reduce the risk of chronic disease by avoiding dietary excesses. A trio of tools devised by governmental agencies to assist consumers with making healthy food choices are the Dietary Guidelines for Americans; its companion illustration, the Food Guide Pyramid; and the Nutrition Facts label.

DIETARY GUIDELINES FOR AMERICANS

The *Dietary Guidelines for Americans* consists of the three basic messages of "Aim," "Build," and "Choose" (ABCs) with 10 guidelines to promote wellness and prevent chronic disease in healthy Americans 2 years of age and older. The guidelines focus on food patterns and the total diet, not on individual foods or numeric nutrient goals which are meaningless to the general public. The guidelines recognize that good health can be achieved by a variety of different dietary patterns and that food choices are influenced by culture, history, environment, and taste, in addition to energy and nutritional needs. Included with each guideline is advice for the present and suggestions for implementation.

Aim for Fitness

Aiming for fitness involves two guidelines: Aim for a healthy weight and be physically active each day.

- Aim for a healthy weight. Excess weight increases the risk of heart disease, hypertension, stroke, certain types of cancer, arthritis, breathing problems, and type 2 diabetes. A healthy weight is key to a long, healthy life. Body mass index (BMI) is used to evaluate weight in adults. People who are at a healthy weight should strive to avoid weight gain. People who are overweight should first prevent additional weight gain and then gradually lose weight to improve their health.

- Be physically active each day. Being physically active reduces the risk of heart disease, colon cancer, and type 2 diabetes; helps manage weight; increases fitness, endurance, and muscular strength; helps build and maintain healthy bones, muscles, and joints; helps manage blood pressure; promotes psychological well-being and self-esteem; and reduces feelings of depression and anxiety. Adults can achieve health benefits by participating in a moderate amount of physical activity for a total of at least 30 minutes most days of the weeks. Children need at least 60 minutes of moderate physical activity daily.

Build a Healthy Base

To build a base for healthy eating, Americans are urged to let the Pyramid guide their food choices; choose a variety of grains daily; especially whole grains; eat a variety of fruits and vegetables daily; and keep food safe to eat.

- Let the Pyramid guide your food choices. The USDA's Food Guide Pyramid, the official food guide for the United States, is a complex graphic designed to illustrate the Dietary Guidelines for Americans. People should choose the appropriate number of daily servings from each of the five major food groups, based on their total caloric needs. People who eliminate a food group should seek guidance to ensure that adequate amounts of all essential nutrients are consumed. For more on the Food Guide Pyramid, see the section below.
- Choose a variety of grains daily, especially whole grains. Foods made from grains form the foundation of a healthy diet. Whole grains are especially beneficial in that they provide more fiber, vitamins, minerals, and phytochemicals than refined grains. Grains are also generally low in fat. Whole-grain foods include whole wheat bread, whole-grain ready-to-eat cereal, oatmeal, corn tortillas, whole wheat pasta, whole barley in soup, tabouli salad, brown rice, and popcorn.
- Choose a variety of fruits and vegetables daily. Fruits and vegetables provide vitamins, minerals, fiber, and phytochemicals. Generally the more the better, the less preparation the better, and the greater the variety the better. Best bets are dark green leafy vegetables, bright orange fruits and vegetables, and cooked dried peas and beans.
- Keep food safe to eat. "Safe" means the food is not likely to cause illness due to bacteria, toxins, parasites, viruses, or chemical contaminants. See the section on Foodborne Illnesses.

Choose Sensibly

To choose a sensible diet, Americans are advised to choose a diet that is low in saturated fat and cholesterol and moderate in total fat, choose beverages and foods that limit their intake of sugars, choose and prepare foods with less salt, and drink only moderate amounts of alcoholic beverages.

- Choose a diet low in saturated fat and cholesterol and moderate in total fat. Saturated fats increase the risk of coronary heart disease by raising blood cholesterol levels. Sources of saturated fat include high-fat dairy products, fatty and processed meats, poultry skin and fat, and palm and coconut oils. *Trans*-fatty acids, found in foods made with partially hydrogenated vegetable oils, also raise blood cholesterol levels. Total fat intake should provide no more than 30% of total calories.
- Choose beverages and foods to moderate your intake of sugars. Foods high in added sugar are often "empty calories," meaning they provide few nutrients other than sugar. Many foods high in added sugar are also high in fat, such as pies, cakes, candy, and cookies. Sugars and starches, especially when consumed between meals, promote tooth decay. To reduce the risk of tooth decay, people are urged avoid snacking on foods and beverages containing sugars or starches, rinse after eating dried fruit, brush with a fluoride toothpaste regularly, floss regularly, and ask a dentist about the need for a fluoride supplement if drinking water is not fluoridated.
- Choose and prepare foods with less salt. A high salt intake is associated with higher blood pressure. Although there is no way to predict who might develop high blood pressure from eating too much salt, eating less salt is not harmful and is recommended for healthy people. Excess sodium also increases urinary calcium excretion, which may increase the risk of osteoporosis and bone fractures. Processed foods provide the largest percentage of sodium in the typical American diet.
- If you drink alcoholic beverages, do so in moderation. Moderate drinking may lower the risk for coronary heart disease, mainly in men over age 45 and women over age 55. However, higher levels of alcohol intake raise the risk for high blood pressure, stroke, certain cancers, accidents, violence, suicides, birth defects, and overall mortality (deaths). Too much alcohol may cause social and psychological problems, cirrhosis of the liver, inflammation of the pancreas, and damage to the brain and heart. Moderation is defined as no more than 1 drink per day for women and no more than 2 drinks per day for men. Each of the following count as 1 drink: 12 ounces of regular beer, 5 ounces of wine, 1.5 ounces of 80-proof distilled spirits. Alcohol should not be consumed by children, adolescents, and women who are trying to conceive or who are pregnant, because a safe level of alcohol intake during pregnancy has not been established. Also, alcohol should not be used with certain prescription and over-the-counter medications because it may alter the drug's effectiveness or toxicity. People who plan to drive, operate machinery, or take part in other activities that require attention or skill should not use alcohol. Lastly, alcohol is contraindicated in people who cannot limit their drinking to moderate levels.

THE FOOD GUIDE PYRAMID

The Food Guide Pyramid represents a new generation of food guides that addresses both undernutrition and overnutrition by suggesting a range of daily servings from each major food group, instead of minimum recommendations (Figure 8-1). Concepts emphasized in the Food Guide Pyramid are variety, balance, and moderation.

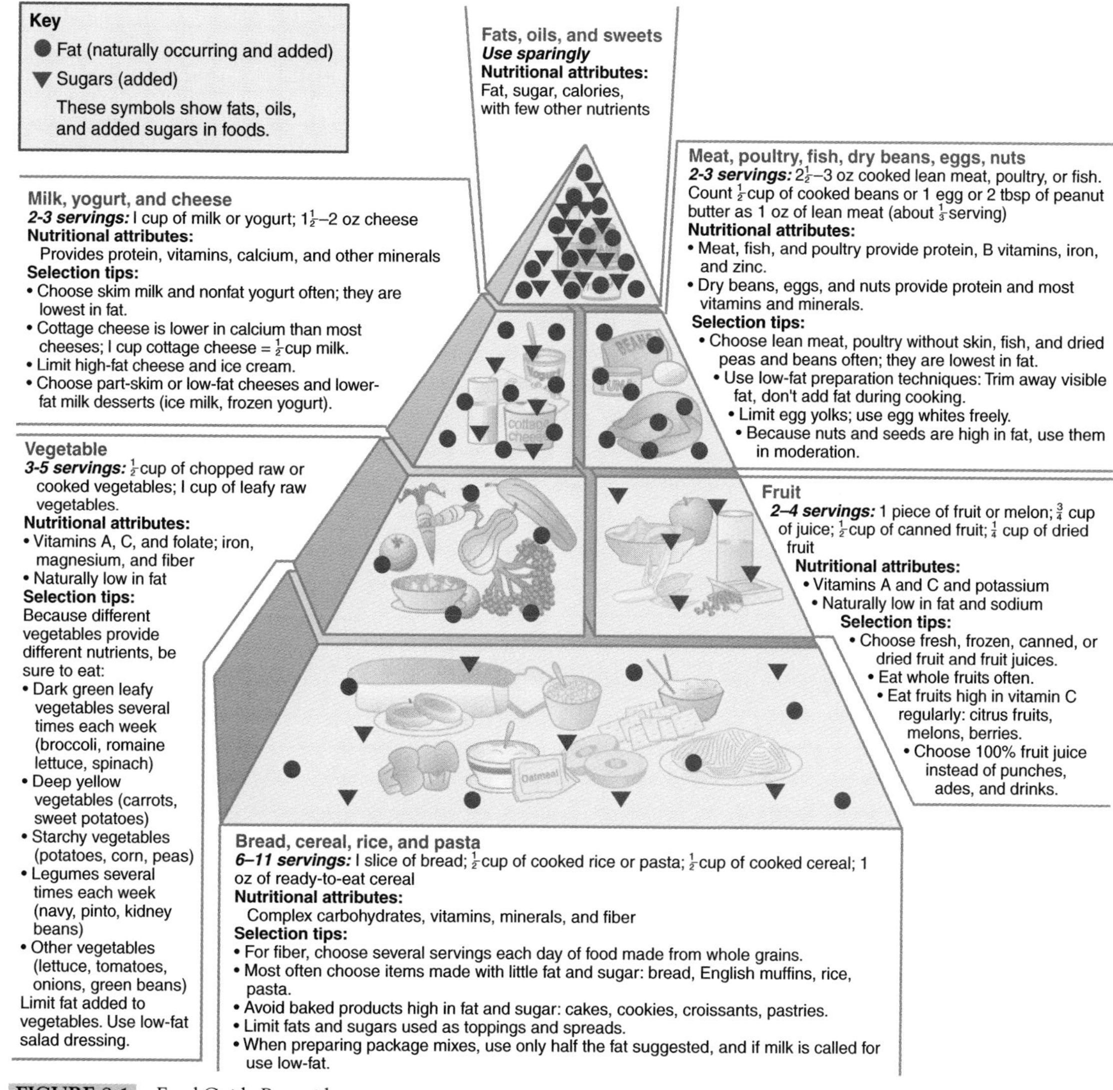

Key
Fat (naturally occurring and added)
Sugars (added)
These symbols show fats, oils, and added sugars in foods.
Fats, oils, and sweets
Use sparingly
Nutritional attributes:
Fat, sugar, calories, with few other nutrients
Milk, yogurt, and cheese
2-3 servings: I cup of milk or yogurt; 1½–2 oz cheese
Nutritional attributes:
Provides protein, vitamins, calcium, and other minerals
Selection tips:
• Choose skim milk and nonfat yogurt often; they are lowest in fat.
• Cottage cheese is lower in calcium than most cheeses; I cup cottage cheese = ½ cup milk.
• Limit high-fat cheese and ice cream.
• Choose part-skim or low-fat cheeses and lower-fat milk desserts (ice milk, frozen yogurt).
Meat, poultry, fish, dry beans, eggs, nuts
2-3 servings: 2½–3 oz cooked lean meat, poultry, or fish. Count ½ cup of cooked beans or 1 egg or 2 tbsp of peanut butter as 1 oz of lean meat (about ⅓ serving)
Nutritional attributes:
• Meat, fish, and poultry provide protein, B vitamins, iron, and zinc.
• Dry beans, eggs, and nuts provide protein and most vitamins and minerals.
Selection tips:
• Choose lean meat, poultry without skin, fish, and dried peas and beans often; they are lowest in fat.
• Use low-fat preparation techniques: Trim away visible fat, don't add fat during cooking.
• Limit egg yolks; use egg whites freely.
• Because nuts and seeds are high in fat, use them in moderation.
Vegetable
3-5 servings: ½ cup of chopped raw or cooked vegetables; I cup of leafy raw vegetables.
Nutritional attributes:
• Vitamins A, C, and folate; iron, magnesium, and fiber
• Naturally low in fat
Selection tips:
Because different vegetables provide different nutrients, be sure to eat:
• Dark green leafy vegetables several times each week (broccoli, romaine lettuce, spinach)
• Deep yellow vegetables (carrots, sweet potatoes)
• Starchy vegetables (potatoes, corn, peas)
• Legumes several times each week (navy, pinto, kidney beans)
• Other vegetables (lettuce, tomatoes, onions, green beans)
Limit fat added to vegetables. Use low-fat salad dressing.
Fruit
2–4 servings: 1 piece of fruit or melon; ¾ cup of juice; ½ cup of canned fruit; ¼ cup of dried fruit
Nutritional attributes:
• Vitamins A and C and potassium
• Naturally low in fat and sodium
Selection tips:
• Choose fresh, frozen, canned, or dried fruit and fruit juices.
• Eat whole fruits often.
• Eat fruits high in vitamin C regularly: citrus fruits, melons, berries.
• Choose 100% fruit juice instead of punches, ades, and drinks.
Bread, cereal, rice, and pasta
6–11 servings: I slice of bread; ½ cup of cooked rice or pasta; ½ cup of cooked cereal; 1 oz of ready-to-eat cereal
Nutritional attributes:
Complex carbohydrates, vitamins, minerals, and fiber
Selection tips:
• For fiber, choose several servings each day of food made from whole grains.
• Most often choose items made with little fat and sugar: bread, English muffins, rice, pasta.
• Avoid baked products high in fat and sugar: cakes, cookies, croissants, pastries.
• Limit fats and sugars used as toppings and spreads.
• When preparing package mixes, use only half the fat suggested, and if milk is called for use low-fat.

FIGURE 8-1 Food Guide Pyramid.

Variety

Variety is important because no single food supplies all 40+ essential nutrients in amounts needed. For instance, milk was once promoted as "nature's most nearly perfect food," yet it lacks iron, vitamin C, fiber, and other essential nutrients. Another benefit of variety is that it helps mitigate the natural toxins and food contaminants by diluting the impact a single food has on overall intake. For instance, vegetables of the cabbage family contain goitrogens, "antinutrients" that can induce goiter by their antithyroid action.

Limiting vegetable intake to only members of the cabbage family makes a person more susceptible to the effects of goitrogens than when a variety of vegetables are eaten. Variety helps ensure an adequate intake while minimizing the likelihood of imbalances.

Variety is achieved by choosing different colors, different textures, and different items from within each group day to day. For instance, variety in the grain group is achieved by eating whole wheat bread, corn tortillas, brown rice, kasha, and oatmeal, not by eating white bread, plain bagels, hamburger rolls, refined pasta, and puffed wheat, which are basically different forms of the same food. Day-to-day variety means not eating the same breakfast everyday, the same lunch everyday, and the same dinner everyday.

Balance

The Food Guide Pyramid visually depicts balance by portraying the size contribution each food group makes to the total figure. For instance, the Bread, Cereal, Rice, and Pasta group is the foundation of the pyramid and corresponds to the foundation of a healthy diet. The largest range of servings is recommended from this group. Conversely, the apex, Fats, Oils, and Sweets, occupies the smallest portion of the pyramid and should occupy the smallest portion of a healthy diet. The recommendation regarding foods from the apex is to use them "sparingly."

Moderation

Moderation means that "all foods can fit" into a healthy eating plan when used in moderation. For instance, it is not necessary to limit food selections to only those that are low in fat. For example, a high-fat burger for lunch is "moderated" by baked fish for dinner. Moderation is achieved by making conscious decisions about food choices, not by eating whatever and whenever.

The Food Guide Pyramid as a Teaching Tool

The Food Guide Pyramid is a versatile teaching tool because it can be adapted to the client's educational, cultural, and ethnic background. Points to keep in mind while using the Food Guide Pyramid as a teaching tool are as follows:

- No group is more important than any other. Each group supplies some essential nutrients, but no group supplies adequate amounts of all essential nutrients. Even though some groups should be eaten in greater quantity than others, it does not mean that those groups are more important to overall health than the smaller groups. For instance, even though more daily servings are recommended from the Vegetable group than the Milk, Yogurt, and Cheese group, the Milk group is vital for supplying adequate calcium. Without the recommended servings from the Milk group, clients are not likely to consume enough calcium.

- The apex is not a major food group. The apex of the pyramid is a category (Fats, Oils, and Sweets), not a major food group. Although no foods are illustrated there, it contains items that basically provide only calories, such as butter, jelly, and honey. A surprise to many people is that foods commonly thought of as "junk," such as hot dogs, French fries, doughnuts, cakes, and pies, are not in this category.
- Not all foods neatly fit into one particular category. Many clients get discouraged when they do not know how to classify mixed dishes like casseroles, burritos, and sushi. Any food can be mentally reduced to its component parts to determine its food group value. For instance, pizza crust is from the Bread, Cereal, Rice, and Pasta group; tomato sauce and vegetables are from the Vegetable group; cheese comes from the Milk, Yogurt, and Cheese group; and sausage, pepperoni, anchovies, and other meats come from the Meat, Poultry and Fish group.
- Vegetables and Fruit are two separate food groups. Separate groups for vegetables and fruit is significant in that it underscores the emphasis of a plant-based diet: Of the five major food groups depicted in the Food Guide Pyramid, the bottom three are plant-based, and the two highest groups contain animal products. The Vegetable group is placed to the left of the Fruit group and occupies a bigger space than fruit, signifying more servings are recommended from vegetables than fruit. Although both groups are rich in vitamins, phytochemicals, and fiber, vegetables have the additional benefit of providing minerals.
- The number of recommended servings a person needs is based on his or her total calorie needs. A common misconception about the number of recommended servings is that it is appropriate to eat any amount within the range for each group on any given day. In truth, the number of servings from each group that an individual should consume is dependent on his or her total calorie requirements. People who need approximately 1600 calories daily (eg, many sedentary women and some older men) should eat the minimum number of servings from each group. Eating the maximum number of servings recommended for each group supplies approximately 2800 calories, an amount appropriate for teenage boys, many active men, and some very active women. See Table 8-1, How many servings do you need each day?

TABLE 8.1 ***How Many Servings do you Need Each Day?***

	Calorie Level (Approximate)*		
Servings per Food Group	1600	2200	2800
Bread	6	9	11
Vegetable	3	4	5
Fruit	2	3	4
Milk	2–3†	2–3†	2–3†
Meat	2, for total 5 oz	2, for total 6 oz	3, for total 7 oz

*These are the calorie levels if you choose low-fat, lean foods from the five major food groups and use foods from the Fats, Oils, and Sweets group sparingly.

†Women who are pregnant or breast-feeding, teenagers, and young adults to age 24 need three servings.

- The serving size puts everything in perspective. Many clients are shocked when they hear they should consume six or more servings from the Bread, Cereal, Rice, and Pasta group until they understand the concept of portion size. For instance, an entree of spaghetti from a restaurant typically contains 2½ to 3 cups of pasta, which is not one serving even though it is one portion. The Food Guide Pyramid serving size for pasta is ½ cup, so 3 cups of spaghetti actually provides six serving from the Bread, Cereal, Rice, and Pasta group. The serving sizes used by the pyramid are not meant to represent the portion a person should eat at any one time or meal. If someone eats six servings of pasta for dinner and goes over their recommended amount of grain for the day, they can compensate by eating fewer grains the next day.

Food models or pictures of foods in common portion sizes may be helpful. Another way to convey the concept of serving sizes is to correlate portion sizes to other common objects that are relatively the same size. For instance, 3 ounces of meat is approximately the size of a deck of cards. Other useful correlations are:

- Two tablespoons of peanut butter are approximately the size of a ping-pong ball.
- One-and-one-half ounces of cheese are approximately the size of three dominoes.
- One-half cup cooked pasta, rice, or cereal looks like a scoop of ice cream.
- One medium-sized piece of fruit is the size of a baseball.
- Eight cherry tomatoes are approximately ½ cup of vegetable, as are seven packaged, peeled baby carrots.
- Fifteen grapes are approximately ½ cup of fruit.

Another important detail is that the serving sizes on the pyramid may differ from the serving sizes on food labels. The serving sizes used by the pyramid sizes are familiar and easy to use, whereas the serving sizes on food labels represent the amount of food customarily eaten at one time. For example, the pyramid serving size of ready-to-eat cereal is 1 ounce (28 g), but the serving size listed on the Nutrition Facts label of many cereals is 1 cup (approximately 55 g, double the pyramid size).

- Differences among individual selections within each group are not apparent on the pyramid. The icons in the background of each group represent added sugars (inverted triangle) and natural and added fat (circle). The greater the concentration of icons, the greater the amount of fat or sugar in the group. The icons help people make comparisons between groups, but not among items within any group. For instance, the icons indicate that the Milk group contains more fat than the Fruit group. However they do not indicate which items in the Milk group may have fat (eg, skim milk versus whole milk), nor do they show that avocados in the Fruit group do provide fat. Nutrient density is also not readily discerned by looking at the pyramid. For instance, consumers cannot tell that broccoli provides more nutrients and fiber than lettuce, both of which are pictured in the Vegetable group. The concept of quality must be explained.
- Not all of the guidelines are translated onto the Food Guide Pyramid. Dietary Guideline issues that are not conveyed on the Food Guide Pyramid include aim for a healthy weight, be physically active each day, keep food safe to eat, choose

and prepare foods with less salt, and if you drink alcoholic beverages, do so in moderation.

- Positive is always more effective than negative. Rather than empowering people to make doable changes in their eating habits, nutrition guidelines have provoked negative feelings about food and diets in many people, especially the recommendation to choose a diet low in saturated fat and cholesterol. A poll conducted by the International Food Information Council revealed that the vast majority of women (as primary nutrition keepers of the family) have negative feelings about their food choices. Many feel guilty about eating foods they "shouldn't," eat; they worry that they will develop a disease from poor food choices and feel overwhelmed with nutrition information. Replace negative messages (eg, "don't eat fat") with positive ones ("if you eat all the recommended servings of fruits and vegetables, the end result is likely to be a diet moderate in fat.").

Food Guide Graphics in Other Countries

The Food Guide Pyramid is pervasive in the United States, appearing on food packages, grocery bags, and nutrition education materials. Yet because of cultural differences in communicating symbolism and other cultural norms, the pyramid shape is not necessarily superior or even appropriate for food guides in other countries. A wheel or dinner plate, with each section depicting relative proportion to the total diet, is used by many countries, including the United Kingdom, Germany, and Norway. The Philipines' food guide is illustrated by a six-pointed star. Israel's food guide is the shape of a chalice, with water occupying the largest and topmost portion to represent the importance of water for overall health. Canada's nutrition guidelines and food guide are discussed below.

DIETARY GUIDELINES FOR CANADIANS

Canada's nutrition history is similar to that of the United States. During World War II, a national food guide was developed to ensure that Canadians ate enough protein, vitamins, and minerals. It was not until the 1970s and 1980s, when the link between nutrient excess and the risk of developing certain chronic diseases became apparent, that the focus expanded to include avoiding over-consumption of food and nutrients. Hence the goal of the current guidelines is twofold: 1) help consumers obtain adequate amounts of protein, vitamins, and minerals, and 2) to control body weight and reduce the risk of developing nutrition-related problems.

Nutrition Recommendations for Canadians

A report called *Nutrition Recommendations: The Report of the Scientific Review Committee* was published by Health and Welfare Canada in 1990. It contains a review of nutrition research and describes the desired characteristics of the diet in Canada. As a technical report, it expresses nutrition recommendations in scientific terms, with quantities of nutrients and food components specified. It provides useful background information for dietitians and physicians; it is not intended to be used by consumers. It recommends that the Canadian diet:

- Provide energy consistent with the maintenance of body weight within the recommended range.
- Include essential nutrients in amounts specified in the Recommended Nutrient Intakes.
- Include no more than 30% of energy as fat (33 g/1000 cal) and no more than 10% as saturated fat (11 g/1000 cal).
- Provide 55% of energy as carbohydrate (138 g/1000 cal) from a variety of sources
- Be reduced in sodium content.
- Include no more than 5% of total energy as alcohol, or 2 drinks daily, whichever is less.
- Contain no more caffeine than the equivalent of 4 cups of regular coffee per day.
- Community water supplies containing less than 1 mg/L or fluoride should be fluoridated to that level.

Canada's Guidelines for Healthy Eating

The Nutrition Recommendations for Canadians were translated into a set of statements for use by the general public called Canada's Guidelines for Healthy Eating. The straightforward, simple messages to promote healthy eating are to:

- Enjoy a variety of food.
- Emphasize cereals, breads, and other grain products, vegetables, and fruits.
- Choose lower-fat dairy products, leaner meats, and food prepared with little or no fat.
- Achieve and maintain a healthy body weight by enjoying regular physical activity and healthy eating.
- Limit salt, alcohol, and caffeine.

Canada's Food Guide to Healthy Eating

Canada's Food Guide to Healthy Eating is a consumer-friendly tool that illustrates how Canadians can achieve the guidelines for healthy eating. It can be used to help plan and evaluate daily meals for Canadians 4 years of age and older.

The Food Guide to Healthy Eating depicts a four-banded rainbow of foods, with different colors representing each of its four food groups (Figure 8-2). Grain Products occupy the largest arc, followed by Vegetables and Fruit. Milk Products and Meat and Alternatives form the smallest arcs. The rainbow conveys the concept that all four groups are important but that the amounts of foods needed from each group varies. For instance, five to 12 servings are recommended daily from the Grain Products group, whereas the

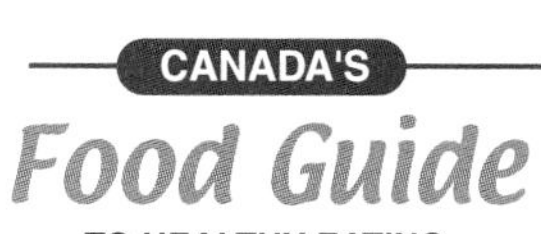

TO HEALTHY EATING
FOR PEOPLE FOUR YEARS
AND OVER

Enjoy a variety of foods from each group every day.

Choose lower-fat foods more often.

A RAINBOW GUIDE

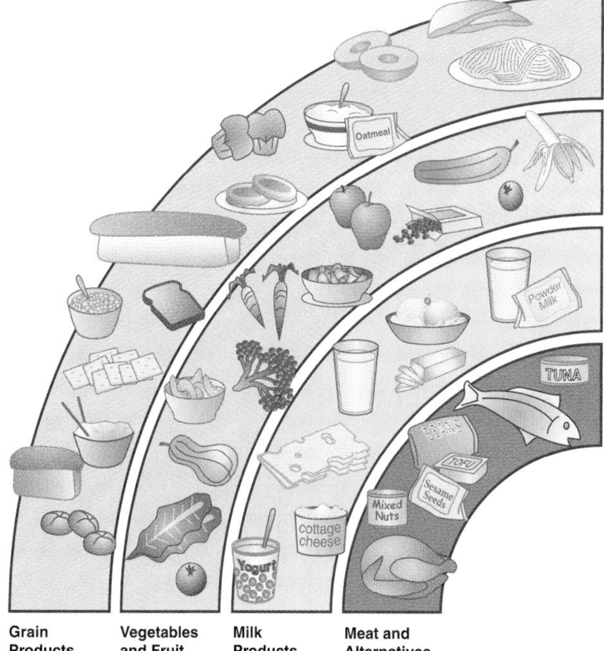

Grain Products Choose whole grain and enriched products more often.

Vegetables and Fruit Choose dark green and orange vegetables and orange fruit more often.

Milk Products Choose lower-fat milk products more often.

Meat and Alternatives Choose leaner meats, poultry and fish, as well as dried peas, beans and lentils more often.

B BAR GUIDE

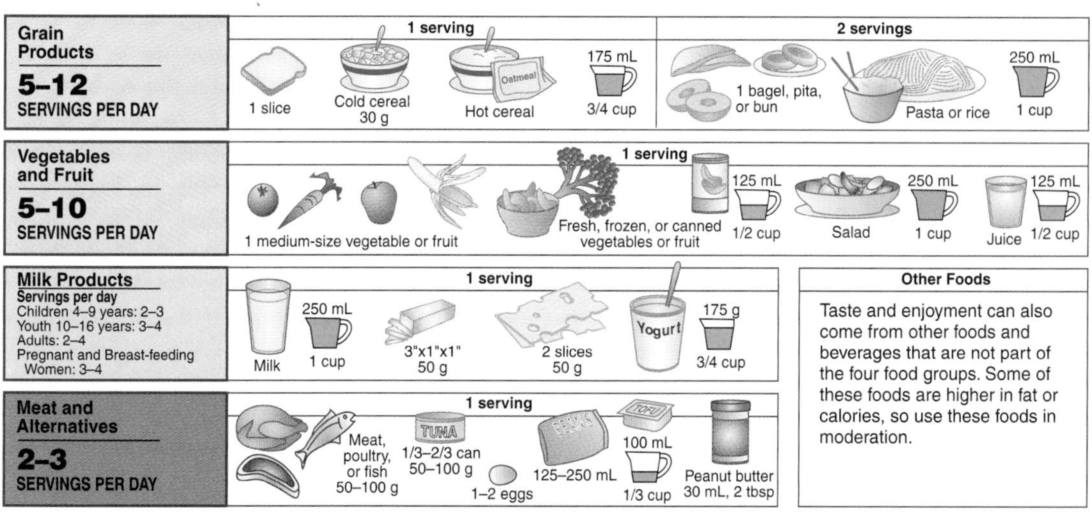

Different People Need Different Amounts of Food

The amount of food you need every day from the four food groups and other foods depends on your age, body size, activity level, whether you are male or female, and if you are pregnant or breast-feeding. That's why the Food Guide gives a lower and higher number of servings for each food group. For example, young children can choose the lower number of servings, while male teenagers can go to the higher number. Most other people can choose servings somewhere in between.

FIGURE 8-2 Canada's Food Guide to Healthy Eating. Four-banded rainbow of foods (*A*). Suggested servings per day (*B*).

recommended daily servings from the Meat and Alternatives group are two to three. The number of daily calories provided ranges from 1800 to 3200, depending on the types and amounts of foods selected from the four groups plus the "Other Foods" category. The guide recommends that sedentary adults choose from the lower end of the range and active adolescents choose from the higher end. Simple statements are included on the food guide to help consumers make healthy choices. For instance, the message to "Choose lower-fat milk products more often" under the Milk Products heading helps Canadians meet the recommendation to lower total fat and saturated fat intake.

NUTRITION FACTS LABEL

The Nutrition Labeling and Education Act of 1990 resulted in the Nutrition Facts label (Figure 8-3) and sweeping nutrition labeling reforms that shifted focus away from avoiding nutrient deficiencies and toward avoiding nutrition-related chronic diseases. For instance, this legislation decreed that it is no longer necessary to list the amount of thiamine, riboflavin, and niacin on food labels because deficiencies of these vitamins are no longer a public health concern. To help people avoid nutrient excesses, some previ-

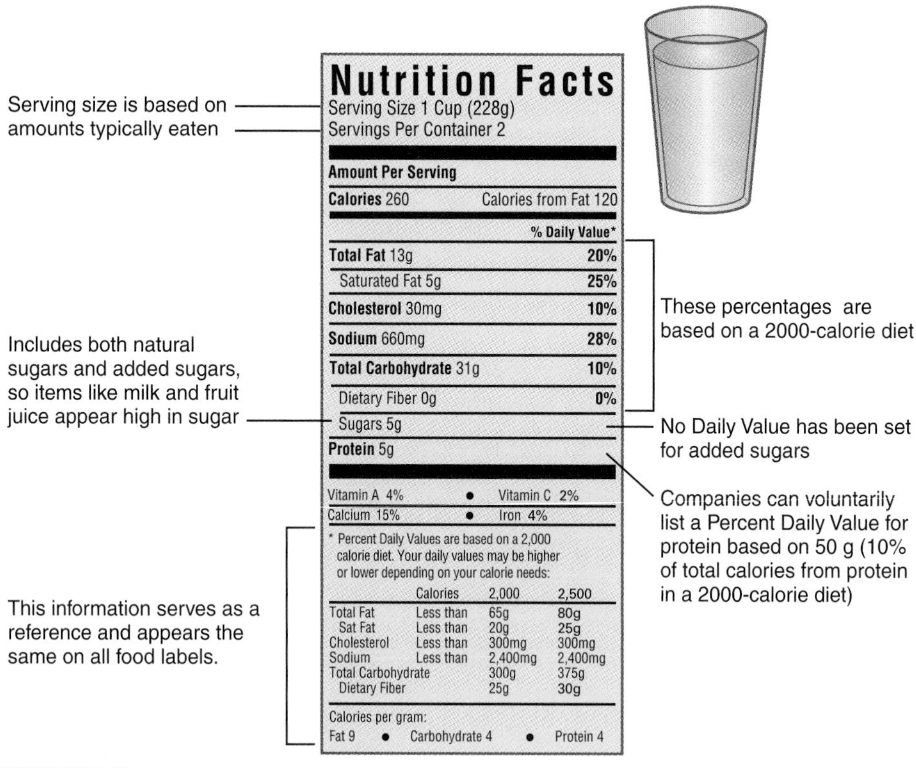

FIGURE 8-3 Nutrition Facts label format.

ously unavailable information is now required, such as the number of calories from fat, and the amount of saturated fat, cholesterol, sugars, and dietary fiber per serving. Even the sequence of information must conform to regulations. The serving size and number of servings per container is specified, after which comes the following information listed per serving:

- Calories
- Calories from fat
- Total fat (g)
- Saturated fat (g)
- Cholesterol (mg)
- Sodium (mg)
- Total carbohydrate, which includes starch, natural sugars, added sugars, and fiber (g)
- Dietary fiber (g)
- Sugars, both natural and added (g)
- Protein (g)

Also, labels must state the percent of Reference Daily Intakes in a serving for vitamin A, vitamin C, iron, and calcium. Labels may voluntarily include other information, such as the amount of polyunsaturated fat, monounsaturated fat, and potassium in a serving. If a food is fortified or enriched with any optional components, or if a health claim is made about any of them, the pertinent information then becomes mandatory.

Almost all processed foods require mandatory labeling. Only plain coffee and tea; some spices, flavorings, and other foods that contain no significant amounts of nutrients; ready-to-eat food prepared primarily on site, such as deli and bakery items; restaurant food; bulk food that is not resold; and food that is produced by small businesses is exempt. Manufacturers of foods in small packages are not required to list nutrition information on their labels unless they make a nutrition claim. Nutrition information is voluntary (point-of-purchase) for many raw foods, including frequently eaten raw fruits, vegetables, fish, and major cuts of meat and poultry.

Daily Value

Daily Value is a reference created by the FDA for labeling purposes. Daily Value actually is a group name for two distinct, behind-the-scenes sets of reference values: Daily Reference Values (DRVs) and Reference Daily Intakes (RDIs).

Daily Reference Values

Daily Reference Values are established for nutrients and food components that have important health implications, but no RDA. For some nutrients, they are amounts that should not be exceeded, while for others, they are amounts to strive toward. For nutrient intakes that are based on the percentage of calories consumed, 2000 calories is the standard used. Most labels list the DV for 2000 calories and 2500 calories on the bottom of the Nutrition Facts label. Nutrients that have DRVs that are independent of calorie intake are appropriate amounts for adults and children older than 4 years of age.

Food Component	DRV	What the DRV Is Based On
Fat	65 g	30% of total calories
Saturated fatty acids	20 g	10% of total calories
Cholesterol	300 mg	Expert recommendations*
Sodium	2400 mg	Expert recommendations†
Total carbohydrate	300 g	60% of total calories
Fiber	25 g	11.5 g/1000 cal
Potassium	3500 mg	Expert recommendations‡
Protein§	50 g	10% of total calories

*Recommendation for total cholesterol intake is independent of calorie intake.

†Recommendation for total sodium intake is independent of calorie intake.

‡Recommendation for total potassium intake is independent of calorie intake.

§An RDI for protein, not a DRV, has been established for infants and children under 4 years of age, pregnant women, and lactating women.

Reference Daily Intake (RDI)

The Reference Daily Intakes replace U.S. RDAs, which are based on National Academy of Sciences' 1968 Recommended Dietary Allowances. They represent amounts of nutrients people should strive to consume.

Nutrient	Amount
Vitamin A	5000 IU, or 875 μg RE
Vitamin D	400 IU, or 10 μg
Vitamin E	30 IU, or 9 mg α-tocopherol equivalents
Vitamin K	80 μg
Thiamine	1.5 mg
Riboflavin	1.7 mg
Niacin	20 mg NE
Vitamin B_6	2.0 mg
Folic acid	400 μg
Vitamin B_{12}	6 μg
Biotin	300 μg
Pantothenic acid	10 mg
Vitamin C	60 mg
Calcium	1.0 g
Iron	18 mg
Iodine	150 g
Magnesium	400 mg
Zinc	15 mg
Copper	2 mg

Percent Daily Value

The Percent Daily Value (%DV) is intended to help consumers determine the contribution a serving of a particular food makes to their overall intake. In theory, a person could add the %DV of a nutrient for all the foods eaten over the course of a day to determine how closely the total intake came to 100% DV. In reality, this is impractical because people do not measure portion sizes and may unknowingly eat more or less than the amount specified on the label, people don't have access to food labels for prepared foods (eg, restaurant or take-out food), and not all foods come with labels, such as fresh meats and vegetables. However the %DV is useful for making comparisons between different brands and types of food. For instance, the %DV for fiber is 4% in ready-to-eat cereal "A" and 20% in cereal "B." The consumer quickly determines that cereal "B" is a better source of fiber than cereal "A."

The Nutrition Facts Label as a Teaching Tool

The Nutrition Facts label is a useful teaching tool, with the following points noted.

Again, Portion Size is Everything

All of the information that appears on the Nutrition Facts label is specific for the size portion listed. Eating twice as much as the serving size listed doubles the amount of calories and nutrients provided.

The %DV May Under- or Overestimate the Contribution to an Individual's Diet

For people who require more or less than 2000 calories daily, the %DV is not accurate for nutrients whose amounts are based on a percent of total calories (eg, carbohydrates, protein, fat, saturated fat). For instance, the figure upon which %DV for fat is based for food labels is 65 g (2000 cal x .30 = 600 cal divided by 9 cal/g = approximately 65 g). Yet for a 1600 calorie diet, 30% or less of total calories from fat translates to approximately 53 g (1600 cal x .30 = 480 cal divided by 9 cal/g = 53 g). Therefore a food that supplies 100% of the DV for fat (eg, some frozen entrees) contains 65 g, which actually provides 123% of the fat recommended for someone consuming 1600 calories daily.

To make the %DV meaningful for calorie levels other than 2000, the endpoint is adjusted downward or upward from 100%. People consuming 1600 calories (which is 80% of 2000 calories) need to eat to a total of 80% DV. People who need 2800 calories need to eat to a total of 140%. But remember, this is only for nutrients whose total is depends upon total calories consumed—not for nutrients whose intake is independent of calorie intake, such as sodium, cholesterol, vitamins, and minerals.

Percent of Calories From Fat is Not Listed on the Label

Many people are aware of the 30%-or-less suggestion for fat intake. Many people mistakenly think that the %DV for fat on the label is the percentage of calories from fat in a serving, not the percentage of total recommended fat intake provided in a serving. For example, the %DV for a serving of corn oil is 22% even though 100% of the calories in the oil come from fat (eg, calories: 120, calories from fat: 120).

The Nutrient Claims, Such as "Low," "Free," and "High," are Reliable and Valid

Terms such as "low," "free," and "high" as well as others like them are legally defined. Any term used to describe the nutrient content of a food is uniform on all products on which the term appears. For example, "good source of fiber" means a serving of the product provides 10% to 19% of the DV for fiber (approximately 2.5 g to 4.5 g) regardless of whether the product is canned beans or dry cereal. Box 8-1 defines the terms used in nutrient claims.

Health Claims are Also Trustworthy

The FDA allows certain health claims about the relationship between certain nutrients or foods and the risk of a disease or healthrelated conditions. All products that have health claims must 1) not exceed specific levels for total fat, saturated fat, cholesterol, and sodium and 2) contain at least 10% of the Daily Value (before supplementation) for

BOX 8.1

Definitions of Terms Used in Nutrient Claims

Free means the product contains virtually none of that nutrient. "Free" can refer to calories, sugar, sodium, salt, fat, saturated fat, and cholesterol.

Low means there is a small enough amount of a nutrient that the product can be used frequently without concern about exceeding dietary recommendations. Low sodium, low calorie, low fat, low saturated fat, and low cholesterol are all defined as to the amount allowed per serving. For instance, to be labeled low cholesterol a product must have no more than 20 mg cholesterol/serving.

Very low refers to sodium only. The product cannot have more than 35 mg sodium/serving.

Reduced or less means the product has at least a 25% reduction in a nutrient compared to the regular product.

Light or lite means the product has ⅓ fewer calories than a comparable product or 50% of the fat found in a comparable product.

Good source means the product provides 10% to 19% of the Daily Value for a nutrient.

High, rich in, or excellent source means the product has at least 20% of the Daily Value for a nutrient.

More means the product has at least 10% more of a desirable nutrient than does a comparable product.

Lean refers to meat or poultry products with less than 10 g fat, less than 4 g saturated fat, and less than 95 mg cholesterol per standardized serving and per 100 g.

Extra lean refers to meat or poultry products with less than 5 g fat, less than 2 g saturated fat, and less than 95 mg cholesterol per standardized serving and per 100 g.

any one or all of the following: protein, dietary fiber, vitamin A, vitamin C, calcium, and iron. Additional health claim criteria are specific for the claim made. For instance, the claim regarding calcium and osteoporosis is only allowed on foods that have at least 20% DV for calcium. The following claims are all approved for use if they meet the proper specifications:

- Calcium and osteoporosis
- Fat and cancer
- Saturated fat and cholesterol and risk of coronary heart disease
- Fiber-containing grain products, fruits, and vegetables and cancer
- Fruits, vegetables, and grain products that contain fiber (particularly soluble fiber), and risk of coronary heart disease
- Fruits and vegetables and cancer
- Sodium and high blood pressure
- Soy protein and reduced risk of coronary heart disease
- Folic acid and neural tube defects
- Soluble fiber from psyllium seed husk or whole oats and coronary heart disease

Ingredients are Listed in Order by Descending Weight

Buyer beware that products stating they contain certain ingredients do have those ingredients, but they may not be present in large enough amounts to be nutritionally significant. For instance, analysis of a frozen vegetable and chicken pot pie found only 10 peas, 1/20 of a raw carrot, and 1/9 of a potato. On the ingredient list, items that appear near the top of the list are present in larger concentrations than those near the end.

Nutrition in Cancer Prevention

Many health agencies publish guidelines or recommendations for healthy eating, such as the American Heart Association and the American Cancer Society. Even though they are written from different health perspectives, the recommendations are remarkably similar. The diet to prevent (and treat) heart disease is presented in Chapter 18. The American Cancer Society's Guidelines on Diet, Nutrition, and Cancer Prevention are discussed in this section.

It is estimated that approximately 1/3 of cancer deaths that occur in the United States are related to dietary factors. Some diet-related cancers may be due to nutritional excesses or deficiencies that alter the body's ability to defend against cancer (altered immunocompetence), or that may alter enzymes, gastrointestinal flora, and hormone levels to create an environment favorable to cancer promotion.

Cancer risk may be reduced by eating more of the foods known to protect against cancer and eating less of the foods associated with an increased cancer risk. A varied diet and moderation in all things seem prudent. Although they are not guaranteed to prevent cancer in all people, the following guidelines are intended to reduce the risk of diet-related cancers.

CHOOSE MOST OF THE FOODS YOU EAT FROM PLANT SOURCES

Plant foods contain a variety of antioxidant vitamins, minerals, and fibers that are believed to be protective against cancer. Plants also contain hundreds of phytochemicals (plant chemicals) that appear to be protective against cancer. Different plants have different types and combinations of protective substances. Because it is not known which substances have the greatest impact on cancer prevention, variety is important. The guidelines recommend:

- Five or more servings of fruits and vegetables daily
- Grain products at every meal and choice of whole grains over refined grains
- Dried peas and beans as an alternative to meat. Of particular interest are the phytochemicals in soy products, which appear to reduce the risk of hormone-related cancers of the breast and prostate. Soy experts suggest that as little as one serving per day of soy-base foods can provide important health benefits.

LIMIT THE INTAKE OF HIGH-FAT FOODS, PARTICULARLY FROM ANIMAL SOURCES

High-fat diets are associated with an increased risk of cancers of the colon and rectum, prostate, and endometrium. Although the correlation exists, it is not known how fat impacts cancer risk. For instance, it is not known whether the risk is related to the amount of total fat consumed or due to the particular type of fat eaten. Also unknown is whether fat alone is to blame for the increased cancer risk, or if the problem is in the excess calories provided by fat.

In addition, people who tend to eat high-fat diets tend to eat fewer fruits and vegetables, which may add to cancer risk. Much has yet to be learned about the role of fat in cancer. The guidelines recommend:

- Choose foods low in fat. This can be accomplished by replacing high-fat foods with fruits, vegetables, grains, and dried peas and beans; eating smaller portions of high-fat foods; choosing baked and broiled foods in place of fried foods; using nonfat and reduced-fat milk and dairy products; and choosing convenience and restaurant foods that are low in fat.
- Limit meat intake, especially the intake of high-fat meats

BE PHYSICALLY ACTIVE: ACHIEVE AND MAINTAIN A HEALTHY WEIGHT

Physical activity may reduce cancer risk by promoting weight management or avoiding obesity, which is linked to an increased risk for cancers of the colon, prostate, endometrium, kidney, and breast (in postmenopausal women). Physical activity may also reduce risk by other mechanisms. For instance, it may reduce colon cancer risk by stimulating peristalsis, which decreases the amount of time potentially harmful substances are in the bowel. Physical activity may reduce the risk of breast and prostate cancer by influencing hormone levels. The recommendations are to:

- Be at least moderately active for 30 minutes or more on most days of the week. This recommendation is consistent with the recommendations made by the Centers for Disease Control and Prevention, the American College of Sports Medicine, and the *1996 Report of The US Surgeon General*.
- Maintain a healthy weight range for height and gender. This guideline uses the "healthy weight" range depicted in the *Dietary Guidelines for Americans*.
- Limit alcohol intake, if you drink at all. The risk of cancer increases with the amount of alcohol consumed and may begin to rise with as few as two drinks daily. In women, one alcoholic drink daily increases the risk of breast cancer. Alcohol and tobacco combined produce a greater risk of cancers of the oral cavity, esophagus, and larynx than the sum of their individual effects.

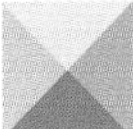

Food Quality and Safety Considerations

Planning an adequate diet relates not only to nutritional adequacy, but also to food quality and safety concerns. Proper storage and preparation are vital to ensure that the vitamin and mineral content of a food is retained. Foodborne illness represents a threat when food is improperly handled or stored, and naturally occurring toxicants may be a much greater threat to health than manmade pesticides.

RETAINING THE NUTRIENT CONTENT OF FOOD

Even when it is carefully planned, an eating plan affords no guarantees that it will provide optimal amounts of all nutrients, especially if the food that is eaten has been improperly stored or overly processed. Generally, food begins to lose its nutrients the moment that harvesting or processing begins, and the more that is done to a food before it is eaten, the greater the nutrient loss. Heat, light, air, soaking in water, mechanical injury, dry storage, and acidic or alkaline food processing ingredients can all hasten nutrient losses. Vitamins, minerals, and fiber are particularly vulnerable to the effects of food processing. Tips to minimize nutrient losses are as follows:

- Don't buy produce that is damaged or wilted, or that has been improperly stored. Produce picked when fully ripe is higher in nutrients than produce picked when green.
- Whenever possible, buy frozen foods instead of canned foods. Canning procedures (blanching, sterilizing, and soaking) destroy nutrients.
- Avoid storing foods for a long time.
- Avoid exposing food to light, especially milk. As little as 2 hours of light can decrease the riboflavin content of milk by 20% to 80%. Keep milk cold and covered.
- Refrigerate fruits and vegetables immediately to slow enzyme activity and retain nutrients. Keep produce in the refrigerator crisper or in moistureproof bags.

- Wash produce, but don't soak, to avoid leaching nutrients.
- Avoid peeling and paring vegetables before cooking because a valuable layer of nutrients is stored directly beneath the skin. If necessary, scrape or pare as thin a layer as possible.
- Avoid cutting produce into small pieces: The more surface area exposed, the greater the nutrient loss.
- Prepare vegetables as close to serving time as possible to avoid excessive exposure to light and air. Don't thaw frozen vegetables before cooking.
- Eat some fruits and vegetables raw.
- Cook produce in as little water as possible to avoid leaching vitamins. Stir-fry, steam, microwave, or pressure-cook vegetables to retain nutrients. If water is used in cooking, save and use it as stock for soups, gravies, or sauces.
- Shorten cooking time as much as possible. Cook vegetables to the tender crunchy, rather than to the mushy stage of doneness; cover the pan to retain heat; and preheat the pan or water before adding foods to speed heating time.
- Cook only as many vegetables as are needed at a time because reheating causes considerable loss of vitamins.

FOODBORNE ILLNESS

As many as 81 million illnesses and 9000 deaths per year are attributed to consumption of contaminated food or water. The microorganisms that cause foodborne illness are found widely in nature. They are transmitted to people from within the food (eg, meat and fish), on the food (eg, eggshell or vegetables), from unsafe water, or from human or animal feces. Bacteria are responsible for approximately ⅔ of all food borne illnesses. To spread, bacteria simply need food, moisture, a favorable temperature, and time to multiply. The remainder of cases are blamed on viruses, parasites, food toxins, and unknown causes. Although foodborne illness can be caused by any food, animal products are the most frequent vehicles. Table 8-2 outlines common pathogens that cause foodborne illness.

The major cause of foodborne illnesses is unsanitary food handling. To reduce the risk of contamination, proper personal hygiene and handwashing must be practiced by all food handlers. Steps must be taken to prevent cross-contact between raw and cooked foods and through food handlers. Because heat kills most bacteria, thorough cooking of meat and fish is vital, as is pasteurization of all milk products. Adequate refrigeration inhibits the growth of bacteria. Basic rules to keep food safe are as follows:

- Keep hot foods hot (>140°) and cold foods cold (<40°).
- Do not buy cans or glass jars with dents, cracks, or bulges.
- Never eat raw or undercooked meat, poultry, seafood, or eggs.
- Cook meat, poultry, seafood, and eggs to at least 165° to kill any bacteria present.
- Promptly refrigerate leftovers after serving.
- Avoid cross-contact between raw meat and poultry and other ready-to-eat foods. All surfaces (hands, cutting boards, countertops, dishes, utensils) that have been

TABLE 8.2 ***Common Pathogens That Cause Foodborne Illness***

Organism	Common Food Vehicles	Onset	Symptoms	Preventive Measures	Other
Bacillus cereus (bacillus)	Meat products, soups, vegetables, puddings, sauces, milk and milk products	8–16 hours	Abdominal pain, watery diarrhea, nausea, vomiting	Cook foods thoroughly; reheat foods thoroughly; prevent cross-contact	
Campylobacter jejuni (campylobacter enteritis)	Untreated water, raw milk, undercooked poultry and meats	1–7 days	Diarrhea, muscle pain, fever, nausea, vomiting, headache	Use pasteurized milk; cook foods thoroughly; prevent cross-contact; use sanitary practices; wash hands after handling pets	Leading cause of diarrhea in the United States: rarely life threatening
Clostridium botulinum (botulism)	Underheated, low-acid canned foods (corn, peppers, green beans, mushrooms, tuna), vacuum-packed meats, sausage, fish	Usually 18–36 hours after ingesting toxin, but onset may range from 4 hours to 8 days	Nausea, vomiting, diarrhea, fatigue, headache, dry mouth, double vision, difficulty speaking and swallowing, muscle paralysis	Follow recommended procedures when canning foods; cook food thoroughly; refrigerate packaged meats and fish	Fatal in 3–10 days if not treated
Clostridium perfringens (perfringens food poisoning)	Meat, poultry, stuffing, and gravy held or stored at inappropriate temperature	8–22 hours	Mild diarrhea, nausea, vomiting that may last 1 day or less	Cool food rapidly after cooking; hold hot foods > 140°; reheat food to 165°	The "cafeteria germ," associated with steam table foods not kept hot enough
Cryptosporidium parvum (intestinal, tracheal, or pulmonary cryptosporidiosis)	Any food touched by an infected food handler, raw vegetables fertilized with contaminated manure or irrigated with contaminated water	Approximately 2 days	Intestinal: severe watery diarrhea Pulmonary/tracheal: coughing, low-grade fever, usually accompanied by intestinal distress	Use treated water	Water must be filtered to remove this pathogen; it is not killed by chlorine
Cyclospora cayetanesis (cyclosporidiosis)	Food or water contaminated with infected stool	1 week	Severe watery diarrhea, fatigue, nausea, vomiting, muscle aches, fever, abdominal cramping, anorexia, weight loss	Avoid contaminated water and food	

(continued)

TABLE 8.2 *Common Pathogens That Cause Foodborne Illness (continued)*

Organism	Common Food Vehicles	Onset	Symptoms	Preventive Measures	Other
Escherichia coli (*E. coli* 0157-H7; hemorrhagic colitis)	Undercooked beef, especially ground beef; raw milk; unpasteurized apple juice; alfalfa sprouts; plant foods fertilized with raw manure or irrigated with contaminated water	2–5 days	Severe abdominal cramps and diarrhea Hemorrhagic colitis may lead to hemolytic-uremic syndrome (severe anemia and renal failure)	Cook meat thoroughly; avoid cross-contact; use sanitary practices; drink pasteurized milk and apple juice	
Hepatitis A virus (hepatitis)	Food contaminated by infected food handlers, water, shellfish, and salads are the most common vehicles	10–50 days (average is 28–30 days)	Fever, malaise, nausea, vomiting, muscle pain, jaundice	Use sanitary practices; avoid eating raw shellfish	
Listeria monocytogenes (listeriosis)	Improperly refrigerated milk, deli-type salads, processed meats, soft cheese, undercooked poultry	2 days to 3 weeks	Sudden fever, chills, headache, backache, occasional abdominal pain, and diarrhea Septicemia and meningitis may lead to death	Cook foods thoroughly; avoid cross-contact; use sanitary practices; keep interior of refrigerator clean	This bacterium thrives in cold temperatures and appears to be able to survive short-term pasteurization
Norwalk virus (food poisoning; viral gastroenteritis)	Untreated water, shellfish, raw or undercooked clams, and oysters	24–48 hours	Nausea, vomiting, diarrhea, abdominal pain, headache, low-grade fever	Avoid raw shellfish; use sanitary practices	Severe illness is rare
Salmonella species (salmonellosis)	Raw and undercooked eggs, poultry, meats, milk and dairy products, frog legs	6–48 hours	Nausea, vomiting, chills, fever, diarrhea Arthritic symptoms may occur 3–4 weeks after onset of acute infection	Cook foods thoroughly; avoid cross-contact; use sanitary practices	Can be fatal
Shigella species (shigellosis)	Salads (potato, tuna, shrimp, macaroni,	12–50 hours	Severe diarrhea that may be bloody,	Use sanitary practices; cook foods thoroughly; store/	Most frequently occurs in children 1–4 years

	chicken), untreated water Foods are usually contaminated by food handler		nausea, headaches, chills, dehydration	hold foods at <40° or >140°	of age
Staphylococcus aureus (staphylococcal food poisoning)	Custard- or cream-filled baked goods, ham, tongue, cooked poultry, dressing, gravy, eggs, potato salad, cream sauce, sandwich fillings	1–6 hours	Severe nausea, vomiting, diarrhea, abdominal cramps	Use sanitary practices; refrigerate foods	Of healthy people, 40%–50% are carriers. Most frequently found in the nose, throat, on skin, and in infected boils, pimples, cuts, and burns
Vibrio vulnificus (vibrio infection)	Raw shellfish, especially oysters	Abrupt	Fever, chills, skin lesions, nausea, vomiting, diarrhea, hypotension, shock May lead to septicemia	Avoid eating raw seafood (organism is easily killed by cooking)	Infection rarely occurs in healthy people; those at risk include people with compromised immune systems, achlorhydria, and chronic liver disease Mortality rate ranges from 46%–75%
Yersinia enterocolitica (yersiniosis)	Pork, raw milk, meat, poultry, tofu	1–3 days	Diarrhea (may be bloody), fever, severe abdominal pain that mimics appendicitis	Use pasteurized milk; cook foods thoroughly; avoid cross-contact; use sanitary practices	

exposed to raw meat and poultry must be thoroughly washed before coming into contact with ready-to-eat foods.
- Never defrost meat, fish, or poultry at room temperature.
- Do not partially precook food and then finish later.
- When basting during grilling or broiling, apply sauce to cooked surfaces only.
- Meat and poultry can be recontaminated when brushed with bristles that have been in contact with raw or undercooked foods.
  - Reheat leftovers thoroughly.
  - Serve cooked food on clean plates with clean utensils.
  - Keep work surfaces clean. Wash hands, utensils, and cutting boards in hot soapy water before preparing food and after handling raw meat or poultry.
  - Use a plastic or other nonporous cutting board. Wash cutting boards in the dishwasher after use.
  - Do not drink unpasteurized milk or untreated water.
  - When in doubt, throw it out.

The most common symptoms of foodborne illness may be mistaken for the flu: diarrhea, nausea, vomiting, fever, abdominal pain, and headaches. Most cases are self-limiting and run their course within a few days. Symptoms that warrant medical attention include bloody diarrhea (possible *E. coli* 0157:H7 infection), a stiff neck with severe headache and fever (possible meningitis related to *Listeria*), excessive diarrhea or vomiting (possible life-threatening dehydration), and any symptoms that persist for more than 3 days. Infants, pregnant women, the elderly, and people with compromised immune systems (people with acquired immunodeficiency syndrome [AIDS] or cancer, organ transplant recipients, people taking corticosteroids) are particularly vulnerable to the effects of food poisoning.

Questions You May Hear

Are "natural" foods safer than synthetic foods? "Natural" ingredients in food include the energy nutrients (carbohydrates, protein, fat, and alcohol), essential nutrients (vitamins and minerals), dietary fiber, and naturally occurring compounds like caffeine and sterols. However, certain toxins and antinutrients may also be natural ingredients in foods; therefore, "natural" foods are not synonymous with "safe" foods. Even though it is estimated that we consume 10,000 times more natural toxins by weight than manmade pesticides, the quantity of natural toxins consumed is generally so small that health is not endangered. A varied diet is the best assurance against untoward effects of both natural and "unnatural" toxins.

KEY CONCEPTS

- Dietary excesses play a role in five of the leading causes of death in the United States.
- Dietary advice from numerous health and government agencies advocate moderation and balance for disease prevention.
- The RDAs are amounts of essential nutrients that are considered to be adequate to meet the nutritional needs of most healthy people. The RDA are currently being revised to the Dietary Reference Intakes, which include new RDAs plus three other sets of reference values.

- The purpose of the *Dietary Guidelines for Americans* is to help the public choose diets that are nutritionally adequate, promote health and wellbeing, and reduce the risk of chronic disease.
- The Food Guide Pyramid is a graphic illustration of the Dietary Guidelines for Americans. It recommends ranges of servings for each of the food groups. The underlying concepts of the pyramid are variety, balance, and moderation.
- The Nutrition Facts label format is intended to provide consumers with reliable and useful information to help them make better food choices.
- The Percent Daily Value listed for fat, saturated fat, carbohydrate, and dietary fiber on food labels is based on a 2000-calorie diet. The %DV for these nutrients underestimates the contribution in diets containing fewer than 2000 calories.
- A seemingly nutritionally adequate diet may provide suboptimal levels of certain nutrients if the food was improperly handled or overprocessed. The more that is done to a food, the greater the nutrient losses.
- Food processing has the greatest impact on water-soluble vitamins, minerals, and fiber.
- Bacteria are blamed for the majority of foodborne illnesses. Viruses, parasites, toxins, and unknown causes are blamed for the remainder of cases.
- Unsanitary food handling is responsible for most of foodborne illness.
- Groups most susceptible to foodborne illness include pregnant women, infants, older adults, and people with compromised immune systems.

Focus on Critical Thinking

Assess your own intake according to the Food Guide Pyramid Guidelines

1. Record everything you ate and drank yesterday. Be sure to specify estimated portion sizes.

FOOD	PORTION SIZE
English muffin	1
Butter	2 tsp
______	______
______	______
______	______

2. Analyze all food and beverages for their contribution to the appropriate Food Guide Pyramid food groups.

GRAINS	VEGETABLES	FRUIT	MILK	MEAT	OTHER
2					2

(continued)

Focus on Critical Thinking (continued)

3. Tally total number of servings for each food group.

GRAINS	VEGETABLES	FRUIT	MILK	MEAT	OTHER

4. Indicate appropriate number of servings you think you should eat from each food group.

GRAINS	VEGETABLES	FRUIT	MILK	MEAT	OTHER

5. List ways you could improve upon yesterday's intake to meet the Food Guide Pyramid recommendations.

___

___

___

___

___

ANSWER KEY

1. **TRUE** The RDAs are intended for healthy people only.
2. **TRUE** In response to criticism that RDAs should be set at levels to promote optimal health, not merely to prevent deficiencies, they are being revised and expanded.
3. **FALSE** Tolerable Upper Intake Level is the level at which nutrients can be tolerated with chronic daily use. It is not a recommended level of intake.
4. **TRUE** Nutrient deficiency diseases are rare in the United States. On the other hand, 5 out of 10 leading causes of death in the United States are associated with dietary excess.
5. **FALSE** The Food Guide Pyramid emphasizes the total diet. Each group provides some essential nutrients, but no one group provides adequate amounts of all essential nutrients.
6. **FALSE** Serving sizes on the Food Guide Pyramid may differ from serving sizes on food labels, which represent the amount of food customarily (although not necessarily wisely) eaten at one time.
7. **FALSE** The number of servings from each group on the Food Guide Pyramid should be dictated by an individual's total calorie requirement.
8. **TRUE** Vitamins, minerals, and fiber are particularly vulnerable to the effects of food processing.

9. TRUE Bacteria are responsible for approximately two thirds of all food borne illnesses.

10. TRUE Food borne illness can be caused by any food; however, animal products are the most common vehicles.

REFERENCES

American Cancer Society. (1996). *Guidelines on diet, nutrition, and cancer prevention*. Dallas: American Cancer Society.

Achterberg, C. (1992). A perspective: Challenges of teaching the Dietary Guidelines Graphic. *Food and Nutrition News*, 64(4), 2326.

Achterberg, C., McDonnell, E., & Bagby, R. (1994). How to put the Food Guide Pyramid into practice. *Journal of the American Dietetic Association*, *94*(10), 1030–1035.

Food and Drug Administration (1999). FDA approves new health claim for soy protein and coronary heart disease. *FDA Talk Paper*, October 20, 1999. [On-line]. Available: www.fda.gov/bbs/topics/ANSWERS/ANS00980.html.

Food and Drug Administration. (1993). Focus on food labeling. Read the label, set a healthy table. FDA consumer. (DHHS Publication No. [FDA] 932262). Rockville, MD: Author.

Hogbin, M., & Hess, M. (1999). Public confusion over food portions and servings. *Journal of American Diet Association*, 99(10), 1209–1211.

International Food Information Council Foundation. (1999). Are you listening? What consumers tell us about dietary recommendations. *Food Insight*, September/October, 1, 4–5.

International Food Information Council Foundation. (1999). Picture this! Communicating nutrition around the world. *Food Insight*, January/February, 1, 4–5.

International Food Information Council Foundation. (1998). It's a small world after all. Dietary guidelines around the world. *Food Insight*, March/April, 3–4.

International Food Information Council Foundation. (1998). Nutrient requirements get a makeover: The evolution of the Recommended Dietary Allowances. *Food Insight*, September/October, 1, 4–5.

International Food Information Council (1998). *A consumer's guide to microbiological risks to food safety*. [On-line]. Available: ificinfo.health.org/resource/microbiorisks.htm.

International Food Information Council. (1998). Backgrounder—Food safety and foodborne illness. [On-line]. Available: ificinfo.health.org/backgrnd/bkgr10.htm.

Morreale, S., & Schwaartz, N. (1995). Helping Americans eat right: Developing practical and actionable public nutrition education messages based on the ADA Survey of American Dietary Habits. *Journal of American Diet Association*, 95(3), 305–308.

National Research Council. (1989). *Recommended Dietary Allowances* (10th Ed.). Washington, DC: National Academy Press.

U.S. Department of Agriculture, & U.S. Department of Health and Human Services. (2000). Nutrition and your health: Dietary guidelines for americans. (6th ed.). [On-line]. Available: www.usda.gov/cnpp.

U.S. Department of Agriculture, Human Nutrition Information Service. (1992). The Food Guide Pyramid. *Home and Garden Bulletin No. 252*.

CHAPTER 9

Assessing Nutritional Status

TRUE	FALSE	Check your knowledge of assessing nutritional status.
⬭	⬭	1 Nutritional status is the balance between nutrient intake and requirements.
⬭	⬭	2 The sole purpose of evaluating a person's nutritional status is to determine whether there is a protein deficiency.
⬭	⬭	3 A person can be malnourished without being underweight.
⬭	⬭	4 Changes in weight reflect acute changes in nutritional status.
⬭	⬭	5 Albumin responds quickly to changes in protein status.
⬭	⬭	6 A low albumin concentration is specific for protein malnutrition.
⬭	⬭	7 "Significant" weight loss is 5% of body weight in 1 month.
⬭	⬭	8 People who take five or more prescription or over-the-counter medications or dietary supplements are at risk for nutritional problems.
⬭	⬭	9 Any amount of daily alcohol intake is considered a risk factor for nutritional problems.
⬭	⬭	10 Laboratory data reveal changes before the physical signs and symptoms of nutritional problems develop.

Upon completion of this chapter, you will be able to

- Explain the differences between nutritional screening and nutritional assessments.
- Describe health conditions that have the potential to affect nutritional status.
- List six intake screening questions to help identify potential problems with a client's usual intake.
- Describe how to calculate percent weight change.
- Describe the "rule of thumb" formula for calculating ideal body weight for men and women based on height.
- Discuss disadvantages of using albumin as an indicator of nutritional status.
- Explain the difficulties of using physical signs and symptoms to diagnose nutritional problems.

Tools to Evaluate Nutritional Status

Nutritional status is loosely defined as the state of balance between nutrient supply (intake) and demand (requirement). Imbalances between intake and requirement have the potential to alter nutritional status, resulting in overnutrition or undernutrition. In clinical settings where the focus is recovery from illness or surgery, the nutritional priority is often to ensure that intake meets requirement. In other words, the emphasis is on getting enough calories and protein. In wellness settings, where the focus is health promotion and disease prevention, the nutritional priority is frequently to ensure that intake does not exceed requirement. The emphasis is on avoiding excesses of calories, fat, saturated fat, cholesterol, and sodium. However, these settings do not have mutually exclusive nutritional priorities. Some hospital patients require restrictive diets (eg, low-sodium diet), and some wellness clients have nutrient intakes below their requirements (eg, not enough calcium or fiber). In all settings, it is appropriate to determine the client's nutritional status so that appropriate goals and interventions can be devised to correct actual or potential imbalances.

This chapter describes tools used to evaluate nutritional status, namely nutritional screening and comprehensive nutritional assessment, including historical data, physical findings, and laboratory data.

Nutritional status can be evaluated by looking at a few or many criteria. Exactly which criteria are evaluated and how the results are interpreted depend on the particular population and setting, as well as the availability of time and resources. Although everyone agrees that it is important to identify actual and potential nutritional problems, there is no universally accepted, definitive tool to do so. Often, professional judgment is as important as objective criteria.

NUTRITIONAL SCREENING

A nutritional screening is a quick look at a few variables to judge a client's relative risk for nutritional problems. Screening can be custom designed for a particular population (eg, pregnant women) or for a specific disorder (eg, cardiac disease). Screens may be completed by a dietitian, diet technician, or other qualified health care professional. Often, a routine screening occurs during the initial nursing history and physical examination.

To be both useful and efficient, screening tools must rely on data that are routinely available. A routine hospital screen is likely to focus on height, weight, significant unintentional weight loss, and serum albumin. Other variables may also be considered, such as skin integrity, appetite, diagnosis, diet order, and the client's functional status. In wellness settings, a screening tool such as that featured in Figure 9-1 may be used to measure nutritional risk in elderly clients, based on body weight, eating habits, living environment, and functional status.

After the appropriate data have been gathered, a judgment is made as to the client's relative risk for nutritional problems based on the number or severity of abnormal findings (Table 9-1). Clients who are found to be at moderate or high risk are given a com-

Name: ______________________ **Date:** ______________

Body Weight

Measure height to the nearest inch and weight to the nearest pound. Record the values below and mark them on the body mass index (BMI) scale to the right. Then use a straight edge (ruler) to connect the two points and circle the spot where this straight line crosses the center line (body mass index). Record the number below.

Healthy older adults should have a BMI between 24 and 27.

Height (in): ______________________

Weight (lbs): ______________________

Body Mass Index: ______________________
(number from center column)

Check any boxes that are true for the individual:

❑ Has lost or gained 10 pounds (or more) in the past 6 months

❑ Body mass index < 24

❑ Body mass index > 27

For the remaining sections, please ask the individual which of the statements (if any) is true for him of her and place a check by each that applies.

NOMOGRAM FOR BODY MASS INDEX

WEIGHT
LB | KG
340, 320, 300, 280, 260, 240, 220, 200, 190, 180, 170, 160, 150, 140, 130, 120, 110, 100, 95, 90, 85, 80, 75, 70, 65, 60, 55, 50 (LB)
150, 140, 130, 120, 110, 100, 95, 90, 85, 80, 75, 70, 65, 60, 55, 50, 45, 40, 35, 30, 25 (KG)

BODY MASS INDEX
[WT/ (HT)^2]
70, 60, 50, 40, 30, 20, 10

WOMEN: OBESE / OVERWEIGHT / ACCEPTABLE
MEN: OBESE / OVERWEIGHT / ACCEPTABLE

HEIGHT
IN | CM
50, 55, 60, 65, 70, 75, 80, 85 (IN)
125, 130, 135, 140, 145, 150, 155, 160, 165, 170, 175, 180, 185, 190, 195, 200, 205, 210 (CM)

Eating Habits

❑ Does not have enough food to eat each day
❑ Usually eats alone
❑ Does not eat anything on one or more days each month
❑ Has poor appetite
❑ Is on a special diet
❑ Eats vegetables two or fewer times daily
❑ Drinks milk or eats milk products once or not at all daily
❑ Eats fruit or drinks fruit juice once or not at all daily
❑ Eats breads, cereals, pasta, rice, or other grains five or fewer times daily
❑ Has difficulty chewing or swallowing
❑ Has more than one alcoholic drink per day (if woman); more than two drinks per day (if man)
❑ Has pain in mouth, teeth, or gums

Living Environment

❑ Lives on an income of less than $6000 per year (per individual in the household)
❑ Lives alone
❑ Is housebound
❑ Is concerned about home security
❑ Lives in a home with inadequate heating or cooling
❑ Does not have a stove and/or refrigerator
❑ Is unable or prefers not to spend money on food (<$25–30 per person spent on food each week)

Functional Status

Usually or always needs assistance with (check all that apply):

❑ Bathing
❑ Dressing
❑ Grooming
❑ Toileting
❑ Eating
❑ Walking or moving about
❑ Traveling (outside the home)
❑ Preparing food
❑ Shopping for food or other necessities

FIGURE 9-1

TABLE 9.1 *Assigning Risk: A Sample Protocol*

Factor	Level of Risk*			
	Low	*Mild*	*Moderate*	*High*
Weight (%IBW)	>90	80–90	70–80	<70
Serum albumin (g/dL)	>3.4	3.0–3.3	2.5–2.9	<2.5
Intake	Adequate	Fair to good	Poor to fair	Poor to fair
Skin (pressure ulcers)	Intact	Stage I or II	Stage III or IV	Stage III or IV
Diet	Solid	Solid; stable enteral nutrition	NOP; clear liquid; unstable enteral nutrition; parenteral nutrition	
Action	Monitor, provide basic nutrition care	Provide supplements; assist with food choices; teach/counsel	Refer to dietitian	Refer to dietitian

*Patients determined to be at no or low risk of malnutrition are not dismissed. Because nutritional status tends to deteriorate over the course of hospitalization, patients should be mointored regularly to detect changes in status.

prehensive nutritional assessment, usually by a dietitian. Clients who are identified to be at no or mild risk may need only to be periodically reevaluated to monitor for any deterioration in nutritional status. It is important to remember that nutritional risks may exist that simply were not evaluated and that a person's relative risk can change.

COMPREHENSIVE NUTRITIONAL ASSESSMENT

Comprehensive nutritional assessments use additional data for the purposes of quantifying the degree of malnutrition, providing effective nutritional care, and establishing a baseline for subsequent nutritional interventions. Data that may be included in an assessment appear in Box 9-1. Nutritional assessments are usually the responsibility of the dietitian, because extensive training is required to ensure accuracy of results. In the clinical setting, nutritional assessments focus on moderate- to high-risk patients with suspected or confirmed protein-calorie malnutrition.

FIGURE 9-1 Wellness screen. If you have checked one or more statements on this screen, the individual you have interviewed may be at risk for poor nutritional status. Please refer this individual to the appropriate health care or social service professional in your area. For example, a dietitian should be contacted for problems with selecting, preparing, or eating a healthy diet, or a dentist if the individual experiences pain or difficulty when chewing or swallowing. A physician should be contacted if the individual has gained or lost 10 pounds unexpectedly or without intending to during the past 6 months. A physician should also be notified if the individual's body mass index is above 27 or below 24. Those individuals whose income, lifestyle, or functional status may endanger their nutritional and overall health should be referred to available community services: home-delivered meals, congregate meal programs, transportation services, counseling services (eg, for alcohol abuse, depression, bereavement), home health care agencies, day care programs, and so forth. Please repeat this screen at least once each year—sooner if the individual has a major change in his or her health, income, immediate family (eg, a spouse dies), or functional status. (These materials were developed by the Nutrition Screening Initiative, a project of the American Academy of Family Physicians, the American Dietetic Association, and the National Council on the Aging, Inc.)

BOX 9.1

Possible Nutritional Assessment Parameters

HISTORICAL DATA

Current and past health history
- Nausea/vomiting
- Gastrointestinal integrity

Diagnosis
Treatment plan
Prognosis
Intake information
- 24-Hour food recall including portion sizes, usual meal and snack patterns, and usual meal timing
- Food frequency record
- Food record
- Diet history, including
  - Food likes, dislikes, intolerances, and allergies
  - Past/present use of a therapeutic diet and diet counseling received
  - A calorie count or nutritional intake study to determine adequacy of intake
  - Information on who purchases and prepares food
  - Adequacy of food storage and preparation facilities

Weight history
- Percent usual body weight
- Percent weight change

Medication uses: prescription drugs, over-the-counter medications, and dietary supplements
Other pertinent information
- Living situation
- Socioeconomic status

PHYSICAL FINDINGS

Signs and symptoms suggestive of nutritional problems
Anthropometric data
- Height
- Weight
- Triceps skinfolds
- Midarm circumference
- Midarm muscle circumference

LABORATORY DATA

Serum albumin
Serum transferrin

(continued)

BOX 9.1

Possible Nutritional Assessment Parameters (continued)

Prealbumin
Retinol-binding protein
24-hour urinary creatinine excretion, creatinine height index
Urinary urea nitrogen, state of nitrogen balance
Hemoglobin/hematocrit
Cholesterol
Lipid profile
Fasting blood glucose
All abnormal values
Total lymphocyte count

Criteria for Evaluation

Just as a blindfolded person's description of an elephant is limited to the part of the body felt, evaluations of nutritional status are limited by the criteria chosen. Limiting an evaluation to one or two criteria may not produce as valid a judgment as using more data. For instance, if evaluation is limited to weight only, a person of normal weight would be labeled adequately nourished; yet if the criteria are expanded to reveal other data, such as a recent unintentional weight loss, difficulty swallowing, and a low serum albumin, adequacy of nutritional status is not so certain. Likewise, in trying to determine whether a client usually consumes enough protein, focusing on the type of fat used and how many vegetables are consumed is not likely to produce the information needed to judge protein intake. It is important to know what to look for and how to interpret the results when evaluating nutritional status.

No single criterion can definitively and completely elucidate a person's nutritional status; however, it is not necessary to gather all available information on every client. Weight, recent weight change, health history, and questions about intake are appropriate for all people, regardless of the setting. Additional laboratory data, anthropometric measurements, and more objective intake data may be used, depending on the individual client and setting.

Although facility policies and procedures may stipulate what information to gather and how often, it is important to recognize that a myriad of factors have the potential to affect a person's nutritional status. Because nurses are more likely to be involved in nutritional screening and monitoring than in comprehensive nutritional assessments, this section focuses on routine data collected during a nursing history and physical examination, as well as routine laboratory data that relate to nutritional status.

HISTORICAL DATA

Relevant historical data are retrieved from the medical record or through a patient interview.

Health History

The client's health history, both current and past, helps identify conditions that may affect nutritional status by altering nutrient supply or demand. Health impairments that have the potential to negatively affect nutritional status include conditions that:

1. Impair nutrient intake, such as:
   - Chewing and swallowing problems, which may result from ill-fitting dentures, missing teeth, mechanical problems (eg, obstruction, inflammation, edema), or neurologic problems (eg, amyotrophic lateral sclerosis, myasthenia gravis, cerebral palsy, Parkinson's disease, multiple sclerosis, sequelae of cerebrovascular accident, or traumatic brain injury)
   - Anorexia, or lack of desire to eat, which may occur secondary to general illness, difficulty breathing, nausea and vomiting, pain, anxiety, depression, fear, or certain drug therapies
   - Anorexia nervosa, the eating disorder characterized by self-imposed starvation
   - Cognitive impairments, which may result from drug abuse, alcoholism, Alzheimer's disease, dementia, or mental illness
   - Impaired sensory function, such as loss of taste, smell, or vision
   - Paralysis or physical disabilities (eg, arthritis) that impair activities of daily living, such as the ability to feed oneself
2. Are characterized by an excessive nutrient intake, such as bulimia nervosa or obesity
3. Impair nutrient digestion and absorption, such as inflammatory, obstructive, or functional disorders of the gastrointestinal tract (eg, lactose intolerance, cystic fibrosis, pancreatic disorders, inflammatory bowel diseases, short-gut syndrome, radiation enteritis, liver disorders)
4. Accelerate metabolism (hypermetabolism), for example, pregnancy, fever, sepsis, thermal injuries, decubitus ulcers, cancer, acquired immunodeficiency syndrome (AIDS), major surgery, or trauma
5. Alter nutrient metabolism (eg, diabetes mellitus, hormonal imbalances, starvation)
6. Increase nutrient excretion (eg, diarrhea, malabsorption syndromes)
7. Impair nutrient excretion (eg, renal insufficiency)

Whether any of the above impairments actually have a negative impact on nutritional status depends on their severity and how long ago they occurred. For instance, inflammatory bowel disease in remission may have no impact on a client's current nutrient requirements or intake. Conversely, the impact of acute renal failure on nutritional status is dramatic.

Intake Information

Whenever possible, observe what the client eats to judge the adequacy of current intake. In clinical settings, patients who are receiving nothing by mouth (NPO), who are restricted to a clear liquid diet, or who are receiving enteral or parenteral nutrition are at risk for nutritional problems.

Historical information about what and how much a person usually eats can help identify nutritional problems and eating behaviors in need of improvement. This information serves as a basis for providing patients and clients with guidance on how to improve their usual intake. The following questions can be used to screen patients and clients for nutritional problems. More formal tools used to obtain intake information appear in Box 9-2.

BOX 9.2

Tools for Obtaining Intake Information

TWENTY-FOUR HOUR FOOD RECALL

The 24-hour food recall is the easiest and quickest way to evaluate a client's usual intake. Through a questionnaire or by interview, the client is asked to recall the types and amounts of all foods and beverages consumed during the previous or any typical 24-hour period. Food models may help to define portion sizes, and probing is often needed to obtain specific details, such as how the food was prepared, what the client put in his or her coffee, and the type of milk used. Open-ended questions, such as questions that begin with "what," "when," "how," "where," "why," or "who," usually provide more information than questions that can be answered with a simple "yes" or "no."

The client's 24-hour food recall data can then be evaluated according to the Food Guide Pyramid to estimate overall adequacy (see Chapter 8). The data generally are considered incomplete or too imprecise to evaluate according to the RDAs. Another drawback is that the 24-hour recall relies on memory and accurate interpretation of portion sizes, so underreporting of food consumption may occur. The underlying assumption in using the 24-hour recall method is that a single day closely represents the usual pattern of intake over an extended period; however, in reality, it may not.

FOOD FREQUENCY RECORD

Sometimes dietary intake is assessed by the use of a food frequency record either alone or in combination with a 24-hour recall. The food frequency record is a checklist that indicates how often specific foods or general food groups are eaten, such as times per day/week/month, or frequently/seldom/never. It provides information about the types of foods eaten but does not usually report the quantities. A selective food frequency record may focus on specific foods or nutrients that are suspected of being deficient or excessive in the diet. Presented is an example of a self-administered, self-scoring food questionnaire that focuses on fat and fruit, vegetable, and fiber intake. Also illustrated is a general tool that serves as a food frequency record based on major food groups. The client can complete the questionnaires relatively quickly and easily, or the clinician can complete them using an interview technique.

Because portion size is generally not emphasized, a food frequency record may be less intimidating than a 24-hour recall. When they are used together, a food frequency record and a 24-hour recall

(*continued*)

Screening questionnaire for fat and fruit/vegetable/fiber intake. Think about your eating habits over the past year or so. About how often do you eat each of the foods listed? Mark an "X" in one box for each food.

	(0) Less than once per MONTH	(1) 2–3 times per MONTH	(2) 1–2 times per WEEK	(3) 3–4 times per WEEK	(4) 5+ times per WEEK	Points Score
Hamburgers or cheeseburgers	☐	☐	☐	☐	☐	____
Beef, such as steaks, roasts	☐	☐	☐	☐	☐	____
Fried chicken	☐	☐	☐	☐	☐	____
Hot dogs, franks	☐	☐	☐	☐	☐	____
Cold cuts, lunch meats, ham, etc.	☐	☐	☐	☐	☐	____
Salad dressings, mayo (not diet)	☐	☐	☐	☐	☐	____
Margarine or butter	☐	☐	☐	☐	☐	____
Eggs	☐	☐	☐	☐	☐	____
Bacon or sausage	☐	☐	☐	☐	☐	____
Cheese or cheese spread	☐	☐	☐	☐	☐	____
Whole milk	☐	☐	☐	☐	☐	____
French fries	☐	☐	☐	☐	☐	____
Potato chips, corn chips, popcorn	☐	☐	☐	☐	☐	____
Ice cream	☐	☐	☐	☐	☐	____
Doughnuts, pastries, cake, cookies	☐	☐	☐	☐	☐	____
					Meat/Snacks Score =	____

Orange juice	☐	☐	☐	☐	☐	____
Not counting juice, about how often do you eat any fruit?	☐	☐	☐	☐	☐	____
Green salad	☐	☐	☐	☐	☐	____
Potatoes	☐	☐	☐	☐	☐	____
Beans, such as baked beans, pintos, kidney beans or in chili	☐	☐	☐	☐	☐	____
About how often do you eat any other vegetables?	☐	☐	☐	☐	☐	____
High-fiber or bran cereal	☐	☐	☐	☐	☐	____
Dark bread, such as whole wheat, rye	☐	☐	☐	☐	☐	____
White bread, including french, Italian, biscuits, muffins	☐	☐	☐	☐	☐	____
					Fruit/Vegetable/Fiber Score =	____

To score:

For each food, write the number that is at the top of the column you checked, in the box at the far right. Add up the numbers in the boxes to get your total scores for Meat/Snacks and Fruit/Vegetable/Fiber.

For Meat/Snacks Score:
If Your Score Is:

more than 27	Your diet is high in fat. There are many ways you can make your eating pattern lower in fat. You should look at your highest scores above to find areas in which to begin.
25–27	Your diet is quite high in fat. To make your eating pattern lower in fat, you may want to begin in the areas where you scored highest.
22–24	You are generally eating a typical American diet, which could be lower in fat.
18–21	You are making better low-fat food choices.
17 or less	You are making the best low-fat food choices. Keep up the great work!

If you scored 17 or less, you're doing well! This is the desirable score on this screener.

For Fruit/Vegetable/Fiber Score:
If Your Score Is:

30 or more	You're doing very well. This is the desirable score on this screener.
20 to 29	You should include more fruits, vegetables, and whole grains.
less than 20	Your diet is probably low in important nutrients. You should find ways to increase the fruits and vegetables and other fiber-rich foods you eat every day.

BOX 9.2

Tools for Obtaining Intake Information (continued)

complement each other and present a more complete dietary intake picture than either method used alone. The major limitation of the food frequency record is that many details of dietary intake are not measured. Also, this method relies on memory.

Food Frequency Checklist

Directions: Indicate how often you eat each food item listed below, in terms of number of times consumed per week, number of times per month, seldom, or never. List the type of food, where appropriate.

Food Item	Type	How often
Meat		
Fish		
Poultry		
Eggs		
Lunch meats		
Pizza		
Peanut butter		
Dried peas and beans		
Nuts		
Milk		
Yogurt		
Cheese		
Milk desserts		
Citrus fruit or juice		
Dried fruit		
Other fruit		
Leafy green vegetables		
Dark yellow vegetables		
Potatoes		
Other vegetables		
Bread		
Cereal		
Pasta		
Rice		
Other grains		
Butter/margarine		
Oil/salad dressing		
Bacon and sausage		
Fried foods		
Cream (sweet or sour)		
Sweets		
Sugar/sugar substitute		
Snack foods		
Salt/salt substitute		
Carbonated beverages/fruit drinks		
Alcoholic beverages		
Coffee/tea		
Other foods not listed that you eat regularly		

General food frequency record.

(*continued*)

BOX 9.2

Tools for Obtaining Intake Information (continued)

FOOD RECORD

A food record is a detailed diary of all foods and beverages consumed and measurements of portion sizes taken during a specified period, usually 3 to 7 days, depending on the regularity of food habits. In theory, an average daily intake can be calculated by totaling the nutrients that were consumed during the entire period and dividing by the total number of days. In practice, food records tend to become unreliable after the first few days because the accuracy of recording deteriorates. However, food records are useful self-monitoring tools for clients who are trying to change their food habits. For instance, a 3-day food record that includes not only what and how much was eaten but the times at which each food was consumed and the client's thoughts, mood, or feelings while eating are useful for clients who are trying to identify problem eating behaviors.

- **How many meals and snacks do you eat in a 24-hour period?** This question helps establish the pattern of eating and identifies unusual food habits, such as pica, food faddism, eating disorders, and meal skipping. People who consume the majority of their calories during the evening and night may be at increased risk for obesity. People who skip breakfast may overeat later in the day. Older adults who skip meals are at increased risk of malnutrition.
- **How many meals per week do you eat away from home?** Generally, foods eaten away from home are higher in fat and cholesterol and lower in other nutrients compared with foods eaten at home. Restaurant portions are often larger than home-cooked portions, and selections of fruits, vegetables, and fiber-rich grains are limited.
- **How many servings of fruits and vegetables do you eat daily?** Not only do fruits and vegetables provide an array of essential nutrients, fiber, and phytochemicals, but eating recommended amounts of plant foods helps ensure a moderate fat intake.
- **What types of bread and cereals do you use?** Without whole-grain bread and high-fiber cereal, it is difficult to get enough fiber in the diet.
- **How often do you eat red meat (beef, lamb, veal), and what is the usual portion size?** A "rule of thumb" assumption is that people who eat red meat more than four times per week are least likely to be following a low-fat eating plan. Because all animal proteins contain saturated fat and cholesterol, consumption of meat, poultry, and fish should generally be limited to 6 ounces or less daily.
- **How often do you eat poultry, and what is the usual portion size?** The skinless, white meat of turkey and chicken has less saturated fat and cholesterol than red meat does. More frequent consumption of poultry instead of red meat generally means a lower fat intake.
- **How often do you eat fish and shellfish, and what is the usual portion size?** Fish and shellfish are lower in fat and saturated fat than red meat and poultry are, and they provide omega-3 fatty acids, which may help lower blood pressure and

triglyceride levels and decrease the propensity of blood to clot. Clients should be encouraged to eat fish or shellfish once per week.

- **How often do you have meatless meals?** For well clients, occasional meatless meals are an effective strategy to help control fat and saturated fat intake. For people who are ill or elderly, meatless meals may signal an inadequate protein intake.
- **How many hours of television do you watch daily?** The longer the time spent watching television, the less time available to participate in physical activities. There is a correlation between television watching and obesity, especially among children who watch for longer than 2 hours daily.
- **How much milk do you drink daily, and what type do you consume?** Without adequate dairy products in the diet, it is difficult to meet calcium requirements from food alone. Calcium intake is important throughout life, not just during childhood. In fact, the DRI for people age 51 years and older (1200 mg) is higher than the DRI for children up to the age of 9 years (800 mg). The highest DRI (1300 mg) is for people 9 to 18 years of age. Clients who avoid milk because of lactose intolerance should be encouraged to use lactose-free products or to take Lactaid. Many lactose-intolerant people are able to tolerate moderate amounts of milk as part of a meal. Because full-fat milk and cheeses provide significant amounts of fat and saturated fat, reduced-fat varieties are recommended.
- **How often do you eat desserts and sweets?** Desserts and sweets tend to be hidden sources of fat and calories. Find out whether the client eats angel food cake, non-fat frozen yogurt, pudding made with skim milk, and sherbet—or pies, chocolate cake, cheesecake, and pastries.
- **What types of beverages do you consume?** Carbonated beverages and sweetened juices provide "empty calories." Clients who are trying to lose weight can save hundreds of calories daily by substituting water for these beverages.
- **How frequently and how much alcohol do you drink?** Although moderate alcohol consumption may help protect against heart disease, higher intakes are associated with increased risks of cancer, liver diseases, and accidental death. From a nutritional standpoint, heavy alcohol consumption interferes with nutrient intake, metabolism, and excretion, and therefore, is a risk factor for nutritional problems.
- **Do you have any food allergies or intolerances, and, if so, what are they?** The greater the number of foods restricted or eliminated in the diet, the greater the likelihood of nutritional deficiencies. This question may also shed light on the client's need for nutrition counseling. For instance, clients with hiatal hernia who are intolerant of citrus fruits and juices may benefit from counseling on how to ensure an adequate intake of vitamin C.
- **What types and amounts of dietary supplements do you take, and why?** Dietary supplements, such as vitamins, minerals, herbs, botanicals and other plant-derived substances, and amino acids and concentrates, are neither drugs nor foods but have the potential to affect nutrition as well as health. The use of supplements is increasingly popular, yet much is unknown about their benefits, health risks, and interactions with drugs and nutrients. It is important to find out what the client takes, what dosage is taken, and why the product is used.

These questions represent only a minimum for obtaining an intake history. Additional questions may be necessary based on the client's response or on the purpose of the nutritional evaluation. For instance, for patients with suspected protein-calorie malnutrition, it is important to find out how much and how frequently protein foods are eaten and whether total calorie intake is adequate.

Weight History

Weight history refers to recent changes in weight, both intentional and unintentional. Rapid intentional weight loss and any unintentional weight loss are risk factors for poor nutritional status. From the weight history, criteria such as percent usual body weight and percent weight change can be calculated and evaluated.

Percent Usual Body Weight

Percent usual body weight (UBW) compares present weight with usual weight to evaluate the degree of weight change.

$$\%UBW = (\text{present weight} \div \text{usual weight}) \times 100$$

For unintentional weight loss, the %UBW is evaluated as follows:

Mild depletion	85%–95% of UBW
Moderate depletion	75%–84% of UBW
Severe depletion	<75% of UBW

Percent Weight Change

Percent weight change is equal to:

$$(\text{usual weight} - \text{present weight}) \div \text{usual weight} \times 100$$

Unintentional weight loss can be evaluated to assess its significance. "Significant" weight loss is that greater than:

1%–2% in 1 week
5% in 1 month
7.5% in 3 months
10% in 6 months (risk factor for malnutrition)

Medication Use

Both prescription and over-the-counter drugs have the potential to affect, and be affected by, nutritional status. Sometimes drug-nutrient interactions are the intended action of the drug. At other times, alterations in nutrient intake, metabolism, or excretion may be an unwanted side effect of drug therapy. Although well-nourished individuals on short-term drug therapy may easily withstand the negative effects of drug-nutrient interactions, malnourished clients and those on long-term drug regimens may experience significant nutrient deficiencies and decreased tolerance to drug therapy. Clients at greatest risk for development of drug-induced nutrient deficiencies include those who:

- Habitually consume fewer calories and nutrients than they need
- Have increased nutrient requirements, including infants, adolescents, and pregnant and lactating women
- Are elderly
- Have chronic illnesses
- Take large numbers of drugs (five or more), whether prescription drugs, over-the-counter medications, or dietary supplements
- Are receiving long-term drug therapy
- Self-medicate
- Are substance abusers

Other Pertinent Information

Other information that may relate to nutritional requirements and intakes or to nutrition counseling includes a history or evidence of:

- Illiteracy
- Language barriers
- Limited knowledge of nutrition and food safety
- Altered or impaired intake related to culture
- Altered or impaired intake related to religion
- Lack of caregiver or social support system
- Social isolation
- Lack of or inadequate cooking arrangements
- Limited or low income
- Limited access to transportation to obtain food
- Advanced age (>80 years)
- Lack of or extreme physical activity
- Use of tobacco or recreational drugs
- Limited use or knowledge of community resources

PHYSICAL FINDINGS

Height and Weight

Height and weight are used to indirectly assess undernutrition and overnutrition in adults. Periodic measurements of weight help monitor a client's progress. However, because changes in weight and other anthropometric measurements may be slow to occur, they are more reflective of chronic, not acute, changes in nutritional status.

Accurate equipment and standardized procedures must be used to ensure accurate and precise data collection. Inexperience on the part of the assessor, an uncooperative client, and inaccurate equipment are all frequent sources of error. However, self-reported height and weight are usually unreliable and should be used only when actual measurements cannot be obtained. Fluid retention and dehydration skew measurements. Also, reference standards may not be appropriate for all populations, because anthropological differences exist among people of different races.

If possible, adults should be weighed on a beam-balance scale (or on a metabolic scale if the client is bedridden) that is checked frequently for accuracy. Bathroom scales are inaccurate and should not be used. Be sure to weight the client on the same scale each time and at approximately the same time of day, preferably before breakfast and after the client has voided. The client should not wear shoes and should wear approximately the same amount of clothing each time. Record the weight immediately.

Weight for height can be used to determine body mass index (BMI; see Chapter 14). Classification of weight based on BMI is as follows:

Underweight	<18.5
Normal	18.5–24.9
Overweight	25.0–29.9
Obesity class 1	30.0–34.9
Obesity class 2	35.0–39.9
Extreme obesity	40.0

Weights at either end of the spectrum (underweight and all classes of obesity) are associated with higher health risks than are BMIs of 18.5 to 29.9.

A frequently used "rule of thumb" reference standard for estimated ideal body weight (IBW) is as follows:

Men: 106 lb for 5 ft plus 6 lb for each additional inch
Women: 100 lb for 5 ft plus 5 lb for each additional inch

The IBW can be 10% higher or lower, depending on body size. To evaluate a person's actual body weight according to the calculated IBW reference, the following formula is used:

$$\%IBW = \text{actual weight} \div IBW \times 100$$

Generally accepted standards based on %IBW are as follows:

Obese	>120% of IBW
Overweight	110%–120% of IBW
Normal	90%–110% of IBW
Mildly underweight	80%–90% of IBW
Moderately underweight	70%–79% of IBW
Severely underweight	<70% of IBW

Although weight is considered to be an important indicator of nutritional status, it does not provide qualitative information about body composition (ie, fat and muscle tissue). Also, a client can be malnourished without being underweight. Measurements that reflect body composition, such as skinfold, midarm circumference, and midarm muscle circumference, are usually reserved for comprehensive nutritional assessments (Box 9-3).

BOX 9.3

Measurements of Body Composition

Each of the following measurements of body composition is evaluated by (1) comparing the measurement with a previously obtained measurement to identify any change and (2) comparing the measurement with a reference standard. Findings lower than 90% of the reference standard may indicate the need for nutritional support.

TRICEPS SKINFOLD

Triceps skinfold (TSF) measures subcutaneous fat stores and is, therefore, an index of total body fat, because approximately half the total body fat is stored directly under the skin. Studies indicate that assessments of subcutaneous body fat by skinfold measurements are accurate.

While the client's arm is hanging freely, grasp a fold of skin and subcutaneous fat between the thumb and forefinger slightly above the midpoint mark. Gently pull the skin away from the underlying muscle, apply the calipers, wait 2 to 3 seconds, and read the measurement to the nearest 1.0 mm. Repeat the procedure two more times; add the three readings, divide by 3, and record the average measurement.

90% of standard = 11.3 mm for men, 14.9 mm for women

Because the chance exists that fat on the arm may not accurately reflect fat in other areas of the body, taking skinfold measurements from other sites may improve validity. Other appropriate sites include the biceps, thigh, calf, and subscapular and suprailiac skinfolds.

MIDARM CIRCUMFERENCE

Midarm circumference (MAC) measures muscle mass and subcutaneous fat. Although it is not a useful measurement by itself, it is used as part of the procedure for calculating arm muscle circumference.

Place a nonstretchable tape, preferably an insertion tape for easy reading (available from Ross Laboratories, Columbus, OH), at the midpoint of the client's nondominant arm between the top of the acromion process of the scapula and the olecranon process of the ulna with the forearm flexed at 90°. With the arm in the dependent position, gently and firmly draw the tape around the midupper arm; do not compress the soft tissue. Record the reading to the nearest millimeter.

90% standard = 26.3 mm for men, 25.7 mm for women

(continued)

BOX 9.3

Measurements of Body Composition (continued)

MIDARM MUSCLE CIRCUMFERENCE

Midarm muscle circumference (MAMC), which is calculated from the MAC and TSF measurements, provides an index of muscle mass (somatic protein stores). It is calculated in centimeters:

$$MAMC = MAC \times (3.14 \times TSF)$$

Although the measurement is not sensitive to small changes in muscle mass, it does provide a quick estimation of muscle mass and is minimally affected by edema.

90% of standard = 22.8 cm in men, 20.9 cm in women

Appearance

Physical signs and symptoms of malnutrition may be visually apparent on inspection (Table 9-2). Abnormal findings should be closely scrutinized to determine whether they are caused by, or are related to, a nutritional deficiency. Most signs cannot be considered

TABLE 9.2 ***Physical Signs and Symptoms of Nutritional Status***

Body Area	Signs of Good Nutritional Status	Signs of Poor Nutritional Status
General appearance	Alert, responsive	Listless, apathetic, and cachectic
General vitality	Endurance, energetic, sleeps well, vigorous	Easily fatigued, no energy, falls asleep easily, looks tired, apathetic
Weight	Normal for height, age, and body build	Overweight or underweight
Hair	Shiny, lustrous, firm, not easily plucked, healthy scalp	Dull and dry, brittle, loss of color, easily plucked, thin and sparse
Face	Uniform skin color; healthy appearance, not swollen	Dark skin over cheeks and under eyes, flaky skin, facial edema (moon face), pale skin color
Eyes	Bright, clear, moist, no sores at corners of eyelids, membranes moist and healthy pink color, no prominent blood vessels	Pale eye membranes, dry eyes (xerophthalmia), Bitot's spots, increased vascularity, cornea soft (keratomalacia), small yellowish lumps around eyes (xanthelasma), dull or scarred cornea
Lips	Good pink color, smooth, moist, not chapped or swollen	Swollen and puffy (cheilosis), angular lesion at corners of mouth or fissures or scars (stomatitis)

(continued)

TABLE 9.2 *Physical Signs and Symptoms of Nutritional Status (continued)*

Body Area	Signs of Good Nutritional Status	Signs of Poor Nutritional Status
Tongue	Deep red, surface papillae present	Smooth appearance, beefy red or magenta colored, swollen; papillae hypertrophied or atrophied
Teeth	Straight, no crowding, no cavities, no pain, bright, no discoloration, well-shaped jaw	Cavities, mottled appearance (fluorosis), malpositioned, missing teeth
Gums	Firm, good pink color, no swelling or bleeding	Spongy, bleed easily, marginal redness, recessed, swollen and inflamed
Glands	No enlargement of the thyroid, face not swollen	Enlargement of the thyroid (goiter), enlargement of the parotid (swollen cheeks)
Skin	Smooth, good color, slightly moist; no sign or rash, swelling, or color irregularities	Rough, dry, flaky, swollen, pale, pigmented, lack of fat under the skin, fat deposits around the joints (xanthomas), bruises, petechiae
Nails	Firm, pink	Spoon-shaped (koilonychia), brittle, pale, ridged
Skeleton	Good posture, no malformations	Poor posture, beading of the ribs, bowed legs or knock knees, prominent scapulas, chest deformity at diaphragm
Muscles	Well developed, firm, good tone, some fat under the skin	Flaccid, poor tone, wasted, underdeveloped, difficulty walking
Extremities	No tenderness	Weak and tender, presence of edema
Abdomen	Flat	Swollen
Nervous system	Normal reflexes, psychological stability	Decrease in or loss of ankle and knee reflexes, psychomotor changes, mental confusion, depression, sensory loss, motor weakness, loss of sense of position, loss of vibration, burning and tingling of the hands and feet (paresthesia)
Cardiovascular system	Normal heart rate and rhythm, no murmurs, normal blood pressure for age	Cardiac enlargement, tachycardia, elevated blood pressure
Gastrointestinal system	No palpable organs or masses (liver edge may be palpable in children)	Hepatosplenomegaly

diagnostic; rather, they must be viewed as suggestive of malnutrition, because evaluation of "normal" versus "abnormal" findings is subjective and the signs of malnutrition may be nonspecific. For instance, dull, dry hair may be related to kwashiorkor (severe protein depletion) or to overexposure to the sun. In addition, physical signs and symptoms of malnutrition can vary in intensity among population groups because of genetic and environmental differences. Finally, physical findings occur only with overt malnutrition, not with asymptomatic, subclinical malnutrition.

LABORATORY DATA

Laboratory tests can objectively detect nutritional problems in their early stages, before changes in weight occur or physical signs and symptoms develop. In clinical settings, most routine tests are aimed at assessing protein-calorie status. Serum albumin is the laboratory measurement most frequently used to screen for nutritional problems. Box 9-4 lists other laboratory tests that are used to assess protein status. Measures of immune system functioning appear in Box 9-5.

BOX 9.4

Measurements of Protein Status

When the primary objective of nutritional therapy is to preserve or restore body protein, assessment of this nutritional component is essential. Laboratory tests can be used to measure byproducts of protein catabolism (eg, urea, creatinine) and products of protein anabolism (eg, albumin, transferrin, prealbumin, retinol-binding protein). From these measurements, the adequacy of body protein stores can be inferred.

MEASUREMENTS OF PROTEIN CATABOLISM

- **Urinary urea nitrogen.** Urea, a byproduct of amino acid deamination, circulates in the blood (blood urea nitrogen or BUN) and is excreted in the urine (urinary urea nitrogen, or UUN). Urea accounts for 60%–90% of urine nitrogen and is reflective of current protein intake. Mean daily excretion of urea is 15.0–49.0 g. Both blood and urine values of urea decrease during protein deficiency.

  The state of nitrogen balance can be determined by comparing nitrogen intake (grams of protein divided by 6.25) with nitrogen output over a 24-hour period. Total nitrogen output equals grams of UUN collected over 24 hours plus 4 g, which is the approximate amount of nitrogen lost daily through the lungs, hair, skin, and feces, and nonurea nitrogen. A positive nitrogen balance (anabolism) exists when intake exceeds nitrogen output. Conversely, negative nitrogen balance (catabolism) is indicated when output exceeds nitrogen intake. For a UUN measurement to be valid, the protein intake must be accurately recorded and the kidney function must be normal.

(*continued*)

BOX 9.4

Measurements of Protein Status (continued)

- **Urinary creatinine.** Every day, about 2% of the creatine phosphate in muscle tissue undergoes an irreversible conversion to creatinine. Creatinine circulates in the blood and is excreted in the urine at a constant rate that depends on the amount of muscle mass: the more muscle mass, the greater the excretion of creatinine. Urinary creatinine is considered to be a measure of long-term protein intake because it provides an indirect measure of skeletal muscle mass. Usual ranges for adults are 20 to 26 mg/kg per 24 h for men and 14 to 22 mg/kg per 24 h for women. Because urinary creatinine excretion varies considerably from day to day, a 3-day average calculation is more reliable than measurement of a single day's collection. Factors that influence urinary creatinine excretion include protein intake, exercise, age, renal function, and thyroid function.

MEASUREMENTS OF PROTEIN ANABOLISM

Ideally, serum proteins that are used to assess protein synthesis should have a short half-life, should respond to a protein-deficient diet, and should be decreased in the bloodstream only in response to calorie and protein deficiency. However, studies indicate that concentrations of serum proteins show significant decline only after protein deficiency is prolonged and severe. In addition, they are not specific indicators of protein deficiency because other factors, such as zinc deficiency, energy deficiency, liver disease, renal disease, and systemic infection, may also contribute to their decline.

BOX TABLE 9.4.1 *Serum Protein*

Serum Protein (Normal Value)	Advantages of Measurement	Disadvantages of Measurement
Serum transferrin (>200 mg/dL)	More sensitive to nutritonal repletion than albumin because of its shorter half-life (8–10 d), smaller body pool, and more rapid response to short-term changes in protein status	Direct measurement is expensive. Although it breaks down in the body more quickly than albumin, it is relatively slow to respond to changes in protein intake. Levels increase from iron deficiency anemia, pregnancy, hepatitis, dehydration, and chronic blood loss. Levels decrease from acute and chronic infection, catabolic stress, overhydration, and nephrotic syndrome.

(*continued*)

BOX 9.4

Measurements of Protein Status (continued)

BOX TABLE 9.4.1 *Serum Protein (continued)*

Serum Protein (Normal Value)	Advantages of Measurement	Disadvantages of Measurement
Prealbumin (16–30 mg/dL)	More sensitive than albumin because of its short half-life (2 d); response to nutritional repletion seen in 2–3 d; not as affected by liver disease and hydration status as albumin	Measurement is expensive. May reflect protein intake rather than protein status. Levels decrease from hemodialysis, hypothyroidism, and surgery. Levels increase from renal failure and corticosteroids.
Retinol-binding protein (2.6–7.7 mg/dL)	Reliable measurement during acute response; responds quickly to nutritional repletion due to small body pool and short half-life (10–12 h)	Levels decrease from vitamin A deficiency, hyperthyroidism, liver disease, and cystic fibrosis. Levels may be elevated in kidney disease.

BOX 9.5

Measurements of Immune Function Status

Malnutrition has a serious effect on immunocompetence; in fact, it is recognized to be the most common cause of secondary immune deficiency. The following tests may be used to measure the body's immunocompetence.

TOTAL LYMPHOCYTE COUNT

Total lymphocyte count (TLC) is obtained from samples that are collected for evaluation of complete blood count (CBC) and differential; therefore, the TLC value is usually available for hsopitalized clients. Malnutrition, especially that resulting from inadequate intake of calories and protein, decreases the total number of lymphocytes, which impairs the body's ability to fight infection. However, TLC is of limited value because it is affected by numerous medical conditions and fluctuates widely. Normal levels range from 1500 to 1800 mm. The TLC is calculated from the leukocyte count (WBC) and the percentage of lymphocytes (% Lymph). Like the WBC, it is reported in cells per cubic millimeter:

$$\text{TLC} = \text{WBC} \times \%\text{Lymph}$$

(*continued*)

BOX 9.5

Measurements of Immune Function Status (continued)

DELAYED CUTANEOUS HYPERSENSITIVITY REACTION

Cellular immunity can be evaluated by placing small quantities of recall antigens, such as *Candida*, mumps, purified protein derivative of tuberculin (PPDP, or streptokinasestreptodornase [SKSD], under the skin. Clients who are immunocompetent exhibit a positive reaction within 24–48 h (a red area of ≥5 mm appears around the test site). Because malnutrition delays antibody synthesis and antibody response to stimulation, clients with malnutrition may experience a delayed reaction, a reaction to only one of the antigens, or no reaction (anergy). A limitation in the use of delayed cutaneous hypersensitivity reaction is that anergy can occur secondary to other conditions (eg, blunt trauma, cancer, acute blood loss, surgery, sepsis, age, recent anesthesia, fever, medications), and therefore. it is not a specific or often used measure of protein status.

Serum Albumin

As the most abundant form of protein in the blood, albumin helps maintain oncotic pressure and helps transport other nutrients, drugs, and hormones through the blood. Albumin synthesis depends on functioning liver cells and an adequate supply of amino acids.

Serum albumin is readily available and may be the best single indicator of nutritional status. Normal serum albumin levels range from 3.5 to 5.0 g/dL. Malnutrition and depletion of visceral protein stores cause serum albumin levels to fall over time. Ranges for "mild" and "moderate" depletion vary. General guidelines are as follows:

Normal	3.5 g/dL
Mild depletion	2.8–3.4 g/dL
Moderate depletion	2.1–2.7 g/dL
Severe depletion	<2.1 g/dL

Because albumin is degraded slowly (half-life: 18–20 days) and because the body has a large extravascular pool that can be mobilized to maintain serum concentrations during periods of protein depletion, serum albumin concentrations are preserved until malnutrition is in a chronic stage. Another drawback is that a low serum albumin concentration may be caused by problems other than protein malnutrition. For instance, serum albumin levels fall during the acute phase after injury, infection, or active chronic disease, regardless of nutritional status. A low serum albumin level may also be caused by liver disease, renal disease, or congestive heart failure.

KEY CONCEPTS

- Nutritional status is the state of balance that exists between nutrient intake and nutrient requirements. Imbalances between intake and requirement have the potential to lead to undernutrition or overnutrition.
- Screening uses a minimum amount of information to identify people who are at moderate or high risk for nutritional problems.
- Clients who are identified through the screening process as being at nutritional risk receive a comprehensive nutritional assessment, from which a nutritional care plan is formulated, implemented, and evaluated.
- A client's current and past health history can help identify problems with intake or alterations in nutrient requirements.
- Intake information should include observations about the client's current intake and diet order for patients in clinical settings. Questions about usual intake can help identify behaviors in need of improvement.
- Significant unintentional weight loss is a risk factor for nutritional problems.
- People who take five or more prescription drugs, over-the-counter medications, and/or dietary supplements are at risk for nutritional problems.
- Underweight and obesity are risks for nutritional problems.
- Serum albumin is commonly used to assess protein status, but it is slow to respond to changes in status and intake.
- Assessment of physical signs of malnutrition that are apparent on visual inspection is highly subjective. Positive clinical findings are considered to be "suggestive" of malnutrition, not a definitive diagnosis.

Focus on Critical Thinking

Conduct a 24-hour recall with a friend or family member. With that same person, complete a general food frequency record (see the example in Box 9–2). Are the results comparable? Which method appears to be more valid? Why?

Complete and score the screening questionnaire for fat and fruit/vegetable/fiber Intake (see the example questionnaire in Box 9–2) according to your own diet. Do you agree with the results? Why or why not?

ANSWER KEY

1. **TRUE** Nutritional status is loosely defined as the state of balance between nutrient supply and demand.
2. **FALSE** In clinical settings, the nutritional emphasis is getting enough calories and protein. In wellness situations, the emphasis frequently is to ensure that intake does not exceed requirement.

3. **TRUE** A person can be malnourished without being underweight. Weight does not provide qualitative information about body composition.
4. **FALSE** Changes in weight and other anthropometric measurements may be slow to occur, and they are more reflective of chronic, not acute, changes in nutritional status.
5. **FALSE** Malnutrition and depletion of visceral protein stores cause the levels of serum albumin to fall over the course of time.
6. **FALSE** Low levels of serum albumin may be caused by problems other than protein malnutrition (eg, injury, infection, liver disease).
7. **TRUE** Weight loss is judged significant if there is a 5% or greater weight loss over the course of a month.
8. **TRUE** People at greatest risk for developing drug-induced nutrient deficiencies include those who take five or more prescription drugs, over-the-counter drugs, or dietary supplements.
9. **FALSE** Heavy alcohol consumption interferes with nutrient intake, metabolism, and excretion, and, thus, is a risk factor for nutritional problems. Moderate intake may help protect against heart disease.
10. **TRUE** Laboratory tests can objectively detect nutritional problems in their early stages before changes in weight occur or physical signs and symptoms develop.

REFERENCES

Chicago Dietetic Association & the South Suburban Dietetic Association. (1992). *Manual of clinical dietetics*. (4th ed.). Chicago: American Dietetic Association.

Hark, L., & Deen, D. (1999). Taking a nutrition history: A practical approach for family physicians. *American Family Physician*, 59, 1521–1536.

Simko, M., Cowell, C., & Gilbride, J. (1995). *Nutrition assessment: A comprehensive guide for planning intervention*. (2nd ed.). Gaithersburg, MD: Aspen.

Whitney, E., Cataldo, C., & Rolfes, S. (1998). *Understanding normal and clinical nutrition*. (5th ed.). Belmont, CA: Wadsworth.

CHAPTER 10

Cultural Influences on Food Choices

TRUE	FALSE	Check your knowledge of cultural influences on food choices.
⬭	⬭	1 Culture defines what are normal food behaviors.
⬭	⬭	2 Race and ethnicity are synonymous with culture.
⬭	⬭	3 Staple foods tend to be from the bottom of the Food Guide Pyramid.
⬭	⬭	4 Ethnocentrism is the belief that one's own culture is superior to all others.
⬭	⬭	5 The hot-cold theory of health and diet refers to the temperature of the food eaten.
⬭	⬭	6 First-generation Americans tend to adhere more closely to their cultural food patterns than subsequent generations.
⬭	⬭	7 For many ethnic groups who move to the United States, breakfast and lunch are more likely than dinner to be composed of new "American" foods.
⬭	⬭	8 People who eat out or get take-out food many times a week tend to eat more calories, fat, and sodium than people who eat out less often.
⬭	⬭	9 Before herbs can be marketed, dietary supplement manufacturers must prove the safety of the herb to the U.S. Food and Drug Administration (FDA).
⬭	⬭	10 Because herbs are natural, they are safe.

Upon completion of this chapter, you will be able to

- Describe how culture influences food choices.
- Name the general ways in which people's food choices change as they become acculturated to a new area.
- Discuss trends in American culture that have nutritional implications.
- List questions appropriate for cross-cultural assessment of food intake.
- Explain the difference in regulation between drugs and herbs.

Introduction

Nutrition is a science, rooted in the disciplines of chemistry, biochemistry, and physiology. But the *delivery* of nutrition is an art, because for most people eating supplies food for the soul as well as the body. The nutritional requirements among people of similar age and gender are essentially the same throughout the world, yet an infinite variety of food and food combinations can satisfy those requirements. How a person chooses to satisfy nutritional requirements is influenced by many variables, including culture, religion, socioeconomic status, and personal factors. To ignore the art of nutrition is to undermine its scientific basis.

This chapter addresses the impact of culture on food choices. Traditional food practices of major cultural subgroups in the United States and selected religious groups are presented. Trends in American culture that have nutritional implications are discussed, including the growing popularity of herbal supplements.

The Significance of Culture

Culture encompasses the total way of life of a particular population or community at a given time. Every culture has an inherent value system that dictates behavior by defining what is normal and teaching that those norms are right. Thus culture is learned, not instinctive, and it is passed from generation to generation. Because its influence on its members is unconscious, members may not be aware of the unwritten rules governing their behavior. Culture resists change, but it is not static. For instance, food habits are basically stable and predictable, but paradoxically they undergo constant and continuous change in response to changes in lifestyle, attitudes, technology, and environment.

Each culture has its own socially standardized food behaviors that dictate what is edible, the role of certain foods in the diet, how food is prepared, the use of foods, the number and timing of daily meals, how food is eaten, and health beliefs related to food. Yet within any culture, individuals or groups of individuals behave differently, based on age, gender, and socioeconomic status. Race, ethnicity, and geographic region are often inaccurately assumed to be synonymous with culture. This misconception leads to stereotypic grouping, such as assuming that all Jews adhere to orthodox food laws or that all Southerners eat sausage, biscuits, and gravy. Subgroups within a culture display a unique range of cultural characteristics that affect food intake and nutritional status.

WHAT IS EDIBLE

Culture determines what is edible and what is inedible. To be labeled a food, an item must be readily available, safe, and nutritious enough to support reproduction. However, cultures do not define as edible all sources of nutrients that meet those criteria. For instance, in the United States, horse meat, insects, and dog meat are not considered food, even though they meet those criteria. Culture overrides flavor in determining what is offensive or unacceptable. For example, you may like a food (eg, rattlesnake) until you know what it is, disliking the *idea* of the food rather than the actual food itself. An unconscious food selection decision process appears in Figure 10-1.

THE ROLE OF CERTAIN FOODS IN THE DIET

Every culture has a ranking for its foods that is influenced by cost and availability. Major food categories include staple foods, protective foods, and status foods.

Staple Foods

Staple foods are typically bland, relatively inexpensive, and easy-to-prepare foods that form the foundation of the diet. They provide a significant source of calories and are considered an indispensable part of the meal. Staple foods usually come from the bottom of

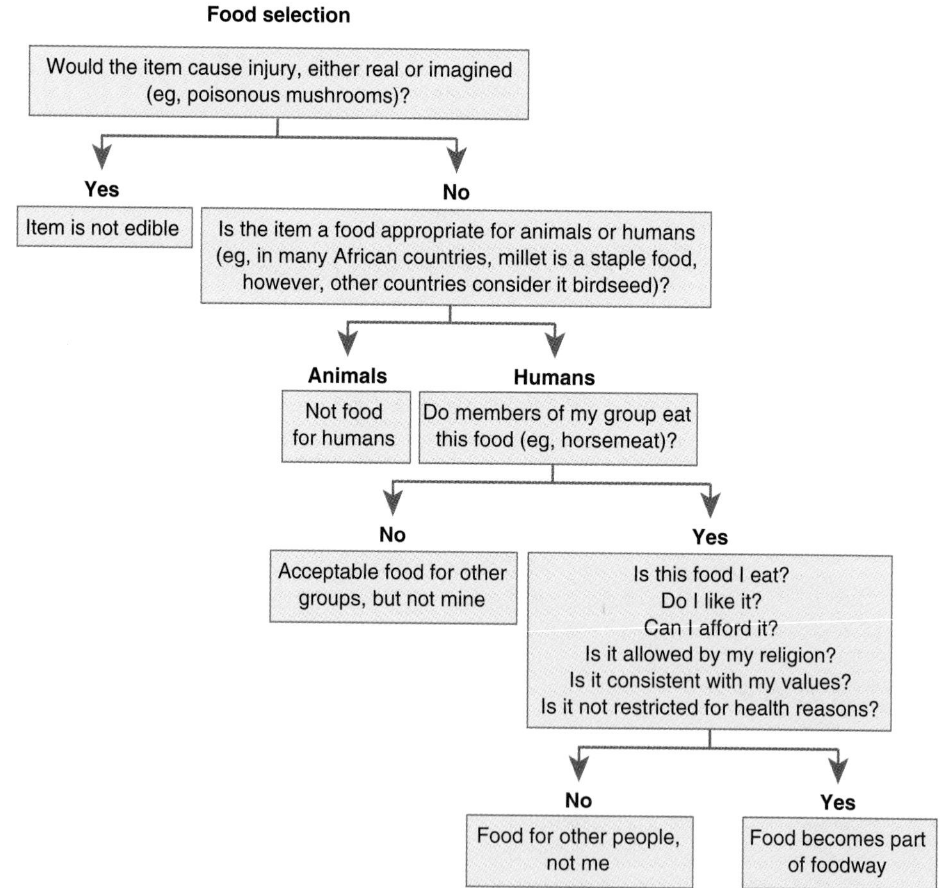

FIGURE 10-1 Food selection decision making.

the Food Guide Pyramid (see Chapter 8). Examples are cereal grains (rice, wheat, millet, corn), starchy tubers (potatoes, yams, taro, cassava), and starchy vegetables (plantain or green bananas).

Protective Foods

Vegetables, legumes, nuts, fish, eggs, and meat are protective foods that are used in various combinations and with various seasonings to give flavor and ethnic identity to meals. Protective foods are generally rich in nutrients. Protective foods used by a culture vary with availability. For instance, the types of legumes used in the Chinese culture include mung beans and soybeans, whereas those used in the Latin American culture include black beans and pinto beans.

Status Foods

Status foods are usually rare and relatively expensive in a culture. They are not part of the usual intake and may be reserved for special occasions. Sometimes foods are considered status foods based on how they are prepared. For instance, in Haitian cultures "shining rice and beans," which is prepared with a lot of oil or pork fat, signifies good financial status, whereas rice and beans prepared with little or no fat is considered food fit for prisoners.

FOOD PREPARATION

Traditional methods of preparation vary between and within cultural groups. For instance, vegetables are stir-fried in Asian cultures but boiled in Hispanic cultures. Traditional seasonings also vary among cultures and may be the distinguishing feature between one culture's foods and another's. The choice of seasonings varies among geographic regions and between seasons, based on availability. For instance, fresh hot peppers are widely used in the tropics because they are plentiful.

USE OF FOODS

Each culture has food customs and bestows symbolism on certain foods. Custom determines what foods are served as meals versus snacks and what foods are considered feminine versus masculine. Symbolically, food can be used to express love, to reward or punish, to display piety, to express moral sentiments, to demonstrate belongingness to a group, or to proclaim the separateness of a group. Culture also determines which foods are used in celebration and which provide comfort.

Celebrations

All cultures use food during celebrations. Special foods may be reserved for or associated with certain celebrations, such as birthdays, national holidays, religious holidays, or family get-togethers. Celebration foods in the United States include birthday cake, Christmas cookies, Halloween candy, and Valentine's Day chocolates. Families within a culture may establish their own food traditions for celebrations.

Comfort Foods

Comfort foods vary among cultures and individuals. In the United States, a child who falls might be offered cookies and milk for comfort, and warm milk at bedtime is used to soothe and relax. People who move from other cultures may retain their own cultural comfort foods as a link with the past.

NUMBER AND TIMING OF MEALS

All cultures eat at least once a day. Typically, Americans have three meals daily; the British have four meals daily; and in some European countries five to six meals daily is the norm. In some places in Africa, one meal per day is standard.

When meals are eaten is also dictated by culture. Dinner takes place between 7 and 9 p.m. in Kenya and at approximately 6 p.m. in Australia. A Lebanese custom is to arrive anytime when invited for dinner, even as early as 9 or 10 a.m.

HOW FOOD IS EATEN

In China, food is usually eaten with chopsticks. In England, almost all foods are eaten with a knife and fork, even sandwiches. In the United States, bad manners in eating may be associated with animal behavior, as in "He eats like a pig," "She chews like a cow," or "Don't wolf down your food."

HEALTH BELIEFS RELATED TO FOOD

Food may be thought to promote wellness, to cure disease, or to have medicinal properties. For instance, hot oregano tea seasoned with salt is used to treat an upset stomach in Vietnamese culture. In Hispanic cultures, raw chopped onions with honey are believed to be good for a cold and other respiratory infections. In Caribbean cultures, chayote and papaya are used to treat high blood pressure.

Asian cultures believe that health and illness are related to the balance between yin and yang forces in the body. Yin represents female, cold, and darkness; yang represents male, hot, and light. Digested foods turn into air that is either yin or yang. Diseases caused by yin forces are treated with yang foods, and diseases caused by yang forces are treated with yin foods. For instance, pregnancy is considered a yang or "hot" condition, so women following traditional practices during pregnancy eat yin foods such as most fruits and vegetables, seaweed, cold drinks, juices, and rice water. Yang foods include chicken, meat, pig's feet, meat broth, nuts, fried food, coffee, and spices. There is also the hot-cold theory of foods and illness in Puerto Rico; it is similar to the Asian view, but the food groupings are somewhat different.

Not all cultural groups view slimness as attractive and desirable. For instance, African-American women have a greater tolerance for heavier body weights than Caucasian women do, and they do not necessarily consider overweight and obesity unattractive. In cultures where thinness is associated with poverty, overweight is a symbol of wealth and success.

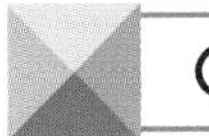

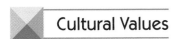

Cultural Values

Underlying a culture's behavior patterns are cultural values that identify what is desirable and what is undesirable. **Ethnocentrism** is the belief that one's own values and behaviors are "right," "normal," and "superior" compared with those of all other cultures, which are "wrong," "odd," or "inferior." An understanding of cultural values fosters more effective communication and can help determine culturally appropriate interventions. A contrast between selected American cultural values and values of more traditional cultures follows.

PERSONAL CONTROL VERSUS FATE

Whereas many Americans have a sense of personal control over their future, members other traditional cultures may accept what happens to them as fate. When illness is perceived as an affliction for sins, spiritual atonement and forgiveness are the ways to cure, not medical interventions. Certain cultural food practices provide a way for spiritual atonement and forgiveness. On Yom Kippur, for example, the Jewish people atone for their sins of the past year by fasting for 24 hours.

INDIVIDUALISM VERSUS GROUP WELFARE

Individualism is the belief that the interests of the individual have preference over the interests of the group. Individual will and personality are valued. In contrast, group welfare values the group over the individual. Food intake decisions may not be made by the individual but rather by the consensus of the group or family.

CLOCK-FOCUSED VERSUS EVENT-FOCUSED ORIENTATION

Americans tend to be ruled by time and schedules. "Being on time" and "not wasting time" are valued. Time-related misunderstandings can occur when fast-paced American culture encounters traditional cultures that are dominated by events or human interactions. This difference is particularly important when determining when and how to convey nutrition information.

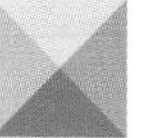

Traditional Diets of Selected Subcultural Groups in the United States

A subculture is defined as a unique cultural group that coexists within a dominant culture. The major cultural subgroups in the United States are African-American, Asian-American, Hispanic-American, and Native-American. Within each of these subgroups are smaller subgroups. For instance, there are 530 federally recognized Native-American nations. Generalizations can be made about traditional eating practices, but actual food choices vary greatly among nations, regions, and individuals within a subcultural group. Traditional food practices of African-Americans, Asian-Americans, Mexican-Americans, and Native-American/Alaska Natives are featured below.

AFRICAN-AMERICANS

"Soul food" describes the traditional food choices of African-Americans. It is a mixture of foods and cooking techniques brought from Africa with foods available in the southern United States and restrictions imposed by slavery. Soul food has become a symbol of African-American identity and African heritage. However, the food choices of African-American families may not differ from the conventional American diet. In such cases, soul food may be reserved for special occasions and holidays.

A food guide pyramid emphasizing foods preferred by African-Americans appears in Figure 10-2. Common foods eaten include biscuits, corn bread, grits, ready-to-eat cereals, corn, hominy, okra, green leafy vegetables, sweet potatoes, dried beans and beans, pork, fruit drinks, and rich desserts. Frying and cooking with added fat, such as lard, bacon, shortening, and fatback or salt pork, are common.

Traditional soul foods tend to be high in fat, cholesterol, and sodium. The prevalence of chronic, diet-related diseases such as coronary heart disease, stroke, hypertension, diabetes, and obesity is higher among African-Americans than in other ethnocultural groups. Nutritional interventions to reduce the risk of chronic disease are aimed at reducing the intake of fat, cholesterol, and sodium. Ways to make soul food "healthier" include the following:

- Use reduced-fat mayonnaise in place of regular mayonnaise.
- Use turkey ham or smoke flavoring instead of bacon.

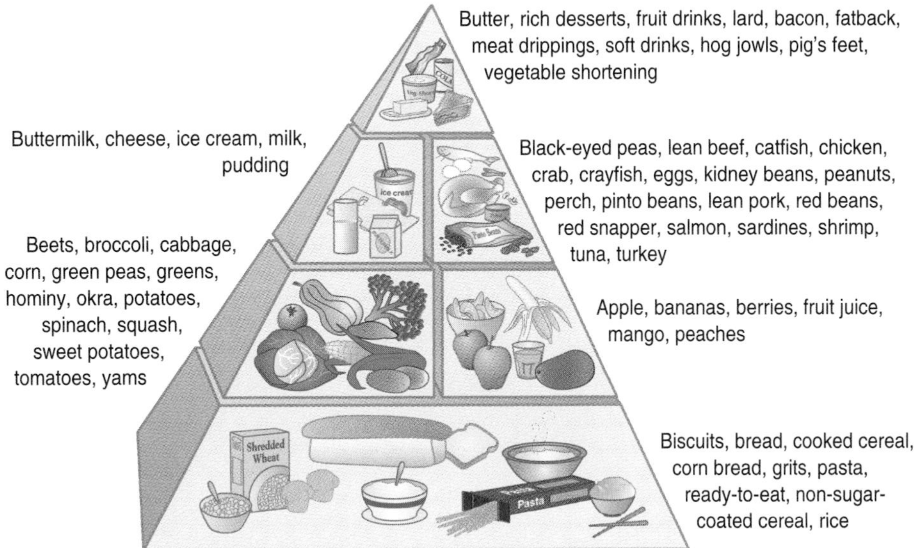

FIGURE 10-2 African-American foods and the Food Guide Pyramid. Source: Kittler P.G., Sucher K. Reprinted with permission from the Penn State Nutrition Center.

- Use sugar-free sweetened drinks.
- Limit the amount of fats added to foods.
- Use small amounts of canola or olive oil, or vegetable oil sprays, in place of shortening or bacon drippings when frying.
- Reduce salt as a seasoning (use onion, garlic, pepper, or hot sauce instead).

ASIAN-AMERICANS

The term "Asian-Americans" encompasses a diverse population originating from at least 17 Asian and 8 Pacific countries, including China, Japan, South Korea, India, Thailand, Vietnam, Cambodia, Indonesia, Malaysia, the Philippines, and other Pacific Rim areas. Just as traditional diets differ among these countries, so do individual variations exist based on the degree of assimilation to the United States. The food choices of descendants of Chinese workers who immigrated to the United States during the California Gold Rush of 1849 to 1924 differ from the food choices of Vietnamese people who immigrated here after the Vietnam War.

The traditional Asian diet is a plant-based diet. Common foods consumed include rice, noodles, flat breads, potatoes, fruits, vegetables (including sea vegetables), nuts, seeds, beans, soyfoods, vegetable and nut oils, herbs and spices, tea, wine, and beer. Poultry and eggs are used in small amounts, and red meat is used sparingly. With the exception of India, milk and dairy products are absent from traditional Asian diets. The use of fish and seafood depends on availability. For instance, people who live in the interior of China or India consume little or no seafood, whereas people who live in seacoast and island areas (eg, Japan, Vietnam) consume large amounts. The food guide pyramid featuring Chinese-American foods appears in Figure 10-3.

The traditional Asian diet is low in fat, saturated fat, and cholesterol and rich in fiber and many nutrients. Asian-Americans have a lower prevalence of cardiovascular disease than other ethnocultural groups do. Moderation is valued, and obesity is rare. Asian-Americans are at high risk for osteoporosis related to:

- Their lighter, less dense bone structure
- Low calcium intake
- High prevalence of lactose intolerance

To reduce the risk of osteoporosis, Asian-Americans should:

- Include nondairy sources of calcium in their diet, such as tofu, canned salmon, canned sardines, and dark green leafy vegetables (eg, broccoli, bok choy).

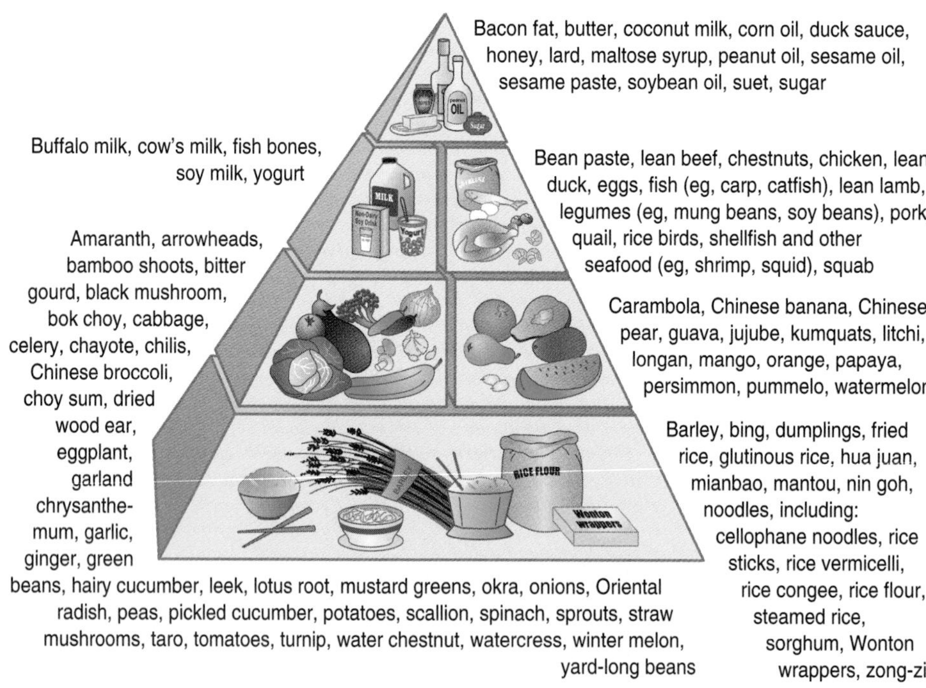

FIGURE 10-3 Chinese-American foods and the Food Guide Pyramid. Source: Kittler P.G., Sucher K. Reprinted with permission from the Penn State Nutrition Center.

- Use calcium-fortified orange juice.
- Participate in weight-bearing exercise on most days of the week.
- Avoid excessive alcohol consumption.

MEXICAN-AMERICANS

Mexican-Americans represent a diverse group with distinct subgroups. The traditional Mexican diet, influenced by Spanish and Indian cultures, is basically vegetarian with an emphasis on corn, beans, and squash (Fig. 10-4). It is high in complex carbohydrates and is composed of mostly unprocessed foods. However, high-fat meats are preferred, and cooking techniques rely heavily on frying and stewing with liberal amounts of oil or lard.

Mexican-Americans have a high prevalence of obesity, high serum triglyceride levels, and diabetes. The intake of fat and cholesterol, especially among men, is high. Because cultural sensitivity is crucial to effective nutritional intervention, the following points are important when counseling Mexican-Americans:

- Promote the positive aspects of the traditional diet, namely the liberal intake of complex carbohydrates, fruits, and vegetables.

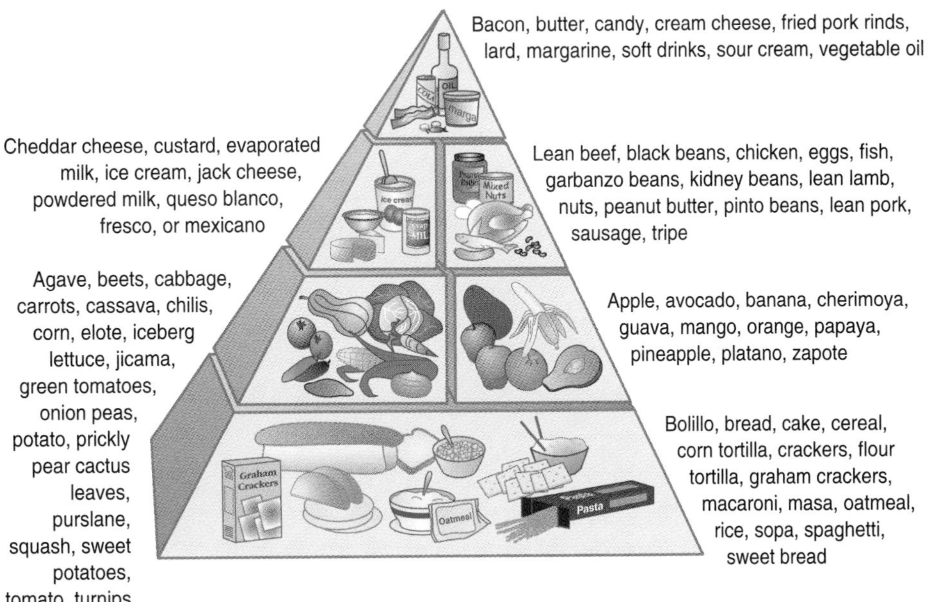

FIGURE 10-4 Mexican-American foods and the Food Guide Pyramid. Source: Algert S.J., Ellison, E.H. (47) and Visiting Nurse Association. Reprinted with permission from the Penn State Nutrition Center.

- Encourage lower-fat cooking techniques; recommend "heart-healthy" alternatives to lard, bacon, and margarine.
- Mexican-Americans encourage interdependence rather than independence in families. Therefore it is more effective to target the message by emphasizing the good of the entire family rather than individual benefits.
- Verbal and written messages in Spanish are important.

NATIVE-AMERICANS/ALASKA NATIVES

Native-Americans/Alaska Natives represent a heterogeneous group of more than 500 tribes and villages with wide diversity in eating patterns. The Navajo tribe is the largest tribe in the United States. The Navajo diet has been influenced by the Pueblo people, who introduced farming, which led to the adoption of corn and other cultivated crops as dietary staples. The Spaniards introduced sheep and goats. Many Navajo people try to live off the land but need assistance from the Food Stamp Program or the Food Distribution Program on Indian reservations. Poverty is widespread. A food guide pyramid showing current Navajo foods appears in Figure 10-5.

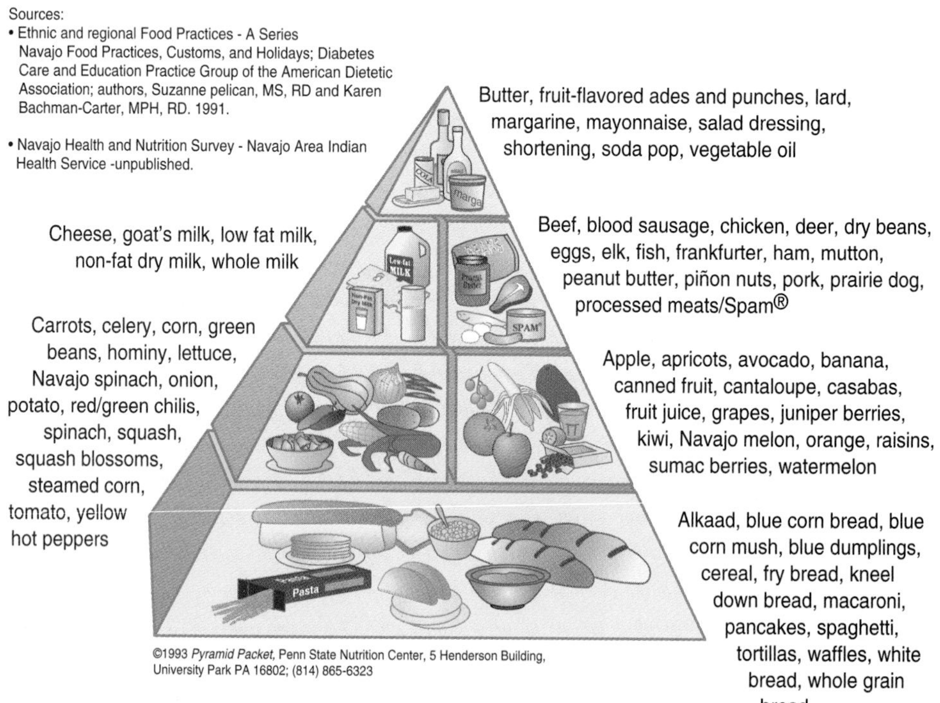

FIGURE 10-5 Navajo foods and the Food Guide Pyramid. Reprinted with permission from the Penn State Nutrition Center.

The prevalence of obesity is high among Native-Americans. Diabetes has reached epidemic proportions, and diabetes complications are the leading cause of illness and death in many Native-American populations. For instance, rates of kidney failure, blindness, and amputations are three to four times higher than in the general population.

Lack of understanding of Native-American/Alaska Native cultures is cited as a major barrier to nutritional intervention. Ways to become more familiar with the culture and lifestyle of a particular population include the following:

- Become familiar with the community by reading the local newspaper and walking around the area.
- Seek out community leaders.
- Visit local restaurants, supermarkets, and schools to identify traditional food sources.
- Seek out community groups, such as senior citizen groups and school parent organizations.
- Attend open community functions such as powwows and feast days.
- Visit local craft fairs and flea markets.
- Ask questions.

Traditional Food Practices of Selected Religious Groups

Religion tends to have a greater impact on food habits than nationality or culture does (eg, Orthodox Jews follow kosher dietary laws regardless of their national origin). However, religious food practices vary significantly, even among denominations of the same faith. National variations also exist. How closely an individual follows dietary laws is based on his or her degree of orthodoxy. An overview of religious food practices follows.

JUDAISM

In the United States there are three main Jewish denominations: Orthodox, Conservative, and Reform. Hasidic Jews are a sect within the Orthodox. These groups differ in their interpretation of the precepts of Judaism. Orthodox Jews believe that the laws are the direct commandments of God, and they adhere strictly to dietary laws. Reform Jews follow the moral law but may selectively follow other laws; for instance, they may not follow any religious dietary laws. Conservative Jews fall between the other two groups in their beliefs and adherence to the laws. They may follow the Jewish dietary laws at home but take a more liberal attitude on social occasions. Because Jews have diverse backgrounds and nationalities, their food practices vary widely.

Kosher is a word commonly used to identify Jewish dietary laws that define "clean" foods, "unclean" foods, how food animals must be slaughtered, how foods must be prepared, and when foods may be consumed (eg, the timing between eating milk products and meat products). Orthodox Jews eat only kosher meat and poultry that has been slaughtered according to ritual, soaked in water, salted, and washed. All crustaceans, shellfish, and fishlike mammals, such as catfish, shark, frog, crab, shrimp, lobster, scallops, oysters, and clams, are forbidden, as are all pork products. Milk and dairy products are used widely but cannot be consumed at the same meal with meat or poultry. Dairy products are not allowed within 1 to 6 hours after eating meat or poultry, depending on the individual's ethnic tradition. Meat and poultry cannot be eaten for 30 minutes after dairy products have been consumed. Margarine labeled *pareve* (dairy-free), nondairy creamers, and oils may be used with meats. Fruits, vegetables, plain grains, pastas, plain legumes, and eggs are considered kosher and can be eaten with either dairy or meat products. Separate utensils must be used for preparing and serving meat and dairy products.

Food preparation is prohibited on the Sabbath. Religious holidays are celebrated with certain foods. For example, only unleavened bread is eaten during Passover, and a 24-hour fast is observed on Yom Kippur. Because dietary laws are rigid, Orthodox Jews rarely eat outside the home, except at homes or restaurants with kosher kitchens.

CHRISTIANITY

The three primary branches of Christianity are Roman Catholicism, Eastern Orthodox Christianity, and Protestantism. Dietary practices vary from none to explicit.

Roman Catholics do not eat meat on Ash Wednesday or on Fridays of Lent. Food and beverages are avoided for 1 hour before communion is taken. Devout Catholics observe several fast days during the year.

Eastern Orthodox Christians observe numerous feast and fast days throughout the year.

The only denominations in the Protestant faith with dietary laws are the Mormons (Church of Jesus Christ of Latter-Day Saints) and Seventh-Day Adventists. Mormons do not use coffee, tea, alcohol, or tobacco. Followers are encouraged to limit meats and consume mostly grains. Some Mormons fast one day a month. Most Seventh-Day Adventists are lacto-ovovegetarians, and those who do eat meat avoid pork. Overeating is avoided, and coffee, tea, and alcohol are prohibited. An interval of 5 to 6 hours between meals is recommended, with no snacking between meals. Water is consumed before and after meals. Strong seasonings, such as pepper and mustard, are avoided.

ISLAM

Muslims eat as a matter of faith and for good health. Overindulgence is discouraged. Islamic dietary laws are called *halal*, which is also the term used to describe all permitted foods. *Haram* are foods that are prohibited, such as pork in any form or birds of prey. Meats must be properly slaughtered. Alcohol is prohibited, and devout Muslims avoid stimulants such as coffee and tea. Muslims are required to fast during the entire month of Ramadan and on certain other days during the year.

HINDUISM

Generally, Hindus avoid all foods that are believed to inhibit physical and spiritual development. Eating meat is not explicitly prohibited, but many Hindus are vegetarian because they adhere to the concept of *ahimsa*, which is nonviolence as applied to foods. Those who eat meat do not eat beef, because cows are considered sacred. Pork is often avoided. Other food prohibitions vary by region and may include snails, crabs, fowl, cranes, ducks, boars, fish with ugly forms, and the heads of snakes. Devout Hindus may avoid alcohol. Those seeking spiritual unity may avoid garlic and onions.

The concept of purity influences Hindu food practices. Products from cows (eg, milk, yogurt, ghee-clarified butter) are considered pure. Pure foods can improve the purity of unpure foods when they are prepared together. Some foods are innately polluted and can never be made pure, such as beef or alcohol. Numerous feast and fast days are observed.

Jainism, a branch of Hinduism, also promotes the nonviolent doctrine of *ahimsa*. Devout Jains are complete vegetarians and may avoid blood-colored foods (eg, tomatoes) and root vegetables (because harvesting them may cause the death of insects).

SIKHISM

Sikhs participate in many Hindu practices. They abstain from beef, and alcohol is prohibited. Pork is allowed.

BUDDHISM

Buddhist dietary practices vary widely depending on the sect and country. Most Buddhists subscribe to the concept of *ahimsa*, so many are lacto-ovovegetarians. Some eat fish, and some avoid only beef. Feast days vary regionally. Buddhist monks avoid eating solid food after the noon hour.

Acculturation

To varying degrees, people who move to a different cultural area adopt the beliefs, values, attitudes, and behaviors of the dominant culture. This process, called **acculturation,** is not limited to immigrants but affects anyone who moves from one community to another.

Acculturation is influenced by many factors, including the length of time the individual or group has been in the new culture. Usually, first-generation Americans adhere more closely to cultural food patterns than subsequent generations do, and they may cling to traditional foods to preserve their ethnic identity. Subsequent generations may follow cultural patterns only on holidays and at family gatherings, or they may give up ethnic foods but retain traditional methods of preparation. Another factor that influences acculturation is the individual's age and exposure to new ideas. Children tend to adopt new ways quickly as they learn from other children at school. People seeking higher education tend to have greater exposure to new ideas than those who remain more closely tied to their native cultural group.

There are three types of interrelated changes in food habits that occur as part of acculturation: New foods are added to the diet, substitutions are made for some traditional foods, and some traditional foods are rejected. In addition, as part of acculturation in the United States, individuals begin to adopt growing food trends in American culture, such as changes in food purchasing and preparation methods and fewer meals eaten at home. Some changes in food choices have a positive health outcome, and some have a negative effect.

NEW FOODS

Status, economics, information, taste, and exposure are some of the reasons why new foods are added to the diet. For instance, eating "American" food may symbolize status and make people feel more connected to their new culture. Frequently, new foods are added because they are relatively inexpensive and widely available.

FOOD SUBSTITUTIONS

Traditional foods may be replaced by new foods. This often occurs because traditional foods are difficult to find, are too expensive, or have lengthy preparation times. For many ethnic groups who move to the United States, breakfast and lunch are most likely to be composed of convenient American foods, whereas traditional foods are retained for the major dinner meal, which has greater emotional significance.

REJECTION OF TRADITIONAL FOODS

Children and adolescents are more likely than older adults to reject traditional foods so as to become more like their peers. Traditional foods may also be rejected because of an increased awareness of the role of nutrition in the development of chronic diseases. For instance, one reason why Asian Indians who have resided in the United States for a relatively long period tend to eat significantly less ghee (clarified butter served with rice or spread on Indian breads) may be that they are trying to decrease their intake of saturated fat.

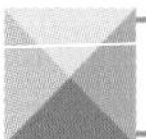

Changes in American Culture

CHANGES IN FOOD PURCHASING AND PREPARATION

The growing number of women in the workforce and the increasing number of single-parent families contribute to the increased use of convenience foods. In fact, lack of time is the impetus behind the trend to use fully or partially prepared ingredients to make meals. Americans want simple recipes with few ingredients that can be prepared in a minimum amount of time. The food industry is responding to this demand by developing products that are fully assembled and cook quickly. Unfortunately, convenience may take precedence over nutritional considerations when food choices are made. Many "convenience" products are high in sodium and relatively low in fiber (eg, frozen meals consisting of vegetables, pasta, meat, and seasonings that come in a bag). Nutrition counseling should address how to evaluate food labels and comparison shop between different brands of the same item (eg, comparing the sodium content between different bottled spaghetti sauces) (Fig. 10-6). The use of "healthy" convenience products, such as bagged fresh salad mixtures, fresh fruits and vegetables from the in-store salad bar, and whole-grain breads from the bakery section, should be encouraged.

FEWER MEALS EATEN AT HOME

A greater percentage of Americans are eating away from home than ever before. In 1997, more than half of all adults ate in a restaurant on a typical day. In an average month, 78% of American households ordered carry-out or delivered food. People who eat at restaurants or buy take-out food tend to eat more calories, fat, and sodium than people who eat home-prepared meals. Nutrition counseling should address how to eat a healthy diet while eating out, with an emphasis on portion sizes, the significance of food preparation techniques, and sources of hidden fat (eg, cream sauces) and sodium (eg, fast food fruit "pies").

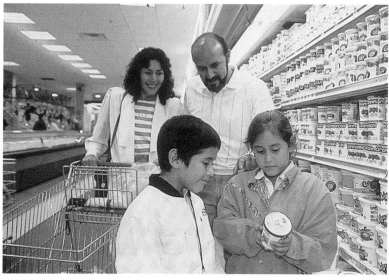

FIGURE 10-6 Parents and children can choose foods that are culturally appealing and nutritionally beneficial by learning to read food labels. Copyright: Jeff Greenberg/Science Source/Photo Researchers.

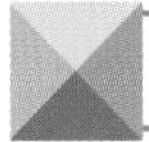

Cultural Sensitivity in Nursing Care

By the year 2050, it is estimated that only half of Americans will be Caucasian. The nutritional implications of this shift in cultural predominance is that cultural sensitivity will become increasingly important to nursing care. The key to cross-cultural assessment and counseling is an understanding of the client's cultural values and their impact on health and food choices. From this awareness, nutrition information can be tailored to the client's needs, desires, and lifestyle. Nutrition information that is technically correct but culturally inappropriate is not likely to produce behavior change.

ASSESSING USUAL FOOD BEHAVIORS

In assessing usual food behaviors, it is important to determine how tradition and acculturation have influenced the client's intake.

- What traditional foods does the client eat daily? Weekly? How often does the client currently eat traditional foods? What traditional foods does the client no longer eat? Why? Are there similar foods available? Does the client substitute new foods for traditional foods?
- What were the client's favorite cultural foods? Does the client still eat those foods? Are they still the client's favorite foods? If not, why not? Are similar foods available? Does the client substitute new foods for favorite foods?
- What new foods has the client tried? Which new foods did the client like? Which new foods did the client dislike? Does the client eat new foods regularly?
- What are the client's health beliefs related to food? Does the client use herbs or other dietary supplements?
- Who is responsible for procuring, storing, and preparing food? Does the client shop at grocery stores or ethnic specialty markets? Are refrigeration and cooking facilities adequate?
- Is the client intent on becoming "Americanized" or on trying to retain his or her ethnic identity?

CROSS-CULTURAL NUTRITION COUNSELING

In counseling clients from other cultures about nutrition, it is important to remember that eating is a very personal matter. Be respectful and understanding of other cultures without being judgmental, especially regarding foods that you may personally find distasteful, such as turtle eggs or lizards. No one likes to have their food choices criticized. Clients may tell you what you want to hear to avoid the risk of being chastised. Other considerations include the following:

- Determine the client's level of fluency before beginning counseling. Obtain an interpreter if needed. Speak directly to the client, even if an interpreter is used.

- Ask how the client wishes to be addressed.
- Avoid body language that may be misinterpreted.
- Determine reading ability before giving out written material.
- Reinforce positive eating habits. Promote change only in harmful practices. Remember that knowledge does not necessarily lead to behavior change.

Herbal Supplements

Herbs are plants or parts of plants used to alleviate health problems or promote wellness. Within recent years, sales of herbal products in the United States have soared. Despite the unknown and known risks, it is estimated that one third of American adults use herbs. This trend is attributed to several cultural factors. Current issues surrounding the health care industry include a distrust of traditional medicine and inadequate medical insurance coverage. An increase in ethnic populations who traditionally use herbs has influenced the use of herbal supplements. The American culture's sense of freedom of choice and personal control, the value placed on youth, and a growing desire to promote health and well-being with "natural" products has contributed to the popularity of herbal supplements. It should be noted that "natural" is not synonymous with "healthful." For instance, arsenic is natural but poisonous.

HERBS VERSUS TRADITIONAL DRUGS

In their medicinal sense, herbs are technically unapproved drugs. In fact, some drugs used today originated from plants (eg, Taxol, aspirin, digoxin). Yet compared to drugs, herbs are more dilute because they contain a myriad of other active and inert ingredients. They may also contain substances that counteract the action of the active ingredient, thereby reducing its effectiveness. Herbs differ greatly from conventional drugs in how they are marketed and regulated.

Herbs are Self-Prescribed

In the United States, the use of herbs is self-prescribed. A major concern with self-medicating is that consumers may misdiagnose their condition or forsake effective conventional medical care to treat themselves "naturally." Another problem with self-medicating is that patients may not inform their physicians about their use of herbs, so that side effects and herb-drug interactions go undiagnosed.

Claims on Packaging for Herbal Products do not Require FDA Approval

Although herbs cannot claim to be used for the diagnosis, treatment, cure, or prevention of disease, herbs can be labeled with statements explaining their purported effect on the structure or function of the human body (eg, "alleviates fatigue") or their role in promoting well-being (eg, "improves mood"). Unsuspecting consumers may be misled by herbal claims.

Herbs are not Regulated for Purity

Government standards of quality for herbs are nonexistent in the United States. Lack of quality standards means that contamination is a risk. For instance, in the past, cases of atropine poisoning occurred because preparations of the herb burdock were contaminated with belladonna. The contamination occurred because the two plants have similar-looking roots.

Herbs are not Regulated for Potency

The concentration of active compounds in different batches of supposedly identical plant material is highly variable. The difference in concentration may be related to different plant varieties, differences in harvesting techniques, the environmental conditions under which the plants were grown (eg, fertility of the soil, amount of moisture), or how they were processed (eg, temperature and length of time used to dry plant materials). Labels listing the content of active ingredients are not always valid or reliable.

Herbs do not Have to Prove Safety and Efficacy Before Being Marketed

Before a drug can be marketed, the FDA must authorize its use based on the results of clinical studies performed to determine safety, effectiveness, possible interactions with other substances, and appropriate doses. In contrast, dietary supplement manufacturers that want to market a new ingredient (an ingredient not marketed in the United States before 1994) must submit information to the FDA that supports their conclusion that a new ingredient can reasonably be expected to be safe. After a dietary supplement is marketed, the FDA can take action to restrict its use only after it shows that the product is unsafe. The responsibility lies with the FDA to prove danger, rather than with the manufacturer to prove safety. Examples of herbs that have been linked to health problems include the following:

- Chaparral can cause liver disease that may be irreversible.
- Comfrey can cause liver damage.
- Ephedra can cause high blood pressure, rapid heartbeat, muscle injury, and nerve damage.
- Lobelia can cause breathing problems, sweating, rapid heartbeat, and low blood pressure; coma and death are possible with high doses.
- Sassafras (safrole) has been shown to be carcinogenic in rats and mice.
- Yohimbine can cause nervous disorders, paralysis, fatigue, and death.

Herb Dosages are not Standardized

The most common way to consume herbs is as a tea or tisane made from the dried plant material. The recommended amount of herb to use is usually imprecise (eg, "a heaping teaspoon"). When making tea, steeping times are also important, especially when the active ingredients are not highly water soluble.

COMMON HERBAL SUPPLEMENTS

The five top-selling herbs in the United States are St. John's wort, echinacea, *Ginkgo biloba*, garlic, and ginseng. For more information on herbs and dietary supplements, visit the National Institutes of Health web site at www.nih.gov.

St. John's Wort

St. John's wort is purported to be a "natural" treatment for mild to moderate depression, anxiety, seasonal affective disorder, and sleep disorders. It is the leading treatment of depression in Germany, where it is prescribed about 20 times more often than Prozac, one of the most widely prescribed antidepressants in the United States.

St. John's wort contains many biologically active compounds. One of its active ingredients is hypericin, which may act as a monoamine oxidase inhibitor. In vitro studies show that St. John's wort extract inhibits serotonin, dopamine, and norepinephrine reuptake; low levels of serotonin are associated with depression. Another proposed mechanism by which the active compounds in St. John's wort treat depression is by reducing levels of interleukin-6, which prevents increases in adrenal hormones associated with depression. More research is needed to precisely identify the active ingredients and how they work. Large-scale, controlled clinical trials are underway in the United States to assess whether St. John's wort has a significant therapeutic effect in patients with clinical depression.

Compared with antidepressant drugs, St. John's wort produces fewer and less severe side effects, is far less expensive, and does not require a prescription. However, some users complain of dry mouth, dizziness, gastrointestinal symptoms, increased sensitivity to sunlight, and fatigue. Also, clinical depression is a serious medical disorder, and to treat it with an herb that has not been proven effective could be dangerous. St. John's wort should not be used with antidepressants. Adverse interactions may occur when St. John's wort is used with Crixivan (indinavir), and possibly with other protease inhibitors used in the treatment of human immunodeficiency virus infection, or with cyclosporine or other immunosuppressant drugs.

Echinacea

Echinacea, also known as the purple coneflower, is a native North American wildflower. Native-Americans used echinacea to treat wounds and respiratory infections. Many people today take echinacea to prevent or treat colds and the flu.

The echinacea plant contains several active compounds that appear to stimulate the production and activity of white blood cells whose function is to attack and destroy bacteria and other microbes in the bloodstream. Echinacea may also increase the production of cytokines, chemicals that help control immune system function.

Echinacea can help relieve colds and infections caused by bacteria, viruses, and yeast, and it may help reduce inflammation. However, dosage levels are not established, and knowledge about the potential toxic effects of the plant is incomplete. Studies are underway to determine whether echinacea is effective against cancer in humans. Clients should be advised to consult with a physician before using echinacea, especially if the client has an autoimmune illness or progressive disease such as acquired immunodeficiency syndrome.

Ginkgo Biloba

Ginkgo, also known as the maidenhair tree, is the oldest living species of tree on earth. The leaves of the ginkgo are fan-shaped and have two distinct lobes—hence the term, "biloba."

Ginkgo biloba extract contains two types of active ingredients. One is antioxidants, which help prevent cell damage from free radicals and appear to inhibit platelet aggregation, thereby reducing the risk of blood clots. The other active ingredients may work by improving circulation and by repairing damage to nerve cells. The combination of improved blood flow (especially to the brain) and improvements in nerve cell function may account for the belief that ginkgo helps prevent or relieve senile dementia.

Ginkgo does seem to relieve symptoms of blood vessel insufficiency related to aging and atherosclerosis. It may improve blood flow through the head, thus increasing the supply of oxygen to the brain. In older adults, ginkgo may reduce symptoms of vertigo, ringing in the ears, and headache. Some people report that ginkgo reduces leg pain from intermittent claudication and enables them to walk for longer distances. It has a moderate effect on memory loss and only in people with dementia.

Some people complain of mild headaches or upset stomach from ginkgo. *Ginkgo biloba* may interact with aspirin or warfarin (Coumadin), increasing the risk of spontaneous bleeding in the brain. People who take garlic, vitamin E, warfarin, aspirin, or other drugs with antiplatelet or anticoagulant effects should be warned about the potential interactions with ginkgo. Clients using ginkgo should be advised to contact their physician if they experience unusual bleeding or bruising, new-onset headaches, or vision changes.

Garlic

Garlic is a member of the onion family and has been used for thousands of years as both a food and an herbal remedy. Ancient Greek physicians believed that garlic could help numerous problems, such as parasitic infections, colds, poor digestion, and low energy. The active compound in garlic is allicin, which is converted into other active ingredients when it is acted on by enzymes.

Studies confirm that garlic helps prevent atherosclerosis and lowers blood levels of cholesterol and triglycerides. It helps prevent blood clot formation by reducing platelet aggregation. It is mildly effective in preventing infections by bacteria, viruses, fungi, and perhaps intestinal parasites. Garlic extracts stimulate the immune system by triggering the proliferation of lymphocytes, boosting the release of cytokines, and promoting the activity of natural killer cells. Some studies suggest that people who eat high amounts of garlic have a lower risk of cancers of the stomach, esophagus, and colon.

There is no consensus regarding which form of garlic is best: whole raw garlic in table form; aged or fresh; with odor or "deodorized." Too much garlic can cause heartburn and flatulence and can interfere with normal blood clotting.

Ginseng

Ginseng refers to a group of plants of which there are approximately 700 species. Ginseng is common in the Americas and in Asia. The root is believed to have medical properties.

The scientific name for ginseng is *Panax*, which means "cure-all" in Greek. Chinese ginseng has been used as a medical treatment for more than 2000 years to improve mental alertness and increase energy. Some people believe ginseng is an aphrodisiac and a stress reliever.

The active ingredients in ginseng are believed to increase energy, relieve stress, and enhance physical and intellectual performance. Ginseng may also lower blood sugar and enhance immune system functioning. Siberian ginseng is used to prevent colds and the flu. Some people claim it increases stamina and endurance. In test-tube studies, ginseng appeared to stimulate immune cells and activate natural killer cells to inhibit the growth of tumors.

Despite its popularity among many cultures for many years, little scientific evidence is available to show that it is effective for any purpose. Scientific studies have not produced data to confirm ginseng's supposed biologic activity. Because it is a stimulant, ginseng may cause nervousness or agitation. People with high blood pressure or headaches should avoid ginseng because it may aggravate those conditions. Ginseng can potentiate the action of warfarin. Large amounts of ginseng can cause vomiting, bleeding, and even death.

TIPS FOR USING HERBAL PRODUCTS

Discuss Herbal use With the Physician

Physicians need to be aware of herb use so they can monitor for side effects and herb-drug interactions. People who take medications for high blood pressure, heart disease, or Parkinson's disease should consult their physician before using herbs.

Beware of People who Give Unqualified Advice

"Herbalist," "herb doctor," and "master herbalist" are unregulated job titles that can be used by anyone. Also beware of a product that claims to be "magical," a "new discovery," or "miraculous."

Take Measures to Prevent and Manage Adverse Side Effects and Herb-Drug Interactions

Stick to single herb products and start with a small dose. Side effects and interactions are less likely to occur and easier to pinpoint when single herbs are used at low doses. Be alert to adverse side effects such as allergy, stomach upset, skin rash, or headache. Take herbs at different times from prescribed medications to help reduce the potential for herb-drug interactions. Herbs taken with drugs have the potential to reduce the drug's effectiveness.

Herbs should be discontinued immediately if adverse side effects or herb-drug interactions occur. Notify the physician so that a report can be filed with FDA MedWatch at 1-800-FDA-1088 or www.fda.gov/medwatch/report.hcp.ht. Consumers can file their own report at the same telephone number or through www.fda.gov/medwatch/report/consumer/consumer.htm.

Avoid Herbs During Pregnancy and Lactation and in Children Younger Than Six Years of Age

Herbs, like drugs, have the potential to cross the placenta to some degree, exposing the fetus to potential teratogenic effects. Herbs may also enter breast milk, resulting in adverse effects in the nursing infant. The distribution of herbs in children's body tissue may be different than in adults because of differences in relative body composition.

Learn to Read Herbal Supplement Labels

Buy products that have the "USP" notation on the label. This indicates that the manufacturer follows standards established by the U.S. Pharmacopoeia. Chose products whose labels show the scientific name of the herb, the name and address of the actual manufacturer, a batch or lot number, the date of manufacture, and the expiration date.

Questions You May Hear

What are "regional food practices"? Regional food practices are certain behaviors associated with specific areas of the country. Advances in food technology and transportation have diluted regional food practices by vastly increasing the variety and availability of foods across the country. The following "regional" foods are available anywhere:

- New England: Boston baked beans, clam chowder, lobster, and clam cakes
- Pennsylvania Dutch Country: shoofly pie, scrapple, and German-style sausage
- The South: grits, fried chicken, hot biscuits, greens, sweet potatoes, and corn bread
- Louisiana: French and Creole-style cooking
- Texas: chili con carne

- The Southwest: Mexican foods such as tortillas, tamales, enchiladas, and refried beans
- The Far West: citrus fruit, fresh produce, salads, and Oriental cooking
- The Midwest: dairy products and beef

How has the increase in minority populations influenced the "American" diet? As cultural groups migrate to the United States, they introduce new foods into the mainstream culture. Not so long ago, foods such as yogurt, green tea, and salsa were considered exotic. Today, ethnic restaurants and ethnic foods sections in grocery stores are commonplace and popular. In fact, it is difficult to ascertain which foods are truly American foods and which are an adaptation from other cultures. Swiss steak, Russian dressing, and chili con carne are American inventions. Cross-cultural food creations include Tex-Mex wontons and tofu lasagna.

KEY CONCEPTS

- Although culture defines what is edible; how food is handled, prepared, and consumed; what foods are appropriate for particular groups within the culture; the meaning of food and eating; attitudes toward body size; and the relationship between food and health, food habits vary considerably among individuals and families within a cultural group.
- Staple foods are an indispensable part of the diet and come from the bottom of the Food Guide Pyramid. Protective foods are nutrient rich and add variety and ethnic identity to meals.
- It is important to understand a client's cultural values so that appropriate assessment data can be gathered and culturally sensitive interventions can be devised.
- Generalizations can be made about traditional eating practices of subcultures within the United States. However, an individual's food choices deviate from these based on personal preferences, socioeconomic status, and degree of acculturation.
- As people move from one cultural area to another, they change their food habits to some degree. New foods are added to the diet or substituted for traditional foods, and some traditional foods are rejected. Availability and cost influence food choices.
- Americans are cooking less and eating out more, which tends to result in greater intakes of fat, cholesterol, and sodium. Clients need to learn how to use convenience products to prepare healthy meals at home and how to eat a healthy diet while eating out.
- Cultural sensitivity is increasingly important to nursing care. The key to cross-cultural assessment and counseling is an understanding of the client's cultural values and their impact on health and food choices. From this awareness, nutrition information can be tailored to the client's needs, desires, and lifestyle.
- The use of herbs is becoming increasingly popular in the United States. Unlike drugs, herbs can be marketed without first being proved safe. There are no legal standards of quality in effect for herbs.
- Clients should be advised to tell their physicians about their use of herbs so that herb-drug interactions and side effects can be monitored. Clients should stick to low doses

of single herbs and should buy only those with the USP notation on the label. Pregnant women, lactating women, and children younger than 6 years of age should not use herbs.
- Religion tends to have a greater impact on food habits than nationality or culture.
- The "American" diet undergoes change as people from different cultures introduce their traditional foods to the mainstream culture.

ANSWER KEY

1. **TRUE** Each culture has its own socially standardized food behaviors that dictate what is edible, the role of certain foods in the diet, how food is prepared, the use of foods, the number and timing of daily meals, how food is eaten, and health beliefs related to food.
2. **FALSE** Race, ethnicity, and geographic region are often inaccurately assumed to be synonymous with culture. This misconception leads to stereotypical grouping.
3. **TRUE** Staple foods (eg, cereal grains, starchy tubers, starchy vegetables) generally come from the bottom of the Food Guide Pyramid.
4. **TRUE** Ethnocentrism is the belief that one's own values and behaviors are "right," "normal," and "superior" compared to those of all other cultures, which are "wrong," "odd," or "inferior."
5. **FALSE** The hot-cold theory of health and diet refers to the Asian culture's belief that health and illness are related to the balance between yin and yang forces in the body. Yin represents female, cold, and darkness; yang represents male, hot, and light.
6. **TRUE** Usually, first-generation Americans adhere more closely to cultural food patterns to preserve their ethnic identity, compared with subsequent generations.
7. **TRUE** For many ethnic groups who move to the United States, breakfast and lunch are most likely to be composed of convenient American foods while traditional foods are retained for the major dinner meal, which has greater emotional significance.
8. **TRUE** People who eat at restaurants or buy take-out food tend to eat more calories, fat, and sodium than people who eat home-prepared meals.
9. **FALSE** The responsibility lies with the FDA to prove danger after a dietary supplement is marketed, rather than with the manufacturer to prove safety before a dietary supplement is marketed.
10. **FALSE** "Natural" is not synonymous with "healthful." For instance, arsenic is natural but poisonous.

REFERENCES

American Cancer Society. *Popular herbs*. [On-line]. Available: www.cancer.org/alt_therapy/popherbs.html. Accessed November 12, 1999.

Borrud, L. (1996). Eating out in America: Impact on food choices and nutrient profiles [speech]. [On-line]. Available: www.barc.usda.gov/blnrc/foodsurvey/Eatout95.html. Accessed March 29, 1999.

Coulston, A. (1998). Preparing for diversity as dietetics professionals. *Journal of the American Dietetic Association*, *98*, 862.

Cupp, M. (1999). Herbal remedies: Adverse effects and drug interactions. *American Family Physician*, *59*, 1239. Available: www.aafp.org/afp/990301ap/1239.html. Information on religious food practices is available at www.eatethnic.com/Religious%20Foods.html.

Eliades, D., & Suitor, C. (1994). *Celebrating diversity: Approaching families through their food*. [On-line]. Prepared for the USDA/DHHS Nutrition Education Committee for Maternal and Child Nutrition Publications. Available: www.penpages.psu.edu/penpages_reference/12101/121011730.HTML.

Harnack, L., Story, M., Martinson, B., Newmark-Sztainer, D., & Stang, J. (1998). Guess who's cooking? The role of men in meal planning, shopping, and preparation in US families. *Journal of the American Dietetic Association*, *98*, 995–1000.

Higgins, C., Laredo, R., Stollar, C., & Warshaw, H. (1998). *Jewish food practices, customs, and holidays*. Developed by the Diabetes Care and Education Dietetic Practice Group of The American Dietetic Association (Chicago). Alexandria, VA: American Diabetes Association.

Kris-Etherton, P., & Burns, J. (Eds.). (1998). *Cardiovascular nutrition: Strategies and tools for disease management and prevention*. Chicago: The American Dietetic Association.

Lee, S., Sobal, J., & Frongillo, E. (1999). Acculturation and dietary practices among Korean Americans. *Journal of the American Dietetic Association*, *99*, 1084–1089.

National Council for Reliable Health Information. (March/April 1999). DSHEA and the FDA guide to supplements. *NCRHI Newsletter*, *22*. Available: www.ncahf.org/newslett/nl22-2.html.

National Institutes of Health, National Center for Complementary and Alternative Medicine (NCCAM), NCCAM Clearinghouse. St. John's wort. [On-line]. Available: www.nccam.nih.gov/nccam/fcp/factsheets/stjohnswort/ stjohnswort.htm. Accessed: March 16, 2000.

Raj, S., Ganganna, P., & Bowering, J. (1999). Dietary habits of Asian Indians in relation to length of residence in the United States. *Journal of the American Dietetic Association*, *99*, 1106–1108.

Religious food practices. [On-line]. Available: Eatethnic.com. Accessed March 2, 2000.

Robbers, J., & Tyler, V. (1999). *Tyler's Herbs of Choice: the Therapeutic Use of Phytomedicinals*. Binghamton, NY: The Haworth Press, Inc.

Terry, R. (1994). Needed: A new appreciation of culture and food behavior. *Journal of the American Dietetic Association*, *94*, 501–503.

CHAPTER 11

Healthy Eating for Healthy Babies

TRUE	FALSE	Check your knowledge of healthy eating for healthy babies.
		1 Adequate weight gain during pregnancy ensures delivery of a normal-weight baby.
		2 Obese women should maintain their weight, not gain weight, during pregnancy.
		3 The recommended rate of weight gain during the second and third trimesters for normal-weight women is approximately 1 pound/week.
		4 A pregnant woman needs only 400 μg daily of synthetic folic acid to reduce the risk of neural tube defects.
		5 Too much preformed vitamin A from food or supplements can cause birth defects early in pregnancy.
		6 Lactation increases calorie requirements more than pregnancy does.
		7 The vitamin content of breast milk is affected by the mother's vitamin intake.
		8 Thirst is a good indicator for the need for fluid in most lactating women.
		9 American women with human immunodeficiency virus (HIV) infection should be advised not to breast-feed.
		10 Women with type 1 diabetes should not breast-feed.

Upon completion of this chapter, you will be able to

- Discuss the recommended pattern and rate of weight gain during pregnancy for underweight, normal-weight, and obese women.
- Describe the number of servings recommended from each Food Guide Pyramid food group during pregnancy.
- List nutritional interventions for problems during pregnancy, such as nausea, constipation, and heartburn.
- Discuss nutritional interventions during pregnancy for women with phenylketonuria (PKU), diabetes, or pregnancy-induced hypertension.

- Describe criteria for assessing nutritional needs during pregnancy.
- List benefits of breast-feeding.
- Discuss variables that affect the composition of breast milk.
- Describe the number of servings recommended from each Food Guide Pyramid food group during lactation.
- List foods to avoid while breast-feeding.
- Describe criteria for assessing nutritional needs during lactation.
- List ways to promote breast-feeding.

Introduction

Maternal diet and nutritional status have a direct impact on the course of pregnancy and its outcome. Malnutrition that occurs in the early months of pregnancy affects development and the capacity of the embryo to survive; poor nutrition in the latter part of pregnancy affects fetal growth. At no other time is the welfare of one so dependent on another.

This chapter discusses the effects of pregnancy on a woman's nutritional requirements and how the Food Guide Pyramid can be used to help women choose a balanced and adequate diet. Tips on healthy eating during pregnancy are presented. Problems and complications of pregnancy with nutritional implications are discussed. The advantages of breast-feeding and nutritional needs to support lactation are explained.

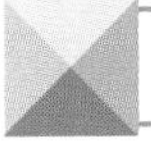

Nutrition and Pregnancy

PHYSIOLOGIC CHANGES

Pregnancy produces physiologic changes that affect all of the mother's body systems. Alterations in metabolism, gastrointestinal function, blood volume, and weight account for some of the changes that influence nutrient requirements and use of nutrients in the body.

Altered Metabolism

The basal metabolic rate increases by the fourth month of gestation and rises to 15% to 20% above normal by term. This increase reflects the increased oxygen demands of the fetus and maternal tissues. Calorie requirements increase proportionately.

In addition to the increased metabolic rate, the metabolism of nutrients is altered. Because the fetus' primary fuel for meeting energy requirements is glucose, fat becomes the major source of maternal fuel, making glucose available for the fetus. A decrease in insulin efficiency occurs during the latter part of pregnancy, which may be a compensatory mechanism to increase glucose availability for the fetus. Some women develop gestational diabetes, a type of diabetes that resolves itself after delivery.

Gastrointestinal Changes

Nausea and vomiting are common in the first trimester and may be related to hypoglycemia, decreased gastric motility, relaxation of the cardiac sphincter, or anxiety. Increases in appetite and thirst are also common.

Increased progesterone production has the effect of relaxing smooth muscle cells. This action helps the uterus expand to accommodate the growing fetus and also slows gastrointestinal motility. An advantage of slowed motility is that nutrient absorption increases. The disadvantages are an increased risk of esophageal reflux, heartburn, and constipation. As pregnancy progresses, the displacement of the stomach and intestines caused by the enlarging uterus contributes to heartburn and constipation.

Blood Volume Changes

Total body water increases throughout pregnancy and accounts for a large percentage of weight gain at term. The increase in blood volume exceeds the increase in red blood cell production, resulting in hemodilution or a physiologic anemia of pregnancy. Minor edema may be considered normal if it is not accompanied by hypertension and proteinuria.

Weight Gain

Weight gain during pregnancy results from the growth of the fetus, placenta, and maternal blood volume and tissues. Many women fail to understand that the increase in maternal fat tissue is a physiologic mechanism designed to prepare women for the energy demands of labor and lactation. Typical weight gain distribution in normal pregnancy is detailed in Box 11–1.

Weight Gain Parameters

The amount of weight a woman gains during pregnancy, especially during the second and third trimesters, is an important indicator of fetal growth. Inadequate weight gain during pregnancy increases the risk of giving birth to a **low-birth-weight (LBW)** infant (a baby weighing less than 2500 g or 5.5 pounds). LBW babies tend to be malnourished, especially if born full-term, and they have a high incidence of postnatal complications and mortality. In fact, birth weight may be the most important predictor, not only of mortality, but also of subsequent development. However, adequate weight gain during pregnancy cannot by itself ensure the delivery of a normal-birth-weight infant.

A growing body of evidence shows that the mother's prepregnancy weight in relation to her height influences fetal growth beyond the effect of gestational weight gain.

BOX 11.1

Weight Gain Distribution in Normal Pregnancy (Pounds)

Birth weight of baby	7.5
Placenta	1.5
Increase in maternal blood volume	4
Increase in maternal fluid volume	4
Increase in uterus	2
Increase in breast tissue	2
Amniotic fluid	2
Maternal fat tissue	7
	30

Women who are thinner before pregnancy tend to have smaller babies, compared with heavier women with the same gestational weight gain. Women who begin pregnancy while underweight and poorly nourished are at higher risk for delivering LBW infants and for experiencing preterm labor of small, underdeveloped infants. Current recommendations for weight gain during pregnancy stress the importance of individualizing weight gain goals based on an accurate assessment of prepregnancy weight. It appears that underweight women may reduce their risk of adverse pregnancy outcome by attaining a higher prepregnancy weight, or by gaining extra weight during pregnancy, or both.

Conversely, very high weight gain during pregnancy increases the incidence of high birth weight, which is associated with some increase in the risk of fetopelvic disproportion and other complications. The effect seems to be greatest in women who are shorter than 62 inches. Some studies also indicate that excessive weight gain during pregnancy contributes to maternal obesity.

Currently, the Weight Gain Subcommittee of the Institute of Medicine sets forth the following desirable ranges of total weight gain based on prepregnancy weight status using body mass index (BMI).

Prepregnancy BMI	Category	Gestational Weight Gain (lb)
<19.8	Underweight	28–40
19.8–26.0	Normal weight	25–35
>26.0–29.0	Overweight	15–25
>29.0	Obese	≥15

Within each weight category, adolescent and African-American mothers should be encouraged to strive for weight gains toward the upper range. The Weight Gain Subcommittee of the Institute of Medicine recommends that women carrying twins gain 35 to 45 pounds; however, some studies suggest gains of 40 to 45 pounds by 35 to 38 weeks' gestation for ideal twin outcome. Length of gestation, BMI, and weight have been shown to be positive factors in twin birth weight.

Pattern of Weight Gain

The pattern of weight gain can also be an indicator of increased risk during pregnancy. Adult women who fail to gain 10 pounds by 20 weeks' gestation appear to be at greater risk for delivering a LBW infant. During the first trimester, a 2- to 5-pound weight gain is considered normal. Thereafter, the recommended weight gain for normal-weight women is approximately 1 pound/week. Underweight women should gain slightly more than 1 pound/week, overweight women should gain about 0.66 pounds/week, and women pregnant with twins should be encouraged to gain at least 1 pound/week. The rate of weight gain for severely obese women should be determined on an individualized basis. However, weight reduction should never be undertaken during pregnancy. Although slightly higher or lower rates of weight gain can be considered normal, obvious or persistent deviations warrant further investigation. For example, after the 20th week of gestation, a sudden sharp weight gain, accompanied by generalized edema and increased blood pressure, may signal preeclampsia. Figures 11–1, 11–2, and 11–3 are provisional weight gain graphs based on prepregnancy BMI.

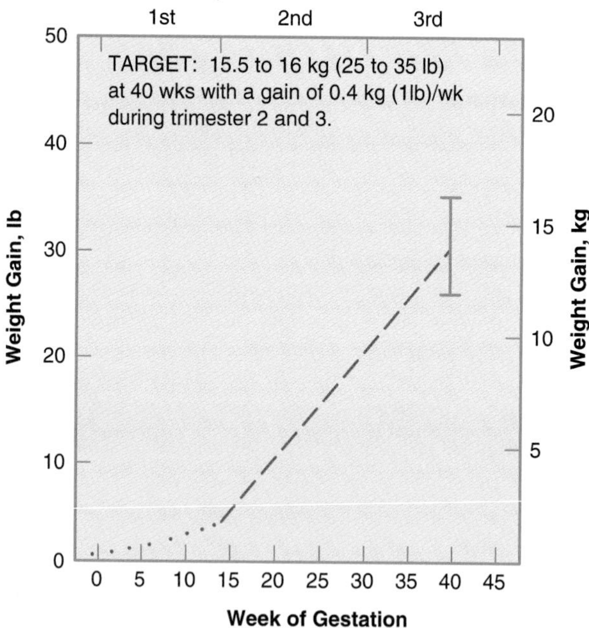

FIGURE 11-1 Provisional weight gain graph for normal-weight women with BMIs of 19.8 to 26.0 (metric).

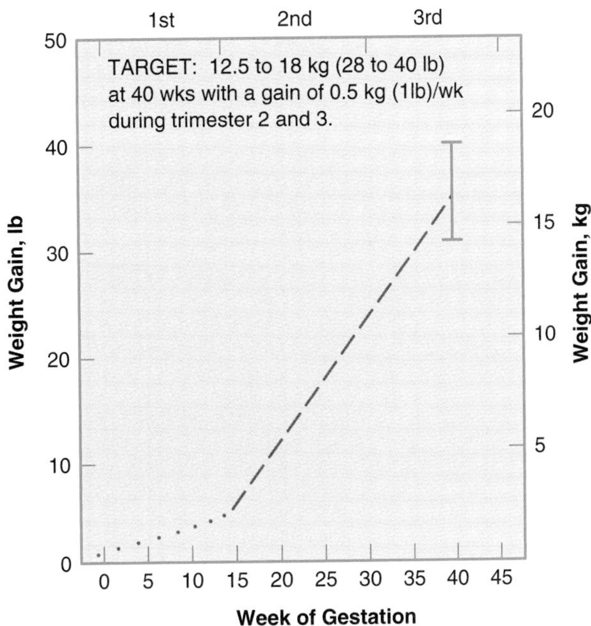

FIGURE 11-2 Provisional weight gain graph for underweight women with BMIs less than 19.8 (metric).

NUTRIENT REQUIREMENTS DURING PREGNANCY

The requirements for most nutrients increase during pregnancy (Table 11–1). However, not all nutrient needs increase proportionately. For instance, the need for iron triples during pregnancy, yet the requirement for vitamin B_{12} increases by only about 10%. Note that among the nutrients cited in Table 11–1, some have the 1989 Recommended Dietary Allowances (RDAs) and some have the new Daily Reference Intake values (RDAs or Adequate Intake [AI] levels). For all reference standards, the following points are notable:

- Actual requirements during pregnancy vary among individuals and are influenced by previous nutritional status and health history, including chronic illnesses, multiple pregnancies, and closely spaced pregnancies.
- The requirement for one nutrient may be altered by the intake of another. For instance, women who do not meet their calorie requirements need higher amounts of protein.
- Nutrient needs are not constant throughout the course of pregnancy. Nutrient needs change little during the first trimester and are at their highest during the last trimester.

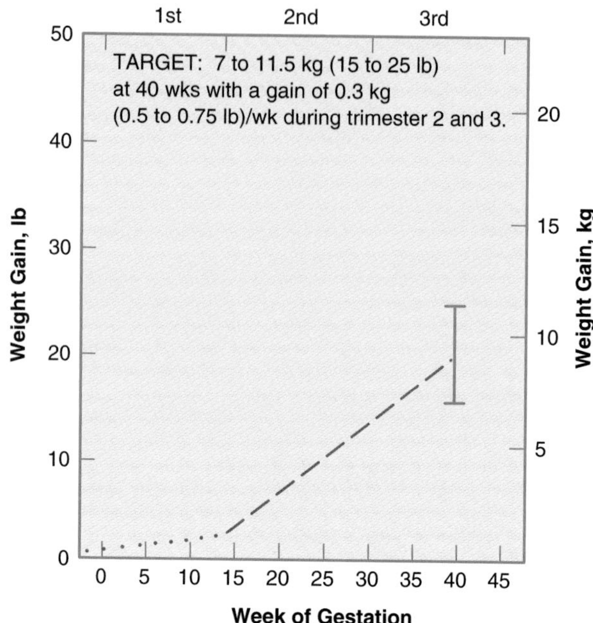

FIGURE 11-3 Provisional weight gain graph for overweight women with BMIs of more than 26.0 to 29.0 (metric).

- Reference standards are usually meaningless to the general public. The Food Guide Pyramid (see later discussion) can be used to teach women how to make food choices that will provide the balanced intake they need.

Calories

Calorie needs increase because of the increase in basal metabolic rate and because weight gain increases the amount of calories burned during activity. The body also uses additional calories to store energy in preparation for lactation after delivery. Adequate intake of carbohydrate calories ensures that protein is "spared" instead of being burned for energy and thus is available for synthesis of new tissue.

The increased need for calories is surprisingly small—a mere 300 extra calories per day, which is approximately 15% of a woman's normal calorie requirement. Also, the increased need for calories does not occur until the beginning of the second trimester. Because calorie needs increase relatively little compared with the increased requirements for other nutrients (eg, iron, folic acid), nutrient density is important.

TABLE 11.1 ***Nutritional Needs for Women (19–30 Years Old) During Pregnancy and Lactation***

Nutrient	Nonpregnant Women	Pregnancy	Lactation
Calories*	2200	1st tri: +0 2nd tri: +300 3rd tri: +300	+500
Protein (g)*[†]	46	60	65
Vit A (μg)*	800	800	1300
Vit D (μg)	5.0*	5.0*	5.0*
Vit E (mg)	15	15	19
Vit K (μg)*	60	65	65
Vit C (mg)	75	85	120
Thiamine (mg)	1.1*	1.4*	1.5*
Riboflavin (mg)	1.1*	1.4*	1.6*
Niacin (mg)	14*	18*	17*
Vit B_6 (mg)	1.3*	1.9*	2.0*
Folate (μg)	400*	600*	500*
Vit B_{12} (μg)	2.4*	2.6*	28*
Pantothenic acid (mg)	5*	6*	7*
Biotin (μg)	30*	30*	35*
Calcium (mg)	1000*	1000*	1000*
Phosphorus (mg)	700*	700*	700*
Magnesium (mg)	310*	350*	310*
Iron (mg)*	15	30	15
Zinc (mg)*	12	15	19
Iodine (μg)*	150	175	200
Selenium (μg)	55	60	70

tri, trimester; Vit, Vitamin.
*1989 Recommended Dietary Allowance.
[†]RDA for protein is 46 g for 19–24-year-olds and 50 g for 20–50-year-old women.

Protein

Protein needs increase to support fetal growth and development, the formation of the placenta and amniotic fluid, the growth of maternal tissues, and the expanded blood volume. The RDA for protein increases by 10 g for pregnant women ages 25 and older. Women who fail to consume adequate protein may be at increased risk for development of toxemia, anemia, poor uterine muscle tone, abortion, decreased resistance to infection, and shorter, lighter infants with low Apgar scores. However, most Americans, including vegetarians, consume more protein than they need, so most women do not need to adjust their usual protein intake. Eating more protein than is necessary offers no benefits and is potentially harmful.

Folic Acid

Women who consume adequate amounts of folic acid before conception and throughout the first month of pregnancy reduce their risk of having a baby with a neural tube defect (eg, spina bifida, anencephaly). Foods rich in the natural form of folic acid (folate) include orange juice, other citrus fruits and juices, green leafy vegetables, dried peas and beans, broccoli, asparagus, and whole-grain products. Synthetic folic acid is found in multivitamins, fortified breakfast cereals, and enriched grain products. Because 50% of pregnancies in the United States are unplanned, the March of Dimes recommends that all women who are capable of becoming pregnant consume a multivitamin containing 400 μg of synthetic folic acid daily in addition to eating foods rich in natural folate. The Institute of Medicine recommends that synthetic folic acid intake increase to 600 μg daily once pregnancy is confirmed. Most prenatal vitamins contain at least this amount of folic acid.

Other B Vitamins

Requirements for the B vitamins thiamine, riboflavin, and niacin increase in proportion to the increase in calories. Most women consume adequate amounts of these nutrients in their usual diet. The increased requirement for vitamin B_6 is proportional to the increase in protein because it is involved in protein metabolism. Because vitamin B_{12} is necessary for the metabolism of folate, a slight increase in intake is recommended.

Calcium

The AI for calcium for pregnant women 19 years of age and older is 1000 mg. The reason why the AI is not higher for pregnant women compared with nonpregnant women is that calcium absorption more than doubles early in pregnancy; in addition, the AI for calcium is higher for adults than the level previously recommended in the RDA. If calcium intake was adequate before pregnancy, the amount consumed does not need to increase. However, 1300 mg/day of calcium is recommended for pregnant adolescents, and intakes higher than this may be beneficial. Women who do not consume enough calcium through foods require calcium supplements.

Iron

Despite the increased rate of iron absorption and iron "saving" that occurs with the cessation of menstruation, the need for iron increases significantly during pregnancy. An estimated 30 mg/day of iron is needed to support the increase in maternal blood volume and to provide iron for fetal liver storage, which will sustain the infant for the first 4 to 6 months of life.

Based on dietary intake studies, the Subcommittee on Nutritional Status and Weight Gain During Pregnancy of the Food and Nutrition Board, NAS, determined that iron is the only nutrient for which requirements *cannot* be met by diet alone. A daily supplement of 30 mg of ferrous iron is recommended for all women during the second and third trimesters. It is preferably taken between meals or at bedtime on an empty stomach to maximize absorption. The simultaneous consumption of vitamin C does not enhance absorption from supplements because the iron is already in the ferrous form.

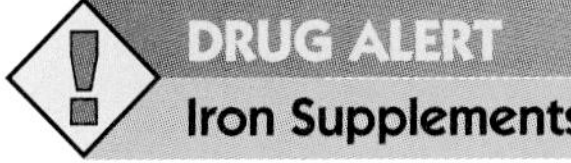

Use: Prevention and treatment of iron deficiency anemia.

Possible adverse side effects: May cause diarrhea, constipation, dark-colored stools, and gastrointestinal upset. Although better absorbed when taken between meals, iron supplements are less irritating to the gastrointestinal tract when taken with food.

Actions: Observe for diarrhea and constipation. If constipation is not alleviated with a high-fiber diet, consider reducing the dosage or frequency. If supplements are irritating to the gastrointestinal tract when taken between meals, advise the client to take them with food. Advise the client that a change in stool color is to be expected.

USING THE FOOD GUIDE PYRAMID TO CHOOSE A HEALTHY DIET DURING PREGNANCY

The Food Guide Pyramid (see Chapter 8) can be used to help women choose healthy diets. A general guide is described in Table 11–2. Tips for healthy eating during pregnancy based on the Food Guide Pyramid are discussed in this section.

Concentrate on Variety

Eating a varied diet increases the likelihood that adequate amounts of all essential nutrients—but not excessive amounts of any nutrients, additives, or contaminants—will be consumed. Variety means selecting different items within each food group and varying meal selections. (For example, one should not eat a plain bagel with cream cheese and orange juice every morning for breakfast.)

TABLE 11.2 *Food Guide Pyramid for Pregnancy*

Food Group	Number of Daily Servings
Bread, cereal, rice, and pasta	10 or more
Vegetable	3–4
Fruit	3–4
Milk	4 or more
Meat, poultry, fish, dry beans, eggs, and nuts (ounces)	6
Fats, oils, and sweets	3–5 or more

Eat in Moderation

Moderation means that no foods are forbidden, based on their nutritional value. However, it does not mean eating anything one wants in any amount. All foods can fit... it is a matter of frequency and portion size.

Aim for Balance

Use the recommended number of servings as a guide to balance, keeping in mind that the number varies somewhat for women whose calorie needs are lower or higher than average. No food groups should be excluded. Women who are strict vegans should be encouraged at least to include milk in their diets to meet calcium and protein requirements. A sample lacto-ovovegetarian menu appears in Box 11–2.

Women who cannot or will not consume enough milk products need to supplement their diet with calcium.

BOX 11.2

Sample Lacto-ovovegetarian Menu for Pregnant Women

Breakfast
Orange juice
Peanut butter and banana on wheat toast
1% milk

Snack
Fresh pear

Lunch
Baked corn tortillas with cheese
Black bean salad
Strawberries with yogurt
1% milk

Snack
Graham crackers
1% milk

Dinner
Veggie burger with lettuce and tomato on whole wheat bun
Baked sweet potato
Spinach salad
Apple crisp

Snack
Bran muffin
1% milk

Eat Three Meals Daily Plus Two or Three Snacks

Fasting, especially after midgestation, can result in hypoglycemia, hyperketonemia, acetonuria, and other signs of metabolic acidosis within 24 hours. Although ketonuria and acetonuria may occur normally in pregnancy (eg, after overnight fasting) and probably do not threaten the fetus, the more serious condition of ketoacidosis, which results from severe calorie restriction, can pose a risk for the developing fetus. Therefore, women are advised to avoid periods of hunger by eating three meals and two or three nutritious snacks each day. Small, frequent meals may also help to alleviate nausea in the first trimester and heartburn during the second half of the pregnancy.

Drink Adequate Fluids

Women are encouraged to drink six to eight 8-ounce glasses of fluid daily in the form of either water, fruit juice, or milk. Empty-calorie drinks like carbonated beverages and fruitades provide little more than calories.

Do Not Restrict Salt Intake

Sodium needs increase during pregnancy to maintain normal sodium levels in the expanded blood volume and tissues. Restriction of sodium intake may adversely affect both mother and fetus. A moderate intake of iodized salt is recommended.

Moderate Caffeine Consumption Does Not Pose a Problem

Studies show no association between moderate caffeine consumption and adverse pregnancy outcomes such as miscarriage, LBW, and short gestation. Moderate use of coffee and caffeine (the equivalent of 2–3 cups of coffee daily) does not appear to pose any risk.

If You Use Artificial Sweeteners, Do So Judiciously

The use of artificial sweeteners during pregnancy has been studied extensively. Even though there is no evidence that it is harmful to the fetus, women should consider carefully the use of saccharin during pregnancy, because it crosses the placenta and remains in fetal tissues owing to slow fetal clearance. Except for women with PKU, aspartame is safe during pregnancy at levels within the U.S. Food and Drug Administration (FDA) guidelines (50 mg/kg body weight). The use of acesulfame-K also appears to be safe for use during pregnancy when consumed within FDA guidelines (15 mg/kg body weight).

Avoid Alcohol

Because alcohol is a potent teratogen and a "safe" level of consumption is not known, women are advised to avoid alcohol during pregnancy. Alcohol can cause damage by dehydrating fetal cells, leaving them dead or functionless, or by causing secondary nutrient deficiencies related to poor intake, decreased absorption, altered metabolism, or increased excretion.

Chronic alcohol consumption can result in **fetal alcohol syndrome (FAS),** a condition that is characterized by varying degrees of physical and mental growth failure and birth defects. Unlike other small-for-gestational-age infants, infants with FAS do not experience normal "catch-up" growth. Some degree of intellectual impairment is also frequently reported in children with FAS.

Not all alcoholic mothers deliver FAS infants, yet even alcoholics who abstain during pregnancy have a higher incidence of LBW infants than women who do not have a history of alcoholism. Although chronic alcohol abuse clearly increases the risks of growth failure and birth defects and the effects of alcohol appear to be dose related, there are no established guidelines to indicate when consumption is safe and how much alcohol can be consumed safely. Studies on the effects of low doses of alcohol on fetal growth have been limited and inconsistent. Although an occasional drink may not cause damage, abstinence is recommended.

Be Aware of Foodborne Risks During Pregnancy

Foodborne risks are more dangerous for pregnant women than for other adults. For instance, listeriosis in pregnant women can cause meningitis in the mother and infection in the fetus that results in miscarriage or stillbirth. To reduce the risk of listeriosis, pregnant women should avoid certain soft cheeses (eg, feta, Brie, Camembert); cook all meat, poultry, and seafood thoroughly; wash raw vegetables thoroughly before cooking; and cook leftover foods or ready-to-eat foods (eg, hot dogs) until steaming hot. It may also be prudent to avoid delicatessen counter foods or to thoroughly reheat coldcuts.

The FDA recommends that pregnant women and women who may become pregnant limit their intake of swordfish or shark to no more than one meal per month, because the flesh may contain high levels of mercury. The fetal brain is highly susceptible to mercury damage, which can range from learning delays in walking or talking to more severe problems such as cerebral palsy, seizures, and mental retardation. Other types of fish that may be contaminated with mercury or with polychlorinated biphenyls (PCBs) are bluefish, striped bass, and freshwater fish (eg, salmon, pike, trout, walleye) from contaminated lakes and rivers. Women should consult with the local health department or Environmental Protection Agency to determine which fish from local waters are safe to eat.

SUPPLEMENT USE DURING PREGNANCY

Use of vitamin and mineral supplements or dietary supplements during pregnancy should be carefully considered.

Vitamin and Mineral Supplements

The Subcommittee on Dietary Intake and Nutrient Supplements During Pregnancy considers food to be the ideal source of required nutrients. Except for iron and folic acid, a balanced diet can meet the needs of most pregnant women. The Committee stated that the use of supplements "should be based on evidence of a benefit as well as a lack of harmful effects." They recommended that multivitamin and mineral supplements not be used routinely, nor should they replace food. However, supplements may be appropriate for certain nutrients and in certain population groups. For instance, a low-dose multivitamin and mineral supplement is recommended for pregnant women in high-risk categories, such as heavy smokers, drug abusers, and those carrying twins, and for pregnant women who are unlikely to consume an adequate diet despite nutritional advice or nutrition counseling. Other indications for supplements are as follows:

- Women who do not receive adequate exposure to sunlight may need a vitamin D supplement. The AI for vitamin D is 5 μg, the same as for nonpregnant women. The amount of vitamin D in prenatal supplements is 10 μg, an amount that is not excessive.
- Women who do not consume adequate calcium (eg, the equivalent of about three 8-ounce glasses of milk daily) need calcium supplements. For maximum absorption, calcium supplements should be taken in doses of 500 mg or less and not at the same time as iron supplements.
- Complete vegans need daily supplements of vitamin B_{12}.
- Women who take more than 30 mg of iron to treat iron deficiency anemia should take supplements of zinc and copper, because iron interferes with the absorption and utilization of these trace elements.

There are instances in which vitamin or mineral supplements are dangerous. For example, accumulating data show that excessive consumption of vitamin A (retinol) poses a teratogenic risk to the developing fetus. In the early weeks of pregnancy, excess preformed vitamin A from over-the-counter supplements or from the drug isotretinoin results in a variety of birth defects. The FDA recommends that women of childbearing age limit their intake of preformed vitamin A to 100% of the Daily Value (5000 IU). Women should check their supplements to make sure they are not taking too much vitamin A from retinol, and they should limit their intake of liver and cereals fortified with preformed vitamin A (but not beta-carotene, the vegetable precursor of vitamin A).

Dietary Supplements

Because little is known about the risks and benefits of dietary supplements, it is generally recommended that they not be used during pregnancy and lactation. Herbal products are technically unapproved drugs. Most drugs cross the placental barrier to some degree, exposing the fetus to potentially teratogenic effects.

NUTRITIONAL INTERVENTION FOR PROBLEMS DURING PREGNANCY

Nausea and Vomiting

Nausea and vomiting, common during the first trimester, may be related to hypoglycemia, decreased gastric motility, relaxation of the cardiac sphincter, or anxiety. Interventions that can help lessen nausea include eating small, frequent meals every 2 to 3 hours. Carbohydrates may be especially helpful because they leave the stomach quickly and readily raise blood glucose levels. Women should also be advised to:

- Eat carbohydrate foods such as dry crackers, melba toast, dry cereal, or hard candy before getting out of bed in the morning.
- Avoid drinking liquids with meals.
- Avoid coffee, tea, and spicy foods.
- Limit high-fat foods, because they delay gastric emptying time.
- Eliminate individual intolerances.

Constipation

Constipation during pregnancy may be caused by relaxation of gastrointestinal muscle tone and motility related to increased progesterone levels, or it may result from pressure of the fetus on the intestines. Other contributing factors may include a decrease in physical activity and an inadequate intake of fluid and fiber. Constipation is also a common side effect of the consumption of iron supplements. If iron supplementation is contributing to constipation, the dosage or frequency should be reduced, if possible.

Encourage the client to:

- Increase fiber intake, especially intake of whole-grain breads and cereals high in bran (see Chapter 17).
- Drink at least eight 8-ounce glasses of liquid daily.
- Try hot water with lemon or prune juice upon waking to help stimulate peristalsis.
- Participate in regular exercise.

Heartburn

A decrease in gastric motility, relaxation of the cardiac sphincter, and pressure of the uterus on the stomach are contributing factors to heartburn.

Encourage the client to:

- Eat small, frequent meals and eliminate liquids immediately before and after meals to avoid gastric distention.
- Avoid coffee, high-fat foods, and spices.
- Eliminate individual intolerances.
- Avoid lying down or bending over after eating.

Inadequate Weight Gain

Inadequate weight gain may occur secondary to a poor appetite related to nausea, vomiting, heartburn, or smoking, or from an inadequate intake related to lack of knowledge or fear of gaining weight. Women who mistakenly believe that the fetus is a perfect parasite and will be adequately nourished regardless of maternal intake may also experience inadequate weight gain. If an inadequate food budget is responsible for the inadequate intake, refer the client to social services. Determine whether the client is eligible for the Women, Infants and Children (WIC) subsidy program (discussed later).

Although a short-term goal is to promote weight gain, the timing and the source of the weight gain are equally important. On a long-term basis, an improvement in overall eating habits benefits both the health of the family and any subsequent pregnancies.

Encourage the client to continue good eating practices and recommend specific ways to improve other habits. Depending on the cause, make appropriate dietary modifications to improve appetite. Advise the client to quit smoking, not only to improve appetite but because smoking is detrimental to both maternal and infant health.

Counsel the client on the recommended rate and quantity of weight gain associated with optimal maternal and infant health and successful breast-feeding. Explain how the weight gain is distributed among the fetus, placenta, and maternal tissues. Encourage the client to ask questions and verbalize feelings. Advise the client that extra weight gained during pregnancy is quickly lost during lactation or through dieting *after* pregnancy. Set mutually agreeable weight gain goals.

Advise the client that:

- If her diet is inadequate in calories, it probably is also inadequate in other nutrients.
- Although the fetus can use maternal nutrient stores if the mother's diet is inadequate, many nutrients are not stored by the body and require a daily dietary intake.
- An inadequate intake can adversely affect maternal health (eg, poor iron intake leading to anemia) and infant health (eg, LBW, anemia, other postnatal complications).

Excessive Weight Gain

Sudden weight gain may signal preeclampsia. Notify the physician if other signs are observed, such as hypertension, fluid retention, albuminuria, and complaints of headaches, blurred vision, or visual disturbances.

Women who experience excessive weight gain related to overeating may do so because they lack knowledge concerning recommended weight gain, or they may believe that a pregnant woman must "eat for two." Other factors contributing to excessive weight gain are stress and a decrease in physical activity.

Although it is prudent to prevent excessive weight gain, weight reduction diets should *never* be undertaken during pregnancy, because of the risk of ketonemia and its potential damage to the fetus. Likewise, counting calories should not take priority over the nutritional values of foods which could result in a nutrient-poor diet. Again, a long-term objective of diet counseling is to improve eating habits for family health and any subsequent pregnancies.

Counsel the client on the recommended rate and quantity of weight gain associated with optimal maternal and infant health and successful breast-feeding. Explain that the weight gain is distributed among the fetus, placenta, and maternal tissues. Set mutually agreeable weight gain goals. Recommend specific ways to limit the rate of weight gain without compromising nutrient intake, such as to:

- Substitute skim or low-fat milk for whole milk.
- Bake, broil, or steam foods instead of frying.
- Eliminate empty calories: carbonated beverages, candy, rich desserts, and traditional snack foods.
- Limit portion sizes to those recommended by the Food Guide Pyramid.
- Use fats and oils sparingly.

Pica

Pica is a psychobehavioral disorder characterized by the ingestion of nonfood substances; dirt, clay, starch, and ice are the most common items ingested. Eating of these items may displace the intake of nutritious foods or interfere with nutrient absorption. Other potential complications vary with the items ingested and include lead poisoning, fecal impaction, parasitic infections, toxemia, prematurity, perinatal mortality, LBW, and anemia in the infant.

Iron deficiency was commonly considered to be a risk factor for pica, but studies suggest it is more likely a consequence. Pica can be a strongly rooted social tradition and is more prevalent among African-Americans and rural residents. Other suggested risk factors include low socioeconomic status, inadequate nutritional status, and a childhood or family history of pica.

Pica is surrounded by misconceptions about pregnancy and childbirth. Some women who practice pica claim that it "helps" babies, cures swollen legs, relieves nausea and vomiting, ensures beautiful children, helps infants "slide out" more easily, and prevents birthmarks. Pica may also be used to relieve tension or hunger, and some women claim they are merely satisfying cravings for clay or starch.

It is important to determine not only what is being ingested, but also why. *Remain nonjudgmental*, but stress the importance of an adequate diet, the use of iron supplements during pregnancy, and the potential dangers of pica. Offer economical ways to obtain an adequate diet, and refer the client to social services or the WIC program if appropriate. Encourage women who experience constipation to consume a high-fiber, high-fluid diet. Women who experience diarrhea and vomiting may have a parasitic infection or lead poisoning.

NUTRITIONAL INTERVENTIONS FOR MEDICAL COMPLICATIONS DURING PREGNANCY

Maternal Phenylketonuria

PKU is an inborn error of the metabolism of phenylalanine (an essential amino acid) that results in retardation and physical handicaps in newborns if it is not treated with a low-phenylalanine diet beginning shortly after birth. Before the 1980s, the low-phenylalanine diet was discontinued when the child began school because it was thought that high levels of phenylalanine were not damaging once brain growth was completed. Current practice is to continue a restricted diet for people with PKU throughout childhood and adolescence and possibly for life, because high levels of phenylalanine in children and adolescents can cause a decrease in IQ, learning disabilities, and behavioral problems in most children with PKU.

Women who have PKU and who consume a normal diet during pregnancy have very high blood levels of phenylalanine, which are safe for the mother but devastating to the developing fetus. As many as 90% of babies born to PKU mothers have mental retardation, and many also have microcephaly, heart defects, and LBW. Most of these infants do not inherit PKU and cannot benefit from a low-phenylalanine diet after birth.

To prevent mental retardation and other problems associated with maternal PKU, a rigid low-phenylalanine diet is necessary before conception and throughout the duration of the pregnancy. With a low-phenylalanine diet, blood levels of phenylalanine are controlled to very low levels, eliminating risks to the developing fetus. Maternal PKU may present a bigger problem for an adolescent girl with an unexpected pregnancy, who may hide the pregnancy until late in gestation.

Clients who have a history of PKU should be advised that:

- Complete understanding and strict adherence to the diet are vital.
- Protein foods are high in phenylalanine and must be eliminated: meat, fish, poultry, eggs, dairy products, and nuts.
- The special PKU formula is expensive and often offensive to adult palates, but it must be consumed in adequate amounts both to support fetal growth and to prevent maternal tissue breakdown, which would have results similar to those caused by cheating on the diet.
- An adequate calorie intake is necessary for normal protein metabolism.
- Close monitoring of blood phenylalanine levels is essential.

Diabetes Mellitus

Diabetes mellitus, characterized by abnormal glucose tolerance, requires dietary management regardless of whether it was present before conception (established diabetes) or developed during gestation (gestational diabetes) as a result of the metabolic changes of pregnancy. Diabetes increases the risk of infection, especially urinary tract infection, preeclampsia, and eclampsia. The incidence of spontaneous abortion, hydramnios, extrauterine and neonatal death, and congenital abnormalities is higher among patients with established diabetes. Gestational diabetes does not usually produce maternal complications or birth defects, but it can make delivery difficult, because babies born to gestational diabetics are usually large, which may increase the risk of postpartum hemorrhage.

Monitor the progress and course of pregnancy of established diabetics. Screen all women for gestational diabetes between 24 and 28 weeks of pregnancy. Check for ketonuria regularly. Diabetic management during pregnancy includes nutrition therapy and, possibly, multiple daily doses of insulin. Advise the client that:

- Pregnant diabetics require the same nutrients and weight gain as nondiabetic pregnant women.
- She is not on a "diet." Weight loss and fasting should never be undertaken during pregnancy.
- Calorie requirements are based on prepregnancy weight. Suggested guidelines are as follows:
  - 30 cal/kg for women of normal weight before conception
  - 24 cal/kg for women weighing more than 120% of desirable weight before conception
  - 36–40 cal/kg for women weighing less than 90% of desirable weight before conception
- Adequate food intake prevents ketone formation and promotes proper weight gain. The individualized meal plan should be high in complex carbohydrates and fiber and limited in fat and sugar.
- Three meals plus three snacks daily may promote better glycemic control.
- Close monitoring (ie, daily urine ketone testing for gestational diabetics, blood monitoring for established diabetics) and periodic evaluations are necessary throughout the course of pregnancy to meet nutritional needs and to control blood glucose levels.
- Glucose tolerance returns to normal in gestational diabetics after delivery, although they are at increased risk for development of diabetes later in life.

Pregnancy-Induced Hypertension

Pregnancy-induced hypertension (PIH or toxemia) is a hypertensive syndrome that occurs in approximately 6% to 7% of all pregnancies. Severe cases are associated with increased risks of maternal, fetal, and neonatal death. **Preeclampsia** is characterized by hypertension accompanied by proteinuria, edema, or both. A sudden weight gain (>2 pounds/week after the 20th week of gestation) may indicate preeclampsia. **Eclampsia** develops with the occurrence of one or more convulsions resulting from preeclampsia.

Although the exact cause is unknown, the development of PIH is strongly correlated with maternal poverty and malnutrition, especially inadequate intakes of calories, protein, sodium, and possibly calcium. Good nutrition can prevent toxemia, and prevention is far more effective than treatment. Women at risk include those who are poorly nourished, primigravida, economically deprived, very young or very old, obese and gaining too much weight, or underweight and failing to gain enough weight.

Screen women at risk for toxemia and monitor for signs and symptoms: hypertension, facial edema, proteinuria (especially albumin), headaches, and blurred vision or visual disturbances.

Obtain a 24-hour food intake recall record and evaluate the diet according to the Food Guide Pyramid, paying particular attention to intakes of calories, protein, calcium, and sodium.

Advise clients at risk for preeclampsia to consume a liberal intake of calories, protein, and calcium, and to salt their food to taste. Sodium-restricted diets and diuretics are not advised. Recommend ways to improve the diet that are acceptable to the client. Identify and refer women who are eligible for social service programs or WIC.

ASSESSMENT OF NUTRITIONAL NEEDS DURING PREGNANCY

Initial evaluation of historical data, physical findings, and laboratory data should be performed to identify clients who are at risk for poor nutritional status during pregnancy (Box 11–3) and also to establish baseline data. Ongoing evaluation, performed regularly throughout the course of pregnancy, provides continuing surveillance and helps to identify clients in need of nutrition counseling or community assistance.

Historical Data

- Does the client have a medical condition that may benefit from nutrient therapy, such as diabetes, hypertension, lactose intolerance, or PKU? Does the client have any gastrointestinal side effects of pregnancy, such as nausea, vomiting, constipation, and heartburn? If so, assess onset, frequency, causative factors, severity, interventions attempted, and the results of these interventions.

BOX 11.3

Risk Factors for Poor Nutritional Status During Pregnancy

Historical data

Prepartum weight <85% or >120% of ideal weight
Use of a therapeutic diet for a chronic disease
Use of alcohol, tobacco, or drugs
Food faddism, unbalanced diet, pica
Teens and women older than 40 years of age
Poor obstetric history (LBW, stillbirth, abortion, fetal anomalies), high parity, multipara
Repetitive pregnancies at short intervals
Low socioeconomic status
Chronic preexisting medical problems, such as hypertension, diabetes, heart disease, pulmonary disease, renal disease, maternal PKU
Untimely prenatal care

Physical findings

Inadequate weight gain: <10 lb during the first 20 weeks of pregnancy; <2 lb/mo after the first trimester
Excessive weight gain: >2 lb/wk

Laboratory data

Low or deficient hemoglobin and hematocrit

- Is the client's usual 24-hour intake adequate for pregnancy? Pay particular attention to the total quantity of food consumed; the number of servings consumed from each of the major food groups and from the Fats, Oils, and Sweets group; and the amount of fluid consumed. Because low intakes of iron and folic acid are common in the average American diet, assess food sources of these nutrients.
- Has the client made dietary changes in response to pregnancy or diet-related complications of pregnancy? What foods does the client avoid? What foods does the client prefer? Does the client use alcohol, tobacco, caffeine, or drugs? How frequently does the client eat?
- What cultural, religious, and ethnic influences affect the client's food choices? Does the client practice pica? If so, what items are consumed and how does their consumption affect nutrition?
- Does the client have food allergies or intolerances (especially lactose intolerance)?
- Before pregnancy was the client underweight, normal weight, or overweight? Is her weight gain adequate and appropriate for the length of gestation?
- Does the client take a vitamin and mineral supplement? Is it being used appropriately? Does the client use dietary supplements? What over-the-counter or prescribed medications does the client take?
- Has the client ever been pregnant before now? If so, how long ago was the pregnancy and what was the outcome? Is the client carrying more than one fetus?
- What is the client's knowledge of nutrition, and is she able and willing to implement dietary changes? Is the client's food budget adequate? Women who are at nutritional risk because of inadequate nutrition and inadequate income may be eligible for the WIC program. WIC is a supplemental food program for pregnant women, postpartum women (up to 1 year if breast-feeding, or up to 6 months if bottle-feeding), infants, and children up to 5 years of age. WIC provides nutrition counseling and vouchers for specified foods of high nutritional quality.
- Does the client plan to breast-feed?

Physical Findings

- Measure the client's present height and weight.
- Assess the client's blood pressure.
- Assess for severe dependent edema.
- Assess for abnormal findings of the skin, mucous membranes, gums, teeth, tongue, eyes, and hair. Although these findings (eg, bleeding gums) may be related to normal physiologic changes of pregnancy, they may indicate potential nutritional problems that warrant further investigation.

Laboratory Data

Obtain the client's hemoglobin and hematocrit values to detect abnormal findings. Note that many laboratory values change during pregnancy because of normal adjustments in maternal physiology. For this reason, results of laboratory tests performed during pregnancy cannot be validly compared with nonpregnancy standards.

NUTRITION COUNSELING DURING PREGNANCY

Nutrition counseling is an essential component of prenatal care. For optimal impact on maternal and infant health, nutrition counseling ideally should begin before conception. However, before counseling can begin, it is necessary to identify the client's emotional needs by talking with her to learn about her attitudes, beliefs, and fears.

The most effective approach to nutrition counseling begins by determining the client's usual intake and food preferences and aversions to identify potential nutritional problems. Individualized nutrition counseling, initiated during the first prenatal visit and continued throughout the course of pregnancy, should stress the maintenance of good dietary habits and recommend realistic ways to improve intake. A variety of teaching materials are available. Select those appropriate for the client's level of understanding.

Because the risk of low gestational weight gain is higher among unmarried women, adolescents, African-American and Hispanic women, cigarette smokers, and women with low levels of education, these women should receive additional nutrition counseling to ensure an adequate weight gain during pregnancy.

Instruct the client and family:

- **About the importance of adequate nutrition and weight gain for maternal and infant health.** Describe the optimal rate of weight gain. Explain that weight gain during pregnancy is not synonymous with "getting fat" and that weight reduction should never be undertaken during pregnancy, even by overweight women. Overweight women who require less weight gain than normal should be instructed on how to choose a nutrient-dense diet for a controlled amount of high-quality weight gain.
- **About how to achieve nutritional adequacy by using the Food Guide Pyramid.** Stress the principles of variety, balance, and moderation. Items from the Fats, Oils, and Sweets group should be used sparingly. Counsel the client regarding meal frequency, fluid requirements, and the use of salt, alcohol, caffeine, and artificial sweeteners.
- **To take supplements only as prescribed by the physician.** Discourage the use of supplements that are not prescribed by the physician and stress the importance of taking only the prescribed dosage, because megadoses of some vitamins and minerals can cause fetal malformations. Advise against the use of dolomite and bonemeal as calcium supplements, because they may contain high levels of lead and other heavy metals, which pose a hazard to both mother and fetus.
- **To avoid alcohol, tobacco, and drugs during pregnancy.** These substances pose actual or potential adverse health effects to both mother and baby.
- **To use coffee, caffeine, and artificial sweeteners in moderation, if so desired.** These items are not necessarily contraindicated during pregnancy, but intake should be prudent.
- **That cravings during pregnancy do not appear to have a physiologic basis.** Cravings are likely to be influenced by culture, geography, social traditions, the availability of foods, and previous experience. Satisfying cravings for foods is relatively harmless so long as the overall impact on nutrient intake is not negative. (For example, an occasional dill pickle is okay but eating an entire jar of them is

BOX 11.4

Common Myths About Nutrition During Pregnancy

You can eat anything you want because you're eating for two.
You can eat double portions because you're eating for two.
You should eat whatever you're craving; your body must need it.
If you take prenatal vitamins, you don't have to worry about what you eat.
You must take vitamins to have a healthy baby.
The baby gets what he or she needs first, and the rest goes to the mother.
If you breast-feed, you can lose all the weight you gain in pregnancy.
Obese women don't need to gain weight during pregnancy.
It doesn't matter what you eat, because the baby will take what it needs from your body.
As long as you take vitamins, it's all right to skip meals.
When you are pregnant, you will crave pickles and ice cream.
Gaining lots of weight makes a healthy baby.
You lose a tooth with every baby if you don't drink milk.
Beets build red blood.
Food cravings during pregnancy determine your child's likes and dislikes later in life.
Give in to your cravings, or you will mark the baby.
Do not eat fish and milk at the same meal.
Do not eat egg yolks, because they will rot the uterus.
If you crave sweets, the baby will be a girl; if you crave pickles, the baby will be a boy.

Carruth, B., & Skinner, J. (1991). Practitioners beware: Regional differences in beliefs about nutrition during pregnancy. *Journal of the American Dietetic Association*, *91*, 435.

not.) Cravings for nonfood items should be investigated. Dispel myths about diet during pregnancy (Box 11–4).

- **About how to modify her diet to alleviate or avoid nutrition-related problems and complications of pregnancy,** as appropriate
- **To avoid all medications unless approved by the physician**
- **That once labor begins, no foods or liquids should be consumed.** This is to prevent aspiration if anesthesia must be used.

Adolescent Pregnancy

Each year, 10% of American women between 15 and 19 years of age become pregnant. Compared with infants born to adults, those born to adolescent mothers are more likely to be preterm, to have LBW, to require intensive care, to have physical problems, or to die at birth or just after the newborn period. Pregnancy-induced hypertension, anemia, and sexually transmitted disease are the most common problems seen in pregnant adolescents younger than 16 years of age.

Pregnant adolescents are at increased risk for complications because of psychosocial and economic factors. Adolescents with a **gynecologic age** (age at conception minus age at menarche) of less than 4 years are at high nutritional risk because the nutritional needs of the developing fetus are superimposed on the mother's own needs for growth. Those with gynecologic age of less than 2 years have the highest risk for pregnancy complications. Compared with adult women, pregnant adolescents:

- Are more likely to be physically, emotionally, financially, and socially immature. Low socioeconomic status may be the major reason for the high incidence of LBW infants and other complications of adolescent pregnancy.
- May not have adequate nutrient stores because they need large amounts of nutrients for their own growth and development. Although female adolescent growth is usually complete by the age of 15 years, physical maturity is not reached until 4 years after menarche, which usually occurs by age 17 years.
- Have eating practices that may not provide adequate nourishment to support their own growth, pregnancy, and fetal development. Voluntary calorie restriction to control weight, erratic eating patterns, reliance on fast foods and convenience foods, and meal skipping (especially breakfast) are common adolescent practices.
- Must gain weight early and steadily to maximize the chance of giving birth to an optimal-weight infant. The National Academy of Sciences recommends that pregnant adolescents gain 25 to 40 pounds, depending on their prepregnancy BMI.
- Are more concerned with body image and confused about weight gain recommendations. Many do not understand why they should gain 30 pounds when the average baby weighs only about 7 pounds.
- Are more likely to smoke during pregnancy.
- Seek prenatal care later and have fewer total visits during pregnancy.

NUTRITIONAL REQUIREMENTS

The DRIs for pregnancy are categorized according to maternal age: 18 years of age or younger, 19 to 30 years, and 31 to 50 years. Compared with nonpregnant 18-year-olds, those who are pregnant have higher DRIs for magnesium, thiamine, riboflavin, niacin, vitamin B_6, folate, vitamin B_{12}, pantothenic acid, and biotin. Nutrients whose DRI does not increase in response to pregnancy among 18-year-olds are calcium, phosphorus, vitamin D, and fluoride. For nutrients with 1989 RDAs, requirements for pregnancy are not broken down by age. Obviously, teenagers require more than their normal RDA during pregnancy, but actual nutrient needs depend more on gynecologic age than on chronologic age and should be determined on an individual basis.

Nutrient requirements during pregnancy also are influenced by preconception nutritional status. Nutrients most often lacking in female adolescent diets are calcium, iron, and zinc; vitamins A, C, and B_6; and folate. Like pregnant adults, adolescents need supplements of iron and folic acid in addition to a nutritious diet. It is recommended that adolescents at risk for poor intake take multivitamin and mineral supplements.

NUTRITION COUNSELING

Proper nutrition is one of the most important controllable factors that determine the overall outcome of pregnancy. Good nutrition has the potential to decrease the incidence of LBW infants and to improve the health of infants born to adolescents. Identifying and treating undernutrition in adolescents may be a particularly important way to improve pregnancy outcome. The nutrition counseling and client teaching points outlined previously are appropriate for adolescent pregnancies as well, but counseling methods must take into account teenage lifestyles and the social and cognitive development of the client. To maximize the effectiveness of nutrition counseling for adolescents, it is particularly important to establish a rapport in a relaxed, nonthreatening, nonjudgmental environment. In addition to assessing the client's nutritional needs, her social, emotional, and economic needs, her psychosocial status, and her ethnicity must also be evaluated. Many teens have limited reading skills, so teaching materials must be appropriate for their level of understanding. The Food Guide Pyramid is useful both in assessing dietary strengths and weaknesses and in providing a framework for implementing dietary changes in a way the teenager can understand.

Set mutually agreeable realistic goals for weight gain and food intake. Diet recommendations must be concrete, reasonable, and achievable within the client's financial status and lifestyle. Because teens living with one or more adults may have little control over what food is available to them, parents and significant others should also be encouraged to attend counseling sessions. Compared with pregnant adults, pregnant teens generally need 1 to 2 extra servings from the Milk, Yogurt, and Cheese group and 1 more serving from the Meat, Poultry, Fish, Dry Beans, Eggs, and Nuts group.

Ideally, the client should be counseled early in the pregnancy and monitored frequently throughout gestation to evaluate the effectiveness of the nutritional care plan and to redefine needs as the pregnancy progresses. Prenatal counseling should also include information about infant and child feeding practices.

Lactation

Because of the unquestionable benefits to both mother and infant, exclusive breast-feeding for the first 4 to 6 months of age is recommended for most full-term infants. Breast-feeding with weaning to foods is recommended for at least the first 12 months of age. The benefits of breast-feeding are especially important to infants born of low-income mothers, because they are at higher risk for health problems that could be minimized by breast-feeding. Nevertheless, a large percentage of American women, especially low-income, minority, and younger women, do not breast-feed their babies or do so for only a short period. It is estimated that only about 60% of American infants are breast-fed at birth and that by 5 to 6 months of age only 20% are still being breast-fed. Many benefits are forfeited by early discontinuation of breast-feeding.

BENEFITS OF BREAST-FEEDING

Breast-feeding provides significant nutritional, health, and psychological benefits to both mother and infant.

For the mother:

- Breast-feeding promotes optimal maternal-infant bonding.
- Breast-feeding can mobilize fat stores to help women lose weight, particularly in the lower body.
- Early breast-feeding stimulates uterine contractions to help control blood loss and regain prepregnant size.
- Breast milk is readily available and requires no mixing or dilution.
- Breast-feeding is less expensive than purchasing bottles, nipples, sterilizing equipment, and formula.
- Breast-feeding may decrease the risk of thromboembolism, especially after operative deliveries.
- Childbirth and breast-feeding may be protective against breast cancer.
- Although not reliable for birth control, breast-feeding does afford some contraceptive protection.

For the infant:

- "Breast is best"—breast milk is unique in its types and concentrations of macronutrients (carbohydrates, protein, fat), micronutrients (vitamins and minerals), enzymes, hormones, growth factors, host resistance factors, inducers/modulators of the immune system, and antiinflammatory agents. It contains optimal amounts and forms of nutrients the infant can easily tolerate and digest, and it changes to match the needs of a growing infant.
- Breast milk is a "natural" food that contains no artificial colorings, flavorings, preservatives, or additives.
- Breast milk contains many components that impart active and passive protection to infants against viral and bacterial pathogens, such as specific T and B lymphocytes and nonspecific macrophages and neutrophils.
- Breast milk is sterile, is at the proper temperature, and is readily available.
- Breast-feeding promotes better tooth and jaw development than bottle-feeding because the infant has to suck harder.
- Breast-feeding avoids nursing-bottle caries.
- Breast-feeding is protective against food allergies.
- Overfeeding is not likely with breast-feeding.

- Breast-feeding is associated with decreased frequency of certain chronic diseases later in life, such as non–insulin-dependent diabetes mellitus, lymphoma, and Crohn's disease.

UNIQUENESS OF BREAST MILK

Breast milk is said to have more than 200 known components, with more being identified all the time. Its composition is uniquely suited to support the growth and development of human infants.

Protein

Protein provides a mere 4% to 5% of total calories of mature milk, an amount adequate to support growth and development without contributing to an excessive renal solute load. The majority of the protein is whey, which is easy to digest. Breast milk contains small amounts of amino acids that may be harmful in large amounts (eg, phenylalanine) and high levels of amino acids that infants cannot synthesize well (eg, taurine).

Fat

Approximately 58% of the total calories in mature milk are from fat, yet it is easily digested because of fat-digesting enzymes contained in the milk. The content of linoleic acid (the essential fatty acid) is high. The high level of cholesterol is believed to help infants develop enzyme systems capable of handling cholesterol later in life.

Carbohydrate

Lactose, which stimulates the growth of friendly gastrointestinal bacteria and promotes calcium absorption, provides 35% to 41% of total calories of mature milk. Only trace amounts of glucose and other carbohydrates are present. Breast milk contains amylase (a starch-digesting enzyme), which may promote starch digestion in early infancy, when pancreatic amylase is low or absent.

Minerals

Breast milk contains enough minerals to support adequate growth and development but not excessive amounts that would burden immature kidneys with a high renal solute load. Calcium, phosphorus, chlorine, potassium, and sodium are the major minerals in mature milk. Trace amounts of iron, copper, and manganese are present. Amounts of zinc, magnesium, aluminum, iodine, chromium, selenium, and fluorine are minute. The rate of iron absorption from breast milk is approximately 50%, compared with about 4%

for iron-fortified formulas. Zinc absorption is better from breast milk than from either cow's milk or formula. Breast milk is low in sodium.

Vitamins

All vitamins needed for growth and health are supplied in breast milk, but the vitamin content of breast milk varies with the mother's diet. The amount of biologically active vitamin D is low in breast milk, prompting controversy over the need for routine vitamin D supplementation for exclusively breast-fed infants.

Renal Solute Load

The renal solute load of breast milk is approximately half that of commercial formulas and one quarter that of cow's milk. The low renal solute load is suited to the immature kidneys' inability to concentrate urine.

Other Compounds

Although they are more abundant in colostrum, antibodies and antiinfective factors are present in mature breast milk. Resistance factors are present, including bifidus factor, which promotes the growth of friendly gastrointestinal bacteria (eg, *Lactobacillus bifidus*) that protect the infant against harmful gastrointestinal bacteria. Breast milk also contains several enzymes (eg, lipases, amylase) and numerous hormones and hormonelike substances, such as melatonin, thyroid gland hormones, adrenal gland hormones, estrogen, insulin, and prostaglandins.

VARIABLES AFFECTING BREAST MILK COMPOSITION

The composition of breast milk is constantly changing with the stage of lactation, the mother's diet, and the duration of the feeding.

Stage of Lactation

The composition of breast milk varies considerably with the stage of lactation. **Preterm milk,** which is secreted in small amounts before delivery, is higher in nitrogen (protein) than is milk produced after a term delivery.

Colostrum, which is secreted during the first few postpartum days, is a thick, yellowish fluid that is higher in protein, minerals, and sodium than mature milk, but lower in sugar, fat, and calories. Colostrum is rich in antibodies and antiinfective factors that protect the infant against various gastrointestinal and nongastrointestinal infections.

Colostrum begins to change to transitional milk about 3 to 6 days after delivery as the protein content decreases and the carbohydrate and fat contents increase. Major changes in the milk take place by the tenth day, and **mature milk** is stable by the end of the first month.

Maternal Diet

Almost all women are capable of producing enough high-quality breast milk to promote infant growth and development. When maternal intake is inadequate, the mother's tissues are depleted to maintain nutrient levels in breast milk, especially calcium and folate. Even women with depleted nutrient stores are able to produce milk with adequate protein, carbohydrate, fat, folate, and most minerals. However, the vitamin content of breast milk declines as a result of inadequate maternal intake, especially vitamins B_6, B_{12}, A, and D. Conversely, unusually high intakes of most vitamins, through either food or supplements, do not increase their concentration in breast milk, with the exception of vitamin D.

Duration of the Feeding

Foremilk, the milk secreted as each feeding begins, is significantly lower in fat than hindmilk, the milk secreted at the end of each feeding. The increase in fat content may be a physiologic mechanism designed to provide satiety and to signal the infant to stop nursing.

NUTRITIONAL NEEDS FOR LACTATION

Nutritional needs during lactation are based on the nutritional content of breast milk and the nutritional "cost" of producing milk. In general, women who are lactating have higher nutritional needs than at any other time in their adult lives (Table 11–1).

Calories

Calorie requirements while breast-feeding are proportional to the amount of milk produced and are higher during lactation than during pregnancy. The average calorie content of breast milk that is produced by well-nourished mothers is 70 cal/100 mL, and approximately 85 cal are needed by the mother for every 100 mL produced. The average woman uses approximately 640 cal/day for the first 6 months and 510 cal/day during the second 6 months to produce a normal amount of milk. Women who only partially breastfeed use fewer calories.

Women who gained the appropriate amount of weight during pregnancy should increase their calorie intake by 500 cal/day for both the first and second 6 months of lactation. Because more than 500 cal/day is actually used to produce milk, women draw on fat reserves accumulated during pregnancy to furnish the additional calories needed. This calorie deficit over time may help them to reduce fat stores and body weight to prepregnancy levels. However, because failure to consume enough calories can jeopardize the quantity of milk produced, women should be discouraged from restricting their calorie intake. A daily minimum intake of 1800 cal is recommended to obtain adequate amounts of essential nutrients. The average woman should consume 2300 to 2700 cal daily while breast-feeding.

Women who failed to gain enough weight during pregnancy, or who have inadequate fat reserves, should consume a total of 650 additional calories per day during the first 6 months of breast-feeding.

Protein

Women need an additional 20 g of protein above normal requirements while breast-feeding. This accounts for only 16% of the additional 500 cal recommended. Because the typical American intake of protein greatly exceeds the requirement, most women do not need to adjust their usual protein intake while nursing. An extra 2 cups of milk provide 16 g of protein.

Fluid

Another nutritional consideration during lactation is fluid intake. It is suggested that nursing mothers drink 2 to 3 quarts of fluid daily, preferably in the form of water, milk, and fruit juices instead of carbonated beverages, sweetened fruit drinks, and caffeine-containing beverages. Usually women are urged to drink a glass of fluid every time the baby nurses. Thirst is a good indicator of need, except among women who live in a dry climate or who exercise in hot weather. Fluids consumed in excess of thirst quenching do not increase milk volume.

Vitamins and Minerals

For many vitamins and minerals, requirements during lactation are higher than during pregnancy. The nutrients most likely to be consumed in inadequate amounts by breast-feeding women are calcium, magnesium, zinc, vitamin B_6, and folate. Foods, rather than supplements, are the preferred source of these nutrients, because foods provide a plethora of other nutrients and substances important for good health. To obtain adequate amounts of vitamins and minerals, women are encouraged to choose a varied diet that includes enriched and fortified grains and cereals, fresh fruits and vegetables, and lean meats and dairy products.

Multivitamin and mineral supplements are not recommended for routine use. However, specific supplements may be indicated when maternal intake is inadequate. For instance:

- A balanced multivitamin and mineral supplement may be necessary for women who consume fewer than 1800 cal/day.

- A calcium supplement is indicated for women who are lactose intolerant or who do not consume enough milk and other calcium-rich foods.
- A vitamin D supplement may be appropriate for women who avoid vitamin D–fortified foods (eg, milk, cereals) and have limited exposure to the sun.
- A vitamin B_{12} supplement is necessary for strict vegetarians if they do not regularly consume vitamin B_{12}–fortified plant products.
- An iron supplement may be needed to replace iron deficits during pregnancy and blood loss during delivery.

USING THE FOOD GUIDE PYRAMID TO CHOOSE A HEALTHY DIET DURING LACTATION

Although actual nutrient content of the diet varies with the foods chosen, using the Food Guide Pyramid helps ensure an adequate and balanced intake. Compared with the guidelines for pregnancy, there are few changes during lactation (Table 11–3).

Again, the most notable difference is that consumption of 4 or more servings of milk per day is suggested to meet calcium requirements. The extra servings of milk also provide extra protein to meet the increased requirements. Liberal amounts of fruits and vegetables, whole-grain breads and cereals, and protein-rich foods are encouraged to meet the additional nutrient and calorie requirements that are imposed by lactation.

FOODS TO AVOID

Few foods are contraindicated during lactation except for freshwater fish from water contaminated with dioxin, PCBs, or other chemicals. Women should contact their State Health Department for recommendations regarding fish consumption during lactation. Women who have been exposed to high levels of environmental toxins should have their milk analyzed for contaminants.

Alcohol easily enters breast milk and appears to hinder lactation. Although an occasional drink is within safe limits, lactating women should consume little or no alcohol.

TABLE 11.3 ***Food Guide Pyramid for Lactation***

Food Group	Number of Daily Servings
Bread, cereal, rice, and pasta	12 or more
Vegetable	4
Fruit	4
Milk	4–5
Meat, poultry, fish, dry beans, eggs, and nuts (ounces)	7
Fats, oils, and sweets	5

Caffeine also enters breast milk, but at lower rates. Consumption of one to two cups of coffee daily does not pose any problems. Intakes higher than this may cause the infant to become irritable and restless. It usually is not necessary to eliminate any other foods while breast-feeding unless the infant shows an intolerance. For instance, oils from garlic and onion may flavor the taste of breast milk, but they need not be eliminated from the mother's diet unless the taste of the milk is objectionable to the infant.

LACTATION IN THE DIABETIC MOTHER

Breast-feeding complicates blood glucose control in women with type 1 diabetes by inducing hypoglycemia and lowering insulin requirements. Because successful lactation is dependent on adequate blood glucose control, individualized care is needed to balance intake, insulin, exercise, and lactation. Although optimal calorie requirements for lactation for type 1 diabetics have not been determined, 35 cal/kg is usually recommended to achieve optimal glucose and lipid levels and promote moderate weight loss (4.5 pounds/month). Other points to consider include:

- **Careful and frequent monitoring of blood glucose levels is essential.** Women should be encouraged to check their blood glucose levels immediately before breast-feeding. An acceptable 1-hour postprandial capillary blood glucose level is proposed to be 150 to 160 mg/dL.
- **Frequent snacks are recommended.** Unless breast-feeding occurs within 1 to 2 hours after eating, women should eat a light snack before or during breast-feeding. Milk, fruit, or crackers are sufficient.
- **Medical concerns may keep mother and baby apart during the critical first few hours after birth.** If the child is born with hypoglycemia or the mother has complications, the mother and infant may be separated during the first 60 to 90 minutes after delivery, a time shown to be critical in establishing successful lactation. Mothers can be assisted to pump milk for storage to help initiate lactation and prevent engorgement.
- **Breast care takes on greater importance.** Diabetic women face a higher risk of mastitis because of their elevated blood glucose levels. Measures to prevent mastitis include alternating breasts when feeding, cleaning breasts with water and letting them air dry, making sure the baby's mouth is positioned correctly over the nipple, drinking adequate fluids, and not wearing tight brassieres.
- **Support groups may be especially helpful.** Encourage participation in appropriate programs that provide support and education.

CONTRAINDICATIONS TO BREAST-FEEDING

Breast-feeding is contraindicated when the mother is being treated with certain drugs (or uses addictive drugs) that have the potential to enter breast milk and harm the infant. Examples are antiprotozoal compounds, antineoplastic drugs, some antithyroid drugs, and synthetic anticoagulants. If possible, drugs known to pose a risk for infants should be replaced with safer, more acceptable ones. Street drugs such as amphetamines, cocaine, heroin, marijuana, and phencyclidine (PCP) are contraindicated during lactation.

Colostrum and breast milk can efficiently transmit HIV from infected mothers to their infants. The Centers for Disease Control and Prevention and the American Academy of Pediatrics recommend that HIV-positive women not breast-feed to avoid postnatal HIV transmission. However, in developing countries where infants are at high risk for death from infectious disease and malnutrition, breast-feeding is always recommended, regardless of HIV status.

Other contraindications to breast-feeding include:

- An inborn error of metabolism in the infant (eg, galactosemia, PKU)
- A serious psychiatric disorder in the mother
- Breast milk that is contaminated with environmental pollutants
- Pregnancy, because the combined demands of pregnancy and lactation on maternal tissues are great
- Maternal consumption of more than a minimal amount of alcohol

ASSESSMENT OF NUTRITIONAL NEEDS DURING LACTATION

The reliability and validity of anthropometric and laboratory data for assessing the nutritional status of lactating women have not been proven. The only criteria recommended for routine screening for nutritional problems are maternal weight and dietary intake.

Maternal Weight

- Is the client's weight stable?
- If she is losing weight, how much weight is lost per month? Normal monthly weight loss while breast-feeding is 1 to 2 pounds, an amount that does not adversely affect milk production. Even among overweight women, it is recommended that weight loss not exceed 2 kg/month.

Dietary Intake

- Is the client's usual 24-hour intake adequate for lactation? Pay particular attention to the total quantity of food consumed; the number of servings consumed from each of the major food groups and from the Fats, Oils, and Sweets group; and the amount of fluids consumed.
- What cultural, religious, and ethnic influences affect food choices?
- Does the client adhere to a modified diet to treat a disease?
- Is the client's exposure to sunlight adequate?
- Does the client use alcohol, tobacco, caffeine, drugs, or artificial sweeteners?

PROMOTION OF BREAST-FEEDING

Although almost all women have the potential to breast-feed successfully, lactation may fail because of inadequate knowledge, lack of adequate support, or conflict with lifestyle and career. The partner's beliefs and concerns about breast-feeding also directly influence most mothers. To provide the greatest chance for success, preparation for breast-feeding should begin prenatally with counseling, guidance, and support for both the woman and her partner throughout the gestational period.

Postpartum teaching has been shown to have a significant effect on both the ability to breast-feed successfully and the duration of lactation. Individual or small group counseling sessions should first assess the couple's attitudes, fears, expectations, misperceptions, and knowledge. Information can then be provided on how milk is produced and secreted, factors that impair lactation (Box 11–5), breast care, feeding positions, how to express milk manually, how to stimulate the infant, and how to prevent and manage various breast-feeding problems.

Some studies show that the most vulnerable period for lactation is the immediate postpartum period. To establish lactation and promote the best chance of success, the infant should be offered the breast as soon as possible after birth and at frequent intervals thereafter. Hospital procedures should allow for immediate maternal-infant contact after delivery and for true demand feedings, preferably through rooming-in. Other practices that facilities can use to promote successful breast-feeding include:

- Informing all pregnant women about the benefits and management of breast-feeding

BOX 11.5

Factors That Impair Lactation

Impaired letdown, related to
- Embarrassment or stress
- Fatigue
- Negative attitude, lack of desire, lack of family support
- Excessive intake of caffeine or alcohol
- Smoking
- Drugs

Failure to establish lactation, related to
- Delayed or infrequent feedings
- Weak infant sucking because of anesthesia during labor and delivery
- Nipple discomfort or engorgement
- Lack of support, especially from baby's father

Decreased demand, related to
- Supplemental bottles of formula or water
- Introduction of solid food
- The infant's lack of interest

- Showing mothers how to breast-feed and how to maintain lactation even if they are separated from their infants
- Giving newborn infants no food or drink other than breast milk unless medically indicated
- Giving no artificial teats or pacifiers (eg, dummies, soothers) to breast-feeding infants
- Fostering the establishment of breast-feeding support groups and referring mothers to them upon discharge from the hospital or clinic

Instruct the client and partner:

- **About the benefits of breast-feeding.** Provide assurance that all women have the ability to breast-feed if given proper instruction and encouragement. Emphasize the benefits of breast-feeding for both mother and infant, and point out that even a short period of breast-feeding is better than not nursing at all. Partners who believe that they will miss opportunities to bond with their exclusively breast-fed infant may benefit from developing skills to comfort the infant that do not involve feeding.
- **On the mechanics of breast-feeding.** Women need basic how-to information, especially if they do not have any family members or friends who have successfully breast-fed their infants.
  - Discuss breast care, positioning of the infant, ways to stimulate the infant, and how to end a feeding. Explain that certain factors may inhibit lactation (Box 11–5). Point out that a warm bath, gentle massage, and a relaxed atmosphere may help achieve letdown.
  - Inform the client that the infant should be allowed to nurse for 5 minutes on each side on the first day to achieve letdown and milk ejection. By the end of the first week, the infant should be nursing up to 15 minutes per side.
  - Mothers need to know that the supply of milk is equal to the demand—the more the infant sucks, the more milk is produced. Infants age 6 weeks or 12 weeks who suck more are probably experiencing a growth spurt and hence need more milk.
  - Advise the client that even though the infant will be able to virtually empty the breast within 5 to 10 minutes once the milk supply is established, the infant needs to nurse beyond that point to satisfy the need to suck and to receive emotional and physical comfort.
  - Reassure the client that both feeding the infant more frequently and manually expressing milk will help increase the milk supply.
  - Acknowledge that because breast milk is easier to digest than formula, breast-fed babies usually need to nurse at shorter intervals than bottle-fed babies do.
  - Warn that early substitution of formula or introduction of solid foods may decrease the chance of maintaining lactation.
- **How to pump milk for later use.** Breast pumps are available for manual expression of milk. Milk that is expressed into a sanitary bottle should be refrigerated or frozen immediately. Milk should be used within 24 hours if refrigerated, within 3 months if stored in the freezer compartment of the refrigerator, and within 2 years if maintained at 0°F.

- **About the importance of eating a varied and balanced diet that is adequate in calories, fluid, and calcium.** Use the Food Guide Pyramid to illustrate the food group approach to choosing an adequate diet. Appetite and thirst are generally good indicators of need. Excess consumption of either foods or liquids will not produce "better" or more milk. Women should avoid freshwater fish and alcohol and should limit their intake of caffeine to 1 to 2 cups of coffee a day or less.
- **Not to aggressively diet while breast-feeding.** Reassure the mother that even if she has adequate fat stores, calorie intake should increase during lactation because fat is mobilized slowly. Lean women may be at risk for impaired lactation if calorie intake is restricted.
- **Not to take drugs or medications unless approved by the physician.**
- **Where to find additional information.** The La Lèche League is an international organization that was founded for the purpose of helping nursing mothers. The League prints a bimonthly newsletter, holds conventions and monthly group meetings, and is available as a source of information and advice 24 hours a day. Also, numerous instructional materials and books on breast-feeding are available from community organizations and bookstores.

NURSING PROCESS

Jana is a well-educated professional who is 33-years-old and 20 weeks pregnant with her first baby. Her prepregnancy BMI was 19.2. She has gained 7 pounds and complains of constipation. She plans on returning to work 6 weeks after delivery and wants to limit her weight gain so that she can fit into her clothes by the time she returns to work. She has asked you what she should eat that will be good for the baby but not cause her to get fat.

Assessment

Obtain clinical data:

Current weight
Blood pressure
Laboratory data, including hemoglobin, hematocrit, albumin, glucose

Interview client to assess:

Medical history, such as diabetes, hypertension, anemia, or other chronic disease
Use of prescribed and over-the-counter medications that affect nutrition
Symptoms of constipation including frequency, interventions attempted, and results
Intake information, including:

- Usual 24-hour intake of food and fluid, with focus on calories, protein, calcium, folic acid, fiber, and fluid

- Frequency and pattern of eating
- Pica or unusual eating habits
- Use of vitamin/mineral or dietary supplements: what, how much, and why taken
- Appetite
- Cultural, religious, and ethnic influences on eating habits
- Use of alcohol, tobacco, caffeine, and drugs

Prepregnancy weight history; rate and pattern of 7-pound weight gain
Usual frequency and intensity of physical activity
Psychosocial and economic issues, including:

- Attitude regarding pregnancy
- Living situation, family support
- Understanding of recommended weight gain during pregnancy and nutritional requirements
- Willingness to change eating behaviors

Nursing Diagnosis

1. Constipation, related to pregnancy and the use of iron supplements.
2. Health-Seeking Behaviors, as evidenced by lack of knowledge of appropriate diet for pregnancy and a desire to learn.
3. Altered Nutrition: Less Than Body Requirements, related to voluntary food restriction to limit weight gain.

Planning and Implementation

CLIENT GOALS

The client will:

Explain the importance of diet for her health and for fetal growth and development
Explain the amount and pattern of recommended weight gain
Consume an adequate, varied, and balanced diet based on the Food Guide Pyramid
Gain approximately 1 pound of weight per week
Avoid constipation

NURSING INTERVENTIONS

Nutrition Therapy

Promote the intake of a varied, nutrient-dense diet based on the Food Guide Pyramid.
Increase fiber and fluids to prevent constipation.

Client Teaching

Instruct the client:

On the role of nutrition and weight gain in the outcome of pregnancy

On the role of fiber and fluids in preventing and alleviating constipation

On eating plan essentials, including:

- Choosing a variety of foods within each major food group
- Selecting the appropriate number of servings from each of the major food groups
- Consuming sources of fiber, such as bran and whole-grain breads and cereals, dried peas and beans, fresh fruits, and vegetables

On behavioral matters, including:

- Abandoning the idea of limiting weight gain to fit into clothes after pregnancy
- Eating small, frequent meals
- The importance of maintaining physical activity

On where to find more information:

March of Dimes Birth Defects Foundation
1275 Mamaroneck Avenue
White Plains, NY 10605
914-428-7100
www.modimes.org

La Lèche League International
1400 North Meacham Road
Schaumburg, IL 60173
847-519-7730
www.lalecheleague.org

Evaluation

The client:

Explains the importance of diet for her health and for fetal growth and development

Explains the amount and pattern of recommended weight gain

Consumes an adequate, varied, and balanced diet based on the Food Guide Pyramid

Gains approximately 1 pound of weight per week

Avoids constipation

Questions You May Hear

Is it possible for some infants to be allergic to breast milk? Allergy to breast milk occurs infrequently, and some researchers believe it does not exist. However, the infant may develop an allergic reaction to breast milk if the mother ingests a protein that enters the breast milk intact; if this occurs, the protein can be identified and eliminated from the mother's diet.

KEY CONCEPTS

- Although proper nutrition before and during pregnancy cannot guarantee a successful pregnancy outcome, it does profoundly affect fetal development and birth.
- A woman's prepregnancy weight status and weight gain during pregnancy are correlated to infant birth weight. Underweight women should gain weight before conception or gain more weight during pregnancy to reduce their risk of adverse pregnancy outcomes.
- Most nutrient requirements increase during pregnancy but can be met with an adequate and varied diet.
- Calorie requirements do not increase until the second trimester of pregnancy. During the last two trimesters, normal-weight women need an extra 300 cal/day.
- Women who are capable of becoming pregnant should take a multivitamin containing folic acid or eat folic acid–fortified cereals to ensure an adequate intake.
- Iron is the only nutrient that cannot be adequately obtained from food alone during pregnancy. Women in high-risk categories (smokers, drug abusers, women carrying twins) and those who do not consume an adequate diet should take a multivitamin and mineral supplement.
- Nutrition counseling should be initiated early in prenatal care and continue throughout the pregnancy. It should stress the importance of weight gain, ways to improve overall intake, the adverse effects of smoking, and the benefits of breast-feeding.
- Proper nutrition may help reduce the incidence of preterm births, pregnancy-induced hypertension, and anemia—three problems common to adolescent pregnancies.
- Breast-feeding is recommended as the sole source of nutrition for the first 4 to 6 months of life. In addition to being uniquely suited to infant growth and development, it imparts other significant benefits to both infant and mother.
- Almost all women are capable of breast-feeding.
- The concentration of some nutrients in breast milk is maintained at the expense of maternal stores when the mother's diet is inadequate.
- Neither the volume nor the caloric density of breast milk is influenced by an excessive or inadequate intake of calories.
- For many nutrients, nutritional needs are higher during lactation than during pregnancy.

Focus on Critical Thinking

Ann Wilson is 22-years-old and 6 weeks pregnant with her first child. She is 5 feet 10 inches tall, and her prepregnancy BMI was 22.2. Ann has gained 6 pounds. She is complaining of a voracious appetite despite periodic nausea and vomiting throughout the day. Her typical intake is as follows:

Breakfast: nothing

Snack: jelly doughnut with a can of cola

Lunch: 2 pieces of pepperoni pizza and 1 large cola

Snack: 2 to 3 cookies with cola

(continued)

Focus on Critical Thinking (continued)

Dinner: ¼-pound hamburger on a bun with ketchup, French fries, cola, and cake or cookies for dessert

Snack: chips

Evaluate Ann's diet based on the Food Guide Pyramid for pregnancy. In what food groups is she deficient? What nutrients may she be lacking in her diet?

From what food groups is she consuming too much? What nutrients may she be consuming in excess of need?

What recommendations would you make to help her improve her intake? Design a meal plan, using her typical pattern of three meals with three snacks.

What interventions would you suggest to help relieve nausea and vomiting?

How much weight should she gain throughout the course of her pregnancy? Evaluate her weight gain thus far.

ANSWER KEY

1. **FALSE** The amount of weight a woman gains during pregnancy is an important indicator of fetal growth. However, adequate weight gain during pregnancy cannot by itself ensure the delivery of a normal-birth-weight infant.
2. **FALSE** Obese women should gain at least 15 pounds during pregnancy.
3. **TRUE** The recommended rate of weight gain during the second and third trimesters for normal-weight women is approximately 1 pound/week.
4. **FALSE** The March of Dimes recommends that pregnant women take 600 μg daily of synthetic folic acid and consume foods rich in natural folate to reduce the risk of neural tube defects.
5. **TRUE** In the early weeks of pregnancy, intake of excess preformed vitamin A from over-the-counter supplements or the drug isotretinoin results in a variety of birth defects.
6. **TRUE** Calorie requirements while breast-feeding are proportional to the amount of milk produced and are higher during lactation than during pregnancy.
7. **TRUE** The vitamin content of breast milk varies with the mother's diet.
8. **TRUE** Thirst is a good indicator of the need for fluids, except among women who live in a dry climate or exercise in hot weather.
9. **TRUE** The Centers for Disease Control and the American Academy of Pediatrics recommend that HIV-positive women not breast-feed to avoid postnatal HIV transmission. However, in developing countries where infants are at high risk for death from infectious disease and malnutrition, breast-feeding is always recommended, regardless of HIV status.
10. **FALSE** Women with type 1 diabetes can breast-feed; however, individualized care is needed to balance intake, insulin, exercise, and lactation to ensure adequate blood glucose control.

REFERENCES

American Dietetic Association. (1997). Position of the American Dietetic Association: Promotion of breast-feeding. *Journal of the American Dietetic Association, 97*, 662–666.

American Dietetic Association. (1998). Position of the American Dietetic Association: Use of nutritive and nonnutritive sweeteners. *Journal of the American Dietetic Association, 98*, 580–587.

Carruth, B., & Skinner, J. (1991). Practitioners beware: Regional differences in beliefs about nutrition during pregnancy. *Journal of the American Dietetic Association, 91*, 435–440.

Doran, L., & Evers, S. (1997). Energy and nutrient inadequacies in the diets of low-income women who breast-feed. *Journal of the American Dietetic Association, 97*, 1283–1287.

Fagan, C. (1998). Preparing pregnant women with diabetes for special breast-feeding challenges. *Journal of the American Dietetic Association, 98*, 648.

March of Dimes Birth Defects Foundation. (1999). *Fact sheet: Folic acid.* [On-line]. Available: www.modimes.org/Programs2/FolicAcid/FactSheet.htm. Accessed November 28, 1999.

March of Dimes Birth Defects Foundation. (1999). *Fact sheet: Food-borne risks in pregnancy.* [On-line]. Available: www.modimes.org/HealthLibrary2/FactSheets/Food-Born-Risks.htm. Accessed November 28, 1999.

March of Dimes Birth Defects Foundation. (1999). *Fact sheet: Low Birthweight.* [On-line]. Available: www.modimes.org/HealthLibrary2/factsheets/Low-Birthweight.htm. Accessed November 28, 1999.

March of Dimes Birth Defects Foundation. (1997). *Fact sheet: PKU.* Available: www.modimes.org/HealthLibrary2/factsheets/PKU.htm. Accessed December 8, 1999.

March of Dimes Birth Defects Foundation, International Food Information Council. (1995). *Healthy eating during pregnancy.* White Plains, NY.

Murtaugh, M. (1997). Optimal breast-feeding duration. *Journal of the American Dietetic Association, 97*, 1252–1254.

Murtaugh, M., Ferris, A., Capacchione, C., & Reece, A. (1998). Energy intake and glycemia in lactating women with type 1 diabetes. *Journal of the American Dietetic Association, 98*, 642–648.

National Center for Health Statistics. *New study identifies infants at greatest health risk.* [On-line]. Available: www.cdc.gov/nchswww/releases/98fact/98sheets/linkedbd.htm. Accessed December 8, 1999.

National Research Council. (1989). *Recommended dietary allowances* (10th ed.). Washington, DC: National Academy Press.

Robbers, J., & Tyler, V. (1999). *Tyler's herbs of choice: The therapeutic use of phytomedicinals.* Binghamton, NY: The Haworth Herbal Press.

Sharma, M., & Petosa, R. (1997). Impact of expectant fathers in breast-feeding decisions. *Journal of the American Dietetic Association, 97*, 1311–1313.

Standing Committee on the Scientific Evaluation of Dietary Reference Intakes, Food and Nutrition Board, Institute of Medicine. (1997). *Dietary Reference Intakes for calcium, phosphorus, magnesium, vitamin D, and fluoride.* Washington, DC: National Academy Press.

Subcommittee on Nutrition During Lactation, Food and Nutrition Board, National Academy of Sciences. (1991). *Nutrition during lactation.* Washington, DC: National Academy Press.

Subcommittee on Nutritional Status and Weight Gain During Pregnancy, Food and Nutrition Board, National Academy of Sciences. (1990). *Nutrition during pregnancy.* Washington, DC: National Academy Press.

Trissler, R. (1999). The child within: A guide to nutrition counseling for pregnant teens. *Journal of the American Dietetic Association, 99*, 916–917.

Worthington-Roberts, B. (1997). The role of maternal nutrition in the prevention of birth defects. *Journal of the American Dietetic Association, 97*(Suppl. 2), S184–S185.

Yates, A., Schlicker, S., & Suitor, C. (1998). Dietary Reference Intakes: The new basis for recommendations for calcium and related nutrients, B vitamins, and choline. *Journal of the American Dietetic Association, 98*, 699–706.

CHAPTER 12

Nutrition for Infants, Children, and Adolescents

TRUE	FALSE	Check your knowledge of nutrition for infancy through adolescence.
		1 Infants have higher calorie and protein requirements per kilogram of body weight than adults do.
		2 Early introduction of solid foods into the infant's diet may increase the risk of food allergies.
		3 Formula left in a bottle after a feeding can be refrigerated and used within 2 days.
		4 Preterm breast milk contains sufficient amounts of calcium and phosphorus to meet the needs of low-birth-weight (LBW) infants.
		5 Among young children, serving sizes are approximately 1 teaspoon per year of age (eg, the serving size for a 3-year-old is 3 teaspoons.)
		6 A low-fat diet after the age of 2 years has been proven to lower the risk of atherosclerosis later in life.
		7 Iron deficiency in young children may be related to drinking too much milk.
		8 Obese children tend to eat 25% more calories, on average, than their thin counterparts.
		9 Food additives cause hyperactivity and attention-deficit disorder.
		10 Adolescent males are at risk of iron deficiency anemia.

Upon completion of this chapter, you will be able to

- Discuss how growth and development during the first year of life, during childhood (1–12 years of age), and during adolescence influence nutritional requirements and intake.
- List teaching points for formula feeding.
- Identify factors that place LBW infants at nutritional risk.
- List teaching points for introducing solid foods into an infant's diet.
- Describe two nutritional concerns for each age group: infants, children, and adolescents.
- Discuss the rationale for promoting a low-fat diet during childhood.

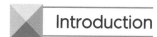

Introduction

Although adequate nutrition cannot guarantee that a child will experience normal growth and development, inadequate nutrition can prevent the child from reaching his or her genetic potential for both physical and mental growth and development. For instance, general undernutrition can cause growth retardation, and iron deficiency can impair cognitive development. *Weight for height* is the foremost standard used to assess whether a child is receiving adequate nutrition.

Although the focus of childhood nutrition has traditionally been on getting enough calories and nutrients, problems related to overconsumption are much more prevalent among today's American children. Nutritional guidance for children has expanded beyond "getting enough" to include recommendations for healthy eating to reduce the risk of chronic disease related to nutritional excesses.

Actual nutrient requirements vary according to health status, activity pattern, and growth rate. The greater the rate of growth, the more intense the nutritional needs. Although a child's growth pattern is individualized, growth predictions and estimates of nutritional requirements can be made based on age.

Infancy (Birth to 1 Year)

Characteristics that influence the type and method of feeding include the following:

- **Growth rate:** Excluding fetal growth, growth in the first year of life is more rapid than at any other time in the life cycle. Although the total amount recommended for most nutrients during infancy is less than the adult requirement, the amount needed per unit of body weight is greater than at any other age.

Nutrient	Daily Requirement for a 174-lb (79-kg) Adult Male	Daily Requirement for a 13-lb (6-kg) Infant
Calories	37 cal/kg Total: 2900 cal/day	108 cal/kg Total: 650 cal/day
Protein	0.8 g/kg Total: 63 g/day	2.2 g/kg 13 g/day

- **Muscular control:** Control of the head, neck, jaw, and tongue; hand-eye coordination; and the ability to sit, grasp, chew, drink, and self-feed all develop over time. Because of inborn reflexes, the most appropriate feeding for an infant is milk (breast milk or commercial formulas). At 4 to 6 months of age, reflexes disappear, head control develops, and the infant is able to sit, making spoon-feeding possible.

- **Kidney function:** At birth, the kidneys are immature and unable to concentrate urine; by 4 to 6 weeks of age, urine concentrating ability approximates adult levels. Excess protein and mineral intake (eg, cow's milk) can tax kidney function and lead to dehydration. Infants need to consume more water per unit of body weight (150 mL/kg) than adults do, related to their immature renal function and the high percentage of body weight from water.
- **Digestive organs:** Stomach capacity is limited to about 90 mL at birth; emptying time is short (2½–3 hours), and peristalsis is rapid. Initially, small, frequent feedings are necessary; the amount of food per feeding increases with age and increased stomach capacity.
- **Digestive function:** Decreased quality and quantity of pancreatic amylase (starch-digesting enzyme), pancreatic lipase (fat-digesting enzyme) and bile (for fat digestion) limits digestion and absorption of nutrients. Infants are unable to digest starch (cereal) until about 3 months of age; bile composition reaches maturity at about 6 months of age.
- **Immune system:** Susceptibility to food allergies decreases between 4 and 6 months as the immune system matures. Introduction of solid foods (beikost) before age 4 to 6 months increases the risk of food allergies.
- **Eruption of teeth:** The texture of food progresses from strained to mashed to chopped fine to regular as the ability to chew improves.

FORMULA FEEDINGS

The American Academy of Pediatrics recommends that infants receive breast milk for the first 6 to 12 months of life (see Chapter 11). If breast-feeding is contraindicated or has failed because of maternal anxiety or misconceptions, the mother should be reassured that infant formula can supply adequate nutrition. The amount of formula provided per feeding and the frequency of feeding depend on the infant's age and individual needs. General parameters are provided in Table 12–1.

Teaching Points for Formula Feeding

- One of the greatest hazards of formula feeding is overfeeding. Never force the infant to finish a bottle or to take more than she wants. Signs that an infant is finished include biting the nipple, puckering the face, and turning away from the bottle. Discourage the misconception that "a fat baby = a healthy baby = good parents."
- Each feeding should last 20 to 30 minutes.
- Formula may be given at room temperature, slightly warmed, or directly from the refrigerator; however, always give formula at approximately the same temperature.
- Spitting up of a small amount of formula during or after a feeding is normal. Feed the infant more slowly and burp more frequently to help alleviate spitting up.

TABLE 12.1 *General Parameters for Formula Feeding*

Age	No. of Feedings in 24 h	Amount per Feeding (oz)	Amount per Day (oz)
1 wk–1 mo	6–8	4–5	21–24
1–3 mo	5–6	5–7	24–32
3–6 mo	4–5	6–7	24–32
6–12 mo (feedings from the cup and bottle if the infant is not completely weaned)	3–4	6–8	16–24

- Hold the infant closely and securely. Position the infant so that the head is higher than the rest of the body.
- Avoid jiggling the bottle and making extra movements that could distract the infant from feeding.
- Never prop the bottle or put the infant to bed with a bottle. Giving the infant a bottle of anything but plain water at bedtime can cause tooth decay **(nursing bottle caries)** once the teeth erupt.
- Check the flow of formula by holding the bottle upside down. A steady drip from the nipple should be observed. If the flow is too rapid because of too large a nipple opening, the infant may overfeed and develop indigestion. If the flow rate is too slow because of too small a nipple opening, the infant may tire and fall asleep without taking enough formula. Discard any nipples with holes that are too large; enlarge holes that are too small with a sterilized needle.
- Reassure caregivers that there is no danger of "spoiling" an infant by feeding him when he cries for a feeding.
- Burp the infant halfway through the feeding, at the end of the feeding, and more often if necessary, to help get rid of air that is swallowed during feeding. Burping can be accomplished by gently rubbing or patting the infant's back as she is held on the shoulder, lies on her stomach over the caregiver's lap, or sits in an upright position.
- During hot weather, provide the baby with supplemental bottles of water.

Formula Composition

Routine infant formulas made from cow's milk are designed to resemble breast milk and to provide comparable nutritional benefits (Table 12–2). Standards for levels of nutrients in formulas were established by the U.S. Congress in the Infant Formula Act (revised in 1982), based mostly on recommendations of the Committee on Nutrition of the American Academy of Pediatrics. Infants who are intolerant of the protein or lactose in cow's milk may be given formulas made with soy isolates or casein hydrolysates.

TABLE 12.3 *Comparisons of Breast Milk, Cow's Milk, and Infant Formula*

Nutrient	Mature Breast Milk	Whole Cow's Milk	Infant Formula	How Cow's Milk is Modified to Resemble Breast Milk
Protein (g/L)	7–9	35	15	Total protein content is reduced.
Whey-casein ratio	60:40	18:82	60:40	Milk is homogenized and treated with heat to reduce curd tension and increase digestibility. Some formulas combine demineralized whey with nonfat milk to approximate the whey-casein ratio of breast milk. Taurine (an amino acid that infants cannot efficiently synthesize) is being added to many milk-based and soy-based formulas to approximate the levels found in breast milk.
Fat				Butterfat (difficult to digest) is replaced by vegetable oils to increase polyunsaturated fat, which is more easily digested by infants.
Total (g/L)	34	37	37	
% Linoleic acid calories	14.7–18.8	1	17.2	
Carbohydrate (g/L)	66	49	71	Lactose is added.
Minerals (mg/L)				Total mineral content is reduced. The calcium-phosphorus ratio is adjusted to be no less than 1.1 and no greater than 2.0.
Sodium	170	580	200	
Calcium	260	1250	470	
Phosphorus	140	960	350	
Ca:P ratio	2.4	1.3	1.1–2.0	
Iron	5	5	12*	Formulas may be fortified with additional iron.
Calories (cal/L)	640	660	670	Standard formulas contain the same amount of calories as cow's milk.

*Iron-fortified formula. Unfortified formula is 1.0.

A variety of formulas have been developed for infants with special needs (Table 12–3). For instance, incomplete formulas are available for infants with inborn errors of metabolism, such as phenylketonuria (PKU) or maple syrup urine disease. These specialized formulas are intentionally lacking or deficient in one or more nutrients and, therefore, do not supply adequate nutrition for normal infants. They must be supplemented with small amounts of regular formula.

Formula Preparation

Most caregivers prepare formula a single bottle at a time. Formula must be prepared using safe food handling practices, which include proper handwashing before making the formula; thorough washing of formula cans, bottles, and nipples; and proper refrigeration. Water must be clean and free of contamination. Care must be taken to prepare formulas to the proper level of dilution. Formulas that are made too dilute can result in inadequate

TABLE 12.3 *Comparisons Among Various Types of Infant Formula*

Type of Formula	Source of Protein	Source of Fat	Source of Carbohydrate
Regular (milk-based, intended for routine use; provides 67–68 cal/100 mL in normal dilution)			
Similac (Ross)	Casein	Soy oil, coconut oil, corn oil	Lactose
Enfamil (Mead)	Reduced mineral whey, casein	Soy oil, coconut oil	Lactose
SMA (Wyeth)	Demineralized whey, casein	Oleo; soybean, safflower, and coconut oils	Lactose
Gerber (Gerber)	Nonfat milk	Soy oil, coconut oil	Lactose
Good Start (Carnation)	Hydrolyzed reduced mineral whey	Palm, safflower, and coconut oils	Lactose, corn syrup
Soy-based (for infants with lactase deficiency or galactosemia; infants born to vegetarian families; and infants recovering from diarrhea; provides 67–68 cal/100 mL in normal dilution)			
Prosobee (Mead)	Soy protein	Soy oil	Corn syrup solids
Isomil (Ross)	Soy protein	Coconut oil, soy oil	Sucrose, corn syrup solids
Casein Hydrolysate (for infants who do not tolerate either cow's milk or soy)			
Nutramigen (Mead)	Casein hydrolysate	Corn oil	Modified tapioca, sucrose
Pregestimil (Mead)	Casein hydrolysate	Corn oil, medium-chain triglycerides	Corn syrup solids, modified tapioca starch
Incomplete Formulas (must be supplemented with regular formula)			
Lofenalac (Mead) (for infants with PKU)	Hydrolyzed casein with most of the phenylalanine removed	Corn oil	Corn syrup solids and modified tapioca starch
MSUD Diet Powder (Mead) (for infants with maple syrup urine disease, a disorder of branched-chain amino acid metabolism)	Amino acids without any branched-chain amino acids	Corn oil	Corn syrup solids and modified tapioca starch

growth and water intoxication; formulas that are made too concentrated can cause hypernatremia, tetany, and excessive weight gain.

Teaching points for formula preparation include:

- Prepare one bottle at a time, immediately before each feeding.
- Before beginning, wash hands thoroughly with soap and hot water.
- Thoroughly wash and rinse all equipment to be used, including formula cans, bottles, and nipples.
- Open can with a clean opener; cover and refrigerate any unused liquid formula.
- Use standard measuring devices to ensure accuracy.
- Fill bottles with just the amount of formula the infant will need at one feeding; discard formula that remains after a feeding.

- Use formula immediately after preparation, or store it in the refrigerator. Formula in a bottle or can that is left at room temperature for more than 1 hour should be discarded (bacteria thrive on warm formula).
- Maintain the refrigerator temperature between 32° and 40°F.
- Discard opened, refrigerated cans of formula if they are not used within 2 days.

Disadvantages of Formula Feeding

Although they have been designed to resemble breast milk, formulas lack the unique nutrient, enzyme, and hormone content; ease of digestibility; and antiinfective properties of breast milk. There is also a greater chance of overfeeding when formulas are used, and they must be properly prepared. Ready-to-use formulas are more expensive than formulas that require mixing.

FEEDING PREMATURE INFANTS

Although the nutrient needs of premature infants differ from those of full-term infants with regard to rate of growth, body composition, and physiologic maturity, the nutritional requirements of LBW infants are not precisely defined.

Nutritional Concerns

Several nutritional concerns associated with LBW can place the premature infant at risk for subsequent health problems.

Increased Calorie and Nutrient Needs Related to Rapid Rate of Growth

Normally, weight gain between 26 and 36 weeks of gestation is greater than at any other time in the life cycle; the earlier the infant is born before term, the greater the impact on nutritional status and requirements. Premature infants are usually expected to "catch up" to normal weight by 24 months of age and to normal height by 36 months. Neonates' postnatal growth should parallel in utero growth at term (ie, a weight gain of approximately 14–36 g/day). After the first week of life, the calorie requirements of premature infants are greater than those of full-term infants. Standard LBW formulas supplying 24 cal/ounce are indicated until the infant weighs 2 kg. Preterm infants need more protein than normal infants do, but their immature kidneys are unable to handle large amounts of nitrogenous waste generated from protein metabolism.

Inadequate Nutrient Reserves

Fat and glycogen reserves are normally deposited during the last weeks of pregnancy. In a premature infant, fat may account for less than 1% of total body weight, compared with 16% in a full-term infant. Inadequate glycogen stores leave the infant at risk of hypoglycemia. Because bone mineralization occurs during the last trimester, preterm infants are at risk for osteopenia, also known as rickets of prematurity.

Maldigestion or Malabsorption Related to Insufficient Amount or Potency of Digestive Enzymes

LBW infants may have impaired fat digestion and subsequent malabsorption of calories and nutrients related to an insufficient amount or potency of fat-digesting enzymes. Because medium-chain triglyceride (MCT) oil is absorbed without the aid of fat-digesting enzymes, it is used as some of the fat source in LBW formulas. To promote ease of protein digestion, LBW formulas have a high ratio of whey protein to casein, 60:40, which is similar to that of breast milk. This ratio also provides adequate amounts of the nonessential amino acids cystine and methionine, which premature infants may have difficulty synthesizing.

Risk of Essential Fatty Acid Deficiency

LBW infants are at increased risk for essential fatty acid deficiency due to impaired fat digestion and because some of the fat in LBW formulas is in the form of MCT oil, which does not contain essential fatty acids. Essential fatty acid deficiency can cause impaired growth, lung changes, altered fluid balance, increased red blood cell fragility, dermatitis, and fatty liver.

Limited Ability to Consume Adequate Amounts of Nutrients

Delayed oral neuromusclar development and small gastric capacity affect oral feedings. Preterm infants are at increased risk for aspiration related to gastric residuals caused by delayed or incomplete gastric emptying. Immature sucking or swallowing reflexes (if <32–34 weeks of gestation) also increase the risk of aspiration.

Dehydration Related to Immature Renal Function and a Low Renal Solute Tolerance

In addition to the immature renal development of the infant, the high osmolalities of concentrated LBW formulas (24 cal/ounce) increase the risk of dehydration. Fluid requirements vary with the infant's condition and treatment.

Increased Risk of Hypoglycemia

Hypoglycemia may be related to immature hepatic function, leading to inadequate enzymes for glycogenolysis and gluconeogenesis; inadequate glycogen reserves; respiratory distress syndrome; or hypothermia, which occurs as a result of inadequate brown fat reserves. To prevent hypoglycemia, frequent and adequate feedings containing a readily usable source of carbohydrate are needed. Blood glucose levels are closely monitored.

Vitamin E Deficiency Leading to Hemolytic Anemia

Deficiency of vitamin E (a fat-soluble vitamin) may occur secondary to fat malabsorption or to excessive iron supplementation, which interferes with vitamin E absorption. Vitamin E deficiency can be prevented by giving water-soluble supplements of vitamin E orally and by avoiding excess iron supplementation. Infants should be monitored for hemolytic anemia (the first sign of vitamin E deficiency) at 6 to 10 weeks of age.

Feeding Options

Breast milk has numerous benefits that are particularly favorable to preterm infants (ie, low renal solute load, antiinfective properties, easily digested fat, high nitrogen content, unique amino acid composition, and high whey-casein ratio). However, even if consumed in large amounts, preterm breast milk lacks sufficient calcium, phosphorus, and, possibly, some essential vitamins. Further compounding the problem is the inability of many preterm infants to consume enough milk to meet their nutritional needs.

To boost its nutritional value, calcium, phosphorus, and vitamins can be added to breast milk through nasogastric or bottle feedings; however, gastrointestinal intolerance often results because of the increase in osmolarity.

Another option is to alternate breast milk feedings with premature formula. Compared with routine formulas for full-term infants, LBW formulas generally contain more whey protein, more vitamins and minerals (except iron), and less lactose. However, a combination of breast milk and LBW formula may not provide adequate amounts of calcium and phosphorus; although LBW formula provides adequate amounts of calcium and phosphorus when used as the sole source of nutrition, it cannot compensate for the low content in breast milk when it is used as a supplemental feeding.

Human milk fortifiers (eg, Enfamil Human Milk Fortifier powder) are designed to supplement preterm breast milk after the first 2 weeks of life (preterm milk during the first 2 weeks is rich in nutrients, so fortification usually is not required). Along with calcium and phosphorus, the human milk fortifiers also provide protein and other nutrients. Because LBW infants are vulnerable to nutrient imbalances, blood nutrient levels (eg, calcium, sodium, urea nitrogen) should be closely monitored when milk fortifiers are used. Human milk fortifiers are not necessary for every preterm infant and are not used once the infant weighs 2 kg.

When possible, premature infants are given small, frequent feedings by mouth. Gavage feedings by continuous infusion or bolus may be needed for very small premature infants. Check for gastric residuals before administering a feeding to avoid distention and possible aspiration. Parenteral nutrition is required if enteral feedings are contraindicated or if growth falls below established minimum standards.

VITAMIN AND MINERAL SUPPLEMENTS

Vitamin D is recommended for infants from birth to 1 year of age who receive the majority of their milk as breast milk. From 6 months through 1 year of age, both breast-fed and formula-fed infants need fluoride supplements, unless their formula is prepared with fluoridated water. Iron-fortified cereal or iron supplements are recommended for infants between 4 to 6 months of age, unless iron-fortified formula is used. Infants should not be given supplements unless prescribed by the physician.

INTRODUCING SOLIDS

Infants usually are not developmentally ready for solid foods until 4 to 6 months of age (Table 12–4). Early introduction of solids should be discouraged, because it can contribute to overfeeding, increase the chance of food allergies, and frustrate both the mother and the infant. There is no evidence to support the belief that solids help the infant sleep through the night. Conversely, to provide a nutritionally adequate intake and

TABLE 12.4 ***Introduction of Solid Foods Based on Development***

Age (Mo)	Feeding Skills	Appropriate Foods to Introduce
0–3	Sucking reflex Rooting reflex Swallowing reflex Tonic head reflex	Breast milk; formula
4–6	Sucking, rooting, and biting (clamping down on spoon) reflexes disappear between 3 and 5 mo Head and neck control Can transfer food to the back of the mouth for swallowing Can sit with support	Introduce iron-fortified infant cereals between 4 and 6 mo for formula-fed infants, after 6 mo for exclusively breast-fed infants
5–8	Brings hand to mouth Grasps and reaches for objects in sight; can self-feed finger foods At 7 mo, grasps spoon, nipple, cup rim Drinks from cup when held to lips Interested in biting and chewing; begins chewing movements Sits alone	At 5–7 mo, introduce strained vegetables, fruits, and fruit juices (noncitrus) and sips of water, juice, formula, from cup At 6–8 mo, introduce the following: Finger foods between 24 to 28 weeks of age: arrowroot biscuits, crackers, dry toast Beginning protein foods: strained meats, egg yolk, cheese, yogurt Rice, noodles, potatoes Citrus juices Plain desserts: pudding, ice cream, plain cookies
9–12	Increased ability to chew Improved pincer grasp	Gradually increase texture by replacing strained foods with finely chopped, mashed, or soft vegetables, fruits, and meat Child prefers finger foods; give smaller-sized finger foods Child can drink from cup alone
12	More refined chewing, especially after molars erupt Increasingly independent Drinks from cup without sucking; blows bubbles in cup	Limit milk to 16–24 oz/day, all by cup Because the risk of allergy is diminished, egg white may be added Using molars, child can eat regular solid foods and teething crackers Continue iron-fortified infant cereal until 18 mo of age, if possible

promote normal development, the introduction of solids should not be delayed beyond 7 to 9 months of age.

Teaching points for introducing solids include the following:

- Always feed the infant in an upright position; do not feed the infant solids from a bottle.
- Offer iron-fortified infant rice cereal as the first solid feeding; follow with other iron-fortified infant cereals.
- Before giving cereal the first few times, give the infant a small amount of formula or breast milk to take the edge off hunger and increase the likelihood of acceptance. After the infant is accustomed to solids, introduce new foods at the beginning of the feeding (when the infant is most hungry) and with a familiar favorite.
- Introduce new foods, in plain and simple forms, one at a time for a period of 5 to 7 days each to observe for possible allergic reactions, which may be exhibited as a rash, fussiness, vomiting, diarrhea, or constipation.
- Infants differ in the amount of food they want or need at each feeding; let the baby determine how much food she needs. The amount of solids taken at a feeding may vary from 1 to 2 teaspoons initially to ¼ to ½ cup as the infant gets older.
- Respect the infant's likes and dislikes; rejected foods may be reintroduced at a later time.
- If there is a positive family history for food allergies, delay introduction of milk, eggs, wheat, and citrus fruits, which tend to cause allergic reactions in susceptible infants.
- Offer infants the same plain, pure fruit juices as the rest of the family drinks, instead of expensive infant juices. Avoid sweetened fruit drinks.
- Except for mixed dinners (little meat content) and desserts (highly sweetened), commercially prepared baby food is nutritious and safe for infant use (sodium was removed in 1976). Read the label to determine whether sugar or fillers have been added.
- Homemade baby food can be prepared by blending, mashing, or grinding food to the proper consistency for the infant's stage of development. Do not salt the food, and do not use spicy or high-fat foods. Do not use canned vegetables, because their sodium content is high and their water-soluble vitamin content is usually lower than that of fresh or frozen vegetables.
- Do not give honey to infants younger than 1 year of age because of the risk of infant botulism.
- Avoid peanuts and peanut butter because of the potential for severe allergic reactions.
- By 6 to 8 months of age, the infant may be ready for three meals with three planned snacks daily.
- When the infant is ready for finger foods, try ripe banana, Cheerios, toast strips, graham or soda crackers, cubes of cheese, noodles, and chunks of peeled apple, pear, or peach.
- To decrease the risk of choking:
    - Avoid foods that are most often the cause of choking: hot dogs, candy, nuts, and grapes. Other offenders include raw carrots, tough meat, watermelon with seeds, celery, biscuits, cookies, popcorn, and even peanut butter.

  - Always supervise meals and snacks.
  - Do not allow the infant to eat or drink from a cup while lying down, playing, or strapped in a car seat.
  - Cook foods well and serve in small pieces.
  - Do not give a child food he cannot chew, or food you are not sure he can chew.
  - Topical teething anesthetics that numb the gums can interfere with the ability to swallow foods that require chewing.
- Avoid foods that may be difficult to digest: bacon, sausage, fatty or fried foods, gravy, spicy foods, and whole-kernel corn.
- Delay the introduction of cow's milk until the infant is 1 year old. Cow's milk is a poor source of iron, can cause occult blood loss (possibly from an allergic response to the protein), and provides an unsuitably high potential renal solute load related to its protein, phosphorus, and electrolyte composition. Use whole milk until the age of 2 years, because skim and 2% milks do not provide adequate fat or sufficient calories for the amount of protein they contain.
- Avoid vegan diets (no animal products) for infants and young children. Vegan diets are not recommended because certain vitamins and minerals are likely to be deficient if not properly supplemented, namely riboflavin, vitamin D, calcium, iron, zinc, and vitamin B_{12}. In addition, the intake of protein, fat, and calories may be inadequate, and the high fiber content may increase satiety (further reducing calorie intake) or interfere with the absorption of some vitamins and minerals.

NUTRITION CONCERNS

Iron Deficiency Anemia

Iron stores present at birth, along with breast milk or fortified infant formula, provide adequate iron for most full-term infants. Even though breast milk is a poor source of iron, its bioavailability and absorption are higher than that of iron from infant formulas, making the risk of iron deficiency among exclusively breast-fed infants rare.

By 6 months or age, infants' liver stores of iron usually become depleted and their requirement for iron increases. Among all age groups, infants age 9 to 18 months are at highest risk for iron deficiency because of their rapid growth rate and often inadequate intake of iron. As the quantity of breast milk or infant formula consumed decreases, the quantity and bioavailability of iron consumed from other sources becomes more important. To prevent iron deficiency among infants, encourage mothers to:

- Give iron-fortified formula to breast-fed infants who are weaned before 1 year of age; iron-fortified formula should be used until the infant is 1 year old.
- Use iron-fortified infant cereals until the infant is 12 to 18 months old, because the iron in these cereals is absorbed more readily than that in other cereals.
- Limit milk consumption to amounts recommended in the infant feeding schedule or the Daily Food Guide for toddlers (see later discussion), because milk can displace iron-rich food from the diet.

Dental Health

Protein; calcium; vitamins A, C, and D; and fluoride are important for dental health. Fluoride has been shown to prevent tooth decay by incorporating itself into the structure of the teeth as they form during infancy and childhood. Sources of fluoride include fluoridated water, concentrated liquid or powdered formula mixed with fluoridated water, and fluoride supplements. Breast milk and ready-to-use formulas may be inadequate sources of fluoride. The American Academy of Pediatrics recommends that fluoride supplements be given to formula-fed infants living in areas with unfluoridated water and to breast-fed infants. Advise parents not to give their infants more than the prescribed dose of fluoride, because it can cause spots to form on the teeth.

Nursing bottle caries occur when infants or children are put to bed with a bottle of milk, juice, or any other sweetened liquid (Fig. 12–1). Advise parents that after the teeth erupt the baby should be given only plain water for a bedtime bottle-feeding.

ASSESSMENT OF INFANT NUTRITION

Adequacy of growth is the best indicator of whether an infant is receiving sufficient nutrition. However, it should be noted that breast-fed infants usually have a slower growth rate than formula-fed infants. Also, infants with impaired growth related to undernutrition or illness experience "catch-up" growth, which usually is completed by 2 years of age. When this occurs, weight gain increases rapidly until the child reaches her normal weight percentile; thereafter, weight and height increase together at a slower rate. Depending on the timing, severity, nature, and duration of the malnutrition, growth may or may not be permanently affected.

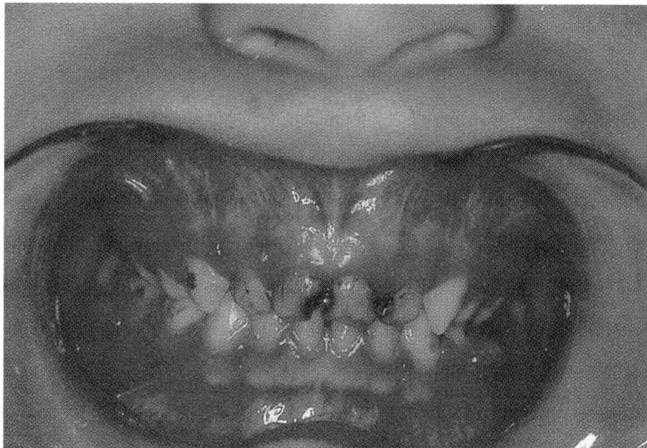

FIGURE 12-1 Nursing bottle caries. Notice the extensive decay in the upper teeth. © K. L. Boyd, DDS/Custom Medical Stock Photo.

Historical Data

- Length of gestation: Determine whether there were complications during pregnancy, labor, or delivery.
- Type of feeding: Determine whether the infant is being formula-fed, breast-fed, fed a combination of breast milk and formula, or fed solids.
- Use of vitamin/mineral supplements: Identify the type, amount, and frequency of supplement use. Determine whether the local water is fluoridated.
- For breast-fed infants, assess the mother's prepregnancy nutritional status, weight gain pattern, and food allergies, as well as adequacy of present intake. Assess maternal use of alcohol, tobacco, caffeine, and drugs.
- For formula-fed infants, assess the type of formula used, the frequency of feeding, and the method of formula preparation. Determine whether the formula is iron-fortified.
- For infants who are receiving solid foods, determine what foods are given, at what age each item was introduced in the diet, the frequency of eating these foods, and whether they are age appropriate. Determine whether any untoward side effects, such as diarrhea, fussiness, or skin rash, occurred after eating any of these foods.
- Sleeping habits: Determine whether the infant is given a bottle at bedtime and, if so, what it contains.
- Familial attitudes: Identify attitudes about food, eating, and body weight.
- Immunizations: Determine whether the infant has received immunizations.

Physical Findings

- Measure height (length) and weight. To assess growth percentile for age, plot height and weight measurements on the appropriate grids, such as on the National Center for Health Statistics growth grids (Appendix 6). Normally, an individual's percentile status for height (length) and weight remains fairly constant throughout childhood. A deviation of more than two percentile channels warrants a more in-depth assessment of growth and nutritional status. An increase in weight percentile may suggest the development of obesity; a decrease may indicate undernutrition, an undiagnosed chronic disease, or the onset of emotional problems.
- Assess growth rate. Usually, birth weight doubles in 4 to 6 months and triples by 12 months. Length increases 50% during the first year.
- Assess dental health.
- Perform a physical examination to identify deviations from normal growth and development for age.

Laboratory Data

- Obtain urine screening results to detect the presence of glucose, protein, and red or white blood cells (may be done at 6 months of age).

- Obtain hemoglobin (Hgb) and hematocrit (Hct) values to detect abnormal findings and iron deficiency anemia (Hgb <10 g/dL and Hct <29% indicate iron deficiency anemia).

(text continues on page 341)

NURSING INTERVENTIONS AND CONSIDERATIONS FOR DISORDERS OF INFANCY AND CHILDHOOD

Failure to Thrive

Failure to thrive is generally defined as an inadequate gain in weight and/or height in comparison with growth and development standards. It can be caused by clinical diseases, such as central nervous system disorders, endocrine disorders, congenital defects, or intestinal obstructions, or it can occur secondary to an inability to suck, chew, or swallow related to neuromuscular problems. An inadequate calorie intake related to inappropriate formula selection, improper formula dilution, or alterations in digestion or absorption (eg, lactose intolerance) can lead to failure to thrive. Family problems, such as inadequate nurturing and infant stimulation, may also be implicated.

Nursing Interventions and Considerations

To develop a plan of care, the cause or causes of failure to thrive must first be identified.

Diet interventions depend on the infant's age and stage of development. Usually, a high-calorie, high-protein diet is indicated.

Physical, emotional, and intellectual growth may be permanently affected if failure to thrive becomes a chronic problem.

Colic

Colic is characterized by intermittent periods of profuse crying lasting 3 hours or longer per day. It is accompanied by symptoms of irritability, gastrointestinal distention, and abdominal cramping. It most often affects the firstborn child, is more common in formula-fed infants than breast-fed infants, and usually resolves itself by the time the infant is 3 months old. The exact cause of colic is unknown, but it may be related to overfeeding, underfeeding, feeding too quickly, swallowed air, or maternal or infant anxiety. Although conclusive evidence is lacking, some studies suggest that cruciferous vegetables (broccoli, cauliflower, brussels sprouts), cow's milk, onion, and chocolate in the diets of women who exclusively breast-feed may be related to colic symptoms in infants.

Nursing Interventions and Considerations

Assess feeding practices: frequency of burping; type of feeding used; volume, concentration, and frequency of feedings; and size of nipple opening (formula-fed infants).

(continued)

NURSING INTERVENTIONS AND CONSIDERATIONS FOR DISORDERS OF INFANCY AND CHILDHOOD (continued)

Assess maternal diet for intake of cruciferous vegetables, cow's milk, onion, and chocolate; advise the mother to eliminate these food items and observe for improvement. Women who eliminate cow's milk may need supplemental calcium.

If no feeding problems are identified, reassure the caregivers that colic is transient and does not indicate health problems or parental ineptness.

Cleft Palate

Numerous combinations of developmental defects involving the lip and palate can occur and result in an opening in the roof of the mouth or incompletely formed lips. Feeding difficulties begin at birth. The cause may be hereditary or unknown.

Nursing Interventions and Considerations

Depending on the type of defects, infants with a cleft palate may be unable to suck. A squeezable cleft lip/palate nurser and a crosscut nipple with rigid bottle are effective methods of feeding.

Infants with cleft palates may achieve normal growth when caregivers are educated about feeding techniques, formula volume goals, and use of energy-dense solids.

Advise caregivers:

- To feed the infant in an upright position and direct the formula to the side of the mouth to prevent formula from entering the nasal passage.
- To feed the infant slowly and burp the infant frequently. Feeding can be a long and tiring process for both infant and caregivers.
- To follow the normal diet progression and introduction of solids based on the child's development and nutritional needs. Reassure the caregivers that children with a cleft palate can handle solids better than liquids.

Pyloric Stenosis

Pyloric stenosis is characterized by an obstructive narrowing of the pyloric opening, which results in projectile vomiting within 30 minutes after feeding, weight loss, dehydration, and poor nutritional status. Excessive thickening of the pyloric muscle or hypertrophy and hyperplasia of mucosa and submucosa cause it.

Nursing Interventions and Considerations

The major goal of nutritional therapy is to achieve fluid and electrolyte balance so that the infant can undergo surgery.

After surgery, the infant is given glucose water and then advanced to full-strength formula as tolerated, after which the infant can be breast-fed, if desired.

(continued)

Vomiting

Vomiting, characterized by the ejection of stomach contents through the mouth, may occur secondary to viral infection, formula contamination, food poisoning, or intestinal obstruction.

Nursing Interventions and Considerations

Food intake is unimportant; the major nutritional concern for prolonged vomiting is fluid and electrolyte replacement.

Advise caregivers:

- To withhold solid food and offer the child small amounts of clear liquids.
- To progress the diet as tolerated after the vomiting subsides.

Mild Diarrhea (1 to 4 days)

Mild diarrhea may be related to numerous causes, such as viral infection, formula contamination, food poisoning, overfeeding, excessive fat intake, excessive fiber intake, and food allergies. Sorbitol (sugar alcohol used as a sweetener) can cause osmotic diarrhea if it is consumed in large amounts. In infants, a frequent cause of mild diarrhea is the introduction of solid food (cereal) before enzyme levels are adequate, which leads to carbohydrate fermentation within the gastrointestinal tract.

Nursing Interventions and Considerations

Obtain a diet history to rule out diet-related causes.

Diarrhea can cause intestinal inflammation, resulting in loss of the enzyme lactase. Without lactase, lactose is maldigested and diarrhea worsens. An irritated intestinal wall may become more permeable, allowing protein to leak through the bowel wall and into the bloodstream, setting up an allergic reaction. An allergy to protein and impaired ability to digest lactose may persist for a few days after diarrhea subsides.

Prolonged or severe diarrhea can be serious in infants and young children; hospitalization may be required to correct fluid and electrolyte imbalances parenterally.

Advise caregivers:

- To withhold all food for 12 to 24 hours, then offer small amounts of clear liquids (avoid iced liquids). However, clear liquids lack the proper balance of electrolytes; therefore, a commercial electrolyte solution (eg, Pedialyte, Resol, Lytren) may be indicated for electrolyte replacement. It is recommended that a total of 1 cup of commercial oral rehydration mixture be given after each loose bowel movement, perhaps 1 teaspoon at a time if necessary, until diarrhea subsides, to prevent dehydration.
- That it may be necessary to withhold milk and lactose-containing formulas for at least 1 week if diarrhea is severe. Soy- or casein-based formulas are used until the infant is able to tolerate lactose.

(continued)

NURSING INTERVENTIONS AND CONSIDERATIONS FOR DISORDERS OF INFANCY AND CHILDHOOD (continued)

- When milk-based formula is reintroduced, dilute it and gradually progress to full strength (ie, 1 part formula to 3 parts water for 1 day, then 1:2, 1:1, and full strength).

Constipation

Formula that is too concentrated or inadequate in carbohydrate may contribute to constipation in formula-fed infants; constipation is rare in breast-fed infants. In older children, an excessive milk intake, inadequate fluid and fiber intake, or irregular bowel habits may be the cause of constipation, or it may be labeled psychogenic constipation related to toilet-training trauma.

Nursing Interventions and Considerations

Daily bowel movements are not necessary so long as the stools are easily passed.
Obtain a diet history to determine the cause of constipation.
Advise caregivers how to modify the diet to prevent constipation, such as:

- Properly diluting the formula.
- Limiting milk intake to the recommended amount for the child's age.
- Adding fiber to the diet, including whole-grain breads and cereals, fresh fruits and vegetables, and dried peas and beans. The American Health Foundation suggests that daily fiber intake during childhood should be approximately equivalent to 1 g per year of age plus 5 g/day to promote normal laxation (see Chapter 17).

Phenylketonuria

PKU is an inborn error of metabolism (autosomal recessive hereditary trait) characterized by a defect in the metabolism of phenylalanine (an essential amino acid) that prevents the conversion of phenylalanine to tyrosine (a nonessential amino acid), which is normally converted to thyroxine, melanin, and catecholamines. Tyrosine becomes an essential amino acid. PKU causes the accumulation of toxic phenylalanine in the tissues, bloodstream, and the central nervous system, resulting in mental retardation and urinary excretion of phenylketones.

Nursing Interventions and Considerations

Because early diagnosis and initiation of the diet can prevent mental retardation, all infants should be tested for PKU immediately after birth. Diet cannot reverse brain damage after it occurs.

The diet for PKU is low in phenylalanine, but it is not phenylalanine-free. Because phenylalanine is an essential amino acid, it must be supplied in the diet for tissue growth and repair to occur. If the phenylalanine content of the diet is inade-

(continued)

quate, the body will catabolize its own protein to supply the missing amino acid; the effect is the same as cheating on the diet, namely an increase in blood and urine phenylalanine levels. Therefore, the phenylalanine content of the diet, as well as the child's blood and urine phenylalanine levels and physical and mental growth and development, must be closely monitored and evaluated. The diet is continuously modified to provide enough phenylalanine to support growth and development without causing a buildup of phenylketones.

The diet must be adequate in protein-sparing calories to prevent the use of protein for energy, which would also result in body protein catabolism.

The age at which the diet can be discontinued is controversial. From a practical standpoint, some physicians recommend discontinuing the diet when the child enters school (4–6 years of age) because brain growth is at least 90% completed. However, a study of school-age children who followed the diet from the first few weeks of life until age 6 showed that, although discontinuation of the diet did not affect baseline IQ, the children performed less well in school, which could be as damaging to overall development as a decrease in IQ. Some researchers recommend that the diet be followed to adolescence or even later.

Women with PKU have a high incidence of aborted pregnancies and infants born with mental handicaps unless they follow a low-phenylalanine diet during pregnancy or possibly before conception (see Chapter 11).

Lofenelac (Mead), the formula specially prepared for infants with PKU, has 95% of the phenylalanine removed. It may need to be supplemented with small, controlled amounts of formula or milk to supply the proper amount of phenylalanine. However, the formula is expensive, and older children and adults find the taste objectionable, although it is usually well accepted by infants.

Once solid foods are added to the infant's diet (at 4–6 months of age), caregivers may be given meal patterns and exchange lists of foods grouped according to their phenylalanine content to aid in diet planning.

Comprehensive and frequent diet counseling is necessary to assess the child's intake, monitor progress, and allay caregivers' fears.

Advise caregivers:

- That following the diet is essential to prevent mental retardation and other problems of PKU.
- That although other infant formulas or milk may be used to *supplement* Lofenalac, they cannot *replace* Lofenalac in the infant's diet.
- That the diet is low in phenylalanine, not phenylalanine-free, and must provide adequate calories.
- That phenylalanine is an amino acid and therefore is found in greatest concentrations in high-protein foods such as meat, fish, poultry, milk, dairy products, and eggs. These products are eliminated or restricted.
- That vegetables, fruits, some cereals, breads, and other starches are low in phenylalanine and are used in measured amounts.

(continued)

NURSING INTERVENTIONS AND CONSIDERATIONS FOR DISORDERS OF INFANCY AND CHILDHOOD (continued)

- That label reading is essential; for example, aspartame (NutraSweet) is not appropriate for phenylketonurics because it contains phenylalanine.

Cystic Fibrosis

Cystic fibrosis (CF), inherited as a recessive trait, is a metabolic disease characterized by excessive exocrine secretions (especially mucus) that form plugs. The sites most commonly affected by mucous plugs are the bronchi, which leads to chronic pulmonary infections and fibrosis of the lung tissue; the intestines, which creates problems with nutrient absorption; and the pancreatic and bile ducts, which impairs pancreatic enzyme secretion and results in protein and fat malabsorption (steatorrhea), secondary nutrient deficiencies, malnutrition with possible growth retardation, and glucose intolerance related to impaired insulin secretion. In addition, sweat gland secretions contain excessive amounts of sodium and chloride. Nutritional interventions should begin as soon as CF is diagnosed.

Nursing Interventions and Considerations

Monitor fluid and electrolyte balances, as well as growth and development.

Fat malabsorption (leading to steatorrhea, malabsorption syndrome, and malnutrition) is the greatest nutritional problem of CF. Fat tolerance varies considerably among individuals.

Clients with CF need to take pancreatic enzyme supplements with all meals and snacks to enhance fat digestion and absorption. Because protein requirements are greatest during the first year of life, infants are particularly susceptible to protein deficiency and malnutrition. Energy requirements may be 120% to 150% of RDA.

Anorexia, nausea, and early satiety may occur during periods of decreased pulmonary function and infection and may impair intake.

Clients with CF excrete high concentrations of sodium in their sweat.

Addition of table salt to formula or food may be needed to prevent hyponatremia, especially in summer months.

Protein-calorie malnutrition impairs immune function and increases the risk of pulmonary infection. Increasing calorie intake and weight seems to improve clinical and respiratory status.

Advise caregivers:

- That good nutritional status can influence long-term survival and quality of life.
- That a high-protein, high-calorie diet is necessary to replace losses. The Daily Food Guide can be used to plan a varied, balanced diet.
- That although fats are a concentrated source of calories and are needed for their essential fatty acids, fat may not be well tolerated and may need to be re-

(continued)

stricted; medium-chain triglycerides (MCTs) are readily absorbed and may be given for additional calories (see Chapter 4).
- That simple sugars are better tolerated than starches
- To give the child water-soluble supplements of the fat-soluble vitamins and a multivitamin, as prescribed.
- To give the child pancreatic enzyme supplements with all meals and snacks.
- That children with CF need more fluid and sodium than other children do; encourage a liberal intake of both.
- When CF is complicated by diabetes, the diet is adjusted. Nutrition guidelines recommend adequate calories (100%–200% of RDA), with 30% to 40% of total calories from fat. Simple sugars are not restricted. Carbohydrate counting may be used to achieve glycemic control without limiting calories or sacrificing preferences.

Nutrition for Children (1 to 12 Years of Age)

Growth and development characteristics during childhood are as follows:

- **Growth rate decreases dramatically by 1 year of age and continues erratically during childhood.** Appetite fluctuates widely because of erratic growth patterns. Interest in food declines, resulting in "physiologic anorexia."
- **Maturation of biting, chewing, and swallowing abilities continues during the preschool period.**
- **Greater mobility and coordination develops.** Self-feeding skills improve so that children can completely self-feed by the end of the second year. They also become able to seek food independently.
- **Autonomy increases.** Food "jags," which may begin at about 15 months of age, are a normal expression of autonomy as the child develops a sense of independence. As long as the diet is adequate but not excessive in water, calories, and all essential nutrients, food jags should not be a cause of concern.
- **Socialization increases.** Parents are the primary gatekeepers and role models of their young children's food intake and habits. Although parents should be encouraged to set a good example, they must also realize that children's individual food preferences have an important impact on their actual intake. As the growing child becomes more social, the parents' role as gatekeepers diminishes.
- **Muscle mass and bone density increase.** Adequate amounts of protein, calcium, and phosphorus are needed to support normal bone growth.
- **Language skills increase.** Between the ages of 1 and 3 years, children become able associate food with its taste and name; between 4 and 6 years, they begin to verbalize food dislikes and preferences.
- **Between the ages of 3 and 5 years, attitudes about food and eating are developed.** Inappropriate use of food (eg, to reward, punish, convey love, bribe) may lead to inappropriate food attitudes.

- **Permanent teeth erupt.** Nutrients important for dental health include fluoride, vitamin A, vitamin D, calcium, and phosphorus.
- **Reserves are laid down for the upcoming adolescent growth spurt.** Toward the end of the school-age period, nutrient needs increase in preparation for the adolescent growth spurt. Girls are usually well into puberty by the end of this period.

NUTRIENT AND FOOD CONSUMPTION

Among children age 2 to 11 years, average intake of most vitamins and minerals exceeds the Recommended Dietary Allowance (RDA) (Tables 12–5 and 12–6). However, it is estimated that 91% of children 6 to 11 years of age do not consume the recommended minimum intake of 5 servings of fruits and vegetables daily. Reported mean calorie intake, which may underestimate actual intake, meets the 1989 RDA for energy, indicating that many children are consuming more calories than required. It is estimated that 70% of American children exceed the current recommendations for limiting total fat intake to less than 30% of total calories and saturated fat to less than 10% of total calories.

Although there are individual differences, usually a larger child eats more than a smaller one, an active child eats more than a quiet one, and a happy, content child eats more than an anxious one. Among young children, appetite is often least at dinner and ritualistic eating may become apparent. School-age children maintain a relatively constant intake in relation to their age group; that is, children who are considered big eaters in second grade are also big eaters in sixth grade.

Although children can generally eat the same foods as adults, they cannot and do not need to eat them in the same amounts. A rule-of-thumb guideline to determine age-appropriate serving sizes is to allow 1 tablespoon of food per year of age (eg, the serving

TABLE 12.5 ***Pediatric Nutrient Needs for Protein, Vitamin A, Iron, and Zinc***

Age (Y)	Protein (g)	Vitamin A (μg RE)	Iron (mg)	Zinc (mg)
Birth–0.5	13	375	6	5
0.5–1.0	14	375	10	5
1–3	16	400	10	10
4–6	24	500	10	10
7–10	28	700	10	10
Boys				
11–14	45	1000	12	15
15–18	59	1000	12	15
Girls				
11–14	46	800	15	12
15–18	44	800	15	12

RE, retinol equivalent.

(Food and Nutritional Board, National Academy of Sciences—National Research Council. [1989]. *Recommended Daily Dietary Allowances*.)

TABLE 12.6 *Pediatric Nutrient Needs for Vitamin D, Vitamin C, and Calcium*

Age (Y)	Vitamin D (μg)*	Vitamin C (mg)	Calcium (mg)
Birth–0.5	5†	40†	210†
0.5–1.0	5†	50†	270†
1–3	5†	15	500†
4–8	5†	25	800†
Boys			
9–13	5†	45	1300†
14–18	5†	75	1300†
Girls			
9–13	5†	45	1300†
14–18	5†	65	1300†

*As cholecalciferol: 10 μg cholecalciferol = 400 IU vitamin D
†Adequate Intakes

size for a 3-year-old is 3 tablespoons). It is better to serve seconds than to overwhelm the child with too much food. Parents should decide *what* young children should eat; the child should decide *how much*. Instead of "clean your plate," the rule should be "try a little bit of everything."

Young children eat an average of five to seven times a day. Among children aged 6 to 11 years, snacks provide 20% of total calorie intake and 19% of total fat and saturated fat intake. Snacks are an excellent way to provide protein, calories, and essential nutrients to children who cannot eat a lot at mealtime, but they should be offered at least 90 minutes before mealtime to avoid interfering with appetite (Fig. 12–2). Suggestions for snacks include:

- Unsweetened cereal, with or without milk
- Meat or cheese on whole-grain bread or crackers
- Graham crackers, fig bars
- Whole-grain cookies or muffins made with oatmeal, dried fruit, or iron-fortified cereal
- Quick breads such as banana, date, pumpkin
- Raw vegetables, vegetable juices
- Fresh, dried, or canned fruits without sugar
- Pure fruit juice as a drink or frozen on a stick
- Low-fat yogurt, with or without fresh fruit added
- Air-popped popcorn (not before age 3), pretzels
- Peanut butter on bread, crackers, celery, apple slices
- Milk shakes made with fruit and ice milk or frozen yogurt
- Low-fat ice cream, frozen yogurt, ice milk, sherbet, sorbet, fruit ice
- Animal crackers, ginger snaps
- Angel food cake
- Skim or 1% milk (after age 2)
- Low-fat cheese, low-fat cottage cheese

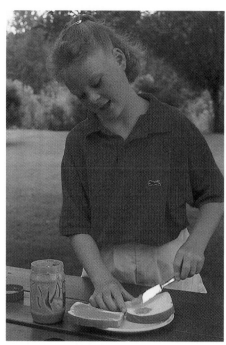

FIGURE 12-2 Good nutritional habits, such as eating healthy snacks, develop early in life. © Bob Kramer.

EATING BEHAVIOR CONCERNS

The most frequent eating behavior concerns of parents of young children are that their children eat a limited variety of foods; dawdle while eating; have a limited intake of fruits, vegetables, and meat; and/or eat too many sweets. However, feeding problems tend to be a product of culture, economic status, and parental nutrition knowledge, and they often occur because parents overestimate the amount of food children need and force them to overeat. Reassure parents that if the child's growth chart shows a consistent and reasonable rate of growth, nutritional intake is probably adequate.

Teaching points on how to foster good eating habits include:

- Offer a variety of nutritious foods, using the Food Guide Pyramid (Chapter 8) as a guide. It is not important if a child refuses to eat a particular food (eg, spinach), so long as the child has a reasonable intake from each of the major food groups.
- Encourage children to taste new foods, but respect individual likes and dislikes. Young children are most likely to reject meats (with the exception of chicken, hamburger, and hot dogs), cooked vegetables, and casseroles or mixed dishes.
- Introduce a small amount of a new food with a familiar favorite.
- Prepare mildly flavored foods, which children usually prefer.
- Avoid encouraging the inborn preference for sweets. Sweets can displace other nutrient-rich foods and contribute to nutrient deficiencies, dental caries, and obesity.

- Make dessert (eg, pudding, fruit, nutrient-rich cookies) a nutritious part of the meal instead of using it as a bribe, reward, or routine bedtime snack.
- Serve nutritious, planned snacks.
- Use child-sized utensils and small, unbreakable cups and plates. Provide comfortable, child-sized tables and chairs.
- Serve colorful foods (eg, red tomatoes, orange slices, green peas) of various textures (eg, smooth mashed potatoes, crunchy raw vegetables, tender meats) that are attractively presented (eg, shaped sandwiches made with cookie cutters, carrot curls).
- Children prefer finger foods. Allow children to explore foods by touching.
- Children who are learning to use utensils often place the food on the utensil by hand.
- Never force a child to eat; if a healthy child is hungry, he will eat.
- Do not use food to reward, punish, bribe, or convey love.
- Mealtime should be relaxed, pleasant, and unhurried. Allow 20 to 30 minutes per meal.
- Eat with the child.
- Minimize confusion and excess noise at mealtime. Keep mealtime conversation pleasant; do not use mealtime as a time for discipline.
- Praise good eating behaviors and do not scold children for not eating.
- Expect occasional table accidents as a part of growing up.
- Avoid common pitfalls. Children may refuse to eat for the following reasons:
  - Too excited or distracted. Allow the child time to calm down before eating, and try to minimize mealtime commotion.
  - Too tired. A brief rest or quiet time before mealtime may help.
  - Not hungry. Remove the child's plate without comment. If the child wants a snack later, make it nutritious. Try spacing meals further apart and limit snacking so the child will be hungry at mealtime.
  - Seeking attention. Provide attention other than at mealtimes. Do not tolerate manipulative behavior.
  - Expressing independence. Accept it as a normal phase of development and do not make it an issue.
- Encourage children to participate in food preparation and cleanup.

NUTRITION CONCERNS

Dental caries and iron deficiency anemia continue to be nutritional concerns into childhood. Additional concerns are the role of preventive nutrition for children, lead poisoning, breakfast skipping, and obesity.

Preventive Nutrition for Children

In adults, excess fat, saturated fat, and cholesterol are implicated in the development of atherosclerosis and coronary heart disease. Because adult risk factors are assumed to apply to children and adolescents as well, several expert panels and health organizations have reached a consensus and issued dietary recommendations directed at the general population including all healthy children older than 2 years of age. The Expert Panel on Blood Cholesterol Levels in Children and Adolescents recommends that nutritional adequacy be achieved by eating a wide variety of foods; that calories be adequate to support growth and development and to reach or maintain desirable body weight; and that intake follow the pattern of no more than 30% of calories from fat, less than 10% of calories from saturated fat, and less than 300 mg/day of cholesterol. The American Academy of Pediatrics recommends that children older than 2 years of age gradually reduce their fat intake so that by age 5 total fat intake is less than 30% but greater than 20% of total calories. It has been suggested that children's fiber intake should be equal to or greater than their age plus 5 g/day. For instance, a 10-year-old child should consume 15 g or more of fiber daily.

Not everyone agrees that a low-fat diet is effective or appropriate for children and adolescents. Fatty streaks are universally present in arteries of infants and children, regardless of national origin, diet, and gender. Some argue that these fatty streaks are reversible, and although some go on to form plaques in adults, most disappear during adolescence. Evidence confirming that a low-fat diet in childhood prevents atherosclerosis in adulthood is lacking. In addition, low-fat, low-cholesterol diets have less of an effect on serum lipids in childhood than in adulthood, and most children grow out of high lipid levels. Whether following a low-fat diet during childhood increases the likelihood that the individual will adhere to a low-fat diet as an adult is unclear. Finally, the safety of low-fat diets in childhood has not been firmly established. Overzealous parents who too tightly control their child's intake of fat may compromise growth, development, and nutritional status. Yet even if a low-fat diet does not influence the development of heart disease later in life, it may help prevent childhood obesity and its comorbidities.

Lead Poisoning

Children younger than 6 years of age are at significant risk for lead poisoning related to their higher rate of intestinal absorption of lead, rapidly developing nervous system, and frequent exposure to lead from mouthing of objects. Lead poisoning can cause permanent growth stunting, cognitive deficits, and other neurologic problems. It appears that inadequate intakes of calories, calcium, phosphorus, iron, and zinc may increase susceptibility to the effects of lead poisoning; the Centers for Disease Control and Prevention recommends that children eat at regular intervals (more lead is absorbed on an empty stomach) and that they consume adequate amounts of iron and calcium.

Breakfast Skipping

Breakfast skipping is a concern of parents of school-age children. Studies suggest that cognition and learning are adversely affected when children skip breakfast. The effect is more striking in children at risk for poor nutritional status than in well-nourished children. Breakfast eating is correlated with improved school attendance; adds significantly to a child's total intake of calories, protein, carbohydrate, and micronutrients; and increases the likelihood of meeting nutritional requirements.

Obesity

In the past several decades, the prevalence of childhood obesity has risen dramatically in the United States. An estimated 25% to 30% of children are obese, which is defined as either 20% or more above the mean weight for children of the same height, or weight for height at or above the 85th percentile. Hispanic, Native-American, and African-American children tend to be more affected.

Several factors affect the chance of whether an obese child becomes an obese adult, including the age at which the child becomes obese, the severity of the obesity, and the presence of obesity in at least one parent. Overweight in children younger than 3 years of age does not predict future obesity unless at least one parent is also obese. After the age of 3 years, the chance that obesity will continue into adulthood increases as the child ages and is higher for children with severe obesity at all ages. After 6 years of age, the probability that an obese child will become an obese adult is 50%. Seventy percent to 80% of obese adolescents become obese adults. At every age, obesity in at least one parent increases the risk of childhood obesity continuing into adulthood.

Obesity results from an imbalance between caloric intake and caloric expenditure. Several studies show that, on average, calorie intake by obese children is not significantly greater than that of thin children. Physical inactivity has been suggested as a major contributor to weight gain in children. Studies show an inverse relation between physical activity and body fatness.

Psychosocial Impact of Obesity

The social and psychological impacts of obesity are greater on children than on adults. Overweight or obese children:

- Tend to have poorer academic performance than normal-weight children of the same intellectual ability
- May be teased and psychologically abused by peers and adults, which leads to social isolation, depression, and low self-esteem
- May actually consume fewer calories than their thin counterparts; however, because they are social outcasts, a perpetuating cycle of weight gain, inactivity, and further weight gain makes weight control difficult.
- May be discriminated against in school and later in college and at work. Studies have found that most preschoolers believe a fat child is ugly, stupid, mean, sloppy, lazy, dishonest, forgetful, naughty, sad, lonely, and poor at sports. Both children and adults ranked a chubby child lower on a scale of preference than a child with crutches and a brace, a child in a wheelchair, a child missing the left hand, or a child with a facial disfigurement.

Assessment of Overweight or Obese Children

Before a child is labeled as obese or overweight, assess

- Age at onset. Because obesity may be easier to prevent than to treat, overweight children (who are likely to become obese adolescents and adults) should be identified and treated.

- Degree and duration of the obesity. Fat stores that increase before puberty in preparation for the adolescent growth spurt may cause transient excess body weight and resolve themselves as the child grows taller while maintaining body weight.
- Family history for genetic or endocrine problems that may be the cause of obesity
- Health status for medical complications. In children, obesity is the major cause of hypertension and increases the risk of cardiovascular disease, diabetes mellitus, joint diseases, and other chronic illnesses.
- Family dynamics. Unresolved crises and conflicts within the family may contribute to eating problems and complicate weight control.
- Body image and attitudes toward body weight. Tolerance toward body weight varies considerably among families and ethnic groups. For instance, African-American women prefer a larger body size. One study found that African-American girls were two times more likely to describe themselves as thinner than other girls their age and seven times more likely to say that they were not overweight. African-American girls were more satisfied with their size than Caucasian girls were.

Nursing Interventions to Prevent Obesity

Because prevention may be more effective than treatment, weight should be monitored among all children. Interventions to help prevent obesity include the following:

- Help caregivers recognize that infants cry for reasons other than hunger and should not be fed every time they cry. Overfeeding is one of the biggest hazards of formula feeding.
- Teach caregivers to properly dilute infant formula. Concentrated formulas are a source of concentrated calories.
- Do not force infants to finish their bottle.
- Instruct caregivers to delay the introduction of solid foods until the infant is developmentally ready (4–6 months old).
- Encourage caregivers to allow children to eat at their own pace in a relaxed atmosphere.
- Encourage caregivers to allow children to stop eating whey they are full; they do not need to eat until their "plate is clean."
- Encourage healthy "thin" eating habits through parental example, because young children tend to imitate their parents.
- Teach caregivers to limit the amount of high-calorie foods kept in the home.
- Instruct caregivers to provide a healthy diet with less than 30% of calories from fat. Provide ample fiber in the form of fresh fruits and vegetables and whole-grain products.
- Advise caregivers not to use food as a reward for good behavior and not to withhold food as punishment. Food should not be used to bribe children or to give them comfort.
- Encourage activity.
- Teach caregivers to limit television viewing to less than 2 hours daily.

Nursing Interventions to Treat Obesity

- Assess the child's normal daily intake, eating behaviors and attitudes, and activity patterns.
- Individualize the plan of care for the child and the family.
- Reduce total fat intake, and increase intake of complex carbohydrates.
- Teach caregivers and children to reduce television time and increase level of activity. Encourage exercise that an obese child will feel comfortable doing, such as exercise that does not require a lot of skill or a change of clothes (eg, walking, bowling).
- If possible, it is best to allow children to "outgrow" obesity by maintaining their weight as they grow taller, rather than actually losing weight. If weight loss is desired, a reasonable goal of 1 to 4 pounds per month should be set, based on the child's age.
- Do not put children under pressure to lose weight; resentment and rebellion may cause extreme behavior, resulting in anorexia nervosa, bulimia, or compulsive eating. Subtle changes such as limiting portion sizes; eating baked instead of fried foods; substituting fresh fruits and nutritious desserts for pies, cakes, and cookies; and eliminating traditional empty-calorie snack foods is more effective than measuring food and counting calories.
- Encourage contractual agreements between parents and children; they may be highly effective.
- Encourage behavior modification techniques, such as self-monitoring, stimulus control, attitude change, and positive reinforcement, that promote positive behavioral changes.
- Recommend group support, which is most effective at achieving and maintaining weight loss in overweight adolescents.

ASSESSMENT OF CHILDHOOD NUTRITION

Historical Data

- Assess adequacy of intake based on the Daily Food Guide (Table 12–7), paying particular attention to variety and to the intake of meat, fruits, vegetables, and sweets.
- Identify the pattern of meals and snacks.
- Determine the use of vitamin or mineral supplements, including the type, amount, and frequency.
- Identify the need for follow-up family diet counseling.
- Determine the frequency and intensity of physical activity.

Physical Findings

- Measure weight and height; assess growth rate, weight status, and weight fluctuations.

TABLE 12.7 ***The Food Guide Pyramid Daily Food Guide for Children and Adolescents***

	Number of Servings (Based on Age)			
Food Group	*1–5 y*	*6–11 y**	*Teen**	*Adult*
Bread, cereal, rice, and pasta	6–11 (¼ to ½ adult-size portions)	6–11	6–11	6–11
Vegetable	3–5†	3–5	3–5	3–5
Fruit	2–4†	2–4	2–4	2–4
Milk, yogurt, and cheese	2 cups	2 cups	4 cups	2–3 servings
Meat, poultry, fish, dry beans, eggs, and nuts‡	2–3 oz	2–3 oz	4–5 oz	5–7 oz

*Serving sizes for children age 6–11 y and teens are about the same size as those for an adult.
†Serving sizes for children age 1–5 y are about 1 level tablespoon per year of age (eg, 3 tbsp for a 3-year-old).
‡Nuts are not recommended for children younger than 4 y because they are a choking hazard.
(Dray, J. [1992]. *Mealtime family time*. Manhattan, KS: Cooperative Extension.)

- Assess dental health.
- Perform a physical examination to identify deviations from normal growth and development for age.

Laboratory Data

- Obtain hemoglobin and hematocrit values to detect abnormal laboratory values indicating iron deficiency anemia (suspected at Hgb <11 g/dL and Hct <33%).
- Obtain urine dipstick measurement to detect the presence of glucose, protein, white blood cells, or red blood cells.

Nutrition and Adolescence (12 to 18 Years of Age)

Growth characteristics and nutritional implications for adolescents include:

- **Rapid period of physical, emotional, social, and sexual maturation.** To support adequate growth and development, nutritional needs increase, especially for calories, protein, calcium, iron, and zinc.
- **Growth begins at different times in different individuals; therefore, physiologic age is a more valid indicator of need than chronologic age.** Because the RDAs are based on chronologic, not physiologic age, they may be invalid for some or many adolescents, depending on when the growth spurt begins (the increase in nutritional requirements depends on the timing and duration of the growth

spurt). Because of varying growth rates, a wide range of weights is considered normal during adolescence. Growth charts are no longer appropriate.

- **Usually, the growth spurt begins in girls at 10 to 11 years of age, peaks at 12 years, and is completed by age 15 years.** Nutritional needs increase earlier for girls than for boys. To replace monthly losses of iron through menstruation, the requirement for iron increases and remains high until menopause. Adolescent girls tend to develop iron deficiency slowly after puberty, related to poor eating habits, chronic fad dieting, and menstrual losses.
- **Girls experience fat deposition, especially in the abdomen and pelvic girdle; the pelvis widens in preparation for childbearing.** Fat requires fewer calories to maintain than does lean body tissue; therefore, girls have lower calorie requirements than boys.
- **Girls experience less growth of lean body tissue and bones than boys do.** Girls tend to become weight and figure conscious and often voluntarily restrict the amounts and types of food eaten.
- **Usually, the growth spurt begins in boys at about 12 to 13 years of age, peaks at 14 years, and is completed by age 19 years.** Nutritional needs increase later for boys than for girls.
- **Boys experience an increase in muscle mass, lean body tissue, and bones.** Lean body tissue requires more calories to maintain than does fat tissue; therefore, boys have higher calorie needs than girls do. During the growth spurt, adolescent boys need the same amount of iron as menstruating girls because of the increase in muscle mass and blood volume; iron need for boys decreases to below the female requirement after the growth spurt is complete. Adolescent boys can develop iron deficiency quickly after the onset of puberty because of their increased need for iron.
- **Period of intense psychosocial growth, family conflict, and social and peer pressures.** Peer and social pressures and enjoyment often have greater impacts on adolescent food choices than do nutritional quality of the food and dietary health implications. Nutritional needs may be difficult to meet because fewer meals are eaten at home, work schedules may interfere with mealtimes, and adolescents may express their independence through their food choices.

NUTRIENT AND FOOD CONSUMPTION

Studies show that adolescents and children eat similar percentages of total calories from carbohydrates, protein, and fat; that is, they exceed recommended intakes for fat. Adolescent girls are most likely to consume inadequate amounts of vitamin A, vitamin B_6, iron, calcium, zinc, and magnesium. Adolescent boys are most likely to consume inadequate amounts of zinc.

Intake data show that carbonated beverage consumption by children and adolescents has increased dramatically over the last two decades. One study showed that almost 25% of adolescents drank more than 26 ounces of carbonated beverages daily, which may contribute to a positive calorie balance and obesity. The calories provided in carbonated beverages are virtually nutrient free. Carbonated beverages appear to displace milk and fruit juice from the diet, and adolescents who have the highest intake of carbonated beverages tend to have low intakes of nutrients found in milk (calcium, riboflavin, vitamin A, and phosphorus) and in fruit juice (folate and vitamin C).

EATING BEHAVIOR CONCERNS

The number of meals missed and eaten away from home increases from early to late adolescence. There is increased intake of fast foods, which tend to be high in fat, calories, and sodium and low in folic acid, fiber, and vitamin A. Girls are more likely to skip meals than boys are, often because they think skipping breakfast or lunch (or both) will help them control their weight. Snacks may contribute 30% or more of adolescents' total calorie intake each day. But snacks are often high in fat, sugar, or sodium and may increase the risk of obesity and dental caries. Adolescents should be encouraged to take responsibility for choosing healthy snacks.

NUTRITION CONCERNS

Childhood nutritional problems tend to intensify during adolescence; dental caries, iron deficiency anemia, breakfast skipping, and obesity continue to be concerns. Additional concerns are dieting; adolescent pregnancy; the use of alcohol, tobacco, marijuana, and oral contraceptives; and nutrition for the growing athlete.

Dieting

Many adolescents are preoccupied with dieting because of concerns about their appearance. Also, many girls do not understand that increases in fat tissue during puberty are necessary for normal growth and development; boys may have the mistaken belief that dieting will improve athletic performance. Counting calories often results in an inadequate intake of nutrients essential for normal growth and development. Adolescents should be counseled on realistic views of desirable weight and on the importance of regular physical activity. (For a discussion of extreme eating disorders, see the sections on anorexia and bulimia in Chapter 14.)

Adolescent Pregnancy

Adolescent pregnancy is associated with increased medical, nutritional, social, and economic risks depending on biologic maturity, ethnic background, economic status, prenatal care, and lifestyle (see Chapter 11).

Use of Alcohol, Tobacco, Marijuana, and Oral Contraceptives

Alcohol, especially in growing adolescents, can produce nutritional deficiencies related to decreased food intake, decreased absorption, increased excretion, decreased storage, and altered metabolism of nutrients. Likewise, tobacco and marijuana can alter food intake. The effect of substance abuse on nutritional status depends on the nature of the substance; the amount, duration, and frequency of use; previous health and nutritional status; stage of physical growth; and nutritional adequacy of the diet consumed. Oral contraceptives alter serum levels of some nutrients and may increase the requirement for folic acid and vitamin B_6, although clinical observations of deficiencies are rare and vitamin supplements usually are unnecessary.

Nutrition for the Growing Athlete

Nutrition guidelines for growing athletes suggest a balanced, varied diet with adequate fluid and calories to meet increased needs. During training, the diet should be composed of about 15% protein, 55% carbohydrate, and 30% fat. Young athletes may develop a transient low hemoglobin value that may be related to a greater increase in plasma volume than in red blood cell mass, or to true iron deficiency anemia. Amenorrhea is common among adolescent female athletes and may be related to the stress of physical training and competition or to a reduction in body fat. Regular menstrual activity returns after intense training is reduced and body fat level increases. Misconceptions regarding the role of nutrition and diet in athletic competition should be dispelled (see Chapter 7).

ASSESSMENT OF ADOLESCENT NUTRITION

Historical Data

- Assess adequacy of intake based on the Daily Food Guide for adolescents (Table 12–7), paying particular attention to intakes of iron, calcium, and protein.
- Identify the pattern of meals and snacks.
- Determine the use of vitamin/mineral supplements, including type, amount, and frequency.
- Determine the use of alcohol, tobacco, and drugs.
- Assess familial attitude toward weight, thinness, and the client's weight.
- Identify the use of any fad diets; assess the age at which dieting began and elicit associated events, methods and patterns of dieting that have been used, and the client's feelings and beliefs about food and dieting.
- Identify the frequency and intensity of physical activity.

Physical Findings and Laboratory Data

- Measure height and weight; assess growth rate, weight status, and weight fluctuations.
- Obtain routine screening tests including hemoglobin and hematocrit for iron deficiency anemia; urine dipstick tests for abnormal presence of glucose, protein, white or red cells; and tuberculin skin testing.

NURSING PROCESS

Amanda is a 24-month-old girl who is regularly brought to the Well Baby Clinic for her checkups and immunizations. At this visit you discover that her height and weight are in the 25th percentile for her age; records indicate that previously she had consistently ranked in the 75th percentile for weight and 50th percentile for height. The change has occurred over the last 6 months. Her mother complains that Amanda is "fussy" and has lost interest in eating.

Assessment

Obtain clinical data:

- Laboratory values, including hemoglobin, hematocrit, serum albumin, and the significance of any other values that are abnormal
- Level of development for age
- Elimination and reflux patterns, if applicable
- Use of medications that can cause side effects, such as delayed gastric emptying, diarrhea, constipation, or decreased appetite
- Length for age, weight for age, head circumference for age, and weight for length
- Food records, if available

Interview the primary caregiver to assess:

- Amanda's usual 24-hour intake, including portion sizes, frequency and pattern of eating, and texture of foods eaten. Assess caloric and nutritional adequacy of usual intake based on the Food Guide Pyramid. Assess appropriateness of texture and meal frequency. Are self-feeding skills appropriate for Amanda's age? Is the mealtime environment positive?
- Weight history
- Pattern of elimination, including history of vomiting or reflux
- Caregiver's attitude about Amanda's current weight, recent weight loss, and eating behaviors. Are the caregiver's expectations about how much Amanda should eat reasonable and appropriate? What is the problem according to the caregiver?
- Caregiver's ability to understand, attitude toward health and nutrition, and readiness to learn
- Medical history, including prenatal, perinatal, and birth history. Specifically assess for gastrointestinal problems, such as slow gastric emptying, constipation, diarrhea, and allergies.
- Cultural, religious, and ethnic influences on the family's eating habits
- Psychosocial and economic issues, such as the living situation, who does the shopping and cooking, adequacy of food budget, need for food assistance, and level of family and social support
- Usual activity patterns
- Use of prescribed and over-the-counter drugs
- Use of vitamins, minerals, and nutritional supplements: what, how much, and why they are given

Nursing Diagnosis

Altered Nutrition, Less Than Body Requirements, related to inadequate intake as evidenced by change of two percentile channels in growth charts.

Planning and Implementation

CLIENT GOALS

The client will:

Experience appropriate growth in height and weight
Consume, on average, adequate calories, protein, vitamins, and minerals for her age
Achieve or progress toward age-appropriate feeding skills

NURSING INTERVENTIONS

Client Teaching

Instruct the caregiver on the role of nutrition in maintaining health and promoting adequate growth and development, including:

The importance adequate calories, protein, and other nutrients to support growth
The importance of frequent feedings of nutrient-dense foods to help maximize intake
Eating plan essentials, including the importance of:

- Providing adequate calories and protein to meet needs for growth
- Choosing a varied diet to help ensure an average adequate intake
- Providing foods of appropriate texture for age
- Providing three meals plus three or more planned snacks to maximize intake
- Providing liquids after meals, instead of with meals, to avoid displacing food intake

The importance of limiting low-nutrient-density foods (eg, fruit drinks, carbonated beverages, sweetened cereals), because they displace the intake of more nutritious foods
The need to modify the diet, as appropriate, to improve elimination patterns
The need to address behavioral matters, including the importance of:

- Providing a positive mealtime environment (eg, limiting distractions, having the child well rested before mealtime)
- Not using food to punish, reward, or bribe the child
- Promoting eating behaviors and skills appropriate for this age

The value in keeping accurate food records
How to modify foods to increase their nutrient density, such as fortifying milk with skim milk powder; using milk in place of water in recipes; melting cheese on potatoes, rice, or noodles; and so on.

CAREGIVER SUPPORT

Provide resources to help support the caregiver. Additional information can be obtained from

Nutrition Resources for Caregivers

Kids Food CyberClub at *www.kidsfood.org*. Connecticut Association sponsors this site for Human Services and Kaiser Permanente and features nutrition information for teachers, kids, and parents.

Nutrition Explorations at *www.nutritionexplorations.org*. Sponsored by the National Dairy Council, this site provides nutrition information for children, teachers, and families.

KidsHealth at *www.kidshealth.org*. This site, created by the Nemours Foundation, offers information for children, teens, and parents on health, food, and fitness.

Evaluation

The client:

- Experiences appropriate growth in height and weight
- Consumes, on average, adequate calories, protein, vitamins, and minerals for her age
- Achieves or progresses toward age-appropriate feeding skills

Questions You May Hear

What foods are most likely to cause allergies? Ninety percent of food allergy reactions are caused by these eight foods: milk, eggs, soy, peanuts, nuts (cashews, almonds), wheat, fish, and shellfish. Most people who have a food allergy are allergic to only one food.

Does chocolate cause or aggravate acne? There is no scientific evidence to correlate any dietary factors with the appearance or severity of acne. Although vitamin A is important for normal skin integrity, vitamin A supplements are not effective in treating acne and are toxic in large amounts. A compound related to vitamin A (13-*cis*-retinoic acid or Accutane) has been approved for treatment of severe cystic acne but is available only through prescription and must be used with caution.

Do food additives cause attention-deficit disorder or hyperactivity? In the 1970s, the late Dr. Ben Feingold proposed that food additives and salicylates may be responsible for about 25% of cases of hyperactivity with learning disability among school-age children. Numerous studies indicate that the Feingold diet (a diet that is devoid of artificial colors and flavors; the preservatives beta-hydroxytheophylline [BHT] and butylated hydroxyanisole [BHA]; and salicylate-containing fruits, vegetables, and spices) rarely helps control hyperactivity. However, the Feingold diet is probably not nutritionally harmful, so long as fruits and vegetables containing vitamin C are allowed, and it may have a placebo effect on behavior.

KEY CONCEPTS

- An optimal diet is necessary to support normal growth and development.
- Because of varying rates of growth and activity, nutritional requirements are less precise for children and adolescents than they are for adults.

- Breast-feeding is the preferred method of infant feeding up to the age of 1 year.
- Formula-feeding is an acceptable alternative.
- Adequacy of growth (height and weight) is the best indicator of whether an infant's intake is nutritionally adequate.
- Solid foods should not be introduced before 4 to 6 months of age. New foods should be introduced one at a time for a period of 5 to 7 days so that, if an allergic reaction occurs, it can be easily identified.
- Iron deficiency and dental health are nutritional concerns during infancy.
- Feeding problems in young children usually result from parents' overestimation of how much food their young child should eat.
- Appetite dramatically decreases after 1 year of age because the rate of growth dramatically decreases.
- Nutritional concerns during childhood include lead poisoning, breakfast skipping, and obesity. The role of a low-fat diet during childhood to prevent heart disease in adulthood is controversial.
- Childhood nutrition problems often intensify during adolescence. Common concerns include dieting, adolescent pregnancy, substance abuse, and optimal diet for athletics.

Focus on Critical Thinking

Karen Thomas is 10-years-old, is 4 feet 10 inches tall, and weighs 101 pounds. Karen has consistently been above the 95th percentile of height and weight since birth. She is concerned that she weighs too much, which has prompted her mother to bring her to the pediatrician for fear her daughter may develop an eating disorder.

What dietary information would you gather to assess Karen's nutritional status and growth?

What is an appropriate weight for Karen?

Develop a nutritionally adequate meal plan for Karen, based on the Daily Food Guide.

What would you tell Karen's mother about:

- Her daughter's growth record
- Her concerns about Karen's snacking
- Activity
- Substituting low-fat foods for high-fat foods
- Weight-loss diets for 10-year-olds
- Karen's upcoming adolescent growth spurt

ANSWER KEY

1. **TRUE** The amount of calories and protein needed per unit of body weight is greater for infants than for adults, because growth in the first year of life is more rapid than at any other time in the life cycle (excluding the fetal period).
2. **TRUE** Early introduction of solids (ie, before the age of 4–6 months) may increase the chance of food allergies.

3. **FALSE** Formula that is left in a bottle after a feeding should be discarded. Opened, unused portions of formula may be refrigerated and used within 2 days.
4. **FALSE** Preterm breast milk lacks sufficient amounts of calcium and phosphorus to meet the needs of LBW infants. Therefore, preterm breast milk must be supplemented with calcium and phosphorus.
5. **FALSE** A rule-of-thumb guideline to determine age-appropriate serving sizes is to allow 1 tablespoon of food per year of age (eg, the serving size for a 3-year-old is 3 tablespoons).
6. **FALSE** Evidence confirming that a low-fat diet in childhood prevents atherosclerosis in adulthood is lacking.
7. **TRUE** Too much milk consumption can displace iron-rich food from the diet.
8. **FALSE** Several studies show that, on average, calorie intake by obese children is not significantly greater than that of thin children.
9. **FALSE** In the 1970s, the late Dr. Ben Feingold proposed that food additives and salicylates may be responsible for about 25% of cases of hyperactivity with learning disability among school-age children. However, numerous studies indicate that the Feingold diet rarely helps control hyperactivity.
10. **TRUE** Adolescent boys can develop iron deficiency quickly after the onset of puberty because of their increased need for iron.

REFERENCES

American Dietetic Association. (1999). Position of the American Dietetic Association: Dietary guidance for healthy children aged 2 to 11 years. *Journal of the American Dietetic Association*, 99, 93–101.

Bronner, Y. (1996). Nutritional status outcomes for children: Ethnic, cultural, and environmental contexts. *Journal of the American Dietetic Association*, 96, 891–900, 903.

Feingold, B. F. (1974). *Why your child is hyperactive*. New York: Random House.

Harnack, L., Stang, J., & Story, M. (1999). Soft drink consumption among US children and adolescents: Nutritional consequences. *Journal of the American Dietetic Association*, 99, 436–441.

International Food Information Council. (1998). *Backgrounder: Child/adolescent nutrition and health*. [On-line]. Available: http://ificinfo.health.org/backgrnd/bkgr3.htm. Accessed December 13, 1999.

Krebs, N., & Johnson, S. (2000). Guidelines for healthy children: Promoting eating, moving, and common sense. *Journal of the American Dietetic Association*, *100*(1), 37–39.

Moran, R. (1999). Evaluation and treatment of childhood obesity. *American Family Physician*. [On-line serial]. 59(4). Available: www.aafp.org/afp/990215ap/861.html. Accessed April 12, 1999.

National Institutes of Health, National Heart, Lung, and Blood Institute. (1992). *Cholesterol in children: Healthy eating is a family affair*. (NIH Publication No. 923099).

Olson, R. (1995). The dietary recommendations of the American Academy of Pediatrics. *American Journal of Clinical Nutrition*, *61*, 271–273.

Olson, R. (2000). Is it wise to restrict fat in the diets of children? *Journal of the American Dietetic Association*, *100*, 28–32.

Satter, E. (2000). A moderate view on fat restriction for young children. *Journal of the American Dietetic Association*, *100*, 32–36.

CHAPTER 13

Nutrition for Adults and Older Adults

TRUE	FALSE	Check your knowledge of nutrition for adults and older adults.
		1 A plant-based diet rich in fruits, vegetables, and whole grains may protect against certain types of cancer.
		2 Differences in biology account for the longer longevity in women compared to men.
		3 Loss of muscle mass that occurs with aging is inevitable.
		4 Older adults have a decreased sensation of thirst.
		5 Older adults absorb natural vitamin B_{12} better than synthetic vitamin B_{12} found in supplements and fortified food.
		6 Older adults need more calcium than younger adults.
		7 Most noninstitutionalized older adults eat an adequate and balanced diet.
		8 Age older than 80 years places people at higher nutritional risk.
		9 Long-term care residents are more likely to be malnourished than independently living older adults.
		10 Obese older adults should be encouraged to lose weight.

Upon completion of this chapter, you will be able to

- Discuss leading health issues for women and men.
- Describe how body composition, gastrointestinal function, metabolism, and the sense of taste and smell change with aging.
- Explain how nutritional requirements change with aging.
- List the number of servings from each food group generally recommended for older adults.
- List risk factors for poor nutrition among older adults.
- Describe a liberal diet for older adults and discuss its advantages over restrictive diets.

Introduction

With the exceptions of Chapters 11 and 12, this book implicitly addresses nutrition as it pertains to adults. Section I (Chapters 1 through 7) and Chapter 8 provide background on what constitutes a "healthy" diet and why. In-depth discussion on the role of nutrition in the treatment of various disorders is covered in Section III (Chapters 14 through 21). It is the intent of this chapter to increase awareness about health issues that concern "well" adult women and men. The second part of this chapter deals with nutrition as it specifically relates to older adults.

Adult Health

Genetic and environmental "life advantages"—such as genetic potential for longevity, intelligence, motivation, curiosity, good socialization, religious affiliation, marriage and family, physical activity, avoidance of substance abuse, availability of health care, adequate sleep, sufficient rest and relaxation, and good eating habits—have a positive effect on both length and quality of life. Studies suggest that good eating habits established early in life promote health maintenance throughout adulthood. Clearly, the development and progression of certain degenerative disorders that are associated with aging, such as diabetes mellitus, atherosclerosis, hypertension, and obesity, are influenced by lifelong eating habits.

WOMEN'S HEALTH ISSUES

It has long been recognized that women have more health problems than men, even though women live approximately 7 years longer than men on average. Women are more likely than men to develop acute symptoms, chronic health problems, and chronic disabilities. Women members of minority groups are at even greater risk for health problems related to higher rates of poverty, lack of education, and limited or no access to health care. For instance, minority women have shorter life expectancies, higher rates of maternal and infant mortality, higher rates of acquired immunodeficiency syndrome (AIDS), and a higher incidence of chronic disease, such as hypertension and diabetes.

The term "women's health issues" refers to the prevention, diagnosis, and management of health concerns that:

- Are unique to women, such as menstruation, pregnancy, and reproductive diseases
- Are more prevalent in women than in men. For instance, women account for 80% of osteoporosis cases and 75% of autoimmune diseases. Diabetes mellitus, eating disorders, breast cancer, and certain gastrointestinal diseases (eg, irritable

bowel syndrome) and psychiatric conditions (eg, depression) also afflict women disproportionately.
- Manifest differently in women than in men, such as heart disease and AIDS

Women's health issues have emerged as both a political and a public health concern. As food and nutrition providers, women influence not only their own health and well-being but also that of their children. Interventions to help women achieve better health through improved nutrition have the potential to positively affect future generations.

According to 1996 data compiled by the National Women's Health Information Center, heart disease and cancer are, respectively, the first and second leading causes of death among American and Canadian women. Diabetes, osteoporosis, and obesity are other leading causes of death and disability with nutritional implications. (For more information, visit the National Women's Health Information Center, a project of the office on women's health in the U.S. Department of Health and Human Services, on the World Wide Web, available at http://www.4women.org.) Although each disorder is distinctly different, dietary recommendations to reduce its risk are remarkably similar from disease to disease: Avoid obesity, eat less fat, and eat more fruits, vegetables, and whole grains.

Heart Disease

Even though heart disease is commonly considered a disease of men, it is the leading cause of death among American and Canadian women. It usually appears 10 to 15 years later in women than in men because of the protective effect of estrogen. As estrogen levels decline during menopause, concentrations of total and low-density lipoprotein ("bad") cholesterol rise and those of high-density lipoprotein ("good") cholesterol decline. The increased ratio of "bad" to "good" cholesterol increases the risk of cardiovascular disease. After 50 years of age, women die from heart disease at the same rate as men. Compared with men, women tend to have poorer outcomes of heart disease. For instance, women have higher mortality rates in the hospital after a myocardial infarction and for 1 year afterward.

A heart-healthy diet that is low in fat and saturated fat; rich in fruits, vegetables, and whole grains; and not excessive in calories is an integral part of the lifestyle advocated for the prevention and treatment of heart disease.

Cancer

Cancer is the second leading cause of death among American and Canadian women. Lung cancer, followed by breast cancer and colorectal cancer, are the three leading causes of cancer deaths. The role of diet in the origin of these cancers is not fully understood. A high intake of fruits and vegetables may protect against lung cancers. A plant-based diet rich in fruits, vegetables, and whole grains is protective against breast and colorectal cancers, whereas heavy alcohol intake appears to increase their risk. Laboratory research shows that isoflavones in soy, commonly called *phytoestrogens*, may block the formation of breast and other hormone-dependent cancers (eg, prostate cancer in men). However, in some animal studies, isoflavones were found to act like estrogen and to actually increase cancer risk. There does not appear to be an unsafe intake level of soyfoods, but the same may not be true of powders and other supplements that contain large amounts of isoflavones. Excessive calories, a high intake of fat and saturated fat from red meat, obesity, and inactivity appear to increase the risk of colorectal cancer. Evidence linking diet with gynecologic cancers (cervical, endometrial, and ovarian) is incomplete but growing. Again, a plant-based diet that is low in fat and not excessive in calories may be protective against these cancers.

Diabetes

Diabetes is the fourth leading cause of death among African-American, Native-American, and Hispanic women and the seventh leading cause of death among white women. Diabetes increases the risk of heart disease more in women than in men. Obesity is implicated in the majority of cases of type 2 diabetes. Weight management and a heart-healthy diet are cornerstones of treatment (see Chapters 14 and 18).

Osteoporosis

Throughout life, bone tissue is constantly being destroyed and rebuilt, a process known as remodeling. In the first few decades of life, net gain exceeds net loss as bone mass is accrued. Between 30 and 35 years of age, *peak bone mass*, which is the most bone mass a person will ever have, is attained. Thereafter, more bone is lost than is gained. During the first 5 years or so after onset of menopause, women experience rapid bone loss that is related to estrogen deficiency. After that, bone loss continues at a slower rate.

Osteoporosis is a disease that is characterized by a decrease in total bone mass and deterioration of bone tissue, which leads to increased bone fragility and risk of fracture. The vertebrae, hip, and wrist are the sites most susceptible to fracture. Decreased stature and deformity reduce lung capacity and abdominal volume, which may lead to chronic back pain, early satiety, and decreased tolerance to exercise. Quality of life is significantly impaired, both physically and emotionally.

Because prevention is more effective than treatment, efforts should focus on maximizing peak bone mass; the greater the peak bone mass, the greater the bone mass in old age. Weight-bearing exercise and an adequate calcium intake are important for building and strengthening bones. Although the peak period for calcium retention—and therefore the period during which measures to prevent osteoporosis can have their greatest impact—is between 4 and 20 years of age, an adequate calcium intake throughout life is important for bone health.

Obesity

Obesity is reaching epidemic proportions in the United States as a result of an abundant food supply and reduced physical activity. Approximately one third of adult women are obese, but among African-American and Mexican-American women the prevalence climbs to more than 50%. Excess weight, especially when located in the abdominal area, increases the risk of coronary heart disease, hypertension, hyperlipidemias, diabetes, gallstones, sleep apnea, osteoarthritis, and reproductive cancers. The dismal success rate of treating obesity highlights the need for prevention and early intervention for the whole family.

Cultural pressures on women to be thin and unrealistic body images increase the risk of disordered eating patterns, such as compulsive eating, binge eating, purging, severe dieting, and fasting. Women comprise 95% of cases of anorexia nervosa and bulimia nervosa (see Chapter 14).

MEN'S HEALTH ISSUES

Men have shorter life spans than women, partly because men are greater risk takers. Rates of accidental death and disability are greater among men, and such outcomes are associated with both voluntary activities (eg, driving) and involuntary activities (eg, serving in combat). Nutritional interventions can do little to change these risks.

At most stages of life men are 88% more likely than women to die from heart disease, 45% more likely to die from cancer, 18% more likely to die from stroke, 69% more likely to die from pneumonia or influenza, and almost eight times more likely to die from AIDS. However, men live as long as women among some groups of Mormons, which points to lifestyle, not biology, as the basis for gender differences in longevity. For instance, Mormons do not use coffee, tea, alcohol, or tobacco, and followers are encouraged to limit meats and consume mostly grains.

Heart disease and cancer are, respectively, the first and second leading causes of death in men. Adding to their risk is the fact that men are more likely to be long-term smokers and heavy drinkers. Also, men's diets tend to be lower in fruits and vegetables and higher in meat (fat).

Heart Disease

The risk factors for heart disease are similar among men and women—namely, high blood cholesterol, smoking, sedentary lifestyle, high blood pressure, and a high-fat diet. Strokes are more common in men than in women. Heart disease and strokes are linked to intakes high in fat and low in fruits and vegetables.

Cancer

After lung cancer, colon and prostate cancer are the most frequent causes of cancer death in men, and both may be linked to high intakes of red meat. It is not known whether the risk is related to the fat content of the meat or to what is missing from a high-meat diet (eg, fruits and vegetables). The incidences of cancer of the lower esophagus and cancer of the lower stomach are rising, and both are higher in men than in women. Lower esophageal cancer appears to be related to obesity and inadequate intake of fruits and vegetables.

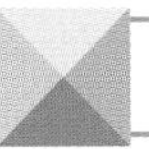

Aging and Older Adults

Aging is a gradual, inevitable, complex process of progressive physiologic, cellular, cultural, and psychosocial changes that begins at conception and ends at death. As cells age, they undergo degenerative changes in structure and function that eventually lead to impairment of organs, tissues, and body functioning. Exactly how and why aging occurs is unknown, although most theories are based on genetic or environmental causes.

Older adults, especially those older than 85 years of age, represent the fastest-growing segment of the American population. By the year 2025, approximately 18.7% of Americans will be 65 years of age or older. Currently, life expectancy is 75 years, compared with 47 years in 1900. The increase can be attributed to improved health care, greater use of immunizations, better hygiene, and the development of nutritional practices that promote well-being.

Despite the misconceptions and stereotypes that people have of older adults, they are a heterogeneous group that vary in age, marital status, social background, financial status, living arrangements, and health status. Eighty percent of adults older than 65 years of age suffer from arthritis, hypertension, heart disease, or diabetes, with 35% having from three or more of these disorders. Yet the majority of older people consider their health to be good to excellent, possibly because people define wellness and illness differently as they age and may accept changes in health as a normal aspect of aging. Certainly, differences exist between the "well" and the "frail" elderly, the latter group consisting of those with defined needs for support for activities of daily living. Only 5% of older adults are institutionalized.

NUTRITIONAL IMPLICATIONS OF AGING

Predictable changes in physiology and function, income, health, and psychosocial well-being are associated with aging, although the rate and timing with which they occur vary among individuals. Changes with a potential impact on diet and nutritional status include the following.

Changes in Body Composition and Energy Expenditure

Loss of lean body mass and an increase in adipose tissue account for the approximate 20% decrease in resting energy expenditure (REE) that occurs between the ages of 20 and 90 years. With the loss of muscle comes a loss of strength and a decrease in aerobic capacity; this causes people to become less active, which contributes to further loss of muscle. Thus the spiral of "normal aging" continues, although it is not inevitable: Strength training exercise can maintain or restore muscle mass and therefore boost the metabolic rate.

Retirement or physical impairments, such as cardiovascular or pulmonary disorders, arthritis, or poor vision, may lead to a decrease in physical activity that contributes to loss of muscle mass and further reduction of REE. Calorie requirements decrease in response to the decrease in REE and the decrease in physical activity.

Oral and Gastrointestinal Changes

Loss of teeth, periodontal disease, and jawbone deterioration related to osteoporosis may create difficulties in chewing. If intake is limited to soft, easy-to-chew foods (eg, meat is eliminated), some essential nutrients may be deficient. As many as 20% of older adults have decreased saliva, often as a side effect of medications. Dry mouth may contribute to difficulty swallowing and altered taste. Constipation is five to six times more frequent in the elderly than in younger adults. It may be related to decreased peristalsis secondary to loss of abdominal muscle tone, inadequate fluid and fiber intake, drug therapy (antihypertensives, diuretics, sedatives, laxative dependence), or a decrease in physical activity. Digestive disorders may develop from a decreased secretion of hydrochloric acid (stomach) and digestive enzymes (pancreatic and intestinal), from decreased gastrointestinal motility, or from decreased organ function. For example, lactose intolerance may develop in older adults owing to decreased secretion of the enzyme lactase, which digests milk sugar. Nutrient absorption may decrease because of decreased mucosal mass and decreased blood flow to and from the mucosal villi.

Metabolic Changes

Altered glucose tolerance is common among older adults. The underlying reason is unclear, but it may be caused by a decrease in insulin secretion or a decrease in tissue sensitivity to insulin. The nutritional implications of this change are not clear.

Central Nervous System Changes

Tremors, slowed reaction time, short-term memory deficits, personality changes, and depression may be related to a decrease in the number of brain cells or decreased blood flow to the brain and nervous system. Between 1% and 6% of people older than 65 years of age have severe dementia, and another 2% to 15% have mild dementia. Central nervous system changes may impair the ability to eat or to purchase and prepare food.

Renal Changes

Factors contributing to impaired excretion of nitrogen and other metabolic wastes include decreased capillary blood flow, decreased glomerular filtration rate, or an inability to regenerate nephrons. Urinary incontinence may develop related to impaired bladder sphincter function. Older adults may voluntarily restrict their fluid intake to cope with incontinence.

Sensory Losses

Gradual progressive sensory losses may be related to impaired nerve cell function. For instance:

- Hearing loss begins at about 30 years of age. Socialized eating may be difficult or intimidating. A lack of socialization can significantly impair appetite and intake among older adults.
- Loss of visual acuity, visual accommodation, ability to see in low light, ability to distinguish color intensities, and depth perception begins at 50 years of age. Vision changes may impair food purchasing and preparation.
- Major olfactory impairments affect as many as 50% of older adults. Elevated odor thresholds, lower perceived odor intensities, and diminished ability to identify odors cause food to become less flavorful and less enjoyable. Many older adults subsequently change their eating habits. Women may compensate by eating more, especially more fat and sugar.
- Taste changes, which begin between 50 and 55 years of age, are related to changes in the sense of smell, a decrease in the number of taste buds and papillae, and decreased flow of saliva. Sweet and salty tastes are lost first, followed by bitter and sour.
- The sensation of thirst is decreased, leaving older adults prone to dehydration. Data suggest that approximately 1 million older adults each year are admitted to acute-care hospitals with isotonic dehydration. Dehydration of as little as 2% loss of body weight results in impaired physiologic and performance responses. This is particularly important among older adults, because an increase in confusion or lethargy related to dehydration may be inaccurately dismissed as a sign of aging.

Economic Changes

An estimated 20% of people older than 65 years of age live in poverty. Milk and meats, which are rich sources of calcium, protein, zinc, iron, and B vitamins, are the first items sacrificed when the food budget is limited. The lower the income, the less likely it is that an adequate and varied diet will be consumed.

Changes in Health

Degenerative diseases such as diabetes, atherosclerosis, hypertension, and cancer are more common among the elderly, as are disabling disorders such as bone fractures, arthritis, and strokes. Changes in health may affect nutrient requirements, intake, digestion, absorption, metabolism, and excretion.

Reliance on Drugs

Older adults account for a disproportionate amount of drugs used. Compared with younger adults, they are more likely to use drugs, to use a combination of drugs, and to take drugs for longer periods.

Drugs may affect nutritional status by altering appetite, ability to taste and smell, or digestion, absorption, metabolism, and excretion of nutrients (see Appendix 7). Likewise, food intake can increase or decrease the effectiveness of some drugs by altering the rate of absorption. If a large percentage of a fixed income is spent on medication, less money is available for food.

DRUG ALERT

Drug Considerations in the Elderly

The elderly, who make up 12% of the population, consume 25% of all prescription drugs in the United States. (Data in this section are from the 1994 Administration on Aging publication *Food and Nutrition for Life: Malnutrition and Older Americans*.) It is estimated that the average noninstitutionalized older adult takes three or more medications daily; those in hospitals and long-term care facilities take an average of eight to 10. The most commonly prescribed medications for the elderly include analgesics, laxatives, cardiovascular medications, vitamins and minerals, diuretics, psycholeptics, antiflatulents, and antihistamines. Large numbers of older adults are also regular users of over-the-counter medications for pain, indigestion, colds, flu, sinus, constipation, gas, and diarrhea.

Because the elderly take more drugs than any other age group, they are particularly prone to nutritional problems related to drug use. Drugs may affect nutrition by inhibiting appetite, altering the sense of taste or smell, altering secretion of saliva, irritating the stomach, or causing nausea. Some drugs contribute directly to dietary deficiencies by altering nutrient absorption, use, or excretion. In a study of residents of long-term care facilities, 41% of those taking one or more drugs that cause anorexia, vomiting, and aversion to food lost more than 10% of their weight over 3 to 12 months. Drugs that are frequently given to long-term care residents may cause deficiencies of vitamins B_6, B_{12}, C, D, and K and the minerals phosphate, potassium, calcium, magnesium, and zinc.

Of the 3% to 8% of all hospital admissions caused by adverse drug reactions, almost one third occur in the elderly. Drug reactions occur more frequently after the age of 60 years and when five or more drugs are used daily. Factors that contribute to an increased incidence of drug reactions in older adults include chronicity and multiplicity of diseases, inability to follow complex medication routines, interactions among prescribed and over-the-counter medications, errors in dosage due to unresolved issues of optimal doses for the elderly, prescriptions written by

(*continued*)

DRUG ALERT

Drug Considerations in the Elderly (continued)

multiple physicians, and age-related body changes (especially in the liver) that alter drug absorption, circulation, or excretion.

To avoid potential problems, older adults should be informed about the side effects of medications they are using (ie, how their medications interact with food, alcohol, and other medicines) and also about the proper dosage and timing of medications. They should be advised to consult their physician or pharmacist if problems arise and to keep all their physicians informed of which prescription and over-the-counter medications they are using.

To reduce instances of nutrient-drug and drug-drug interaction in long-term care facilities, care should be taken to:

- Communicate potential interactions in the resident's medical record.
- Weigh residents frequently.
- Discourage self-medication.
- Administer drugs at the appropriate times.
- Become familiar with potential adverse side effects.

Aspirin may cause gastrointestinal bleeding, which can result in iron deficiency, decreased serum folate levels, and an increased vitamin C requirement.

Diuretics used alone may cause magnesium deficiency.

Potassium-wasting diuretics and **laxatives** used simultaneously increase the risk for severe potassium deficiency.

Digoxin may cause nausea and possibly anorexia and weight loss.

Anticonvulsants used for long periods may cause vitamin D deficiency and can lead to decreased calcium absorption and osteomalacia.

Aluminum-containing antacids may cause phosphate depletion and secondary calcium malabsorption.

Social Changes

Social isolation may arise from the death of a spouse or friends or from impaired mobility. Older adults frequently complain that they do not like to cook for one person or to eat alone, either at home or in a restaurant. Studies indicate that older adults living alone do not make poorer food choices than those living with a spouse, but they do eat fewer calories. Older adults may lack interest in eating because of poor self-esteem related to a change in body image, lack of productivity, or feelings of aimlessness. Generally, older adults who are institutionalized are more likely to have an inadequate diet than are those living independently. An estimated 30% to 50% of nursing home residents are underweight.

NUTRITIONAL NEEDS OF OLDER ADULTS

Knowledge of the nutritional needs of older adults is growing. However, health status, physiologic functioning, physical activity, and nutritional status vary more among older adults (especially people older than 70 years of age) than among individuals in any other age group. Therefore recommendations and generalizations about nutritional needs may be less valid for this age group.

The 1989 Recommended Dietary Allowance (RDA) groups all people 51 years of age and older into a single age category. However, one would expect the nutritional requirements of 51-year-olds to be different from those of 60-, 70-, 80-, and 90-year-olds. The newer standards that replace the RDAs—the Dietary Reference Intakes (DRIs)—have two age groupings for older adults: one for those 51 to 70 years of age, and a group for people older than 70 years.

Calories

Beginning in early adulthood, lean body mass (muscle and bone) declines and the proportion of fat increases, resulting in a decrease in REE. Physical activity also declines with aging, although this is neither desirable nor inevitable. Together, the decline in REE and the reduced physical activity result in decreased energy requirements. However, because these changes occur at varying times among individuals, chronologic age is not a good predictor of energy requirements.

The RDA for calories for men and women of "reference size" who are older than 50 years of age are 2300 and 1900 cal, respectively, or 30 cal/kg of body weight (Table 13–1). The National Academy of Science–National Research Council (NASNRC) Subcommittee noted that calorie requirements of people older than 75 years of age are likely to be lower because of the decrease in lean body mass, REE, and physical activity. However, no specific recommendations were made. As calorie intake declines, it becomes increasingly difficult to consume adequate amounts of all essential nutrients.

Protein

The process of protein metabolism changes with aging, but there is little agreement on protein requirements in older adults. Whereas some studies based on nitrogen balance have shown that older adults require more protein, other studies indicate decreased protein requirements resulting from the reduction in muscle mass and the decrease in renal function that characterize the aging process. Older adults may need more protein than the current recommendation of 0.8 g/kg. A safe intake for people older than 65 years of age may be 1.0 to 1.25 g/kg per day. Although the NASNRC subcommittee acknowledged that aging may alter protein requirements, the RDAs for people 51 years of age and older are not different from those for younger adults (Table 13–1).

TABLE 13.1 ***Nutritional Needs of Older Adults for Selected Nutrients***

	RDA		DRI		
Nutrients	*Age 25–50 y*	*Age ≥51 y*	*Age 31–50 y*	*Age 51–70 y*	*Age ≥70 y*
Calories					
Men	2900	2300			
Women	2200	1900			
Protein (g)					
Men	63	63			
Women	50	50			
Iron (mg)					
Men	10	10			
Women	15	10			
Calcium (mg)					
Men			1000	1200	1200
Women			1000	1200	1200
Magnesium (mg)					
Men			420	420	420
Women			320	320	320
Vitamin D (μg)					
Men			5	10	15
Women			5	10	15
Vitamin B_{12} (μg)					
Men			2.4	2.4*	2.4*
Women			2.4	2.4*	2.4*
Vitamin B_6 (mg)					
Men			1.3	1.7	1.7
Women			1.3	1.5	1.5

*Because many older adults may have impaired absorption of food-bound vitamin B_{12}, it is advisable for people over 50 years to meet their RDA mainly through foods fortified with vitamin B_{12} or a supplement containing B_{12}.

Iron (for Women)

Physiologic data (such as cessation of growth and menstruation) and measurements of body iron stores in the elderly indicate that iron requirements are lowest in old age. The RDA for iron in women decreases from 15 mg for 23- to 50-year-olds to 10 mg for those 51 years of age and older (Table 13–1).

However, some segments of the older adult population may be at risk for development of iron deficiency and iron deficiency anemia because of a decrease in iron availability or absorption. Compared with younger adults, the elderly often eat less red meat, which is the best source of heme iron in the diet. Chewing difficulties and economic factors are often to blame. Iron absorption may be impaired by the decrease in gastric hydrochloric acid secretion that occurs with aging, or deficits in absorption may occur secondary to partial or complete gastrectomy, malabsorption syndrome, or chronic use of antacids. Reliance on "tea and toast" may also be a factor: Tea is a potent inhibitor of iron absorption. Finally, chronic blood loss due to hemorrhoids, ulcers, renal disease, neoplasms, or medications such as aspirin, anticoagulants, and drugs for arthritis may result in iron deficiency anemia.

Calcium

Older adults are at risk for calcium deficiency because both calcium intake and efficiency of calcium absorption decrease with age. Studies suggest a strong relationship between calcium deficiency and the development of osteoporosis, a metabolic bone disease characterized by a negative calcium balance and loss of bone mass.

The DRI for calcium is 1000 mg for both men and women age 35 to 50 years of age; for men and women age 51 to 70 years and for those older than 70 years of age, it increases to 1200 mg (Table 13–1). Although there are rich nondairy sources of calcium—such as calcium-set tofu, Chinese cabbage, kale, calcium-fortified orange juice, and broccoli—calcium requirements are not likely to be met when the intake of dairy products is limited. People who cannot or will not consume the equivalent of at least three 8-ounce glasses of milk daily need calcium supplements to ensure an adequate intake.

Magnesium

The DRI for magnesium for men and women remains constant throughout adulthood (Table 13-1). However, many adults consume less than the recommended amount of magnesium, and magnesium intake tends to decrease among older adults. Aging also reduces magnesium absorption and increases urinary magnesium excretion. Therefore older adults are at risk for magnesium deficiency. Dietary sources include whole grains, dried peas and beans, green leafy vegetables, and hard water.

Vitamin D

Older adults are at high risk for vitamin D deficiency because:

- They tend to consume less vitamin D than they need. There are only a few natural sources of vitamin D: cod-liver oil, fatty fish, and eggs from hens given vitamin D. Almost all vitamin D intake comes from fortified foods, such as milk, but many older adults consume little or no milk. Fortified cereals, margarine, and breads provide smaller amounts of vitamin D.
- Their exposure to sunlight may be limited. This is especially true of older adults who live in nursing homes or who are house bound as a result of physical disabilities. People who live in northern latitudes are also at risk, especially during the winter months.

- Their metabolism of vitamin D is altered. Aging impairs the skin's ability to produce vitamin D. Adults older than 65 years of age have a fourfold decrease in the capacity to synthesize vitamin D, compared with adults 20 to 30 years of age.

The DRI for vitamin D increases from 5 μg for adults age 31 to 50 years to 10 μg for adults age 51 to 70 years. For people older than 70 years of age, the DRI for vitamin D increases to 15 μg (Table 13-1).

Vitamin B_{12}

Vitamin B_{12} deficiency rarely arises from an inadequate intake (eg, pure vegans who do not consume foods fortified with vitamin B_{12}) and is infrequently caused by pernicious anemia (impaired vitamin B_{12} absorption related to lack of intrinsic factor secretion in the stomach). The most common cause of vitamin B_{12} deficiency is an inadequate secretion of gastric acid; without adequate hydrochloric acid, food sources of vitamin B_{12} remain bound to protein and cannot be absorbed. As many as 10% to 30% of adults older than 51 years of age have vitamin B_{12} deficiency related to insufficient gastric acid secretion, which can occur secondary to gastric resection, atrophic gastritis, the use of medications that suppress gastric acid secretion, or gastric infection with *Helicobacter pylori*. However, people with protein-bound vitamin B_{12} deficiency are able to absorb the synthetic (free) vitamin B_{12} that is found in fortified foods and vitamin supplements. The National Academy of Sciences Institute of Medicine recommends that older adults obtain most of their requirement from fortified foods (eg, ready-to-eat cereals) or from supplements (Table 13-1).

Vitamin B_6

Studies suggest that aging alters vitamin B_6 metabolism and therefore increases the vitamin B_6 requirement. The DRI increases from 1.3 mg for younger adults to 1.7 and 1.5 mg, respectively, for men and women older than 50 years of age (Table 13-1). Sources of vitamin B_6 include meat, fish, poultry, shellfish, dried peas and beans, green leafy vegetables, and whole grains.

USING THE FOOD GUIDE PYRAMID TO CHOOSE A HEALTHY DIET

Older adults can used the Food Guide Pyramid (see Chapter 8) to help choose a healthy diet. Most older adults can obtain adequate calories and nutrients by eating the lowest number of servings recommended for each major food group. However, more than the minimum suggestion of two servings from the milk group is needed to ensure an adequate calcium intake. A general guide is as follows:

Food Group	Number of Daily Servings
Bread, cereal, rice, and pasta	6
Vegetable	3
Fruit	2
Milk	3–4
Meat (oz)	5
Fats, oils, and sweets	Use sparingly

Tips for older adults regarding healthy eating include:

- **Concentrate on variety.** Eating a varied diet increases the likelihood that adequate but not excessive amounts of all nutrients will be consumed. Variety means selecting different items within each food group and varying meal selections.
- **Moderation means that no foods are forbidden.** For most age groups, the concept of moderation is intended to help people avoid dietary excesses, particularly of fat, saturated fat, cholesterol, and sodium. However, the benefits of reducing fat and sodium intake in older adults are less obvious, particularly for those who are underweight or who have suboptimal intakes. Among older adults, the nutritional goal of reducing the risk of chronic disease may be replaced by improving the quality of life and maintaining the ability to function. Individualization of nutritional interventions is essential.
- **Aim for balance.** The servings recommended previously are only a guide to balance. A given individual's actual needs vary according to activity level and health status. However, no food groups should be excluded.
- **Choose fiber-rich foods.** Decreased gastrointestinal motility, inactivity, and certain drugs contribute to constipation in older adults. Consuming adequate fluids and rich sources of fiber, such as whole-grain breads and cereals, dried peas and beans, and fresh fruits and vegetables, can promote regularity. Older adults who have difficulty chewing fruits and vegetables should concentrate on soft choices, such as ripe bananas, baked winter squash, mashed potatoes, stewed tomatoes, or baked apples.
- **Drink adequate fluids.** Because the sense of thirst tends to decrease with aging, many older adults do not experience thirst when they need fluid. Older adults may need to make a conscious effort to remind themselves to drink fluid. A total of 8 to 12 glasses of fluid daily are recommended. Older adults should be advised not to voluntarily limit fluids in an attempt to manage incontinence.
- **Watch sodium intake.** Younger adults are advised to reduce their intake of sodium, because excessive sodium may increase the risk of developing hypertension. The appropriateness of limiting sodium in older adults is controversial. For instance, low-sodium diets (2 g sodium per day) limit food choices and may compromise nutrient intake. Also, because taste sensitivity for salt decreases with age, compliance is difficult. Many older adults who live alone rely on convenience

foods, which tend to be high in sodium. Individual considerations should determine sodium allowance.

USE OF SUPPLEMENTS BY OLDER ADULTS

According to the National Institute on Aging, a balanced diet based on the Daily Food Guide is nutritionally adequate for most healthy older adults. However, vitamin and mineral supplements are popular among older adults. Estimates from survey populations indicate that 40% to 60% of older adults use some form of vitamin or mineral supplement, and most of them do so on the recommendation of family, friends, or the media. The elderly are particularly vulnerable to false nutritional claims that promise to restore youth, cure disease, and improve one's sense of well-being. The purchase of unnecessary and ill-advised supplements can displace the purchase of food if funds are limited and may prevent an individual from seeking sound medical advice if the supplements are used to "cure" illness. Unless otherwise directed by a physician, older adults who decide to take supplements should choose a multivitamin and mineral supplement that provides no more than 100% daily value (DV) for nutrients.

RISK FACTORS FOR POOR NUTRITION

As many as two thirds of independently living older adults consume inadequate diets. Those at greatest risk are less educated, live alone, and have low incomes. Inadequate intakes from the meat group often occur in older adults secondary to a limited food budget or difficulty chewing. Many adults avoid milk, which is another source of high-quality protein, because of its association with childhood. The intake of fruits and vegetables may be limited because they are expensive or difficult to chew. Clearly, food choices of the elderly often are based on considerations other than food preferences—such as income; the client's physical ability to shop, prepare, chew, and swallow food; and the occurrence of food intolerances that are related to chronic disease or side effects of medications.

A large proportion of older Americans are at greater risk for nutritional problems than the general population. Nutritional deficiencies exist in as many as 50% of independently living older Americans, and as many as 20% of the elderly skip meals almost daily. Nutrients that are deficient in certain segments of the older population (when compared with the recommended intakes) include calories, calcium, zinc, vitamin B_6, vitamin B_{12}, and vitamin D. Excessive intakes of vitamins A, D, E, and C have been noted in older adults who regularly consume vitamin supplements.

The Nutrition Screening Initiative, a joint effort of the American Academy of Family Physicians, the American Dietetic Association, and the National Council on Aging, has developed the DETERMINE Checklist as a public awareness tool to be used as the first step in identifying older adults who may be at nutritional risk so that the appropriate referrals can be made (Box 13–1).

(text continues on page 377)

BOX 13.1

Determine Your Nutritional Health

The Warning Signs of poor nutritional health are often overlooked. Use this checklist to find out if you or someone you know is at nutritional risk.

Read the statements below. Circle the number in the Yes column for those that apply to you or someone you know. For each Yes answer, score the number in the box. Total your nutritional score.

	YES
I have an illness or condition that made me change the kind and/or amount of food I eat.	2
I eat fewer than two meals per day.	3
I eat few fruits or vegetables, or milk products.	2
I have three or more drinks of beer, liquor, or wine almost every day.	2
I have tooth or mouth problems that make it hard for me to eat.	2
I don't always have enough money to buy the food I need.	4
I eat alone most of the time.	1
I take three or more different prescribed or over-the-counter drugs a day.	1
Without wanting to, I have lost or gained 10 pounds in the last 6 months.	2
I am not always physically able to shop, cook, and/or feed myself.	2
TOTAL	

Total Your Nutritional Score. If it is—

0–2 **Good!** Recheck your nutritional score in 6 months.

3–5 **You are at moderate nutritional risk.** See what can be done to improve your eating habits and lifestyle. Your office on aging, senior nutrition program, senior citizen center, or health department can help. Recheck your nutritional score in 3 months.

6 or more **You are at high nutritional risk.** Bring this checklist the next time you see your doctor, dietitian, or other qualified health or social service professional. Talk with them about any problems you may have. Ask for help to improve your nutritional health.

These materials were developed and distributed by the Nutritional Screening Initiative, a project of:

AMERICAN ACADEMY OF FAMILY PHYSICIANS

THE AMERICAN DIETETIC ASSOCIATION

NATIONAL COUNCIL ON AGING, INC.

Remember that warning signs suggest risk but do not represent diagnosis of any condition. Turn the page to learn more about the Warning Signs of poor nutritional health.

(continued)

BOX 13.1

Determine Your Nutritional Health (continued)

Disease

Any disease, illness, or chronic condition that causes you to change the way you eat or makes it hard for you to eat puts your nutritional health at risk. Four in five adults have chronic diseases that are affected by diet. Confusion or memory loss that keeps getting worse is estimated to affect at least one in five older adults. This can make it hard to remember what, when, or whether you have eaten. Feeling sad or depressed, which happens to about one in eight older adults, can cause big changes in appetite, digestion, energy level, weight, and well-being.

Eating Poorly

Eating too little and eating too much both lead to poor health. Eating the same foods day after day or not eating fruit, vegetables, and milk products daily also causes poor nutritional health. One in five adults skip meals daily. Only 13% of adults eat the minimum amount of fruit and vegetables needed. One in four older adults drink too much alcohol. Many health problems become worse if you drink more than one or two alcoholic beverages per day.

Tooth Loss/Mouth Pain

A healthy mouth, teeth, and gums are needed to eat. Missing, loose, or rotten teeth or dentures that do not fit well or cause mouth sores make it hard to eat.

Economic Hardship

As many as 40% of older Americans have incomes of less than $6,000 per year. Having less—or choosing to spend less—than $25 to $30 per week for food makes it very hard to get the foods you need to stay healthy.

Reduced Social Contact

One third of all older people live alone. Being with people daily has a positive effect on morale, well-being, and eating.

Multiple Medicines

Many older Americans must take medicines for health problems. Almost half of older Americans take multiple medicines daily. Growing old may change the way you respond to drugs. The more medicines you take, the greater the chance for side effects such as increased or decreased appetite, change in taste, constipation, weakness, drowsiness, diarrhea, and nausea. Vitamins or minerals, when taken in large doses, act like drugs and can harm you. Alert your doctor to everything you take.

Involuntary Weight Loss/Gain

Losing or gaining a lot of weight when you are not trying to do so is an important warning sign that must not be ignored. Being overweight or underweight also increases your chance of poor health.

Needs Assistance in Self-Care

Although most older people are able to eat, one in five have trouble walking, shopping, buying, and cooking food, especially as they get older.

Elder Years Above Age 80

Most older people lead full and productive lives. But as age increases, the risk of frailty and health problems increases. Checking your nutritional health regularly makes good sense.

The Nutrition Screening Initiative, 2626 Pennsylvania Avenue, NW, Suite 301, Washington, DC 20037

The Nutrition Screening Initiative is funded in part by a grant from Ross Laboratories, a division of Abbott Laboratories.

ASSESSING THE NUTRITIONAL NEEDS OF OLDER ADULTS

Assessment Data

Assessment data in older adults may be unreliable or invalid because of changes related to aging. For instance, accurate weights are difficult to obtain in clients who are bedridden, and curvature of the spine interferes with accurate measurement of height. Likewise, age-related changes in physiology and function may mimic signs of a nutritional deficiency. For instance, loss of visual acuity in dim light occurs with aging and may not indicate a deficiency of vitamin A. Historical data are difficult to obtain from clients who have hearing loss or cognitive impairments.

Historical Data

- What is the client's usual weight? Has the client experienced significant unintentional weight loss?
- Is the client following a special diet? Is the usual intake adequate? Does the client have difficulty chewing or swallowing? Does the client have food allergies or intolerances? Does the client complain of taste alterations or loss of appetite?
- Does the client do the shopping and cooking? Is the client's food budget adequate?
- What cultural, religious, or ethnic influences affect the client's food choices?
- Does the client have an acute or chronic illness that affects intake, digestion, metabolism, or excretion?
- What over-the-counter and prescription medications does the client use? What nutritional supplements does the client use and for what purpose?
- Does the client use alcohol, tobacco, or caffeine?
- Does the client participate in physical activity?
- Does the client live alone? Are there outside support systems?

Physical Findings

- What is the client's height, weight, and body mass index (BMI)?
- Is the client's blood pressure normal?
- Does the client exhibit signs of malnutrition, such as skin changes, edema, ascites, easy fatigability, loss of subcutaneous fat, and tissue wasting?
- Does the client have missing teeth or ill-fitting dentures?
- Does the client have functional disabilities, such as those seen with arthritis, lung disease, or Parkinson's disease? Is the client able to perform activities of daily living (ADLs)?
- Does the client appear depressed?

Laboratory Data

- Evaluate albumin, hemoglobin, hematocrit, serum lipids, and glucose.
- Evaluate urinalysis for glucose, ketones, protein, and occult blood.

NUTRITION INTERVENTIONS FOR OLDER ADULTS

Rather than using a textbook approach, nutrition therapy for older adults should be client-centered and based on the individual's physiologic, pathologic, and psychosocial condition. Overall goals of nutrition therapy for older adults are to maintain or restore maximal independent functioning and to maintain the client's sense of dignity and quality of life by imposing as few dietary restrictions as possible. Any necessary dietary changes should be incorporated into the client's existing food pattern, because attempting to impose a completely new approach to eating would result in decreased compliance.

Special issues in older adults with nutritional implications include osteoarthritis, Alzheimer's disease, obesity, social isolation, and institutionalization.

Osteoarthritis

As much as 80% of the population older than 55 years of age may be affected with osteoarthritis, a chronic, progressive, noninflammatory joint disorder that is characterized by destruction of joint cartilage, spur and bone cyst formation, pain, and impaired joint movement. It most often affects weight-bearing joints (knees, hips, ankles, and spine) and fingers. Approximately twice as many obese people as people of normal weight have osteoarthritis; however, it is not known whether obesity is an etiologic factor or whether it occurs secondary to reduced activity related to osteoarthritis. For some unexplained reason, weight reduction has been shown to eliminate symptoms of osteoarthritis throughout the body, not just in the weight-bearing joints.

Arthritis has the potential to affect nutrition in several ways. For instance, unorthodox or unproven dietary remedies promoted to "cure" arthritis may endanger nutritional status. Fasting, amino acid supplements, vitamin megadoses, and raw liver are among the many unfounded nutritional treatments for arthritis. Arthritis can affect nutrition when limitation of motion, contractures, or muscle spasms interfere with procuring, preparing, and eating meals. Finally, drugs used to manage arthritis may alter intake or nutrient metabolism.

Alzheimer's Disease

Alzheimer's disease is the most common cause of dementia in Americans 65 years of age and older, affecting an estimated 4 million people. Although researchers do not fully understand what causes Alzheimer's disease, it appears to result from a complex series of events in the brain that occur over time. Disruptions in nerve cell communication, metabolism, and repair eventually cause many nerve cells to stop functioning, lose connections with other nerve cells, and die. Genetic and nongenetic factors (eg, inflammation of the brain, stroke) have been identified in the etiology of Alzheimer's disease. Studies are being conducted to determine whether antioxidants (eg, vitamin E) can slow the course or prevent Alzheimer's disease.

The course of Alzheimer's disease is progressive and nonreversible. Initially, the disease manifests with loss of short-term memory, forgetfulness, and a decrease in social and vocational abilities. The patient may become lost in familiar surroundings, and personality changes may develop. As the disease progresses, the patient can no longer cope without assistance and becomes disoriented to time and place. Delusions, depression, agitation, and language difficulties are noted. Finally, severe intellectual impairment and complete disorientation are seen. Verbal skills are lost, motor skills deteriorate, and self-care activities may be impossible. Urinary and fecal incontinence are common, and clients may become bedridden. Death usually results from infection.

At present, there is no clear evidence that Alzheimer's disease alters nutritional requirements. However, it can have a devastating impact on the nutritional status. Early in the disease, impairments in memory and judgment may make shopping, storing, and cooking food difficult. The client may forget to eat or may forget that he or she has already eaten and, consequently, eat again. Changes in the sense of smell and in food preferences may also develop. A preference for sweet and salty foods is noted, and unusual food choices may occur. Agitation increases energy expenditure, and calorie requirements may increase by as much as 1600 cal/day. Weight loss is common. Choking may occur if the client forgets to chew food sufficiently before swallowing or hoards food in the mouth. Eating of nonfood items may occur, and eventually self-feeding ability is lost.

Nutritional interventions that may be appropriate for clients with Alzheimer's disease include the following recommendations:

- Closely supervise mealtime; check food temperatures to prevent accidental mouth burns.
- Serve meals in the same place at the same time each day, and keep distractions to a minimum.
- Minimize confusion by providing a nonselected menu based on the patient's likes and dislikes, if known.
- Provide one food at a time; a whole tray of foods may be overwhelming.
- Provide between-meal snacks that are easy to consume, such as sandwiches, beverages, and finger foods.
- Modify food consistency as needed, cutting food into small pieces and reminding the client to chew to avoid choking. Physical assistance (eg, lightly stroking the underside of the chin) may be needed to promote swallowing.
- Monitor weight closely.
- Clients in the latter stage of Alzheimer's disease are not only unable to feed themselves but also no longer know what to do when food is placed in the mouth. When this occurs, a decision regarding the use of other means of nutritional support (ie, nasogastric or percutaneous endoscopic gastrostomy tube feedings) must be made.

Obesity

Obesity is common into the sixth and seventh decades of life and then declines. Although early studies suggested that the risk of death might be somewhat lower for moderately overweight older adults than for those of normal weight, studies that have controlled for smoking have found that excess body weight increases the risk of death from any cause. Although a "reserve" of weight may help older adults withstand the metabolic demands of illness, no benefits have been shown for severe obesity. Obesity may significantly diminish quality of life by impairing mobility and function.

Promoting weight loss in obese older adults presents unique challenges. Many older people may not feel a need to make changes at this point in life. Active participation in physical activity may be difficult because of medical problems, financial limitations, or impaired hearing or vision. Diminished sense of taste, living alone, and limited food budget may impede changes in intake. However, small changes in intake and activity can produce significant benefits in terms of function, health, and quality of life, even if weight loss is only modest.

A low-fat diet with adequate protein and fiber is recommended to promote weight loss in older adults. Daily calorie intake should not be less than 1200 to 1500 cal for women and 1500 to 1800 cal for men. A multivitamin and mineral supplement may be indicated. Increasing activity is encouraged. Appetite suppressants and herbal remedies are not recommended.

Social Isolation

Eating alone is a risk factor for poor nutritional status among older adults; therefore, efforts should be made to eat with friends and relatives whenever possible. Other potential options are the federally funded nutrition programs, congregate meals, and Meals on Wheels. These programs are designed to provide low-cost, nutritious hot meals; education about food and nutrition; opportunities for socialization and recreation; and information on other health and social assistance programs. The congregate meal program provides a hot, balanced, midday meal and the opportunity to socialize in senior citizen centers and other public or private facilities. Those who choose to pay may do so; otherwise, the meal is free. Meals on Wheels is a home-delivered meal program for elderly persons who are unable to get to congregate meal centers because they live in an isolated area or have a chronic illness or disability. Usually a hot meal is served at midday and a bagged lunch is included to be used as the evening meal. Modified diets, such as diabetic diets and low-sodium diets, are provided as needed.

Institutionalization

The typical resident of a long-term care facility has numerous psychosocial, functional, and medical problems that often are complicated by poor nutritional status. Seventy percent of nursing home residents have some organic brain disorder, usually accompanied by dementia. Confusion is the most common symptom. Anorexia and involuntary weight loss may also occur. Common medical diagnoses in nursing home residents include diabetes, congestive heart failure, chronic obstructive pulmonary disease, dysphagia, depression, and hypertension.

Malnutrition is a serious problem in long-term care facilities; an estimated 10% to 85% of institutionalized older adults are affected. Common signs of malnutrition among long-term care residents include anemia, low serum albumin, dry skin, brittle hair or fingernails, dehydration, and slow wound healing. Common problems that affect nutritional status include:

- **Anorexia.** Poor appetite is a widespread complaint among residents in long-term care facilities. Limited food choices, unfamiliarity with the foods offered, loss of favorite or familiar foods, altered meal schedules, and a change in serving style may contribute to poor appetite. Restrictive diets may further limit food choices. Chronic disease, medications, sensory losses, dysphagia, and loss of teeth or poor oral health may impair appetite and intake. Depression, anxiety, and feelings of hopelessness contribute to anorexia.
- **Unintentional weight loss.** Numerous physical and emotional factors may contribute to unintentional weight loss among long-term care residents. Two major causes are dental problems and depression. Unintentional weight loss is correlated with increased mortality, decreased resistance to infections, and increased incidence of pressure ulcers.
- **Pressure ulcers.** Poor nutritional status is one of the contributing factors in the development of pressure ulcers. Institutionalized older adults with pressure ulcers have a fourfold increased risk of death.

Therapeutic Diets in Long-Term Care

The use of therapeutic diets as part of medical care in long-term care facilities is controversial. Although carbohydrate- or calorie-controlled diets may be beneficial for older adults with diabetes or obesity, the goals of preventing malnutrition and maintaining quality of life are of greater priority for most long-term care residents. Restrictive diets have the potential to negatively affect quality of life by eliminating personal choice in meals, dampening appetite, and promoting unintentional weight loss, thereby compromising functional status.

Therapeutic diets should be used only when a significant improvement in health can be expected, as in cases of severe hypertension, ascites, or constipation.

Liberal Diet for Older Adults

Many clinicians recommend a liberalized approach to feeding older adults. Residents in long-term care facilities who receive a liberal diet (Box 13–2) similar to what they were eating at home tend to eat better, have fewer bowel problems, enjoy their meals more, are more alert, and are generally happier than residents receiving therapeutic diets. In addition, studies on the effects of liberalizing therapeutic diets in older adults with hypertension (eg, allowing 4 g of sodium per day instead of 2 g) revealed no notable or unacceptable changes in edema, blood pressure, or weight. Other studies support the liberalization of diets for older adults with hyperlipidemia and diabetes.

Nutrition as a Quality-of-Life Issue

Nutritional interventions that are aimed at maintaining quality of life by preventing overt malnutrition are economically, medically, and ethically desirable. Indeed, prevention of unintentional weight loss and pressure ulcers is a key component of meeting the

BOX 13.2

Sample Liberal Diet for Older Adults

Breakfast
- Orange juice
- Oatmeal
- 1 soft-cooked egg
- 1 slice buttered whole wheat toast
- Low-fat milk
- Coffee/tea
- Salt/pepper/sugar*

Lunch
- Grilled cheese sandwich made with two slices whole wheat bread
- Tomato soup
- Sliced strawberries over angel food cake
- ½ cup low-fat milk
- Coffee/tea
- Salt/pepper/sugar*

Dinner
- Baked chicken
- Steamed brown rice
- Baked acorn squash
- Fresh fruit salad
- Low-fat milk
- Iced milk
- Coffee/tea
- Salt/pepper/sugar*

Snack
- ½ cup low-fat milk
- Bran muffin

*Packages of salt or sugar may be omitted if a restriction of either is appropriate.

quality-of-life regulations in the *Omnibus Budget Reconciliation Act* of 1987 (Public Law No. 101239). Prevention and treatment of both problems require adequate calories and protein. Small, frequent feedings or fortified supplements may help maximize intake. For clients with impaired skin integrity, supplemental vitamin C and zinc may be indicated to promote healing. Frequent monitoring of the resident's intake, acceptance and tolerance of supplements, and hydration status is vital. A low serum albumin concentration is associated with both unintentional weight loss and pressure ulcers and should be monitored.

Commercial supplements are often given between meals to increase the calorie and protein content of a resident's diet. Although they may be temporarily useful, they are generally not well accepted or tolerated on a long-term basis. Taste fatigue and lack of hunger for the meal that follows often occur. Use of supplements as a substitute for food deprives residents of the enjoyment of eating foods of their choice. The potential benefits must be weighed against the potential negative consequences. Another option is to increase the nutrient density of foods served with protein or carbohydrate modules.

To promote optimal intake in an institutional setting, the nurse should make mealtime as enjoyable an experience as possible. Encourage independence in eating, and supervise dining areas so that proper feeding techniques are used when residents are assisted or fed by certified nursing assistants. Food preferences should be honored whenever possible. Family involvement increases residents' intake. Encourage adequate fluid intake. Although protein and calories are frequently the focus of intervention efforts, supplemental vitamins and minerals may be needed to ensure optimal intake.

Ongoing monitoring may include intake observations or intake and output records when a problem is suspected. Because weight loss is one of the most important and sensitive indicators of malnutrition, accurate monthly weighing is vital. More frequent weighings may be necessary if a nutritional problem is suspected. Communicate feeding or eating problems, food intolerances, and significant weight changes to the dietitian for further assessment and intervention.

NURSING PROCESS

Harold Hausman is a regular participant of the monthly congregational nursing program sponsored at his church. He is an 80-year-old widower who lives alone. You have noticed that he has lost weight over the last several months. He has asked you to answer a few questions he has about the low-sodium, low-cholesterol diet his doctor gave him.

Assessment

Obtain clinical data:

Because a medical record is not available, clinical data are limited to Mr. Hausman's weight, height, and blood pressure. Determine BMI.

Interview the client to assess:

Understanding of the rationale for the diet the physician gave him and how it can be implemented in his lifestyle

Ability to understand, attitude toward health and nutrition, and readiness to learn

Attitude about his present weight and recent weight loss

Medical history, including hyperlipidemia, hypertension, cardiovascular disease, or gastrointestinal complaints. Does he know his cholesterol level?

Dentition and ability to swallow

Manner of implementing the low-sodium, low-cholesterol diet. For instance, did he simply not use the saltshaker at the table or did he begin reading labels for sodium content? What sources of fat did he eliminate from his usual diet?

Usual 24-hour intake, including portion size, frequency and pattern of eating, and method of food preparation. Assess appropriateness of usual calorie intake and overall nutritional adequacy based on the Food Guide Pyramid. Assess the appropriateness of the low-sodium, low-cholesterol diet.
Cultural, religious, and ethnic influences on eating habits
Appetite
Functional disabilities, such as impaired ability to shop, cook, and eat. Frequent disabling conditions include arthritis, dementia, heart disease, hip fractures, lung disease, Parkinson's disease, and stroke.
Psychosocial and economic issues, such as the client's living situation, who does the shopping and cooking, adequacy of food budget, need for food assistance, and level of family and social support
Usual activity patterns
Use of prescribed and over-the-counter drugs
Use of vitamins, minerals, and nutritional supplements: which ones, how much, and why they are taken
Use of alcohol, tobacco, and caffeine

Nursing Diagnosis

Altered Nutrition: Less Than Body Requirements, related to inadequate intake as evidenced by weight loss.

Planning and Implementation

CLIENT GOALS

The client will:

Attain/maintain a "healthy" weight
Consume, on average, a varied and balanced diet that meets the recommended number of servings from each of the major food groups

NURSING INTERVENTIONS

Client Teaching

Instruct the client:

On the role of nutrition in maintaining health and quality of life (Box 13–3), including:

- That a balanced diet based on the major food groups can help maximize the quality of life
- That avoiding excess salt is prudent for all people; recommendations on sodium intake should be made on an individual basis according to the client's cardiac and renal status, appetite, and use of medications
- That although it is wise to avoid high-fat, nutrient-poor foods such as most cakes, cookies, pastries, pies, chips, full-fat dairy products, and fried foods,

BOX 13.3

Where to get Additional Information

National Institute of Aging Information Office
Building 31
Room 5C-27
31 Center Drive, MSC 2292
Bethesda, MD 20892
301-496-1754
www.nih.gov/nia

American Association of Retired Persons
601 East St NW
Washington, DC 20049
800-424-3410
www.aarp.org

too severe a fat restriction compromises calorie intake and may result in undesirable weight loss

On eating plan essentials, including the importance of:

- Choosing a varied diet to help ensure an average adequate intake; limiting food choices or skipping a food group increases the risk of both nutrient deficiencies and excesses
- Eating enough food to avoid unfavorable weight loss
- Eating enough high-fiber foods, such as whole-grain breads and cereals, dried peas and beans, and fresh fruits and vegetables
- Drinking at least 8 to 12 glasses of fluid daily, even if he does not feel thirsty

On behavioral matters, including:

- That it is important for the client to discuss the rationale for the low-sodium, low-cholesterol diet with his physician, particularly because he has had an unfavorable weight loss
- How to read labels to identify low-sodium foods

On physical activity goals

Evaluation

The client:

Attains/maintains "healthy" weight

Consumes, on average, a varied and balanced diet that meets the recommended number of servings from each of the major food groups

Questions You May Hear

What strategies can help older people improve their intake when they just have no interest in eating? Encourage the client to eat with others whenever possible. When socialization isn't an option, listening to the radio, watching television, or reading while eating can make eating less of a chore, as can eating by a window, on the porch, or out in the yard. Researchers have shown that appetites of older adults improve when they listen to familiar music from their youth at mealtime. Meals that vary in color, texture, temperature, and flavor are more enticing. Older adults with vision changes should eat in an area that is well lit. Encourage the client to experiment with herbs and spices or try a new recipe.

KEY CONCEPTS

- Although women live longer than men, they have more health problems, especially nutrition-related disease such as cardiovascular disease, certain cancers, osteoporosis, diabetes, and weight-control problems.
- Men have shorter life expectancies than women. This may be related to lifestyle, not simply a matter of biology.
- Aging begins at birth and ends in death. Exactly how and why aging occurs is not known.
- Good eating habits developed early in life promote health in old age.
- As a group, older adults are at risk for nutritional problems because of changes in physiology (including changes in body composition, gastrointestinal tract, metabolism, central nervous system, renal system, and the senses), changes in income, changes in health, and psychosocial changes.
- Older adults represent a heterogeneous population that varies in health, activity, and nutritional status. Generalizations about nutritional requirements are less accurate for this age group than for others.
- Goals of diet intervention for older adults are to maintain or restore maximal independent functioning and to maintain quality of life. Except when a significant improvement in health can be expected, therapeutic diets may not be appropriate for older adults and may actually promote malnutrition.
- Institutionalized older adults are at high risk for malnutrition. Preventive efforts should focus on maintaining an adequate intake. Honor special requests, encourage food from home, and provide assistance with eating as needed.
- Weight loss, low serum albumin, and impaired skin integrity increase the need for calories and protein. Increasing nutrient density without increasing the volume of food served (eg, adding protein powder to fluid milk or nonfat dried milk, butter, and sugar to cooked cereal) may be the most effective method of delivering additional nutrients. However, between-meal supplements may also be needed to maximize intake.
- As a group, the elderly are more prone to drug-nutrient interactions and drug-induced nutritional deficiencies.

Focus on Critical Thinking

Bertha Wicks is an 86-year-old, newly admitted resident of a nursing home. She is 5 feet tall, weighs 103 pounds, and has recently been hospitalized for a broken hip, which was surgically repaired. She has a history of glucose intolerance, although her glucose has been within normal limits since she lost 13 pounds while in the hospital. However, her physician has ordered a 1400-calorie diet for her. She is legally blind. Mrs. Wicks is very unhappy about being institutionalized. She complains that the other residents are "old ladies" and refuses to eat with them in the dining room. She hates the food, and her family is concerned that she will continue to lose weight.

- Identify risk factors and major and minor indicators of poor nutritional status that are exhibited by Bertha Wicks.
- Is Mrs. Wicks' current diet order adequate and appropriate? Support your answers.
- What diet would you recommend for Mrs. Wicks?
- What interventions could you try to improve her intake?

ANSWER KEY

1. **TRUE** A plant-based diet rich in fruits, vegetables, and whole-grains appears protective against breast and colorectal cancers. A high intake of fruits and vegetables also may protect against lung cancer.
2. **FALSE** It appears that lifestyle, not biology, is the basis for longevity differences between the genders.
3. **FALSE** Strength training exercises can maintain or restore muscle mass and boost metabolic rate.
4. **TRUE** Older adults are prone to dehydration, because the thirst sensation decreases in old age.
5. **FALSE** Many older adults lack sufficient gastric acid to liberate natural vitamin B_{12} bound to protein in foods. Synthetic vitamin B_{12} in fortified foods and supplements is not bound and is, therefore, readily absorbed.
6. **TRUE** Intake and absorption of calcium decrease with age.
7. **FALSE** As many as two thirds of independently living older adults consume inadequate diets.
8. **TRUE** Actually, the nutritional status of people older than 70 years of age varies more than that of people in any other age group.
9. **TRUE** Institutionalized older adults are at high risk for malnutrition, and anorexia, unintentional weight loss, and pressure ulcers all affect nutritional status.
10. **TRUE** No benefits from severe obesity have been demonstrated. Obesity may significantly alter the quality of life by impairing mobility and function.

REFERENCES

Administration on Aging. (1994). *Food and nutrition for life: Malnutrition and older Americans*. Report by the Assistant Secretary for Aging prepared by National Eldercare Institute on Nutrition. Washington, DC: U.S. Department of Health and Human Services.

Aldrich, J., & Massey, L. (1999). A liberalized geriatric diet fits most dietary prescriptions for long-term-care residents. *Journal of the American Dietetic Association*, 99, 478–480.

American Dietetic Association. (1998). Position of the American Dietetic Association: Liberalized diets for older adults in long-term care. *Journal of the American Dietetic Association*, 98, 201–204.

American Dietetic Association. (1999). Position of the American Dietetic Association and Dietitians of Canada: Women's health and nutrition. *Journal of the American Dietetic Association*, 99, 738–751.

Campbell, W., Crim, M., Dallal, G., Young, V., & Evans, W. (1994). Increased protein requirements in elderly people: New data and retrospective reassessments. *American Journal of Clinical Nutrition*, 60, 501–509.

Gallagher-Allred, C. (1992). OBRA: *A challenge and an opportunity for nutrition care*. Columbus, OH: Ross Laboratories.

Gentry, M. (Ed.). (2000). The straight story on soy. *American Institute for Cancer Research Newsletter*, 67, 5.

Halm, M., & Penque, S. (1999). Heart disease in women. *American Journal of Nursing*, 99, 26–31.

Ho, C., Kauwell, G., & Bailey, L. (1999). Practitioners' guide to meeting the vitamin B_{12} Recommended Dietary Allowance for people aged 51 years and older. *Journal of the American Dietetic Association*, 99, 725–727.

Jackobs, M. (1999). Good nutrition just one health obstacle for the institutionalized elderly. *Journal of the American Dietetic Association*, 99, 722.

Jensen, G., & Rogers, J. (1998). Obesity in older persons. *Journal of the American Dietetic Association*, 98, 1308–1311.

Kerschner, H., & Pegues, J. (1998). Productive aging: A quality of life agenda. *Journal of the American Dietetic Association*, 98, 1445–1448.

National Research Council. (1989). *Recommended Dietary Allowances* (10th ed.). Washington, DC: National Academy Press.

National Women's Health Information Center. [On-line]. Available: http://www.4women.org. Accessed February 17, 2000.

Nutrition Screening Initiative. (1991). *Nutrition screening manual for professionals caring for older Americans*. Washington, DC: Greer, Margolis, Mitchell, Grunwald, & Associates, Inc.

Porter, C., Schell, E., Kayser-Jones, J., & Paul, S. (1999). Dynamics of nutrition care among nursing home residents who are eating poorly. *Journal of the American Dietetic Association*, 99, 1444–1446.

Spangler, A., & Eigenbrod, J. (1995). Field trial affirms value of DETERMINEing nutrition-related problems of freeliving elderly. *Journal of the American Dietetic Association*, 95, 489–490.

Standing Committee on the Scientific Evaluation of Dietary Reference Intakes, Food and Nutrition Board, Institute of Medicine. (1997). *Dietary Reference Intakes for calcium, phosphorus, magnesium, vitamin D, and fluoride*. Washington, DC: National Academy Press.

Vozenilek, G. (1998). Grandma eats like a bird: Helping caregivers improve the nutrition of older persons at home. *Journal of the American Dietetic Association*, 98, 1405.

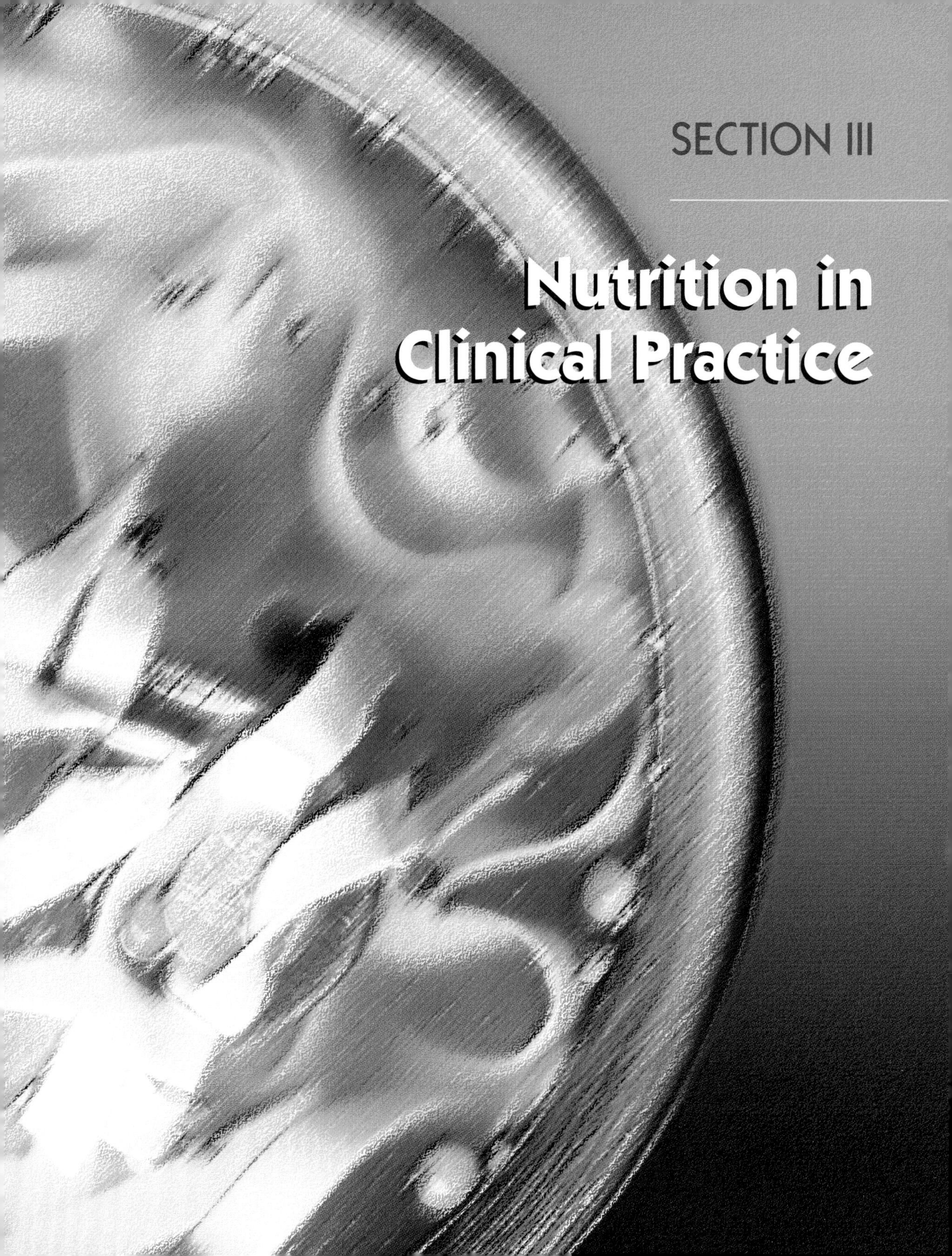

SECTION III

Nutrition in Clinical Practice

CHAPTER 14

Obesity and Eating Disorders

TRUE	FALSE	Check your knowledge of obesity and eating disorders.
		1 It is acceptable to weigh any weight within the appropriate weight range for your height.
		2 People shaped like "apples" have greater health risks than people shaped like "pears."
		3 Anyone with a high body mass index (BMI) is at risk for health problems.
		4 Inactivity is a major cause of obesity in Americans.
		5 The goal for people who are overweight or obese is to lose enough weight to get to the upper limit of their healthy weight range.
		6 If a person will try only one strategy, lowering calories is more effective at promoting short-term weight loss than is increasing activity.
		7 Even if weight loss does not occur, increasing activity helps lower blood pressure and improve glucose tolerance.
		8 People who eat fewer than 1200 cal may need a multivitamin and mineral supplement.
		9 An effective approach to weight loss is to eat less fat, regardless of total calorie intake.
		10 Bulimia poses fewer nutritional problems than anorexia does.

Upon completion of this chapter, you will be able to

- Describe the following standards used to evaluate weight: BMI, waist circumference, and risk status.
- Define overweight and obesity.
- List etiologic factors that may be involved in the development of obesity.
- Discuss the role of each of the following in the treatment of obesity: low-calorie diets, exercise, behavior therapy, medication, and surgery.
- List five tips for controlling calorie intake.
- List five behavior modification ideas.
- Describe nutritional interventions used in the treatment of eating disorders.

Obesity

Issues of weight are a pervasive concern in American culture. According to results from the U.S. Department of Agriculture's tenth nationwide food consumption survey (1994–1996), more than 90% of adults acknowledge that it is important to maintain a healthy weight. Yet the prevalence of obesity continues to grow at an astounding rate. Currently more than half of all American adults are either overweight or obese. Dieting is a national pastime, with approximately 25% of men and 45% of women trying to lose weight at any given time. The proliferation of "diet" foods, "diet" books, and "diet" programs adds up to a business of more than $33 billion annually. A far less common weight issue is disordered eating manifested as anorexia nervosa or bulimia. From the best sellers list to television talk shows, weight is a hot topic in the United States.

This chapter explores the concept of "normal" weight and how weight is evaluated. The complications, prevalence, and treatment of obesity are presented. Eating disorders and their nutritional management are discussed.

"Normal" Weight

Normal weight and *healthy weight* are imprecisely defined terms used to describe weight ranges based on height that are statistically related to good health. Weights lower or higher than these ranges increase the risk of health problems. However, not all weights within a range are appropriate for all individuals, and some people may define their own "normal" weight above or below the recommended range based on how they feel physically or mentally. "Normal" for an individual may differ from "normal" for a population.

Normal weight ranges are a place to begin evaluating a client's weight. Keep in mind that weight tables are imperfect, limited, and often controversial: Overweight people may regard them as overly harsh, whereas people who are underweight may argue that they are inflated.

"HEALTHY" WEIGHT

The Report of Dietary Guidelines Advisory Committee on the *Dietary Guidelines for Americans*, 1995 includes a recommended "healthy" weight range guide that is reproduced in Table 14–1. These weights apply to adult men and women of all ages. Ranges, rather than single weights, are shown because people of the same height may have equal amounts of body fat but different amounts of bone and muscle, which results in different weights for height but does not increase health risks. The ranges are not intended to encourage people at the low end of the range to gain weight.

TABLE 14.1 *Healthy Weight Ranges for Men and Women*

Height*	Weight in Pounds†
4′10″	91–119
4′11″	94–124
5′0″	97–128
5′1″	101–132
5′2″	104–137
5′3″	107–141
5′4″	111–146
5′5″	114–150
5′6″	118–155
5′7″	121–160
5′8″	125–164
5′9″	129–169
5′10″	132–174
5′11″	136–179
6′0″	140–184
6′1″	144–189
6′2″	148–195
6′3″	152–200
6′4″	156–205
6′5″	160–211
6′6″	164–216

*Without shoes.
†Without clothes.
Report of the Dietary Guidelines Advisory Committee on the Dietary Guidelines for Americans, 1995.

METROPOLITAN LIFE INSURANCE TABLES

Another frequently used weight table is the Metropolitan Life Insurance Table (Table 14–2). Although the weights indicated in the most recent edition (1983) of these tables are associated with the lowest mortality rate, they are not labeled "ideal" and are heavier values than were included in previous tables.

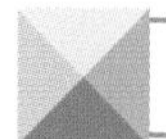

Standards for Evaluating Weight

The relationship between body weight and good health is more complicated than simply comparing the number on the scale to a weight range table. The amount of body fat a person has and how a person's weight is distributed also influence disease risks. For instance, someone may be overweight but not overfat and, therefore, does not have higher

TABLE 14.2 *1983 Metropolitan Life Insurance Company Height and Weight Tables*

Height	Small Frame	Medium Frame	Large Frame
	←	*lb*	→
Men*			
5′2″	128–134	131–141	138–150
5′3″	130–136	133–143	140–153
5′4″	132–138	135–145	142–156
5′5″	134–140	137–148	144–160
5′6″	136–142	139–151	146–164
5′7″	138–145	142–154	149–168
5′8″	140–148	145–157	152–172
5′9″	142–151	148–160	155–176
5′10″	144–154	151–163	158–180
5′11″	146–157	154–166	161–184
6′0″	149–160	157–170	164–188
6′1″	152–164	160–174	168–192
6′2″	155–168	164–178	172–197
6′3″	158–172	167–182	176–202
6′4″	162–176	171–187	181–207
Women†			
4′10″	102–111	109–121	118–131
4′11″	103–113	111–123	120–134
5′0″	104–115	113–126	122–137
5′1″	106–118	115–129	125–140
5′2″	108–121	118–132	128–143
5′3″	111–124	121–135	131–147
5′4″	114–127	124–138	134–151
5′5″	117–130	127–141	137–155
5′6″	120–133	130–144	140–159
5′7″	123–136	133–147	143–163
5′8″	126–139	136–150	146–167
5′9″	129–142	139–153	149–170
5′10″	132–145	142–156	152–173
5′11″	135–148	145–159	155–176
6′0″	138–151	148–162	158–179

*Weights at ages 25 to 59 based on lowest mortality. Weight in pounds according to frame (in indoor clothing weighing 5 lb, shoes with 1″ heels).

†Weights at ages 25 to 59 based on lowest mortality. Weight in pounds according to frame (in indoor clothing weighing 3 lb, shoes with 1″ heels).

Courtesy of Metropolitan Life Insurance Company.

disease risks, as is the case with very muscular athletes. Also, the presence of certain diseases or conditions (comorbidities) affects overall disease risks related to weight. Ideally, BMI (body fat), waist circumference (weight distribution), and overall risk status are all considered when evaluating a client's weight status and identifying who might benefit from treatment. A client's motivation to lose weight should also be assessed.

EVALUATING BODY FAT

Body Mass Index

Body fat can be accurately assessed by several sophisticated methods. For instance, underwater weighing (densitometry) involves submerging the client in water. Computed tomography is an imaging technique that can be used to determine body fat composition. These methods are impractical because they are expensive and not readily available. With bioelectrical impedance analysis (BIA), a mild electric charge is used to estimate lean body mass. The amount of body fat is then calculated by subtracting lean body mass weight from total weight. BIA is safe, inexpensive, easy to perform, and relatively accurate, but it is not sensitive enough to detect short-term changes in body fat. In practice, the BMI has become the medical standard for assessing body fatness.

BMI, defined as the weight in kilograms divided by the square of the height in meters, describes relative weight for height (Box 14–1). It provides an acceptable estimation of total body fat for most people, and it is considered the best method of assessing overweight and obesity. Ultimately, the BMI is used to estimate a client's relative risk for disease compared with people of normal weight. Nomograms and tables have been developed to eliminate complicated mathematical calculations (Table 14–3).

Using BMI to evaluate body weight is inexpensive, nonthreatening, and noninvasive to clients and requires minimal equipment and skill. The major disadvantage of

BOX 14.1

Calculating Body Mass Index (BMI)

Joe is 5 ft 10 in tall and weighs 172 lb. To determine his BMI:

1. Convert weight into kilograms.
   a. 172 lb ÷ 2.2 lb/kg = 78.2 kg
2. Convert height into meters.
   a. 5′10″ = 70″ (5′ × 12″ = 60″ + 10″ = 70″)
   b. 70″ × 2.54 cm/in = 177.8 cm
   c. 177.8 cm ÷ 100 cm = 1.8 m
   1.8 meters squared = 3.2 meters (1.8 × 1.8 = 3.24)
3. Calculate BMI.
   a. 78.2 ÷ 3.2 = 24.43

TABLE 14.3 ***National Heart, Lung, and Blood Institute. Obesity Guidelines Executive Summary BMI Chart***

Body Mass Index Chart

Height (inches)	19	20	21	22	23	24	25	26	27	28	29	30	31	32	33	34	35	36
	Body Weight (pounds)																	
58	91	96	100	105	110	115	119	124	129	134	138	143	148	153	158	162	167	172
59	94	99	104	109	114	119	124	128	133	138	143	148	153	158	163	168	173	178
60	97	102	107	112	118	123	128	133	138	143	148	153	158	163	168	174	179	184
61	100	106	111	116	122	127	132	137	143	148	153	158	164	169	174	180	185	190
62	104	109	115	120	126	131	136	142	147	153	158	164	169	175	180	186	191	196
63	107	113	118	124	130	135	141	146	152	158	163	169	175	180	186	191	197	203
64	110	116	122	128	134	140	145	151	157	163	169	174	180	186	192	197	204	209
65	114	120	126	132	138	144	150	156	162	168	174	180	186	192	198	204	210	216
66	118	124	130	136	142	148	155	161	167	173	179	186	192	198	204	210	216	223
67	121	127	134	140	146	153	159	166	172	178	185	191	198	204	211	217	223	230
68	125	131	138	144	151	158	164	171	177	184	190	197	203	210	216	223	230	236
69	128	135	142	149	155	162	169	176	182	189	196	203	209	216	223	230	236	243
70	132	139	146	153	160	167	174	181	188	195	202	209	216	222	229	236	243	250
71	136	143	150	157	165	172	179	186	193	200	208	215	222	229	236	243	250	257
72	140	147	154	162	169	177	184	191	199	206	213	221	228	235	242	250	258	265
73	144	151	159	166	174	182	189	197	204	212	219	227	235	242	250	257	265	272
74	148	155	163	171	179	186	194	202	210	218	225	233	241	249	256	264	272	280
75	152	160	168	176	184	192	200	208	216	224	232	240	248	256	264	272	279	287
76	156	164	172	180	189	197	205	213	221	230	238	246	254	263	271	279	287	295

To use this table, find the appropriate height in the left-hand column. Move across to a given weight. The number at the top of the column is the BMI at that height and weight. Pounds have been rounded off.

using BMI is that weight can be elevated for reasons other than excess fat, such as large muscle mass or edema. The BMI levels assigned to define overweight and obesity are somewhat arbitrary in that the relationship between increasing weight and risk of disease is continuous. The cutoff points for overweight and obesity have varied over time and among experts. The current guidelines used by the Obesity Education Initiative of the National Heart, Lung, and Blood Institute (NHLBI) to assess BMI are as follows:

Classification	BMI
Underweight	<18.5
Normal	18.5–24.9
Overweight	25.0–29.9
Obesity	≥30.0

TABLE 14.3 ***National Heart, Lung, and Blood Institute. Obesity Guidelines Executive Summary BMI Chart (continued)***

	37	38	39	40	41	42	43	44	45	46	47	48	49	50	51	52	53	54
Height (inches)	*Body Weight (pounds)*																	
58	177	181	186	191	196	201	205	210	215	220	224	229	234	239	244	248	253	258
59	183	188	193	198	203	208	212	217	222	227	232	237	242	247	252	257	262	267
60	189	194	199	204	209	215	220	225	230	235	240	245	250	255	261	266	271	276
61	195	201	206	211	217	222	227	232	238	243	248	254	259	264	269	275	280	285
62	202	207	213	218	224	229	235	240	246	251	256	262	267	273	278	284	289	295
63	208	214	220	225	231	237	242	248	254	259	265	270	278	282	287	293	299	304
64	215	221	227	232	238	244	250	256	262	267	273	279	285	291	296	302	308	314
65	222	228	234	240	246	252	258	264	270	276	282	288	294	300	306	312	318	324
66	229	235	241	247	253	260	266	272	278	284	291	297	303	309	315	322	328	334
67	236	242	249	255	261	268	274	280	287	293	299	306	312	319	325	331	338	344
68	243	249	256	262	269	276	282	289	295	302	308	315	322	328	335	341	348	354
69	250	257	263	270	277	284	291	297	304	311	318	324	331	338	345	351	358	365
70	257	264	271	278	285	292	299	306	313	320	327	334	341	348	355	362	369	376
71	265	272	279	286	293	301	308	315	322	329	338	343	351	358	365	372	379	386
72	272	279	287	294	302	309	316	324	331	338	346	353	361	368	375	383	390	397
73	280	288	295	302	310	318	325	333	340	348	355	363	371	378	386	393	401	408
74	287	295	303	311	319	326	334	342	350	358	365	373	381	389	396	404	412	420
75	295	303	311	319	327	335	343	351	359	367	375	383	391	399	407	415	423	431
76	304	312	320	328	336	344	353	361	369	377	385	394	402	410	418	426	435	443

Skinfold Measurements

Because approximately half of total body fat is located directly under the skin, accurate assessment of subcutaneous fat stores via skinfold measurements provides an index of percent body fat. Skinfolds are measured with a pair of calipers that pinches the skin to the nearest 1.0 mm as the skin is pulled away from the underlying muscle. Sites measured include the triceps, biceps, thigh, calf, and subscapular and suprailiac skinfolds.

Although skinfold measurements may accurately assess percent body fat, they are not widely used to assess or monitor weight status. Validity is one consideration: A client may have a disproportionate amount of fat located in the arm and yet not be an overfat person. That is why it is recommended that multiple sites be measured. Reliability is also a concern, because the test depends on the expertise of the person using the calipers, the accuracy of the calipers, and the appropriateness of the conversion equations used to determine percent body fat. Skinfold measurements are more often used by athletes and ex-

TABLE 14.4 *Classification of Percent Body Fat*

Classification	Appearance	Percent Body Fat	
		Men	*Women*
Very low fat	Skinny	7–10	14–17
Low fat	Thin	10–13	17–20
Average	Normal	13–17	20–27
Above normal	Plump	17–25	27–31
Very high	Fat	>25	>31

ercise enthusiasts working toward optimal fitness than as a tool for assessing percent body fat in the general population. A guide for evaluating percent body fat appears in Table 14-4.

EVALUATING WEIGHT DISTRIBUTION: WAIST CIRCUMFERENCE

Where excess body fat is deposited may be a more important and reliable indicator of disease risk than the degree of total body fatness. Generally, men and postmenopausal women tend to store fat in the upper body, particularly in the abdominal area, whereas premenopausal women tend to store fat in the lower body, particularly in the hips and thighs. Regardless of gender, people with a high distribution of abdominal fat (ie, "apples") have a greater health risk than people with excess fat in the hips and thighs. (ie, "pears") (Fig. 14-1). Although the mechanisms are not clear, increased abdominal fat increases risks for type 2 diabetes, dyslipidemia, hypertension, and cardiovascular disease.

Waist circumference is positively correlated with abdominal fat content and provides an independent prediction of risk over and above that of BMI. A higher relative risk of obesity-related problems occurs when waist circumference exceeds 40 inches in men or 35 inches in women. However, in people with a BMI of 35 or higher, waist measurement is unnecessary because disease risk is already high based on BMI alone. At very high BMIs, waist measurements lose their predictive power.

EVALUATING RISK STATUS

Obesity increases the risk of developing certain diseases and increases the morbidity of certain existing disorders. The presence of existing health problems must be evaluated to determine a person's absolute risk related to weight and to identify interventions necessary to control those risks.

- **Established diseases.** People with the following conditions are classified as being at very high risk for disease complications and mortality related to overweight and obesity: established coronary heart disease, other atherosclerotic diseases, type 2 diabetes, and sleep apnea.

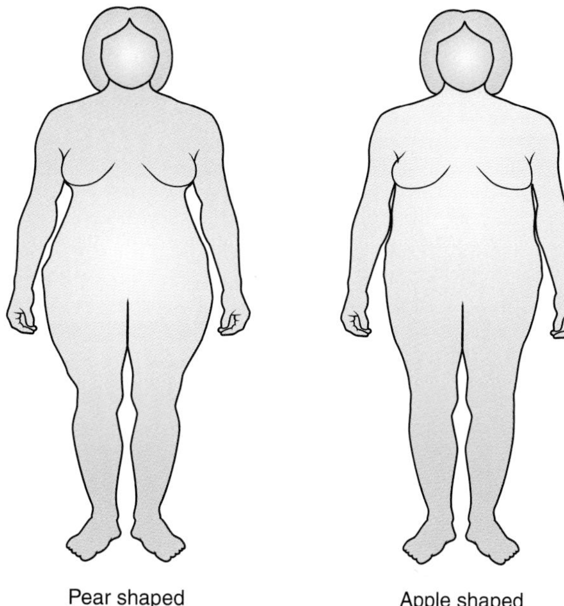

FIGURE 14-1 "Pear" shape versus "apple" shape.

- **Other obesity-related diseases.** The following conditions are not generally life-threatening but require identification and appropriate management: gynecologic abnormalities, osteoarthritis, gallstones and their complications, and stress incontinence.
- **Cardiovascular risk factors that reveal a high absolute risk.** A high absolute risk for obesity-related disorders occurs when a person has three or more of the following risk factors: cigarette smoking, hypertension, high concentration of low-density lipoprotein (LDL)–cholesterol, low concentration of high-density lipoprotein (HDL)–cholesterol, impaired fasting glucose, family history of premature heart disease, and age (45 years or older for men, 55 years or older for women).
- **Other risk factors.** The presence of the following risk factors indicates higher absolute risk above that estimated from the preceding risk factors: physical inactivity and high serum triglycerides.

EVALUATING MOTIVATION TO LOSE WEIGHT

It is essential to assess the client's level of motivation before beginning weight loss therapy. Assess the following factors:

- **Reasons and motivation for weight loss.** Weight loss is not likely to occur in people who are not motivated to lose weight. Is the client ready to make a lifelong commitment to lifestyle change?

- **Previous history of successful and unsuccessful attempts at weight loss.** What does the client see as reasons why previous attempts failed or succeeded?
- **Family, friends, and worksite support.** Determine who may help the client achieve his or her goals.
- **Understanding of the causes of obesity and its impact on disease risk.** Is the client aware of how obesity influences overall health? Is the client concerned about disease risks?
- **Attitude toward physical activity.** Is the client willing to increase activity? Is the client willing to commit time to exercise consistently?
- **Capacity to participate in physical activity.** In what activities is the client physically capable of participating?
- **Time available for weight loss intervention.** Is the client able to commit the time necessary to interact with health professionals for weight loss therapy?
- **Financial considerations.** Is the client able and willing to pay for weight loss therapy that is not covered by health insurance?
- **Barriers to success.** What or who does the client anticipate will hinder his or her ability to succeed? For instance, overweight friends may not support the client's lifestyle change efforts because of their own fears or insecurities.

Overweight and Obesity

Overweight and *obese* are terms frequently used interchangeably, even though they vary by degree. By definition, people with a BMI of 25 to 29.9 are considered overweight and those with a BMI of 30 or higher are obese. The terms are not mutually exclusive, since obese people are also overweight.

ETIOLOGIC FACTORS

The basic mechanism of overweight and obesity is an imbalance between calorie intake and calorie output. When energy consumption exceeds energy expenditure, a positive energy balance results, leading to weight gain over time. This positive balance can be caused by overeating, inactivity, or, most often, a combination of both. For instance, 1 pound of body fat equals 3500 cal; therefore, eating 500 extra calories per day for 7 days will produce a 1-pound weight gain. A person will gain 2 pounds in 1 week if daily intake exceeds expenditure by 1000 cal/day. Even a seemingly insignificant one extra glass of soft drink that supplies 145 cal will produce a 15-pound weight gain in a year if it is consumed daily and is not offset by an increase in activity:

$$145 \text{ cal} \times 365 \text{ d/y} = 52{,}925 \text{ cal/y excess}$$
$$52{,}925 \text{ cal/y} \div 3500 \text{ cal/lb} = 15 \text{ lb/y weight gain}$$

Yet the relationship between calorie intake and weight status is much more complex. For instance, in some people, the body seemingly compensates for variations in calorie intake by adjusting the rate at which it burns calories during inactivity. The "set point" theory of weight control has long proposed that when weight falls below what the body has determined to be "ideal," metabolic rate is adjusted downward to reduce energy expenditure and conserve fat stores. Newer studies show that when calorie intake increases, some people are able to burn hundreds of extra calories in the activities of daily living to help control weight. These results suggest that the reason some people gain weight from overeating and others do not is related to whether this compensatory increase in nonexercise energy expenditure occurs.

Obesity is a complex and multifactorial chronic disease. Exactly how and why obesity develops is not fully understood. It is likely that the imbalance between calorie intake and calorie expenditure leading to the accumulation of fat is related to a combination of the following factors:

- **Genetics.** Understanding of the role of genetics in weight management is incomplete. It is known that a family history of obesity increases the chance of becoming obese by 25% to 30%. Body fat distribution is also influenced by genetics. In addition, genetic defects have been found to alter levels of leptin, a protein that helps regulate metabolism and appetite. It is not known whether alteration of leptin levels can be used to help treat obesity.
- **Nutrition factors.** Excessive food intake contributes to obesity, and diets high in fat contribute to excessive calorie intake. Although the percentage of calories from fat in the average American diet has slightly decreased in recent years, this has resulted from an increase in total calorie intake, not a significant decrease in total fat grams consumed.
- **Level of activity.** Inactivity has been identified as a major cause of obesity among Americans. Only 22% of American adults meet the recommendation to be regularly active for 30 minutes/day. The proliferation of labor-saving devices and decreased leisure time are among the factors contributing to the overall decline in physical activity. Whether inactivity leads to weight gain or weight gain leads to inactivity, the snowball effect perpetuates obesity, that is, inactivity can lead to increased weight, and weight gain can lead to social isolation and further reduction in activity (Fig. 14–2).
- **Environmental influences.** The abundance of food, the frequency of eating out, and technologic advances that save labor contribute to overconsumption of calories.
- **Sociocultural factors.** Sociocultural factors, such as ethnicity, race, gender, income, and education, are important influences on the prevalence of obesity.

PREVALENCE OF OVERWEIGHT AND OBESITY

According to the third National Health and Nutrition Examination Survey (NHANES III) data, 54.9% of Americans aged 20 years and older are overweight or obese. More specifically, 32.6% of adults are overweight (BMI 25–29.9), and 22.3% are obese (BMI ≥30). Generally, overweight and obesity (BMI ≥25):

- Are less common after the age of 70 years.

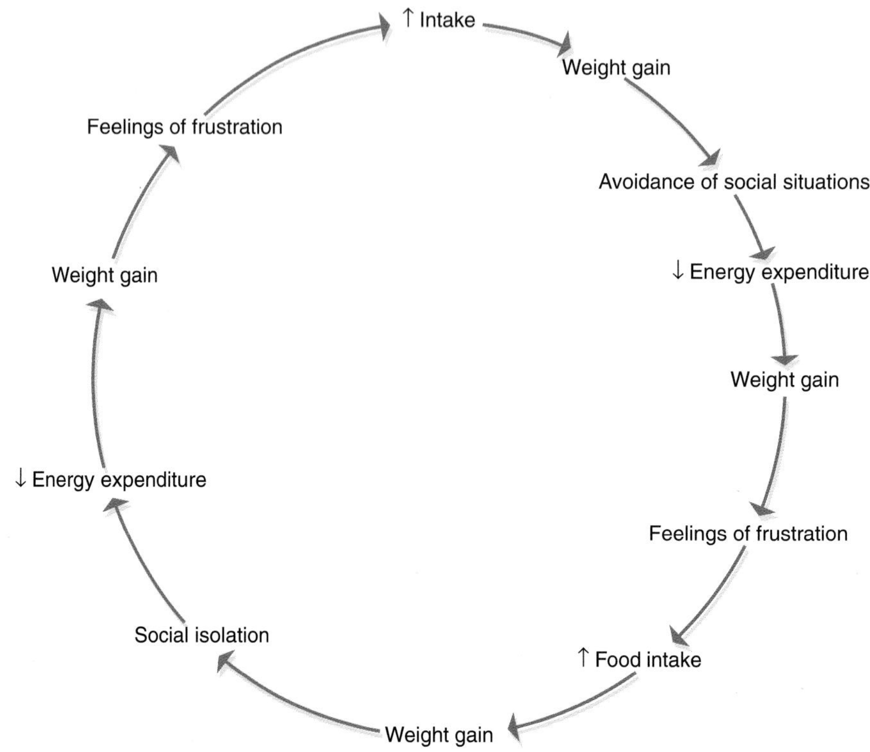

FIGURE 14-2 Perpetuating cycle of inactivity and weight gain.

- Are more prevalent in racial-ethnic minority populations, especially among African-American and Hispanic women, in whom the prevalence of obesity is approximately 60%. The exception to this generalization are Asian-Americans, who have a much lower prevalence of overweight and obesity than the general population.
- Are more prevalent among women with low income or low education than those of higher socioeconomic status. The relationship between socioeconomic status and obesity in men is less consistent.

ECONOMIC AND HEALTH COSTS OF OBESITY

In the United States, the estimated annual health care cost attributed to obesity is approximately $70 billion. A BMI of 25 or higher increases the risk of morbidity from hypertension, dyslipidemia, type 2 diabetes, coronary heart disease, stroke, gallbladder disease, osteoarthritis, sleep apnea and respiratory problems, and cancers of the endometrium, breast, prostate, and colon. Obesity increases surgical risks, and it is associated with complications during pregnancy, labor, and delivery. Higher weights are associated with higher mortality from all causes. Obesity is considered to be a major contributor to preventable deaths in the United States today.

Obesity presents psychological and social disadvantages. In a society that emphasizes thinness, obesity leads to feelings of low self-esteem, negative self-image, and hopelessness. Negative social consequences include stereotyping, prejudice, stigmatization, social isolation, and discrimination in social, educational, and employment settings.

BENEFITS OF WEIGHT LOSS

All people age 18 years and older with a BMI of 25 or higher have the potential to lower their risk of disease by losing weight. Evidence suggests that weight loss in overweight and obese people reduces risk factors for diabetes and cardiovascular disease, which may result in a decrease in morbidity and mortality. Benefits of weight loss include:

- Lower blood pressure in both normotensive and hypertensive people
- Lower serum triglyceride levels
- Higher HDL-cholesterol levels; lower total and LDL-cholesterol
- Lower blood glucose levels in nondiabetics and in some type 2 diabetics

TREATMENT

Health care professionals, including physicians, are not always sufficiently involved in the treatment of obesity. Some fail to recognize obesity as a chronic disease—instead, sharing the societal prejudice that obesity is related to lack of discipline and willpower. Some clinicians are convinced that it is futile to treat obesity because long-term weight loss is poorly maintained by most people. Often, clients treat themselves by using fad diets, over-the-counter appetite suppressants, or fat-burning nutritional supplements or by enrolling in commercial weight loss programs.

Who should be treated for obesity, and how, are topics widely debated. The NHLBI Obesity Education Initiative's Clinical Guidelines Treatment Algorithm is a guide to determining who should be treated for obesity based on BMI, waist circumference, risk factors, and the person's motivation to lose weight (Fig. 14–3). Unfortunately, no single treatment modality or combination of treatment modalities is guaranteed to produce and maintain adequate weight loss in all people.

Weight Loss Goals

The goals of weight loss treatment are to reduce weight and maintain long-term weight loss for the purposes of improving health status and reducing disease risk. Notice that the goal is not to achieve "ideal" weight, even though many clients self-impose that goal for cosmetic reasons or because of societal pressures. Weight loss therapy should refocus to weight management, defined as achieving the best weight possible for the individual in the context of overall health. At the very least, weight loss treatment should prevent further weight gain.

Initial weight loss goals that are unrealistic and overwhelming undermine treatment and are rarely achieved. Fortunately, health benefits can be realized with only a moderate weight loss of 10% of body weight, even if "healthy" weight is not achieved. Compared

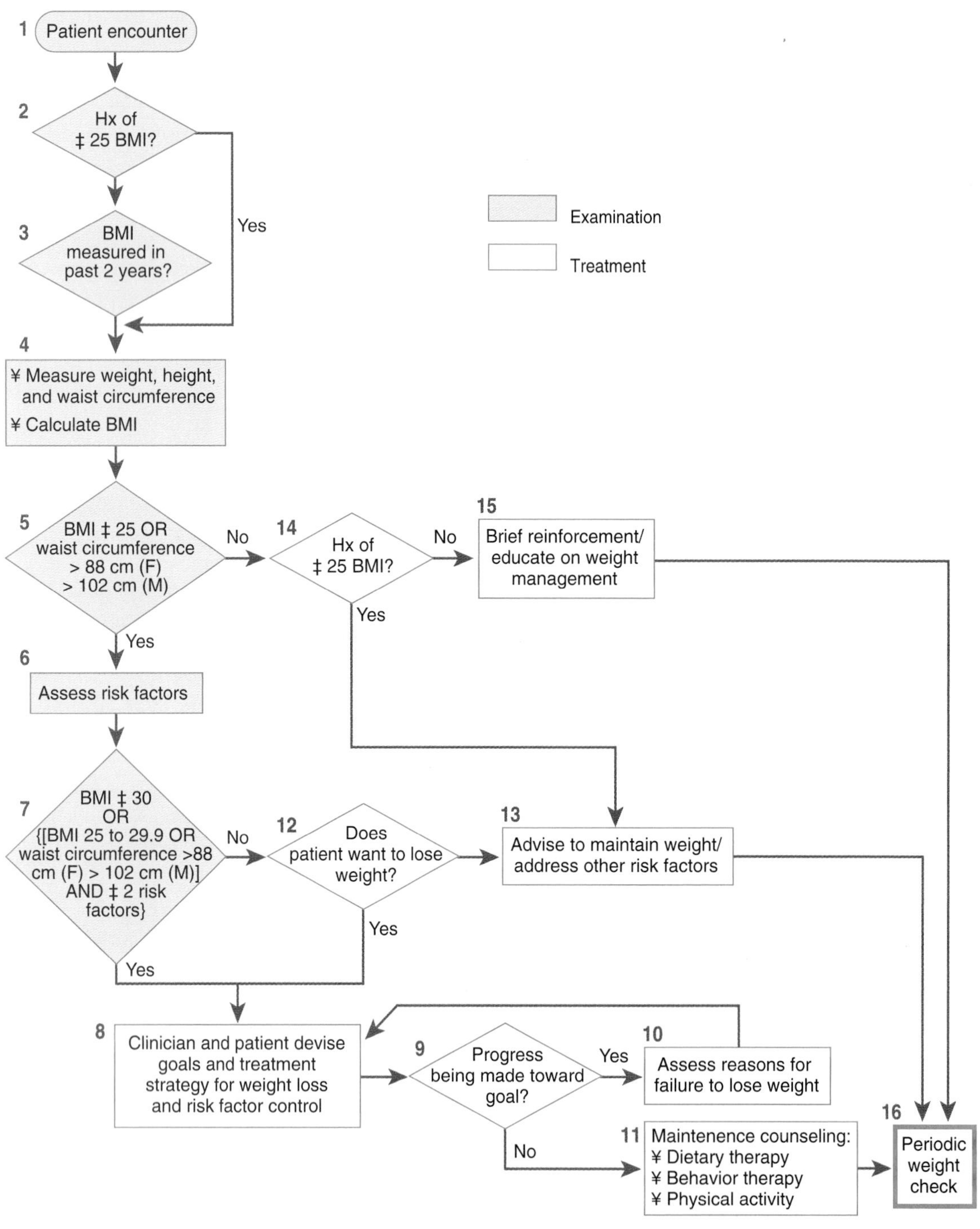

FIGURE 14-3 Treatment algorithm.

with dramatic weight loss, moderate weight loss (1) is more attainable, (2) is easier to maintain over the long term, and (3) sets the stage for subsequent weight loss. An initial weight loss goal of 10% of body weight, or a drop of 1 or 2 BMI units (approximately 10–16 lb below current weight) is achievable and maintainable.

The recommended rate of weight loss is 1 to 2 pounds/week for the first 6 months of weight loss therapy. After 6 months, the rate of weight loss usually decreases and plateaus. It is at this point that the focus should shift to maintenance of weight loss. After weight maintenance has been achieved for 6 months, weight loss efforts can be repeated. Successful long-term weight maintenance is defined by the NHLBI as a weight regain of less than 6.6 pounds in 2 years and a sustained reduction in waist circumference of at least 4 cm.

Clients who are unable to achieve moderate weight loss should strive to prevent additional weight gain. This requires active intervention, not simply maintaining the status quo.

Strategies for Weight Loss and Maintenance

Options to manage weight include nutritional therapy, increased physical activity, behavior therapy, pharmacotherapy, surgery, and combinations of these options.

Nutrition Therapy

DIET APPROACH TO WEIGHT MANAGEMENT

Most weight loss occurs from a decrease in total calorie intake. A nutritionally adequate, individualized eating plan that is mildly restricted in calories and allows for a 1- to 2-pound weight loss per week is the cornerstone of weight loss therapy. The recommended eating plan for weight loss is essentially the Step 1 Diet of the National Cholesterol Education Program with a reduction in total calories (see Chapter 18).

Recommended Eating Plan for Weight Loss

Nutrient	Recommended Intake for Weight Loss
Calories	500–1000 cal/d less than usual intake
Carbohydrates	≥55% of total calories
Protein	~15% of total calories
Fat	≤30% of total calories
Saturated fat	8%–10% of total calories
Monounsaturated fat	≤15% of total calories
Polyunsaturated fat	≤10% of total calories
Cholesterol	<300 mg/d
Sodium	2400 mg/d
Calcium	1000–1500 mg/d
Fiber	20–30 g/d

Generally, calories should not be restricted below 1200 cal/day for adult women or 1500 cal/day for adult men. A sample 1500-cal meal plan and menu appear in Table 14–5. Eating plans that provide less than 1200 cal/day may not provide adequate amounts of essential nutrients. A standard calorie level may be chosen, or calories may be determined on an individual basis by calculating the number of calories needed to maintain healthy body weight and subtracting 500 to 1000 cal/day for a 1- to 2-pound weight loss per week, respectively.

TABLE 14.5 ***Sample Meal Plan and Menu for a 1500-Calorie Intake Based on the American Diabetic Association Exchange Lists***

Exchange	No. of Exchanges (Servings)	Sample Menu
Breakfast		
Fruit	1	½ cup orange juice
Starch	3	½ cup shredded wheat
		1 bagel
Fat	1	2 tbsp reduced-fat cream cheese
Milk, skim	1	1 cup skim milk
Free foods	as desired	coffee, tea
		2 tsp light jelly
Lunch		
Starch	2	1 hamburger bun
Meat, lean	3	3 oz ground-round hamburger
Vegetable	1	1 cup salad made with greens, carrots, onions, mushrooms, and green peppers
Fat	1	1 tbsp regular salad dressing
Fruit	1	1 small apple
Free foods	as desired	1 tbsp ketchup
		mustard
		1 large dill pickle
		coffee, tea
Dinner		
Meat, lean	3	3 oz grilled skinless chicken breast
Starch	2	½ cup rice
		1 cup winter squash
Vegetable	1	½ cup steamed broccoli
Fruit	1	1¼ cup watermelon cubes
Fat	1	1 tsp margarine
Free foods	as desired	sugar-free gelatin
High-starch snack		
Milk, skim	1	1 cup skim milk
Starch	1	3 cups microwave popcorn
Fat	1	

Contains approximately 1482 calories: 54% carbohydrate, 23% protein, 23% fat.

$$500 \text{ cal/d} \times 7 \text{ d/wk} = 3500 \text{ cal/wk deficit}$$
(the equivalent of 1 lb of body weight)
OR
$$1000 \text{ cal/d} \times 7 \text{ d/wk} = 7000 \text{ cal/wk deficit}$$
(the equivalent of 2 lb of body weight)

Lowering fat intake in conjunction with a hypocaloric intake not only promotes greater weight loss but also helps improve blood lipid levels. However, reducing fat intake alone does not cause weight loss unless total calories are also restricted. For instance, substituting low-fat cookies for regular cookies may have no impact on total calorie intake and, therefore, will not promote weight loss.

A hypocaloric intake can be achieved in a variety of ways. Frequently meal plans are devised, similar to those used to manage diabetes. The meal plan specifies the number of servings from each food group "allowed" for each meal and snack. It is used in conjunction with exchange lists that detail items within each food group and appropriate serving sizes. This option provides structure while allowing the client freedom to choose favorite or familiar foods within groups.

A more lax approach recommends total servings to be eaten each day from each of the Food Guide Pyramid food groups based on the total amount of calories desired daily (see Chapter 8). This method produces greater variation in daily calorie intake than use of the exchange lists does, because differences among individual selections within each group are not apparent. For instance, the exchange lists divide the meat group into four parts based on fat content, but no distinctions are made among meat choices in the Food Guide Pyramid.

Table 14–6 represents sample plans for various calorie levels using the Food Guide Pyramid food groups; each plan has fewer than 30% of total calories from fat.

NON-DIET APPROACH TO WEIGHT MANAGEMENT

The virtual obsession Americans have with "dieting" presents many concerns, including:

- The physical and psychological impacts of the pressure to continually diet, especially for women
- The impact of the American ideal of beauty (eg, extremely thin models) on the incidence of eating disorders

TABLE 14.6 ***Plans for Varying Calorie Levels Using Food Guide Pyramid Food Groups***

	Total cal/d			
Food Group	*1200*	*1400*	*1800*	*2000*
Bread, cereal, rice, and pasta (servings)	6	7	8	9
Vegetables (servings)	3	4	5	5
Fruit (servings)	2	3	4	4
Milk and milk products (nonfat servings)	2	2	2	3
Meat and meat alternatives (oz)	4	5	6	6
Fat (from fats, oils, and sweets) (servings)	3	5	6	7

- The changes in food preferences that occur in chronic dieters, namely the increased preference for high-fat, high-sugar foods
- The increased tendency for chronic dieters and restrained eaters to binge eat
- The psychological consequences a failed diet has on the dieter
- Discrimination against fat children and adults
- Long-term health problems associated with certain weight reduction methods

These concerns have led to a relatively new conceptual approach to the nutritional management of obesity: the non-diet paradigm. This approach is based on the fact that most "diets" fail, as evidenced in the growing prevalence of obesity despite the widespread practice of "being on a diet." In fact, research shows that "diets" (food restriction) may lead to binge eating once food is available. Restrictive eating also promotes preoccupation with food and eating and other psychological manifestations. The non-diet approach contends that the negative consequences of "dieting" outweigh the temporary benefits of weight loss. Box 14–2 features the Council on Size and Weight Discrimination's Top Ten Reasons to Give up Dieting.

BOX 14.2

Top Ten Reasons to Give up Dieting

10. **Diets don't work.** Even if you lose weight, you will probably gain it all back and you might gain back more than you lost.
9. **Diets are expensive.** If you did not buy special diet products, you could save enough to get new clothes, which would improve your outlook right now.
8. **Diets are boring.** People on diets talk and think about food and practically nothing else. There's a lot more to life.
7. **Diets don't necessarily improve your health.** Like the weight loss, health improvement is temporary. Dieting can actually cause health problems.
6. **Diets don't make you beautiful.** Very few people will ever look like models. Glamour is a look, not a size. You don't have to be thin to be attractive.
5. **Diets are not sexy.** If you want to feel and be more attractive, take care of your body and your appearance. Feeling healthy makes you look your best.
4. **Diets can turn into eating disorders.** The obsession to be thin can lead to anorexia, bulimia, bingeing, and compulsive exercising.
3. **Diets can make you afraid of food.** Food nourishes and comforts us and gives us pleasure. Dieting can make food seem like your enemy and can deprive you of all the positive things about food.
2. **Diets can rob you of energy.** If you want to lead a full and active life, you need good nutrition and enough food to meet your body's needs.
1. **Learning to love and accept yourself just as you are will give you self-confidence, better health, and a sense of well-being that will last a lifetime.**

 For more information, write: International No Diet, P.O. Box 305, Mt. Marion, NY 12456 or call 914-679-1209.

The non-diet approach is a process-oriented approach to change that addresses size acceptance, disordered eating, eating in response to hunger and satiety, finding pleasure in healthful eating, and enjoying movement without the pressure to follow a precise exercise prescription. It is based on the beliefs that:

- The body will find its natural weight when eating occurs in response to hunger and fullness, not from following a set meal pattern that may not reflect an individual's physiologic state of hunger at any given time.
- All food is acceptable; there are no "good" foods or "bad" foods.
- Eating is self-regulated, internally cued, and nonrestrained.
- Self-esteem and personal power arise from self-regulated eating.
- Bodies come in all shapes and sizes, and being overweight is not synonymous with being in poor health.
- Cultural norms for beauty and size are hazardous.
- A healthy lifestyle that can be maintained indefinitely is the goal, not weight loss or achieving a specific "ideal" weight.

Clients most suited to the non-diet approach are those who are basically healthy and are able to invest time and financial resources in the process. Those who benefit the most are those who:

- Have a history of restrictive dieting and unsuccessful weight loss
- Have food fears
- Do not recognize cues for hunger, satiety, and fullness
- Eat compulsively, binge eat, or restrict food
- Experience food as unsatisfying most of the time
- Have inconsistent activity and exercise patterns
- Relate their self-esteem and self-worth to their weight, food intake, exercise, or appearance

Increasing Physical Activity

Physical activity is a vital component of weight loss therapy, even though it is not likely to produce short-term weight loss unless it used in conjunction with a hypocaloric eating plan. Increasing activity is most helpful in maintaining weight loss.

BENEFITS OF INCREASING ACTIVITY

Physical activity affects obesity in several ways. Increasing activity favorably affects body composition during weight loss by preserving or increasing lean body mass while promoting loss of fat. These changes in body composition result in improved body dimensions and maintenance or an increase in metabolic rate, or both. Activity also reduces abdominal fat, favorably altering the distribution of body fat. Finally, physical activity affects the rate of weight loss in a dose-response manner, based on the frequency and duration of activity.

With or without weight loss, increasing activity lowers blood pressure and triglycerides, increases HDL-cholesterol, and improves glucose tolerance. Subjectively, increased activity improves the sense of well-being, reduces tension, increases agility, and improves alertness. Even without weight loss, an increase in activity improves cardiorespiratory fitness.

RECOMMENDATIONS FOR INCREASING ACTIVITY

Obese clients should change their activity patterns slowly, gradually increasing the frequency, duration, and intensity of exercise. A variety of aerobic activities are suitable, but walking is almost always the most appropriate form of physical activity for obese individuals. An initial goal may be to walk 30 minutes/day for 3 days a week, building to 45 minutes/day of more intense walking at least 5 days/week. This may be accomplished all at once or intermittently throughout the day. In addition, the "everyday" level of activity should be increased, such as taking the stairs instead of the elevator and walking short distances instead of driving. Activity that burns 1500 to 2000 cal/week is suggested as optimal for maintaining weight loss.

Behavior Therapy

Some behavior modification ideas appear in Box 14–3.

BOX 14-3

Behavior Modification Ideas

Think thin

- Make a list of reasons why you want to lose weight.
- Set long-term goals; avoid crash dieting based on getting into a particular dress or weighing a certain weight for an upcoming event or occasion.
- Give yourself a nonfood reward (eg, new clothes, a night of entertainment) for losing weight.
- Don't talk about food.
- Enlist the support of family and friends.
- Learn to distinguish hunger from cravings.

Plan ahead

- Keep food only in the kitchen, not scattered around the house.
- Stay out of the kitchen except when preparing meals and cleaning up.
- Avoid tasting food while cooking; don't take extra portions in order to get rid of a food.
- Place the low-calorie foods in the front of the refrigerator; keep the high-calorie foods hidden.
- Remove temptation to better resist it: "Out of sight, out of mind."
- Keep forbidden foods to a minimum.
- Plan meals, snacks, and grocery shopping to help eliminate hasty decisions and impulses that may sabotage dieting.

Eat wisely

- Wait 10 minutes before eating when you feel the urge; hunger pangs may go away if you delay eating.

(*continued*)

BOX 14.3

Behavior Modification Ideas (continued)

- Never skip meals.
- Eat before you're starving and stop when satisfied, not stuffed.
- Eat only in one designated place and devote all your attention to eating. Activities such as reading and watching television can be so distracting that you may not even realize you ate.
- Serve food directly from the stove to the plate instead of family style, which can lead to large portions and second helpings.
- Eat the low-calorie foods first.
- Drink water with meals.
- Use a small plate to give the appearance of eating a full plate of food.
- Chew food thoroughly and eat slowly.
- Put utensils down between mouthfuls.
- Leave some food on your plate to help you feel in control of food rather than feeling that food controls you.
- Eat before attending a social function that features food; while there, select low-calorie foods to nibble on.
- Don't eat within 3 hours of bedtime.
- Eat satisfying foods and do not restrict particular foods.

Shop smart

- Never shop while hungry.
- Shop only from a list; resist impulse buying.
- Buy food only in the quantity you need.
- Don't buy foods you find tempting.
- Buy low-calorie foods for snacking.

Change your lifestyle

- Keep busy with hobbies or projects that are incompatible with eating to take your mind off eating.
- Brush your teeth immediately after eating.
- Accept "diet" as it really is—a defined way of eating, not a temporary reduction in calories that must be endured before "normal" eating habits can be resumed.
- Trim recipes of extra fat and sugar.
- Don't weigh yourself too often.
- Keep food and activity records.
- Keep hunger records.
- Give yourself permission to enjoy an occasional planned indulgence and do so without guilt; don't let disappointment lure you into a real eating binge.
- Exercise.
- Get more sleep if fatigue triggers eating.

No single strategy or combination of methods has proven best in changing behaviors. One or more of the following strategies may be helpful:

- **Self-monitoring of eating** involves recording the how, what, when, where, and why of eating to provide an objective tool to help identify eating behaviors that need improvement. Also, the act of recording food eaten causes people to alter their intake. Self-monitoring of activity, which includes the frequency, intensity, and type of activity performed, is also useful.
- **Stress management** involves using strategies such as meditation and relaxation techniques to lower stress, which may improve eating behaviors.
- **Stimulus control** involves avoiding or changing cues that trigger undesirable behaviors (eg, keeping "problem" foods out of sight or out of the house) or instituting new cues to elicit positive behaviors (eg, putting walking shoes by the front door as a reminder to go walking).
- **Problem solving** involves identifying eating problems or high-risk situations, planning alternative behaviors, implementing the alternative behaviors, and evaluating the plan to determine whether it reduced problem eating behaviors.
- **Contingency management** involves rewarding changes in eating or activity behaviors with desirable nonfood dividends.
- **Cognitive restructuring** involves reducing negative self-talk, increasing positive self-talk, setting reasonable goals, and changing inaccurate beliefs. Thoughts precede behavior; changing the thoughts can change the behavior.
- **Social support** involves getting others to participate in or provide emotional and physical support of weight loss efforts.

Pharmacotherapy

Historically, drug therapy has been used as a short-term intervention to initiate weight loss in clients with resistant obesity. After weight loss was achieved, drug therapy was discontinued. However, the drugs worked only while they were being taken, so the benefits stopped when drug therapy stopped.

Today drug therapy is considered an adjunct to comprehensive weight loss therapy that includes nutritional therapy, increased activity, and behavior therapy. Although drug therapy is currently reserved for selected obese clients, in the future it is likely that drug therapy will be as standard in the treatment of obesity as it is for other chronic diseases such as hypertension and diabetes. Drug therapy is not effective as a sole treatment, nor do the benefits continue after the drug is stopped.

The use of drug therapy should be considered after 6 months of weight loss therapy that fails to produce a 1-pound weight loss per week. Drug therapy should not be used for "cosmetic" weight loss but only by clients at increased medical risk because of their weight—specifically, those with a BMI of 30 or greater with no concomitant risk factors or diseases and those with a BMI of 27 or greater with certain concomitant risk factors or diseases (ie, hypertension, dyslipidemia, coronary heart disease, type 2 diabetes, and sleep apnea).

Drugs tend to produce a modest weight loss (4.4–22 lb), usually within the first 6 months of use, and may help maintain weight loss. Additional benefits may also be gained, such as improvement in blood lipid levels, lowered blood pressure, and improved glucose tolerance. When drug therapy effectively promotes or maintains weight loss and the adverse side effects are manageable and not serious, it should continue in the long term, given the chronic nature of obesity. However, it is not known how long drug therapy may be safely used, because of the lack of long-term data on the available drugs.

Not all clients benefit from drug therapy. Usually, clients who respond initially continue to respond, and nonresponders are not likely to respond even with higher doses. Clients who fail to lose 4.4 pounds in the first 4 weeks of treatment are not likely to respond to drug therapy. Drug therapy should be discontinued if it is not effective or if the side effects are unmanageable or serious.

Sibutramine is an appetite suppressant that works by inhibiting the reuptake of the neurotransmitters norepinephrine and serotonin. The most common side effects are constipation, dry mouth, headache, and insomnia. It may also increase blood pressure and heart rate. Sibutramine must be used cautiously in clients with hypertension, and it is contraindicated in clients with coronary heart disease, congestive heart failure, arrhythmias, or a history of stroke.

Orlistat has recently been approved for long-term use in weight therapy. It works by inhibiting pancreatic lipase to reduce fat absorption from the gastrointestinal tract; unabsorbed fat means that calories are excreted rather than being absorbed into the body. It is recommended that orlistat be used in combination with a low-calorie diet consisting of approximately 30% of calories from fat. Orlistat has no systemic effects and does not affect appetite. Adverse side effects include decreased absorption of the fat-soluble vitamins, oily and loose stools, and anal leakage. A possible link to breast cancer has been identified.

Surgery

Surgical intervention is an option for clients with severe obesity (BMI ≥40 or ≥35 with comorbid conditions) who fail to lose weight by other methods and who are experiencing complications from obesity. Surgery should be contemplated only when the risk of remaining obese is greater than the risk of surgery. Seventy percent of clients maintain a loss of 50% of their initial excess weight for 5 years. However, long-term success depends mainly on the client's resolve to change his or her behavior and commitment to lifelong follow-up.

Surgical procedures currently used include gastric restriction (vertical gastric gastroplasty) and gastric bypass (Roux-en-Y). A common feature of these procedures is that they reduce the size of the stomach so that the client feels full after eating only small amounts of food. Both of these methods have been proven effective in promoting substantial weight loss but are not without complications.

Gastric restriction is also known as "stomach stapling." A row of staples across the stomach limits the capacity of the stomach to 15 to 30 mL and delays gastric emptying from the upper pouch through the banded opening, which has a diameter of approximately 1 cm (Fig. 14–4). Limiting the stomach capacity does not automatically limit food intake; over time, the pouch stretches to hold more food. Although the incidence of postsurgical complications is low, the staples may burst if too much food or liquid is consumed before the staple line heals. Overindulgence causes the pouch to accommodate

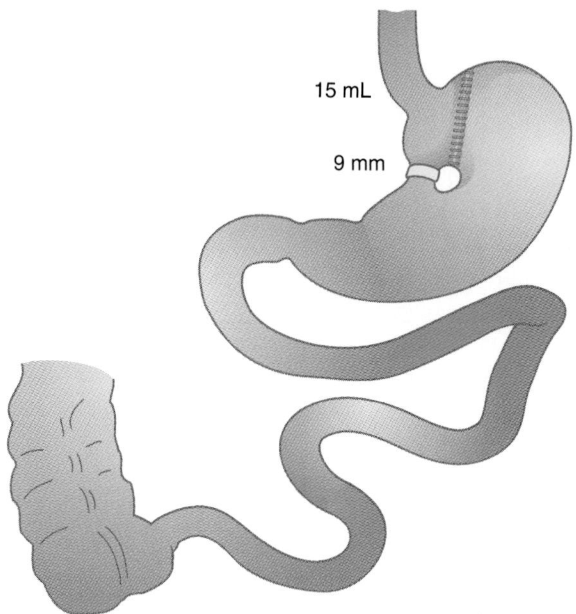

FIGURE 14-4 Vertical gastric stapling.

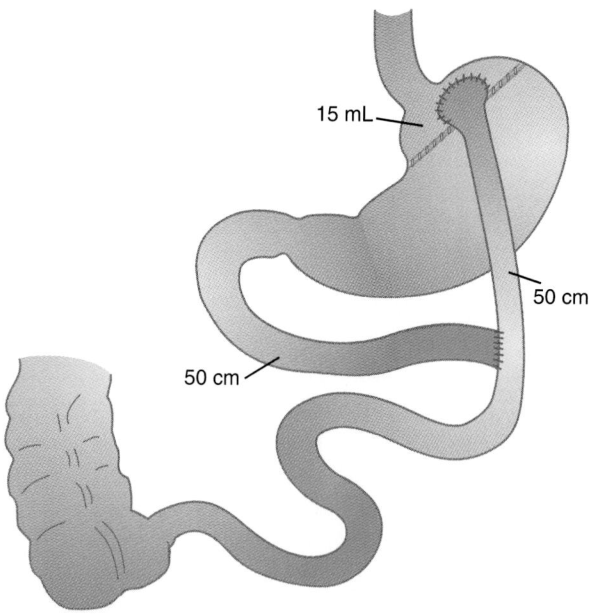

FIGURE 14-5 Gastric bypass.

more food, thereby reducing its effectiveness. Obstruction can occur if food is improperly chewed.

Nutritional complications that have been reported with this procedure include hypoalbuminemia and vitamin deficiencies, in addition to vomiting and nausea. Clients must understand the importance of eating small meals, eating slowly, chewing food thoroughly, and progressing the diet gradually from liquids, to puréed foods, to soft foods.

Gastric bypass combines gastric restriction to restrict food intake with the construction of bypasses of the duodenum and the first portion of the jejunum to cause food malabsorption (Fig. 14–5). Rapid "dumping" of the stomach pouch contents into the small intestine may produce symptoms of nausea, diarrhea, and abdominal cramping that improve over time. Malabsorption of calories and nutrients occurs, particularly of calcium, iron, and vitamin B_{12}. This procedure is superior to gastric resection in both promoting and maintaining weight loss. The amount of weight loss correlates with the severity of the dumping syndrome.

NURSING PROCESS

Thirty-three-year-old Megan Jackson has been "chunky" all her life. She weighs 236 pounds, the heaviest her 5-foot 7-inch frame has ever weighed. Her doctor has advised her to lose weight to bring down her blood glucose levels and blood pressure. She complains of frequent heartburn. She has been on and off "diets" for years, without any long-lasting success at weight control. The doctor wants you to talk to her about dieting.

Assessment

Obtain clinical data:

Current BMI and waist circumference
Recent weight history
Medical history and comorbidities, such as hypertension, dyslipidemia, cardiovascular disease, diabetes, sleep apnea, osteoarthritis, esophageal reflux
Abnormal laboratory values, especially serum cholesterol, triglycerides, glucose, triiodothyronine (T_3), and thyroxine (T_4)
Ability to increase activity
Blood pressure
Medications that affect nutrition, such as oral hypoglycemic agents, antihypertensives, and antacids

Interview client to assess:

Understanding of the relationship between intake, activity, and weight
Understanding of the relationship between obesity and health
Motivation to lose weight, including previous history of successful and unsuccessful attempts to lose weight, social support, and perceived barriers to success

Usual 24-hour intake, including portion sizes, frequency and pattern of eating, method of food preparation, intake of high-fat foods, intake of high-sugar foods, and fiber intake
"Problem" foods that may trigger overeating
Emotional triggers that stimulate overeating, such as depression, boredom, anger, guilt, frustration, or self-hate. People who are identified as compulsive overeaters may benefit from participation in Overeaters Anonymous (OA), a self-help group that uses a 12-step program similar to that of Alcoholics Anonymous.
Cultural, religious, and ethnic influences on eating habits
Psychosocial and economic issues, such as living situation, cooking facilities, finances, employment, education level, and food assistance (if applicable)
Usual activity patterns and attitude toward increasing activity
Sense of body image and weight expectations
Use of vitamins, minerals, and nutritional supplements: what, how much, and why taken
Use of alcohol, nicotine, and caffeine

Nursing Diagnosis

Altered Nutrition: More Than Body Requirements, related to excessive intake in relation to metabolic need.

Planning and Implementation

A positive, supportive approach is needed to establish rapport with the client and develop an atmosphere that is conducive to weight loss therapy. The nurse may not have the opportunity to discuss weight management with the client on a regular, ongoing basis. If time and follow-up opportunities are limited, it is important to focus on one or two changes the client is willing to make.

Remember that the objective of promoting weight loss is to improve health, which can be measured by criteria other than numbers of pounds lost, such as decrease in blood pressure, improvement in serum lipid levels, or subjective improvements in quality of life (eg, increased self-confidence, feeling more energetic). Involve the client in developing eating and exercise goals and plans to increase the likelihood of achieving success.

Goals must be specific, measurable, attainable, and individualized. Small sequential changes in intake and activity are easier to make and usually last longer than a complete overhaul. For instance, an initial goal may be to eat three servings of vegetables daily. After that goal is achieved, a goal of using light margarine in place of regular margarine may be added.

A balanced weight-reduction meal plan should be based on the "normal" recommended pattern of approximately 20% of calories from protein, less than 30% from fat, and the remainder from carbohydrate. All major food groups from the Food Guide Pyramid are included in the plan, but alcohol and items from the Fats, Oils, and Sweets group are discouraged because they provide calories with few nutrients. Encourage the intake of high-fiber foods in place of refined foods, because fiber enhances a feeling of fullness and prolongs gastric emptying time.

Hypocaloric eating plans usually do not provide less than 1200 calories for women and 1500 calories for men. Although extremely low-calorie diets can speed weight loss, they also make compliance more difficult, may be nutritionally inadequate, and may accelerate loss of lean body mass. Multivitamins and mineral supplements are indicated when intake falls below 1200 calories.

Dispel the myth that foods are either "good" or "bad." Forbidden or "bad" foods take on mystical qualities and become increasingly appealing. Rather than forbidding certain foods, emphasize portion control.

Weight-loss plateaus are to be expected because of the temporary increase in body water that results from the oxidation of fat tissue. Eventually, an increase in urine output rids the body of excess water and weight loss continues.

CLIENT GOALS

The client will:

Increase physical activity to ___ minutes daily on ___ days of the week

Explain the relationship between calorie intake, physical activity, and weight control

Consume a nutritionally adequate, hypocaloric diet that contains less than 30% of calories from fat

Practice behavior therapy techniques to change undesirable eating habits

Not skip meals

Lose 1 pound/week on average until ____ pounds of total weight loss is achieved after 6 months

Improve health status, as evidenced by a decrease in total cholesterol, LDL-cholesterol, and glucose; an increase in HDL-cholesterol; and improved blood pressure, as appropriate

Maintain weight loss by regaining less than 6.6 pounds in 2 years and sustaining a reduction in waist circumference of at least 4 cm

NURSING INTERVENTIONS

Nutrition Therapy

Decrease calorie intake by 500 to 1000 cal/day from calculated requirements to promote gradual weight loss.

Individualize the eating plan as much as possible to correspond with the client's likes, dislikes, and eating pattern, because standard plans rarely fit into a person's lifestyle and eating habits.

Limit fat intake to less than 30% of total calories daily; encourage an adequate protein intake and a liberal intake of complex carbohydrates.

Increase fiber intake, because fiber contributes to satiety and is found in foods that are nutrient dense and relatively low in calories. Excellent sources of fiber include whole-grain breads and cereals, especially wheat bran; dried peas and beans; and fresh fruits and vegetables.

Encourage a pattern of three meals plus two to three snacks throughout the day to prevent intense hunger and subsequent overeating. Breakfast is particularly important because it "breaks the fast" experienced while sleeping.

Encourage ample fluid intake to promote excretion of metabolic wastes. Drinking fluid with meals contributes to a feeling of fullness.

Client Teaching

Instruct the client:

On the role of a low-calorie eating plan, increased physical activity, and behavior change in weight loss therapy and maintaining weight loss

On the eating plan essentials, including:

- The importance of eating three to four times per day to avoid hunger, which often leads to snacking and a higher calorie intake
- Low-caloric-density versus high-caloric-density foods, tips for eating out, food preparation techniques, and the basics of food purchasing and label reading (Box 14–4)
- The benefits of reducing fat intake to limit calories and improve blood lipid levels. Foods with a high percentage of calories from fat include fatty meats, whole-milk dairy products, fried foods, butter, margarine, salad dressings, oils, nuts and peanut butter, and rich desserts and pastries.

BOX 14.4

Tips for Controlling Calorie Intake

Rely on low-caloric-density foods for the majority of your calories, such as:

- Baked, broiled, steamed, and boiled foods
- Fresh fruits and vegetables prepared without added fat
- Lean meats, skinless poultry, and fish
- Starchy foods without added fat, such as bread, pasta, rice, potatoes, dried peas and beans, corn, peas, winter squash, and unsweetened cereals; whole-grain products and high-fiber foods are especially good at providing a feeling of fullness without a lot of excess calories.
- Skim or low-fat milk and dairy products

Make sensible choices when ordering from a menu:

- Estimate portion sizes of all foods. If the portion size is too big (eg, a 12-oz steak), eat half and take the rest home for the next day's meal. Consider ordering a la carte (salad and appetizer) for better portion control.
- Stick to plain foods rather than casseroles and stews. When in doubt, ask how the food is prepared; accommodating restaurants will prepare food without added fat, as requested.

(*continued*)

BOX 14.4

Tips for Controlling Calorie Intake (continued)

- Choose tomato juice, unsweetened fruit juice, clear broth, bouillon, or consommé as an appetizer instead of sweetened juices, fried vegetables, seafood cocktail, or creamy or thick soups.
- Choose fresh vegetable salads, and use oil and vinegar or fresh lemon instead of regular salad dressings. If you use regular salad dressing, ask that the dressing be served separately and dip each forkful of salad into the dressing, rather than pouring the dressing on the salad. Avoid coleslaw and other salads with the dressing already added.
- Order plain roasted, baked, or broiled meat, fish, or poultry; avoid items that are au gratin, creamed, sautéed, or fried.
- Order steamed, boiled, or broiled vegetables.
- Choose plain baked, mashed, boiled, or steamed potatoes, rice, or noodles.
- Select fresh fruit for dessert. If you can't resist a high-fat dessert, order one and split it with a friend.
- At fast food restaurants, order the smallest size available; order burgers with lettuce, tomato, onions, pickles, mustard, relish, and ketchup if desired, but skip the cheese and special sauce.
- Order pizza with veggie toppings instead of pepperoni, sausage, other meats, and extra cheese.
- Request milk for coffee and tea, if desired, instead of cream.
- Most airlines will provide low-calorie meals if requested at the time the flight reservations are made.
- Be sure to undereat for the rest of the day if you think you may overeat while you are out.

Trim the fat and sugar while cooking:

- Nonstick sprays are effective and virtually calorie free; you can also sauté foods with a small amount of water or broth instead of margarine or oil.
- Trim all visible fat from meat after cooking, and remove the skin from poultry.
- Prepare soup stock a day ahead; refrigerate and remove the fat that hardens on the surface.
- Whenever possible, replace high-fat ingredients with low-fat substitutes (eg, replace whole or 2% milk with 1% or skim milk).
- When making casseroles or stews, halve the amount of meat called for and double the amount of rice, beans, pasta, or potatoes.
- Use low-fat or diabetic cookbooks for variety.
- Use herbs, spices, cooking wine, and vinegars to enhance flavor with few or no additional calories.

(*continued*)

BOX 14.4

Tips for Controlling Calorie Intake (continued)

Buy smart and read labels:

- Avoid temptation by not buying problem foods.
- Stick to a shopping list.
- Do not shop while hungry.
- Buy only the amount needed.
- "Lite" or "light" foods have one-third fewer calories or no more than one-half the fat of the higher-calorie, higher-fat versions.
- "Low-calorie" foods cannot have more than 40 cal per serving.
- "Calorie-free" items must have less than 5 cal per serving.
- "Sugar-free" and "dietetic" foods are not necessarily low in calories.

- The concept that "all foods can fit," as long as portion size and frequency are considered
- Maintaining adequate fluid intake
- Limiting alcohol consumption

On behavioral matters, including:

- Eating only in one place and while sitting down
- Putting utensils down between mouthfuls
- Monitoring hunger on a scale of 1 to 10, with 1 corresponding to "famished" and 10 corresponding to "stuffed." Encourage clients to eat when the hunger scale is at about 3 and to stop when satisfied (not full) at about 6 or 7.
- Not getting weighed too frequently, because weight losses that are less than anticipated are discouraging. Some clinicians recommend getting rid of the scale because it has too much power to make or break the client's day.
- Periodic record keeping of food and fluid intake
- "Planned" splurges instead of eating on impulse. Planned splurges involve making a conscious decision to eat something, enjoying every mouthful of the food, and then moving on from the experience without feelings of guilt or failure.

On changing eating attitudes:

- Replacing negative self-talk with positive talk
- Replacing the attitude of "always being on a diet" with an acceptance of eating lighter and less as a way of life

To consult her physician or dietitian if questions concerning the eating plan or weight loss arise

Evaluation

The client:

Increases physical activity to ___ minutes daily on ___ days of the week

Explains the relationship between calorie intake, physical activity, and weight control

Consumes a nutritionally adequate, hypocaloric diet that contains less than 30% of calories from fat

Practices behavior therapy techniques to change eating habits that lead to weight gain

Does not skip meals

Loses 1 to 2 pounds/week until ___ pounds total weight loss is achieved after 6 months

Improves health status, as evidenced by a decrease in total cholesterol, LDL-cholesterol, and glucose; an increase in HDL-cholesterol; and improved blood pressure, as appropriate

Maintains weight loss by regaining less than 6.6 pounds in 2 years and sustaining a reduction in waist circumference of at least 4 cm

Eating Disorders: Anorexia Nervosa and Bulimia Nervosa

Historically, the study of obesity and eating disorders has been separate: The former has been rooted in medicine, and the latter has been the focus of psychiatry and psychology. Yet there are commonalities between them, such as questions of appetite regulation, concerns with body image, and similar etiologic risk factors.

Description

Anorexia nervosa is a condition of self-imposed fasting or severe self-imposed dieting that is characterized by dramatic weight loss or maintenance of weight that is at least 15% below the recommended weight for height and by abnormal food intake patterns. Thinness is pursued compulsively through semistarvation and compulsive exercise. Clients with anorexia nervosa are intensely preoccupied with weight and food, and their distorted perception causes them to see themselves as fat when they are emaciated. Anorexics who develop severe malnutrition may experience permanent brain damage, permanent sterility, damage to vital organs, and heart failure. As many as one of every five to seven clients with chronic anorexia dies from complications.

Bulimia nervosa is a variant of anorexia nervosa. It is characterized by recurrent episodes of binge eating, that is, quickly eating large amounts of food (eg, 1200–11,500 cal), during which the client feels unable to stop or control the binge. The gorging is followed by recurrent purging to prevent weight gain, such as self-induced vomiting; excessive exercise; abuse of laxatives, emetics, diuretics, or diet pills; or fasting. Binges may occur several times a day and are frequently planned, with the client stockpiling food for a time when the binge can proceed uninterrupted. Binge foods are easy to swallow and regurgitate and usually consist of the fatty, sweet, high-calorie foods that the client denies himself or herself at other times. Like anorexics, bulimics are preoccupied with body shape, weight, and food, and have an irrational fear of becoming fat. Unlike anorexics, bulimics experience weight fluctuations and are of normal or slightly above-normal weight. Bulimics tend to have fewer serious medical complications than anorexics, because their undernutrition is less severe. Gastric dilation, with its risk of rupture, may be the most frequent cause of death among bulimics.

Eating disorders are considered to be multifactorial in origin. Although numerous psychological, physical, social, and cultural risk factors have been identified, it is not known how or why these factors interact to cause eating disorders. People with eating disorders are prone to depression, irritability, passivity, sadness, and suicidal tendencies. The incidence of alcohol and drug abuse may be four to five times higher among women with eating disorders than in the general population. Psychological and social factors, especially problems with family dynamics, are usually considered to be central to the problem.

Eating disorders are most likely to occur immediately before or after the onset of puberty, and they are almost always preceded by "dieting." Major stressors, such as onset of puberty, parents' divorce, death of a family member, broken relationships, and ridicule because of being or becoming fat, are frequent precipitating factors. Athletes (eg, dancers, gymnasts) may develop eating disorders to improve their performance. Binge eating is often related to anxiety, tension, boredom, drinking alcohol or smoking cannabis, and fatigue. Hunger is rarely cited as a reason for binge eating, even when the gorging follows a 24-hour fast.

Approximately 90% to 95% of cases of anorexia and bulimia occur in girls and women, with two peak ages at onset: 12 to 13 years and 19 to 20 years. Anorexics are often described as "model" children, although they tend to be immature, require parental approval, and lack independence. They typically are from white, middle- to upper-middle-class families that place heavy emphasis on high achievement, perfection, and physical appearance. Bulimia nervosa is more common than anorexia, with as many as one in five female college students admitting bulimic symptoms. Because bulimics are secretive about their binge-purge episodes, the behaviors may go undetected by family members for years and many cases go unnoticed. Eighty-five percent of bulimics are college-educated women. As many as 30% of bulimics have a previous history of anorexia; however, bulimia in persons of normal weight rarely develops into anorexia nervosa.

Assessment

Numerous physical and mental signs and symptoms may be observed in people with eating disorders.

HISTORICAL DATA

- What is the client's current, usual, and ideal weight? What is the client's recent weight history?

- Does the client complain of fatigue, tooth sensitivity, indigestion, nausea, dizziness, intolerance to cold, constipation, or feeling bloated after eating? Does the client self-induce vomiting or abuse laxatives, diet pills, or diuretics? Is menstruation irregular or absent?
- What is the client's usual 24-hour intake? Which foods are best and least tolerated? What cultural, religious, or ethnic influences affect the client's food choices? Does the client admit to food phobias? Does the client practice abnormal eating behaviors? For instance, anorexics may refuse to eat high-calorie foods, cut food into tiny pieces, choose inappropriate utensils, eat extremely slowly, use excessive condiments, drink too much or too little fluid, dispose of food secretly, binge eat, or exhibit ritualistic eating behaviors. Bulimics may eat large amounts of food when not physically hungry, eat rapidly, regurgitate (spit out) food, eat in secrecy, and eat until feeling uncomfortably full.
- What vitamins, minerals, or nutritional supplements does the client use and for what purpose?
- Does the client have a significant medical history?
- What over-the-counter and prescription medications does the client use? Does the client use alcohol or street drugs?
- What is the client's emotional state?
- What is the client's sense of body image? What are her weight expectations?
- What is the client's usual physical activity pattern?
- Does the client have family and social support?

PHYSICAL FINDINGS

- Does the client have edema in the legs and feet?
- Is the client's tooth enamel damaged?
- Does the client have a wasted appearance?
- Is there growth of lanugo hair, alopecia, dry skin, thinning hair, decreased heart rate, or low blood pressure?
- Does the client have puffy cheeks as a result of enlarged salivary glands, particularly the parotid glands?

LABORATORY DATA

Evaluate serum electrolytes, protein status (eg, serum albumin), and abnormal laboratory values.

Management

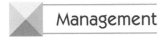

Each person's recovery process is unique; therefore, treatment plans are highly individualized. A multidisciplinary approach that includes nutrition counseling, behavior modification, psychotherapy, family counseling, and group therapy is most effective. Antidepressant drugs effectively reduce the frequency of problematic eating behaviors but do not eliminate them. Most eating disorders are treated on an outpatient basis; however, severe cases of anorexia nervosa may necessitate hospitalization. Bulimia tends to be easier to treat than anorexia, because bulimics know their behavior is abnormal and many are willing to cooperate with treatment. Treatment is often time-consuming and frustrating.

Nutritional intervention seeks to reestablish and maintain normal eating behaviors; correct signs, symptoms, and complications of the eating disorder; and promote long-term maintenance of reasonable weight.

NUTRITION THERAPY FOR ANOREXIA

The goal of nutritional intervention is to gradually restore normal eating behaviors and nutritional status. Step-by-step goals are (1) to prevent further weight loss, (2) to gradually reestablish normal eating behaviors, (3) to gradually increase weight, and (4) to maintain agreed-upon weight goals. Sometimes a lower-than-normal weight is selected as the initial weight goal (ie, enough weight to regain normal physiologic function and menstruation). When this has been achieved, the goal may be reevaluated. Many recovered clients have chronic problems with eating and weight.

Involving the client in formulating individualized goals and plans promotes compliance and feelings of trust. Offer rewards linked to the quantity of calories consumed, not to weight gain. Initially, it may be beneficial to have the client record food intake and exercise activity.

Even though calorie needs are high to restore body weight, the initial eating plan offered is low in calories (approximately 1500 cal/day, or calories for resting energy expenditure plus 300–400 cal). Larger amounts may not be well tolerated or accepted after prolonged semistarvation. Small, frequent meals help maximize intake and tolerance. The diet is advanced only when the client is able to complete a full meal. Calories may eventually be increased to 3000 or more per day.

- Because gastrointestinal intolerance may exist, gassy and high-fat foods should be limited in the early stages of treatment.
- Serve small, attractive meals based on individual food preferences. Foods that are nutritionally dense help to minimize the volume of food needed. Finger foods that are served cold or at room temperature help to minimize satiety sensations.
- Never force the client to eat, and minimize the emphasis on food. Initially, clients may respond to nutritional therapy better if they are allowed to exclude high-risk binge foods from their diet. However, the binge foods should be reintroduced later so that the "feared food" (trigger food) idea is not promoted.
- A high-fiber or low-sodium diet may be helpful in controlling symptoms of constipation and fluid retention, respectively.
- A multivitamin and mineral supplement may be prescribed.
- Because it is both a stimulant and a diuretic, caffeine should be avoided.
- Tube feedings or parenteral nutrition should be used only if they are necessary to stabilize the client medically. Overly aggressive nutritional repletion carries med-

ical risks of fluid retention and electrolyte changes; psychological risks may include a perceived loss of control, loss of identity, increased body distortion, and mistrust of the treatment team. Enteral support should never be used as punishment for difficult clients.

NUTRITION THERAPY FOR BULIMIA

Initially, nutrition therapy for bulimia is structured and relatively inflexible to promote the client's sense of control. Meal patterns similar to those used for diabetics can be used to specify portion sizes, food groups to include with each meal and snack, and the frequency of eating. Having the client record intake *before* eating adds to a sense of control.

- To increase awareness of eating and satiety, meals and snacks should be eaten while sitting down; finger foods and foods that are cold or at room temperature should be avoided; and the meal duration should be of appropriate length.
- Eating strategies that may help to regulate intake include not skipping meals or snacks and using the appropriately sized utensils.
- Encourage clients to introduce forbidden binge foods into their diets.

The initial meal plan is usually not less than 1500 calories distributed among three balanced meals plus snacks. Adequate fat is provided to help delay gastric emptying and contribute to satiety. Calories are gradually increased as needed.

Nutritional counseling focuses on identifying and correcting food misinformation and fears. Bulimics must understand that gorging is only one aspect of a complex pattern of altered behavior; in fact, excessive dietary restriction is a major contributor to the disorder.

Expect minor relapses, especially after therapy is discontinued. When relapse occurs, the structured meal plan should be resumed immediately.

TEACHING POINTS

Promote self-esteem in clients with eating disorders by using a positive approach, providing support and encouragement, fostering decision making, and offering the client choices. Avoid preaching rules and reinforcing the client's preoccupation with food.

Instruct the client:

On the role of calories and nutrition in promoting optimal health and weight management

On the eating plan essentials, including:

- The rationale for the particular eating plan used
- The characteristics of a healthy diet and the recommended servings from each food group. The Food Guide Pyramid or exchange lists may serve as a teaching aid.
- Appropriate food intake patterns, such as not skipping meals

On behavioral matters, including:

- Food- and weight-related behaviors
- Body image
- The dangers of dieting, bingeing, and purging
- How to recognize signs of hunger and satiety
- The likelihood that relapse will occur but should not be viewed as failure

Box 14–5 lists agencies that can be consulted for additional help.

PREVENTION

Prevention may be far more effective than the treatment of eating disorders. Encourage parents, teachers, and significant others:

- To help children and adolescents establish a strong, positive self-image and sense of worth regardless of their weight
- Not to expect perfection and to avoid putting pressure on children to excel beyond their capabilities
- To give adolescents an appropriate amount of independence, responsibility, and accountability for their own actions
- To recognize stresses in the child's life and provide support and encouragement
- To teach the basis of good nutrition and normal exercise

BOX 14.5

Additional Sources of Help for Anorexia and Bulimia

American Anorexia/Bulimia Association, Inc.
165 W 46th St. #1108
New York, NY 10036
212-575-6200
www.AABAInc.org

Anorexia Nervosa and Related Eating Disorders (ANRED)
PO Box 5102
Eugene, OR 97405
541-344-1144
www.anred.com

National Association of Anorexia Nervosa and Associated Disorders
PO Box 7
Highland Park, IL 60035
847-831-3438

- To avoid putting pressure on young people to lose weight. If weight control is really indicated, a medically supervised plan of weight loss and weight maintenance should be followed. Discourage the use of fad diets and diet products.
- To recognize the signs and symptoms of eating disorders
- To seek professional help if eating disorders are suspected

Questions You May Hear

Should clients count calories to stick to their low-calorie diet? Counting calories does not ensure a nutritionally adequate diet. It is possible to lose weight on a diet that consists only of soft drinks and French fries, as long as the total calorie intake is less than total calorie expenditure. In addition, counting calories does not have long-term possibilities. Who would carry around a food composition table, paper, pencil, and calculator indefinitely?

Are commercial weight loss programs effective? Commercial programs, of which Weight Watchers, Jenny Craig, and NutriSystem are the most popular, provide diet and nutrition information and may include behavior modification, exercise, psychotherapy, the provision of food, and group support. The cost of these programs varies widely; programs that require the purchase of prepackaged foods or supplements can cost thousands of dollars. Although these programs are widely used, their effectiveness is relatively unknown: Commercial groups are reluctant to share less than spectacular results for fear of damaging their profitability. Consumer surveys (which may or may not be reliable) indicate that people tend to participate in such programs for about 1 year and to lose 10% to 20% of their initial weight; but the average dieter gains back almost half of that weight within 6 months after ending the program. Within 2 years, most participants regain more than two thirds of their initial weight loss.

How can you tell the difference between a "fad diet" and legitimate advice? Legitimate advice on how to eat to lose weight:

- Is realistic and flexible, that is, easily adaptable to individual lifestyles and based on individual calorie requirements
- Suggests that a doctor be consulted
- Uses food to meet nutritional requirements, rather than vitamin or mineral supplements
- Encourages consumption of foods from each of the major food groups
- Provides adequate amounts of all nutrients
- Promotes nutrition education
- Recommends exercise
- Promotes a weight loss of 1 to 2 pounds/week
- Has long-term possibilities (diets recommended for only short periods obviously are not safe)
- Provides a healthy and reasonable balance of carbohydrates, protein, and fat
- Allows nutritious, low-calorie snacks
- Emphasizes portion control

- Teaches skills and techniques to make permanent changes in eating and activity habits
- Offers a maintenance plan after weight loss is achieved

Are less conventional approaches to weight loss effective, such as fad diets and weight-loss aids? Fad diets and weight-loss gimmicks fail to promote safe, long-term weight loss because they do not address the necessity of making lifelong changes in eating and activity behaviors.

Fad diets, especially those that are high in protein and low in carbohydrates, may produce weight loss, but they tend to be highly restrictive, which leads invariably not only to a decrease in intake and loss of weight but also to boredom and attrition. In addition to their lack of long-term staying power, many of these diets are unbalanced, providing not enough of some nutrients and excessive amounts of others.

Very-low-calorie diets that are medically supervised represent an aggressive, "jump-start" approach for severely obese clients whose health is so jeopardized by obesity that the risk of a modified fast is less than the risk of remaining obese. These diets provide 800 cal, at least 1 g of protein per kilogram of body weight, little or no fat, and little carbohydrate. Meals consist of a small variety of lean meats, a powdered formula available by prescription, or a combination of the two. Although short-term weight loss is dramatic, it is almost certainly regained. Studies suggest that the short-term effectiveness of very-low-calorie diets is related more to the choice-free menu of portion-controlled meals than to their severe calorie restriction. A maintenance program is crucial.

Other weight-loss gimmicks include taking weight-loss pills (appetite suppressants, diuretics, or thyroid pills), fasting for longer than 24 hours, taking laxatives, using weight-loss devices such as body wraps, using meal replacements (liquid drinks or packaged foods), and inducing vomiting after eating. None of these practices are recommended, none produce fundamental changes in eating habits, and most are potentially harmful.

What is Overeaters Anonymous? OA is a self-help group founded on the belief that compulsive overeating is a physical, emotional, and spiritual disease. Its focus is limited to the compulsive nature of overeating. There are no dues or fees, nor is there any weight requirement for entering the program. Like Alcoholics Anonymous, OA regards compulsive overeating as an addiction than can be arrested but not cured. A self-administered questionnaire that focuses on eating behaviors (eg, eating in the absence of hunger, secret binge eating, feelings of guilt after overeating) may be used to help identify a compulsive eating disorder. OA is intended to complement medical and nutritional treatment of obesity. For more information, contact:

Overeaters Anonymous, Inc.
6075 Zenith Ct. NE
Rio Rancho, NM 87124
505-891-4320
www.overeatersanonymous.org

What is "yo-yo dieting"? The repeated loss and regain of weight is known as yo-yo dieting or weight cycling. It was once thought to be more harmful than static obesity; however, there is no convincing evidence that weight cycling has adverse effects on body composition, energy expenditure, risk factors for cardiovascular disease, or the effectiveness of future weight loss attempts. Fears about weight cycling should not deter overweight people from trying to lose weight.

KEY CONCEPTS

- Ideal body weight and healthy body weight are imprecise terms that have not been universally defined.
- The BMI may be the best method of evaluating weight status, but it does not account for how weight is distributed. Overweight is defined as a BMI of 25 to 29.9; obesity is defined as a BMI of 30 or higher.
- Waist circumference is a tool to assess for visceral fatness. "Apples" (people with upper-body obesity) appear to have more health risks than "pears" (people with lower-body obesity).
- Beginning at a BMI of 25, the risk for development of certain diseases increases, as does morbidity from existing disorders.
- Obesity is a chronic disease of multifactorial origin. It is likely that a combination of genetic and environmental factors is involved in its development.
- More than 50% of American adults are overweight or obese. Obesity is more prevalent among members of racial-ethnic minority groups than among whites, with the exception of Asian-Americans. Black and Hispanic women have the highest prevalence of obesity.
- Obesity is resistant to treatment, when success is measured by weight loss alone. Rather than concentrating solely on weight loss to measure success, other health benefits, such as lowered blood pressure and lowered serum lipids, should also be considered. A moderate weight loss of 10% of body weight usually effectively lowers disease risks.
- A hypocaloric intake, increased activity, and behavior therapy are the cornerstones to weight loss therapy. Pharmacotherapy and surgery are additional options for some people.
- Calorie intake should be lowered by 500 to 1000 cal/day to promote a gradual weight loss of 1 to 2 pounds/week. Lowering fat intake in conjunction with a lower calorie intake helps promote weight loss.
- The non-diet approach to weight management promotes self-regulated eating instead of restrained dieting. It is founded on the belief that the body will find its own natural weight as the individual eats in response to internal hunger and satiety cues. Its focus is enhancing total health, not achieving a specific weight.
- An increase in activity helps burn calories and has a favorable impact on body composition and weight distribution. Even without weight loss, exercise lowers blood pressure and improves glucose tolerance and blood lipid levels.
- Behavior therapy is essential to promote lifelong changes in eating and activity habits. It is a process that involves identifying behaviors that need improvement, setting specific behavioral goals, modifying "problem" behaviors, and reinforcing the positive changes.

- Pharmacotherapy is adjunctive therapy in the treatment of obesity. Drugs are not effective in all people, and they are only effective for as long as they are used. Long-term effectiveness and safety are not known.
- The two types of surgery used for weight therapy involve limiting the capacity of the stomach. Gastric bypass also circumvents a portion of the small intestine to cause malabsorption of calories. Both types effectively promote weight loss but have complications.
- Anorexia nervosa and bulimia nervosa are characterized by preoccupation with body weight and food and usually are preceded by prolonged dieting. Although their cause is unknown, they are considered to be multifactorial in origin.
- Anorexia nervosa is a condition of severe self-imposed starvation, often accompanied by a frantic pursuit of exercise. Although they appear to be severely underweight, anorexics have a distorted self-perception of weight and see themselves as overweight. They may have numerous physical and mental symptoms. Anorexia can be fatal.
- Bulimia, which occurs more frequently than anorexia, is characterized by binge eating (consuming large amounts of food in a short period) and purging (eg, self-induced vomiting, laxative abuse). Bulimics usually appear to be of normal or slightly above-normal weight, and they experience less severe physical symptoms than anorexics do. Bulimia is rarely fatal.
- Eating disorders are best treated by a team approach that includes nutritional intervention and counseling to restore normal eating behaviors and adequate nutritional status.

Focus on Critical Thinking

1. Mrs. Edwards is a sedentary 38-year-old woman who is 5 feet 5 inches tall and weighs 160 pounds. She weighed 115 pounds before the birth of her first child 10 years ago and has steadily gained weight ever since. Her goal is to weigh 115 pounds by the end of 2 months, when her high school reunion is scheduled. She is thinking about trying the grapefruit diet.
   - Evaluate Mrs. Edwards's BMI. Is it appropriate for Mrs. Edwards to lose weight?
   - Discuss Mrs. Edwards's weight loss goal, the time frame, and the reason she wants to lose weight.
   - What would you tell Mrs. Edwards about a grapefruit diet? What general guidelines would you suggest she look for in a weight loss plan?
   - What strategies would you recommend Mrs. Edwards try to help promote weight loss?
2. Do you agree that the healthy weight range for your height, as shown in Table 14-1, is appropriate for you personally?

ANSWER KEY

1. **FALSE** Ranges, rather than single weights, are given because people of the same height may have the same amount of body fat but different amounts of bone and muscle. The ranges are not intended to encourage people at the low end to gain weight or people at the high end to lose weight.

2. **TRUE** Although the mechanism is not clear, people of either gender with a high distribution of abdominal fat ("apples") have a greater health risk than people with excess fat in the hips and thighs ("pears").
3. **FALSE** BMI can be elevated for reasons other than excess fat, such as large muscle mass.
4. **TRUE** Physical inactivity, as well as overeating, are major contributors to obesity.
5. **FALSE** The cosmetic advantage of weight loss is only one standard of success; the goal of weight loss is to improve health status and reduce the risk of disease.
6. **TRUE** Most short-term weight loss occurs from a decrease in total calorie intake. Physical activity helps in maintaining weight loss.
7. **TRUE** With or without weight loss, an increase in physical activity helps lower blood pressure and improve glucose tolerance.
8. **TRUE** Eating plans that provide less than 1200 calories may not provide adequate amounts of essential nutrients.
9. **FALSE** Weight loss will not occur unless total calories are cut. Reducing fat intake alone does not promote weight loss.
10. **TRUE** People affected by bulimia tend to have fewer medical complications than those affected by anorexia since the undernutrition is less severe.

REFERENCES

American Dietetic Association. (1997). Position of the American Dietetic Association: Weight management. *Journal of the American Dietetic Association, 97*, 71–74.

American Dietetic Association. (1994). Position of the American Dietetic Association: Nutrition intervention in the treatment of anorexia nervosa, bulimia nervosa, and binge eating. *Journal of the American Dietetic Association, 94*, 902–907.

Aronne, L. (1998). Modern medical management of obesity: The role of pharmaceutical intervention. *Journal of the American Dietetic Association*, 98(Suppl. 2), S23–S26.

Brownell, K., & Fairburn, C. (Eds.). (1995). *Eating disorders and obesity: A comprehensive handbook*. New York: The Guilford Press.

Foreyt, J., & Poston, W. (1998). The role of the behavioral counselor in obesity treatment. *Journal of the American Dietetic Association*, 98(Suppl. 2), S27–S30.

Horn, L., Donato, K., Kumanyida, S., Winston, M., Prewitt, E., & Snetselaar, L. (1998). The dietitian's role in developing and implementing the first federal obesity guidelines. *Journal of the American Dietetic Association, 98*, 1115–1117.

Katrina, K., King, N., & Hayes, D. (1996). *Moving away from diets*. Lake Dallas, TX: Helm Seminars, Publishing.

National Heart, Lung, and Blood Institute Expert Panel on the Identification, Evaluation, and Treatment of Overweight and Obesity in Adults. (1998). Executive summary of the clinical guidelines on the identification, evaluation, and treatment of overweight and obesity in adults. *Journal of the American Dietetic Association, 98*, 1178–1191.

National Research Council. (1989). *Recommended Dietary Allowances* (10th ed.). Washington, DC: National Academy Press.

Polivy, J. (1996). Psychological consequences of food restriction. *Journal of the American Dietetic Association, 96*, 589–592.

Rippe, J., Crossley, S., & Ringer, R. (1998). Obesity as a chronic disease: Modern medical and lifestyle management. *Journal of the American Dietetic Association*, 98(Suppl. 2), S9–S15.

Rippe, J., & Hess, S. (1998). The role of physical activity in the prevention and management of obesity. *Journal of the American Dietetic Association*, 98(Suppl. 2), S31–S38.

Robinson, J., Hoerr, S., Petersmarck, K., & Anderson, J. (1995). Redefining success in obesity intervention: The new paradigm. *Journal of the American Dietetic Association*, 95, 422–423.

Schwartz, M., & Seeley, R. (1997). The new biology of body weight regulation. *Journal of the American Dietetic Association*, 97, 54–58.

U. S. Department of Agriculture, U.S. Department of Health and Human Services. (2000). *Nutrition and your health: Dietary guidelines for Americans*. (5th ed.). Home and Garden Bulletin No. 232. Washington, D.C.: Author.

U.S. Department of Agriculture. (1992). *The Food Guide Pyramid*. (Home and Garden Bulletin No. 252) Washington, D.C.: U.S. Government Printing Office.

U.S. Department of Health and Human Services, Public Health Service, National Institutes of Health, National Heart, Lung, and Blood Institute. (1998). *Clinical guidelines on the identification, evaluation, and treatment of overweight and obesity in adults: The evidence report*. (NIH Publication No. 98-4083). Rockville, MD: Author.

CHAPTER 15

Feeding Patients: Hospital Food and Enteral and Parenteral Nutrition

TRUE	FALSE	Check your knowledge of hospital food and enteral and parenteral nutrition.
		1 Routine hospital diets generally meet the recommendations put forth in the *Dietary Guidelines for Americans*.
		2 Full liquid diets that are planned or supplemented are nutritionally adequate and can be used indefinitely if needed.
		3 Tube feedings can be made more nutrient dense by adding one or more modular products.
		4 The more digested the protein is in a formula, the greater the osmolality.
		5 The terms *fiber* and *residue* are synonymous.
		6 A primary consideration when deciding the type of tube feeding to use is the patient's digestive and absorptive capacity.
		7 Peripheral parenteral nutrition (PPN) is not suitable for patients who need more than 2000 to 2500 cal.
		8 Intermittent feedings should take 20 to 30 minutes to infuse.
		9 Diarrhea in tube-fed patients may be caused by giving too much formula or administering the formula too rapidly.
		10 Coloring tube feeding formulas with food dye helps prevent aspiration.

Upon completion of this chapter, you will be able to

- Describe ways to promote the patient's acceptance of hospital food.
- Describe the characteristics, indications, and contraindications for liquid and soft diets.
- Define enteral nutrition and list indications for its use.
- Describe the categories of enteral formulas.
- Define the two types of parenteral nutrition and list indications for their use.
- Discuss possible causes of and interventions for diarrhea in tube-fed patients.
- Outline teaching points for patients using home enteral nutrition.

Introduction

Feeding patients who are acutely or chronically ill presents many challenges. A widespread problem is inadequate intake, which may occur for a variety of reasons. Appetite may be impaired or lacking owing to the physical or emotional stress of illness or hospitalization. For instance, eating alone, physical pain, and facing an uncertain prognosis all affect appetite. Hospital food may be refused because it is unfamiliar, tasteless (eg, cooked without salt), inappropriate in texture (eg, pureed meat), religiously or culturally unacceptable, or served at times when the patient is unaccustomed to eating. Meals may be withheld or missed because of diagnostic procedures or medical treatments. Inadequate liquid diets may not be advanced in a timely manner.

In addition to inadequate intake, altered nutrient use or increased nutrient requirements may complicate patient feeding. Digestion, absorption, metabolism, or excretion may be impaired by illness or treatments, making it necessary to restrict the intake of certain foods or to provide "artificial" nutrition. Requirements for protein, calories, fluid, and other nutrients may be increased because of stress, illness, fever, infection, or wound healing. It is essential that the nourishment provided be such that the patient is able to consume it, tolerate it, use it, and meet individual nutrient requirements. Figure 15–1 depicts a decision-making model for choosing the appropriate type and method of feeding.

Patients who do not meet their nutritional requirements are at risk for malnutrition, which is seen in all age groups and across the continuum of care. As many as 40% to 55% of hospitalized patients have malnutrition or are at risk for development of malnutrition. Consequences of malnutrition include longer hospital stays, higher costs, and higher rates of complications. Impaired wound healing and susceptibility to infection are well-known outcomes, both of which increase morbidity and mortality. Prevention of malnutrition is easier and more effective than treatment.

This chapter explores hospital diets and how nurses can help promote an adequate intake in their patients. Oral supplements and modular products are discussed. For patients who are unable or unwilling to consume an adequate oral diet, the use of enteral and parenteral nutrition is presented.

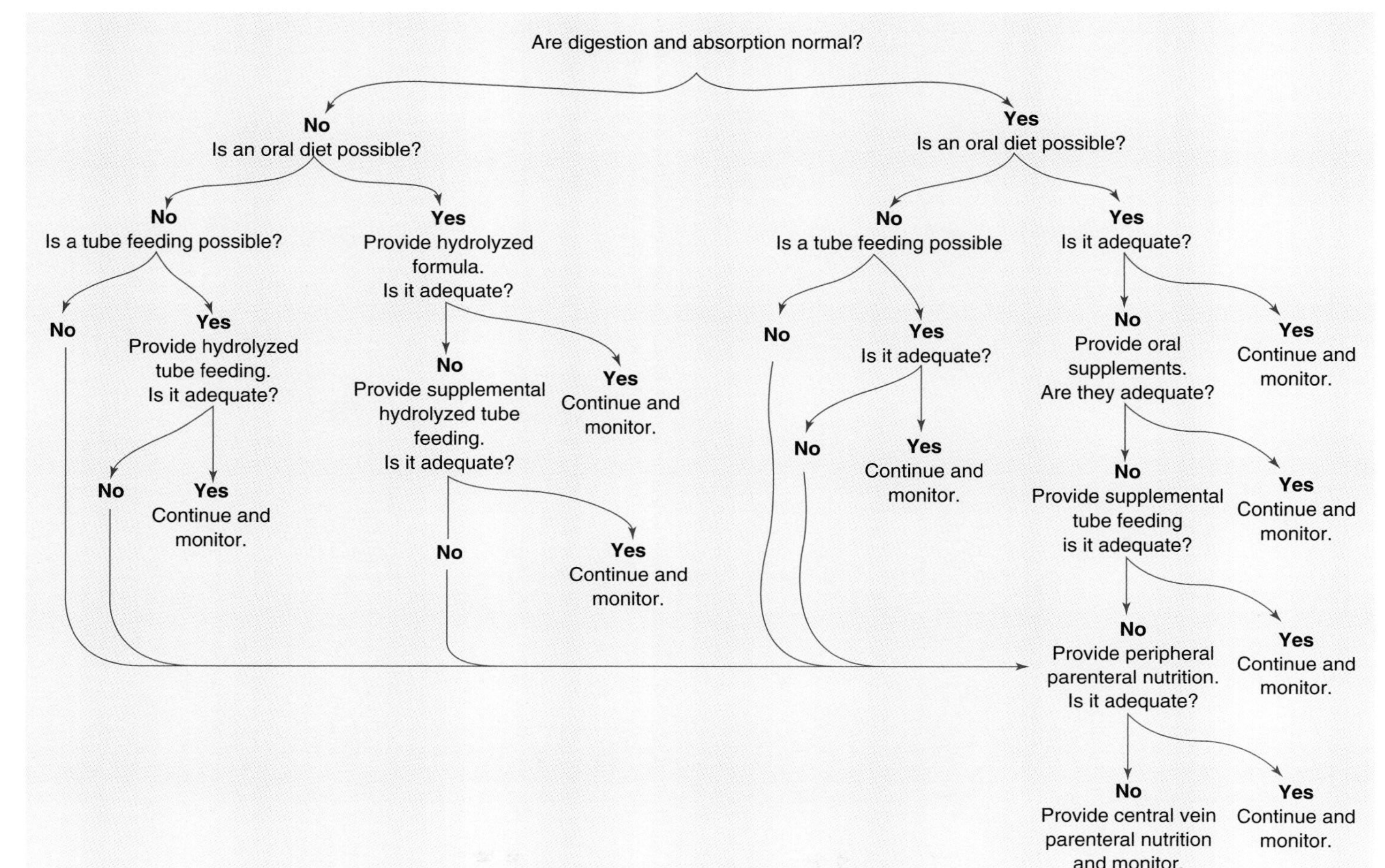

FIGURE 15-1 Selecting the appropriate type and method of feeding.

Hospital Food

Hospital food rarely has a positive image, despite its importance to the patient's health and recovery and overall satisfaction. Although the nurse has no control over the quality of the food, nursing actions can greatly affect the patient's satisfaction with the food. Delivering the tray in a courteous manner, showing a positive attitude toward the food, and explaining the diet to the patient are acts that increase patient satisfaction. Patients who are satisfied are more likely to eat well than patients who are dissatisfied.

Private and government regulatory agencies require that hospital menus be supervised by a qualified dietitian and that they meet the Recommended Dietary Allowances. These stipulations are intended to prevent deficiency diseases, not to prevent chronic diseases. Because of this focus, "regular" diets in hospitals (ie, the default menu sent to patients who do not select their own food) often fail to meet the *Dietary Guidelines for Americans* recommendations to limit fat, saturated fat, cholesterol, and sodium (see Chapter 8). Likewise, the fiber content is often less than recommended. An argument against making routine hospital diets "heart-healthy" is that the objective of feeding patients is to meet increased needs, not to avoid nutritional excesses.

TYPES OF DIETS

Hospital food comes in a variety of regular and modified oral diets. Often combination diets are ordered, such as a 1500-calorie, low-sodium diet or a high-protein, soft diet. Categories of diets include the following.

Normal, Regular, or House Diets

Regular diets are used to achieve or maintain optimal nutritional status in patients who do not have altered nutritional needs related to illness, injury, or impaired health. No foods are excluded, and portion sizes are not restricted on a normal diet. The nutritional value of the diet varies significantly with the actual foods chosen by the patient.

Regular diets are adjusted to meet age-specific needs throughout the life cycle. For instance, a regular diet for a child differs from one for a pregnant woman or an elderly patient. Regular diets are also altered to meet specifications for vegetarian or kosher eating.

Sometimes physicians order a *diet as tolerated (DAT)* on admission or after surgery. This order is interpreted according to the patient's appetite and ability to eat and tolerate food. The nurse has the authority to advance the diet as tolerated.

Modified Consistency Diets

The following diets are modified in consistency and texture: clear liquid, full liquid, soft, mechanical soft, pureed, low-residue, and high-fiber. Usually, after acute illness or when oral intake resumes after a prolonged period, clear liquids are ordered and progressed to full liquids, then to a soft diet, and finally to a normal or modified diet, as appropriate. Depending on the patient's tolerance and condition, this routine progression may be accelerated by eliminating one or more of the transitional diets. Table 15–1 outlines the characteristics, indications, and contraindications for liquid and soft diets.

Calorie-Specific Diets

Diets with specific calorie levels are ordered to promote weight loss or to provide a consistent calorie intake as indicated (eg, in the treatment of diabetes). The specified calorie levels usually range from 1000 to 3000 cal/day. When weight gain is desired, the physician may simply order a "high-calorie" diet without specifying a desired calorie level.

(*text continued on page 440*)

TABLE 15.1 ***Characteristics, Indications, and Contraindications for Liquid and Soft Diets***

Diet Characteristics	Foods Allowed	Indications	Contraindications
Clear Liquid			
A short-term, highly restrictive diet composed only of clear fluids or foods that become fluid at body temperature (eg, gelatin). It requires minimal digestion and leaves a minimum of residue. Although they provide some electrolytes and carbohydrates, clear liquid diets are inadequate in calories and all nutrients (except vitamin C if vitamin C–fortified juices are used). Be sure to include bouillon in the diet if electrolyte replacement is needed; eliminate bouillon if the client requires sodium restriction (one bouillon cube provides 424 mg of sodium).	Clear broth or bouillon Coffee, tea, and carbonated beverages, as allowed and as tolerated Fruit juices, clear (apple, cranberry, grape) and strained (orange, lemonade, grapefruit) Fruit ice made from clear fruit juice Gelatin Popsicles Sugar, honey, hard candy Clear liquid supplements (eg, Enlive!)	Initial feeding after surgery or parenteral nutrition; in preparation for surgery or certain diagnostic tests of the bowel	Long-term use

(continued)

TABLE 15.1 ***Characteristics, Indications, and Contraindications for Liquid and Soft Diets (continued)***

Diet Characteristics	Foods Allowed	Indications	Contraindications
Full Liquid			
Composed of foods that are liquid or liquefy at body temperature (eg, ice cream). Full liquid diets can be carefully planned or supplemented to approximate the nutritional value of a regular of high-calorie, high-protein diet, making them suitable for long-term use. Full liquid diets may be inadequate in folic acid, iron, vitamin B_6, and fiber. If the diet is used longer than 2–3 d, the following modifications may be needed to increase calories and protein: Add sugar and syrups whenever possible. Use whole-fat milk unless the client has hypercholesterolemia. Melt butter or margarine on soup and cereal. Add glucose supplements to fruit juices, milk, and milk drinks. Add skim milk powder to milk, milk drinks, soup, custard, puddings, and cereal. Add instant breakfast mix or commercial supplements.	All items on the clear liquid diet plus: All milk and milk drinks, puddings, and custards All vegetable juices All fruit juices Refined or strained cereals Eggs in custard Butter, margarine, cream	Used as a transition between a clear liquid diet and a soft diet and by clients who have difficulty chewing or swallowing	Severe lactose intolerance (diet relies heavily on milk and dairy products for protein and calories) Unless modified to decrease the cholesterol content, a liquid diet is not suitable for long-term use by clients with hypercholesterolemia.

(continued)

TABLE 15.1 ***Characteristics, Indications, and Contraindications for Liquid and Soft Diets (continued)***

Diet Characteristics	Foods Allowed	Indications	Contraindications
Full Liquid (continued)			
Lactose-reduced milk is available for clients with lactose intolerance. Adapt the diet for clients with diabetes mellitus, renal disease, and other disorders. Low-sodium soups, eggnogs, and custards should be used by clients who require sodium restriction. To avoid salmonella infection, raw eggs should not be used.			
Soft Diet			
An adequate diet that is moderately low in fiber and lightly seasoned. Food textures range from smooth and creamy to moderately crisp. Restrictions vary considerably among institutions, but most raw fruits and vegetables, coarse breads and cereals, and potentially gas-forming foods are excluded.	All items on the full liquid diet plus: Cooked vegetables as tolerated Lettuce in small amounts Cooked or canned fruit Avocado Banana Grapefuit and orange sections without membranes Melon White, refined-wheat, or light-rye enriched breads and cereals Potatoes Enriched rice, barley, pasta All lean, tender meats; fish; poultry Eggs, mild cheese, smooth peanut butter	Used for patients who are unable to tolerate a regular diet after surgery or because of mild gastrointestinal distress Used as a transition between liquids and a regular diet	None

(continued)

TABLE 15.1 *Characteristics, Indications, and Contraindications for Liquid and Soft Diets (continued)*

Diet Characteristics	Foods Allowed	Indications	Contraindications
Soft Diet (continued)			
	Soybeans and other meat alternatives Flavored or plain yogurt Butter, margarine, mild salad dressings Cakes, cookies, and pies made with allowed foods		
Mechanical Soft Diet			
A regular diet modified in texture only. Excludes most raw fruits and vegetables and foods containing seeds, nuts, and dried fruit.	Moist foods that require minimal of chewing Texture may be modified by: Chopping, grinding, puréeing Soaking foods in gelatin or commercial thickener slurry (eg, for breads, cakes, cookies)	Used for patients who have limited chewing ability because they are edentulous or have ill-fitting dentures	None

Modified Nutrient Diets

These diets are *therapeutic*, meaning that they are used in the treatment of disease or illness. They are modified in the concentration of macronutrients (eg, high protein, low fat), in the concentration of micronutrients (eg, low sodium, low potassium), or in fluid.

Diets Restricting or Eliminating Certain Foods

These diets are disease specific. For instance, a gluten-free diet is used only in the treatment of celiac disease, and a phenylalanine-restricted diet is reserved for patients with phenylketonuria, a genetic disorder.

ENCOURAGING INTAKE

Giving the right food to the patient is one thing; getting the patient to eat it (or most of it) is another. The nurse plays a key role in promoting an adequate intake and bridging the gap between the dietary department and the patient. Attention to details can make a big difference in the patient's acceptance of hospital food. Consider the following points:

- **Let the patient select his or her own menu whenever possible.** This gives the patient a greater sense of control, increases the likelihood that the food will be consumed, and may prompt the patient to ask questions about the particular diet or provide information about his or her personal food and nutrition history. The patient's rights and preferences should be respected at all times.
- **Work with the patient to individualize the diet as much as possible to ensure optimal tolerance and compliance.** Patients who do not like menu selections should be offered daily "standby" choices as alternatives. Be aware that "hospital food" is frequently used as a vehicle for patients to vent anger and frustration over their loss of control.
- **Be a patient advocate about diet progressions.** Traditionally, clear liquid diets are given on the first postoperative day if bowel sounds are present and abdominal distention is absent. Once flatus is passed, the diet gradually advances to regular. However, this routine may be based more on history and convention than on science, especially for short-stay patients. Studies show that early introduction of solid food is safe and feasible and can enhance recovery and decrease length of stay for certain types of short-stay postsurgical patients. For these types of patients, a meal of simple fluid and solid items (eg, a sandwich, pudding, dehydrated soup mix that can be prepared later, juice, milk) may be better than traditional liquids. Keep in mind that advancing the diet as quickly as possible allows the patient to meet nutritional requirements sooner and increases patient satisfaction.
- **Set the stage for a pleasant meal.** Be sure trays are delivered promptly to ensure that the foods are at the proper temperatures. Adjust the lighting and make sure the patient is in an appropriate sitting position. Screen the patient from offensive sights and remove unpleasant odors from the room. Encourage family to visit at mealtime, if appropriate. Offer mouth care to improve appetite, if appropriate.
- **Be positive.** Refrain from negative comments about the food. Also be aware of what your body language is saying to the patient. A frown or raised eyebrows can speak volumes.
- **Provide assistance when necessary.** Encourage the patient to self-feed to the greatest extent possible. Some patients may benefit from minor help, such as opening milk cartons or buttering bread; others may need to be completely fed. Monitor the patient's ability to self-feed and adjust the intensity of help accordingly.
- **Gently motivate the patient to eat.** Sometimes encouragement is all that is needed to get the patient to eat. For other patients, motivation comes from being made aware of the importance of food in the recovery process. Thinking of food as part of treatment instead of a social function may improve intake even when appetite is compromised.
- **Identify eating problems.** Patients who feel full quickly should be encouraged to eat the most nutritious items first (meat, milk) and save the less dense items for last (juice, soup, coffee). Patients who have difficulty chewing benefit from a mechanical soft diet. Determine whether the patient would accept between-meal supplements and a bedtime snack to help maximize intake.

IMPROVING NUTRITION WITH SUPPLEMENTS

Some patients are unable or unwilling to eat enough food to meet their requirements, either because intake is poor or because their nutritional needs are so high that it is difficult to meet requirements in a normal volume of food. For these patients, liquid supplements with or between meals can significantly boost protein and calorie intake.

Liquid supplements are easy to consume, are generally well accepted, and tend to leave the stomach quickly, making them a good choice for between-meal snacks. Different brands taste different. If a patient refuses a supplement because of its taste, offer a nutritionally comparable alternative. Studies suggest that patient knowledge of the brand name of the supplement (ie, "the power of advertising") increases acceptability. With any supplement, taste fatigue may occur over time. To maximize acceptance, serve oral supplements cold and experiment with different flavors.

Categories of supplements include clear liquid supplements, milk-based drinks, prepared liquid supplements, and specially prepared foods. Modular products are a special category of single-nutrient supplements that are used to enhance the nutrient density of food or tube feedings. A sampling of products follows.

For more information about various nutritional supplements contact:
Ross Laboratories at www.ross.com (eg, Ensure)
Mead Johnson at www.meadjohnson.com (eg, Boost)
Nestlé InfoLink at 1-800-422-ASK2

Clear Liquid Supplements

Clear liquid supplements are mixed with water to provide protein, calories, or both for patients on clear liquid diets. They are extremely low in fat and have little residue. Although they come in flavors, they are not as well accepted as the other categories of supplements.

Product	Serving Size (oz)	Protein (g)	Calories
Enlive!	8.1	10	300

Milk-Based Supplements

Homemade milk-based supplements may be prepared "from scratch" or with the use of powdered commercial mixes; a few milk-based drinks come prepared and individually packaged. Milk-based drinks provide significant amounts of protein and calories, are palatable, and are relatively inexpensive. However, these drinks are not appropriate for patients with lactose intolerance (ie, those who are unable to digest milk sugar) or for those who need complete nutritional support.

Product	Serving Size (oz)	Protein (g)	Calories
Shake mix in whole milk	8	9.0	263
Instant breakfast mix			
With skim milk	8	12.5	210
With whole milk	8	12.5	280
Eggnog mix in whole milk	8	15.0	290

Commercially Prepared Routine Liquid Supplements

A wide variety of all-purpose, commercially prepared supplements are available that vary in composition, taste, and cost. They are quick and easy, consistent in quality, varied in flavor, and often available in grocery stores. Most are suitable as tube feedings. Standard supplements usually provide 1.0 to 1.2 cal/mL, and 14% to 16% of the total calories are from protein. They are low in residue and lactose free.

Product	Serving Size (oz)	Protein (g)	Calories
Boost	8	10.0	240
Ensure	8	8.8	250
Resource Standard	8	8.8	250

Variations of Routine Supplements

Variations of the standard formulas include high-protein, high-calorie, light, and added-fiber types.

Product	Serving Size (oz)	Protein (g)	Calories	Fiber (g)
High protein: For people who need more protein but not necessarily more calories				
Ensure High Protein	8	12.0	250	—
Boost High Protein Liquid	8	15.0	240	—
High calorie: Concentrated source of protein and calories for people who need to limit volume or fluid				
Ensure Plus	8	13.0	360	—
Boost Plus	8	14.4	360	—
Resource Plus	8	13.0	355	—
Light: Less fat and calories than routine supplements				
Ensure Light	8	10.0	200	—
Added fiber: Routine supplement with fiber				
Boost with Fiber	8	11.0	250	3.0
Ensure with Fiber	8	9.4	260	3.4

Commercially Prepared Supplemental Foods

As an alternative to liquid supplements, manufacturers offer a variety of prepared puddings and bars that provide a concentrated source of protein and calories.

Product	Serving Size (oz)	Protein (g)	Calories
Puddings			
Boost Pudding	5.0	7.0	240
Resource Fortified Pudding (frozen)	5.0	9.0	250
Bars			
Boost Bar	1.6	4.0	190

Modular Products

Modular products are a way of boosting nutrient intake without increasing volume. They are composed of a single nutrient, either carbohydrate (eg, hydrolyzed cornstarch), protein (eg, whey protein), or fat (eg, medium-chain triglycerides [MCT oil]). Used individually or in combination, they increase nutrient density of foods or enteral formulas. For instance, a protein module may be added to a tube feeding to increase protein density without significantly affecting volume. Likewise, clients with chronic renal failure may receive carbohydrate-fortified mashed potatoes and juices to increase calorie intake without increasing protein content. Disadvantages of using modular products are quality control (calculation errors), bacterial contamination, higher costs than standard formulas, and possible nutrient imbalances when modules are added to tube feedings.

Product	Composition	Nutrient Value
Carbohydrate modules		
Modulcal	100% maltodextrins	1 tbsp (8 g) provides 30 cal
Polycose	Glucose polymers derived from hydrolysis of cornstarch	Liquid form: 1 oz provides 60 cal Powdered form: 2 tbsp (12 g) provides 46 cal
Protein modules		
Casec	Calcium caseinate (approximately 95% of calories) and soy lecithin (approximately 5% of calories)	5 g provides 4.5 g protein and 19 cal
ProMod	D-Whey protein concentrate (71% of calories) and soy lecithin (19% of calories)	One 6.6-g scoop provides 5 g protein and 28 cal
Fat modules		
MCT oil	Medium-chain triglycerides derived from coconut oil	1 tbsp (15 mL) provides 115 cal (8.3 cal/g)

Enteral Nutrition

Enteral nutrition is defined as the delivery of nutrients by mouth or tube into the gastrointestinal tract. In practice, the term usually refers to tube feeding.

Tube feedings are the preferred method of feeding whenever oral intake is inadequate and the gastrointestinal tract is at least partially functional, accessible, and safe to use. Enteral nutrition has distinct physical and psychological advantages over parenteral nutrition (ie, feeding by vein). First of all, use of the gastrointestinal tract helps maintain its integrity and function by preventing gut atrophy and reduces the risk of sepsis by preventing bacterial translocation (the movement of gut bacteria from the gastrointestinal tract into lymph nodes and bloodstream). Furthermore, enteral nutrition is safer and significantly less costly than parenteral nutrition. Psychologically, the patient feels somewhat more normal than when fed by vein.

Tube feedings are appropriate for patients who are or will become malnourished because they are not able to consume an adequate oral intake, such as patients who have problems chewing and swallowing; have prolonged lack of appetite; have an obstruction, fistula, or altered motility in the upper gastrointestinal tract; are in a coma; or have very high nutrient requirements. Although they are not routinely prescribed, tube feedings may be beneficial in cases of major trauma, acute or chronic liver failure, malabsorption syndromes, chemotherapy, or radiotherapy and as a transition between parenteral nutrition and an oral diet. Tube feedings are contraindicated when the gastrointestinal tract is nonfunctional, as in gastric or intestinal obstruction, paralytic ileus, intractable vomiting, and severe diarrhea.

TYPES OF FORMULAS

There are a vast number of commercial tube feeding formulas available. One way of categorizing formulas is by the type of protein they contain. Intact formulas contain whole proteins and complex forms of other nutrients. Partially hydrolyzed (partially digested) formulas contain small fragments of proteins in the form of amino acids, dipeptides, and tripeptides, as well as partially digested carbohydrates and fats. Within both categories there are disease-specific formulas.

Intact Protein Formulas

Intact formulas are made from whole complete proteins (eg, milk, meat, eggs) or **protein isolates** (semipurified, high-biologic-value proteins that have been extracted from milk, soybean, or eggs). Because they contain complex molecules of protein, carbohydrate, and fat, intact formulas require normal digestive and absorptive capacity. They are complete with regard to vitamins, minerals, and trace elements. There are several categories of intact formulas designed to meet a variety of needs.

- **Blenderized formulas** provide approximately 1.0 cal/mL and 16% of calories from protein. Unlike other supplements, they are made from regular foods (eg, beef, milk, fruits, vegetables) that are blended to liquid consistency. They contain fiber, and some contain lactose. Examples include Compleat Regular and Vitaneed.
- **Standard formulas** provide approximately 1.0 to 1.2 cal/mL and 14% to 16% of calories from protein. They are low in residue and lactose free. Although they are intended to be used as tube feedings, they are sometimes given orally. Examples include Attain, Isocal, and Osmolite.
- **High-calorie formulas** supply 1.5 to 2.0 cal/mL and have approximately 14% to 17% of calories from protein. They are intended for patients who need to gain weight and those who have volume or fluid restrictions. Examples are Deliver 2.0 and Magnacal.
- **High-protein formulas** provide 1.0 to 2.0 cal/mL and more than 16% of total calories from protein. They are low in residue and are sometimes used orally. Examples are Isocal HN, Osmolite HN, and Promote.
- **Formulas enriched with fiber** provide 1.0 to 1.5 cal/mL and are intended for patients who experience diarrhea or constipation from low-residue formulas. Although high-fiber formulas have been promoted as normalizing bowel function in tube-fed clients, definitive studies on the efficacy of fiber are lacking. Nevertheless, because fiber helps maintain gut mucosal integrity, it may be a desirable component of a standard tube-feeding regimen. Some fiber-enriched formulas are appropriate for oral use. Examples are Fibersource, Jevity, and UltraCal.
- **Intact specialty formulas** are available for a variety of conditions, such as diabetes (Glucerna, Glytrol); pulmonary disorders (Pulmoncare, Respalor); fat malabsorption (Lipisorb Liquid); impaired immune system functioning (Advera, Impact); metabolic stress (TraumaCal); and renal insufficiency (Suplena). They are the equivalent of a therapeutic diet in tube-feeding form.

Hydrolyzed Formulas

Hydrolyzed formulas, also known as *elemental formulas*, contain partially digested nutrients such as monosaccharides and disaccharides (carbohydrate); amino acids, dipeptides, and tripeptides (protein); and medium- and long-chain triglycerides (fat). They are intended for patients with impaired digestion or absorption. These formulas provide 1.0 to 1.5 cal/mL and have 8% to 17% of total calories from protein. They have minimal residue and low viscosity and are lactose free. Most are hypertonic. They are relatively expensive, but they are not well accepted orally and should be used only when digestion and/or absorption is impaired. Examples include Tolerex, Vital HN, and Criticare HN.

- **Stress formulas** are hydrolyzed formulas that are high in branched-chain amino acids, which are metabolized primarily in the peripheral muscle tissue. They may be used preferentially for energy during stress. Examples include Vivonex T.E.N.

- **Specially defined formulas** are hydrolyzed formulas designed for patients with specific metabolic disorders, such as renal failure (AminAid Instant Drink) or hepatic failure (Hepatic-Aid II). Neither of these examples is a complete formula; both lack vitamins and electrolytes.

OTHER CHARACTERISTICS

Besides the complexity of the protein and other nutrients provided, formulas vary in other characteristics. For instance, the amount of protein, calories, and fat provided in a given volume varies among categories (eg, intact versus hydrolyzed formulas), among subgroups within each category (eg, routine versus high-protein varieties), and among individual brands within each subgroup (eg, Osmolite versus Isocal). Cost is another variable. Hydrolyzed formulas and disease-specific formulas are more expensive than routine intact formulas. Other variable characteristics are osmolality and fiber/residue content.

Osmolality

Osmolality is the measure of the number of particles in solution, expressed as milliosmoles per kilogram (mOsm/kg). In enteral formulas, osmolality is determined by the concentration of sugars, amino acids, and electrolytes. Generally, the more digested the protein, the greater the osmolality.

Isotonic formulas have approximately the same osmolality as blood, about 300 mOsm/kg. Osmolalities higher than this are classified as *hypertonic* or *hyperosmolar*. Formulas that are isotonic or mildly hypertonic are well tolerated by most patients. By comparison, hypertonic formulas may not be well tolerated, especially when they are delivered into the intestines at full strength. The high osmolality draws water into the intestines to dilute the particle concentration, which leads to cramping, nausea, and diarrhea **(dumping syndrome)**. Tolerance improves when hypertonic formulas are initiated at a slower rate or strength.

Fiber and Residue

The terms fiber and residue are frequently used interchangeably, but they are not synonymous. **Fiber** is the group name for carbohydrates that are not digested in the human gastrointestinal tract. In addition to stimulating peristalsis and increasing stool bulk, fiber is degraded by gastrointestinal bacteria to short-chain fatty acids, which promote the repair and maintenance of the intestinal lining. Fiber, together with undigested food, intestinal secretions, bacterial cell bodies, and cells shed from the intestinal lining, make up **residue.** Therefore, fiber is a component of residue, but residue encompasses other substances as well.

The residue content of enteral formulas varies greatly. Hydrolyzed formulas are essentially residue free because they are completely absorbed. Most standard intact formulas are low in residue, although some have fiber added. Blenderized formulas contain fiber.

Fiber may help normalize bowel function in people with constipation or diarrhea. Because fiber helps maintain gastrointestinal integrity, formulas with added fiber should be considered when tube feedings are to be used for a long period. However, some patients experience gas and bloating from formulas with fiber. Formulas with added fiber usually are not appropriate as an initial feeding in patients who have been on bowel rest, in patients with certain gastrointestinal disorders, or in patients who have had gastrointestinal surgery.

INDIVIDUAL CONSIDERATIONS

A primary consideration when choosing a formula for tube feeding is whether the patient is able to adequately digest and absorb food. The answer to that question will decide whether an intact formula or a hydrolyzed formula is indicated. This decision only begins the selection process, because within each of these broad categories there are many formulas available. Questions to answer when determining the most appropriate tube feeding are:

- What are the patient's nutritional requirements? Can these needs be met by a reasonable volume of a standard formula, or is a different formula needed? For instance, does the patient need more protein, more calories, or a diabetic formula?
- What is the patient's individual tolerance? Is the patient lactose intolerant, either permanently or secondary to surgery or illness? Would the patient benefit from trying a high-fiber formula because of diarrhea or constipation?
- Which tube feeding formulas are available? Facilities stock only a limited variety of formulas, based on assessment of need, versatility of the product, and cost.

FEEDING TUBE PLACEMENT

The placement of the feeding tube depends on the client's medical status and the anticipated length of time the tube feeding will be used. Transnasal tubes, of which the nasogastric (NG) tube is the most common, are generally used for tube feedings of relatively short duration (ie, <3–4 weeks). Ostomies, or stomas, are surgically created openings made to deliver feedings directly into the stomach or intestines. They are the preferred method for permanent or long-term feedings because they can be hidden under clothing and eliminate irritation to the mucous membranes. Percutaneous endoscopic gastrostomy (PEG) tubes are placed with the aid of an endoscope. The correct placement of any feeding tube should be determined by radiographs of the chest that are taken before the first feeding is initiated. Table 15–2 summarizes the advantages and disadvantages of various feeding routes.

TABLE 15.2 ***Advantages and Disadvantages of Various Feeding Routes***

Route	Indications	Advantages	Disadvantages
Nasogastric (NG)	Inabililty to safely and adequately consume oral intake Short-term feeding (<6 wk) with functional gastrointestinal tract	Easy to place and remove tube Uses stomach as reservoir Can use intermittent feedings Dumping syndrome less likely than with NI feedings	Contraindicated for clients at high risk for aspiration Potentially irritating to the nose and esophagus May be removed by uncooperative or confused patients Not appropriate for long-term use Unaesthetic for patient
Nasointestinal (NI)	Short-term feeding for patients at high risk of aspiration, delayed gastric emptying, or gastroesophageal reflux disease (GERD)	Less risk of aspiration, especially important for patients who have impaired gag or cough reflex, decreased consciousness, ventilator dependence, or a history of aspiration pneumonia	Increased risk of dumping syndrome Not appropriate for intermittent or bolus feedings Not appropriate for long-term use Unaesthetic for patient
Gastrostomy	For long-term use in patients with a functional gastrointestinal tract Frequently used for patients with impaired ability to swallow	Same advantages as NG, but more comfortable and aesthetic for patient Confirmation of tube placement easier Cannot be misplaced into the trachea	PEG insertion contraindicated for clients who cannot have an endoscopy Risk of aspiration pneumonia in clients with GERD Stoma care required Danger of peritonitis Potential for tube dislodgment
Jejunostomy	For long-term use in patients at high risk for aspiration pneumonia and in clients with altered gastrointestinal integrity above the jejunum For short-term use after gastrointestinal surgery	Low risk of aspiration No risk of misplacing tube into the trachea More comfortable and aesthetic for clients than transnasal tubes Because motility resumes more quickly in the intestines than in the stomach after gastrointestinal surgery, feedings can begin sooner than other feedings	Small-diameter tubes easily become clogged Peritonitis can occur from tube dislodgment Cannot be used for intermittent or bolus feedings Stoma care required

HANDLING FORMULA

Improper handling of formulas increases the risk of bacterial contamination, commonly known as *food poisoning*. In a population of patients who are malnourished and therefore compromised immunologically, food poisoning is a serious complication of tube feeding. To reduce the risk of bacterial contamination, closed feeding systems are recommended. Precautions to take when closed systems are not used include:

- Use clean equipment.
- Wash hands thoroughly before handling the formula.
- Clean the top of the formula can before opening.
- Label cans that are not emptied with the date and time of opening.
- Cover opened cans; store mixed or diluted formulas in clean containers.
- Refrigerate unused formula promptly.
- Discard unlabeled formula and all opened cans within 24 hours.
- Rinse the feeding container and extension tubing with water before adding new formula.
- Never add a supply of new formula to old formula.
- Flush the tube with water before and after each use.
- Hang feeding solutions for less than 6 hours.
- Change the feeding container and extension tubing every 24 hours.

ADMINISTRATION

Initiating the Feeding

Before initiating a feeding, tube placement is verified, preferably by radiography, and bowel sounds are confirmed to be present. Elevate the patient's upper body to at least a 30° angle during the feeding and for at least 30 minutes afterward to reduce the risk of aspiration.

Most patients tolerate isotonic and many hypertonic formulas when initiated at full strength. Initial feedings may begin at 50 mL/hour and advance by 25 mL/hour every 12 to 24 hours until the desired rate is achieved. However, patients who are malnourished, who are under severe stress, who have not eaten in a long time, or who are receiving intestinal feedings may not tolerate hypertonic formulas. For these patients, it may be necessary to infuse the formula at a very slow rate (eg, 25 mL/hour). After tolerance is established, the rate is advanced by 25 mL/hour as tolerated every 4 to 12 hours until the desired rate is achieved. Sometimes it is necessary to dilute hypertonic formulas, gradually increase the strength, and then gradually increase the rate. Rate and concentration should never be advanced at the same time, and neither should be progressed until 4 to 12 hours after tolerance is established.

Delivery Methods

Formulas may be given intermittently or continuously over a period of 8 to 24 hours. The rates may be regulated either by a pump or by gravity drip. The type of delivery method to be used depends on the type and location of the feeding tube, the type of formula being administered, and the patient's tolerance.

Intermittent Tube Feedings

Intermittent feedings are administered in equal portions of no more than 250 mL of formula. They offer the advantage of resembling a more normal pattern of intake and allow the client more freedom of movement between feedings. Tolerance of intermittent feedings is optimized by infusing the formula at room temperature by slow gravity drip or by pump over a 20- to 30-minute period. To decrease the risk of aspiration, gastric residuals are checked before each feeding until tolerance is clearly established. Residuals should be less than 150 mL before each intermittent feeding; replace aspirate to reduce the loss of electrolytes and gastric juices.

Bolus feedings are a variation of intermittent feedings. They are poured into the barrel of a large syringe that is attached to the feeding tube. A large volume of formula (300–400 mL) is delivered in a short period. These rapid feedings are given four to six times per day. They are poorly tolerated and often cause *dumping syndrome:* nausea, diarrhea, glucosuria, distention, cramps, vomiting, and increased risk of aspiration.

Continuous Drip Method

Continuous drip feedings are given over an 8- to 24-hour period to maximize tolerance and nutrient absorption. This method is recommended for feeding of critically ill clients and for feedings delivered into the jejunum, and it is frequently used to begin a feeding into the stomach (ie, NG, gastrostomy, or PEG). Infusion pumps are used to ensure consistent flow rates. Feedings should be interrupted every 6 hours so that water can be infused into the line to clear the tubing and hydrate the client. Gastric residuals are measured every 4 to 6 hours. If the volume of gastric residual exceeds the volume of formula given over the previous 2 hours, it may be necessary to reduce the rate of feeding.

WATER FOR THE EQUIPMENT AND THE PATIENT

Periodic flushing of the tube with water helps ensure patency. Intermittent feedings should be followed by an infusion of 40 to 50 mL of warm water, and continuous-feeding tubes should be irrigated every 6 hours with 40 to 50 mL of warm water. Likewise, every time the feeding is interrupted, the tube should be flushed with water.

The water content of tube feedings varies with the caloric concentration. Standard formulas (1.0 cal/mL) provide 850 mL of water per liter. Formulas that furnish 1.5 cal/mL supply approximately 775 mL of water per liter of formula, and 2.0 cal/mL formulas provide approximately 660 mL of water per liter.

Adults in general need approximately 2000 mL of water daily. Patients with fever, vomiting, diarrhea, blood loss, draining fistulas, or burns have higher fluid requirements. Whether the patient needs additional water to meet fluid requirements depends on his or her medical status and how much fluid is given through the tube feeding and flushing.

MEDICATIONS BY TUBE

Although many medications are frequently given through feeding tubes to patients who are unable to swallow, they should never be given while a feeding is being infused. Some drugs become ineffective if added directly to the enteral formula; also, adding drugs to the formula may result in a clogged tube. It is important to stop the feeding before administering drugs and to make sure the tube is flushed with 15 to 30 mL of water before and after the drug is given. If more than one drug is given, flush the tube between doses.

Other drug considerations include the following:

- Drugs that are absorbed from the stomach should never be given through a nasointestinal tube.
- The liquid form of a medication, diluted with 30 mL of water, should be used for feeding tube administration. If there is no alternative, a drug can be crushed to a fine powder and mixed with water before it is administered. Slow-release drugs should never be crushed.
- Drugs should be given orally whenever possible.
- Tube feeding may need to be temporarily stopped to permit drug administration on an empty stomach or to avoid drug-nutrient interaction.

TRANSITION TO ORAL DIET

The goal of diet intervention during the transition period between enteral nutrition and an oral diet is to ensure an adequate nutritional intake while promoting an oral diet. To begin the transition process, the tube feeding should be stopped for 1 hour before each meal. Gradually increase meal frequency until six small oral feedings are accepted. Actual intake should be recorded and evaluated daily. When oral calorie intake consistently includes 500 to 750 cal/day, tube feedings may be given only during the night. When the client consistently consumes two thirds of protein and calorie needs orally for 3 to 5 days, the tube feeding may be totally discontinued.

NURSING PROCESS

The following care plan assumes that the health care team assessed the patient's need for tube feeding and the appropriate order was written to meet the patient's nutritional requirements and goals.

The indicated nursing diagnosis is an example of only one potential problem associated with tube feedings. Other potential problems and their nursing management appear in Box 15–1.

Assessment

Because most patients who are receiving tube feedings have had feeding difficulties or medical problems that place them at increased risk, initial and periodic nutritional assessments are vital to the success of a tube feeding.

Obtain clinical data:

Current nutrition prescription (name of formula, amount, frequency, volume per 24 hours)

(text continues on page 460)

BOX 15.1

Trouble-Shooting for Nutrition-Related Problems in Tube-Fed Patients

Potential Problem	Rationale	Nursing Interventions and Considerations
Regurgitation of stomach contents → aspiration pneumonia	Slowed gastric emptying time (ie, gastric residual >100 mL)	Check gastric residual before each intermittent feeding and every 4 h if continuous feeding is used. Notify physician and evaluate feeding regimen if gastric emptying is consistently delayed. Switch to a continuous drip method of delivery.
	Inhibited cough reflex related to debilitation, unconsciousness, or pulmonary complications	Consider a nasoduodenal, nasojejunal, gastrostomy, or jejunostomy feeding.
	Improper feeding position	Elevate the head of the bed at least 30° during the feeding and for approximately 1 h afterward.
	High fat content of formula (fat delays gastric emptying)	Switch to low-fat formula.
	Relaxed gastroesophageal sphincter related to large-diameter feeding tube	Switch to a pliable, small-diameter feeding tube.
Nausea (Discontinue the feeding. Administer antiemetics if ordered by the physician.)	Malplacement of feeding tube	Check the position of the tube.
	Feeding rate too rapid	Slow the rate of feeding; switch to a continuous drip method of delivery.

(continued)

BOX 15.1

Trouble-Shooting for Nutrition-Related Problems in Tube-Fed Patients (continued)

Potential Problem	Rationale	Nursing Interventions and Considerations
	Volume of formula too great → delayed gastric emptying	Check gastric residual and notify the physician if >100 mL. Reduce the volume, then increase gradually. If distention is contributing to nausea, encourage ambulation.
	Feeding too soon after intubation	Allow approximately 1 h between intubation and the first feeding.
	Anxiety	Explain the procedures to the client and encourage questions. Allow client to verbalize his or her feelings; provide emotional support.
	Intolerance to a specific formula, especially high-fat formulas	Switch to a different formula.
Distention and bloating	High fat content of formula	Switch to lower-fat formula.
	Decrease in gastrointestinal function, especially among critically ill clients	Check for active bowel sounds; switch to a hydrolyzed formula if bowel sounds are hypoactive.
Dehydration	Diarrhea	See Nursing Process section of text.

(continued)

BOX 15.1

Trouble-Shooting for Nutrition-Related Problems in Tube-Fed Patients (continued)

Potential Problem	Rationale	Nursing Interventions and Considerations
	Excessive protein intake → compensatory increase in urine output to excrete nitrogenous wastes	Switch to a formula with less protein. Increase water intake, if possible.
	Inadequate fluid intake	Provide more additional water.
	Glycosuria (glucose in urine)	Test for glucose in the urine; notify physician of glucosuria of 3+ or 4+. Administer insulin if ordered by physician. Switch to a continuous drip method to avoid giving a high-carbohydrate load with each feeding.
Fluid overload	Excessive use of water to flush tube	Use only 30–50 mL of water to rinse tubing after each feeding.
	Formula too dilute	Check formula preparation for proper dilution.
Constipation	Low residue content of formula	Increase residue content if appropriate (ie, change to a formula with added fiber or increase fruits and vegetables in a blenderized diet).
	Inactivity	Encourage ambulation as much as possible.

(continued)

BOX 15.1

Trouble-Shooting for Nutrition-Related Problems in Tube-Fed Patients (continued)

Potential Problem	Rationale	Nursing Interventions and Considerations
	Dehydration	Monitor intake and output. Add free water if intake is not greater than output by 500 to 1000 mL.
	Obstruction	Stop feeding and notify physician.
Gastric rupture	Dangerous retention of feeding in the stomach related to gastric atony or obstruction	Check for residual before beginning each feeding. Observe for signs of impending gastric rupture: distention, epigastric and upper quadrant pain, nausea, a large residual. If observed, discontinue feeding immediately and notify the physician.
Clogged tube	Feeding heated formulas	Do not heat formula.
	Improper cleaning of tube	Replace the feeding tube and bag every 12–24 h. Flush the tube before and after each infusion (regardless of method) with 30–50 mL of water. If flushing fails to remove clog, the tube must be removed and replaced.

(continued)

BOX 15.1

Trouble-Shooting for Nutrition-Related Problems in Tube-Fed Patients (continued)

Potential Problem	Rationale	Nursing Interventions and Considerations
	Formula too thick (Heat can cause changes in the structure of proteins, causing the formula to thicken.)	High-viscosity formulas (ie, blenderized tube feedings or commercial formulas that provide 1.5–2 cal/mL) should be infused by pump and possibly through a large-bore feeding tube to prevent clogging. If possible, consider switching to a less calorically dense formula. Because it is desirable to use the smallest size tube, viscous formulas may be delivered by a pump to help prevent clogging.
Anxiety	Deprivation of food → lack of sensory, social, and cultural satisfaction from eating	Allow oral intake of food that the client requests, if possible. If oral intake is contraindicated, allow the client to chew his or her favorite food without swallowing.

(continued)

BOX 15.1

Trouble-Shooting for Nutrition-Related Problems in Tube-Fed Patients (continued)

Potential Problem	Rationale	Nursing Interventions and Considerations
		If possible, liquefy and add the client's favorite food to the tube feeding. Encourage the client to leave the room when others are eating and find other enjoyable activities. Encourage client and family to view tube feeding as another way of eating, rather than a form of treatment.
	Altered body image	Encourage client to verbalize his or her feelings. Stress positive aspects of tube feeding.
	Loss of control; fear	Encourage client to become involved in preparation and administration of the formula, if possible. Inform client of problems that may occur and how to prevent or cope with them. Encourage socialization with other well-adapted tube-fed clients.

(continued)

BOX 15.1

Trouble-Shooting for Nutrition-Related Problems in Tube-Fed Patients (continued)

Potential Problem	Rationale	Nursing Interventions and Considerations
	Limited mobility	Encourage normal activity. Control gastrointestinal symptoms, such as diarrhea, nausea, vomiting, and constipation, that interfere with normal activity.
	Discomfort related to tube or formula intolerance	Observe for intolerances; alleviate with appropriate interventions. Be sure to inspect and properly care for the tube exit site to avoid potential complications.
Dry mouth	Irritation of the mucous membranes related to lack of oral intake	Encourage good oral hygiene to alleviate soreness and dryness: mouthwash, warm water rinses, regular brushing. Apply petroleum jelly to the lips to prevent cracking. Allow ice chips, sugarless gum, and hard candies, if possible, to stimulate salivation.
	Breathing through the mouth	Encourage client to breathe through the nose as much as possible.

Current height, weight, body mass index (BMI), percentage of usual weight

Laboratory values, especially serum albumin, hemoglobin, hematocrit, glucose, electrolytes, and any other abnormal values for their nutritional significance

Clinical signs and symptoms: bowel function, aspiration risk, blood pressure, lactose intolerance, presence of steatorrhea, difficulty swallowing, clinical signs of malnutrition, signs of dehydration or fluid overload

Fluid status: ability to consume oral liquids, intake and output records

Interview client to assess:

Knowledge, willingness, and readiness to learn tube feeding regimen

Ability to perform activities of daily living

Physical complaints associated with oral food intake or tube feeding, such as fatigue, constipation, diarrhea, nausea, vomiting, early satiety, cramping, or bloating

Psychosocial and economic issues, especially for patients who are candidates for home enteral nutrition: living situation (availability of running water, electricity, refrigeration), cooking and storage facilities, employment, social support system, and financial status

Nursing Diagnosis

Altered Nutrition: Less Than Body Requirements, related to diarrhea secondary to tube feeding.

Planning and Implementation

Although properly administered tube feedings do not cause diarrhea, diarrhea frequently develops in tube-fed clients. Clients fed low-residue formulas cannot be expected to have firm stools; rather, their stools are likely to be pasty or gruel-like. However, if it is established that the client is truly having diarrhea, investigate the probable cause, which could be:

- **Infusion of formula that is cold.** Give canned formulas at room temperature. Warm refrigerated formulas to room temperature in a basin of warm water.
- **Bacterially contaminated formula.** Handwashing and strict sanitation are required for formula preparation. Equipment and utensils used in preparation should be washed in an automatic dishwasher or cleaned with hot, soapy water; rinsed thoroughly in boiling water; and dried upside down. Practice proper techniques for handling formula (see previous discussion).
- **Lactose intolerance,** if milk-based formula is used. Switch to a lactose-free formula.
- **Feeding rate too rapid.** Adhere to facility protocol when initiating and advancing tube feedings. For existing feedings, decrease the rate to the level tolerated and then advance the feeding at a rate of half the original increment (eg, by 12 instead of 25 mL/hour).
- **Volume of formula too great.** Feed smaller volumes of formula at more frequent intervals or switch to a continuous drip method of feeding. Consider a high-calorie formula if problem persists.
- **Dumping syndrome related to hypertonic formula.** Decrease the feeding rate to a

level tolerated by the client; then gradually increase as tolerated. Use the continuous drip method. Switch to an isotonic formula, if possible.

- **Nasogastric feeding tube misplaced into the duodenum, causing dumping syndrome.** Check the position of the tube before administering the formula.
- **Low serum albumin** causing decreased oncotic pressure, which increases water within the bowel, resulting in diarrhea. A low serum albumin concentration, which may indicate malnutrition, may also be accompanied by a decrease in intestinal border enzymes (protein molecules) and/or a decrease or flattening of the microvilli lining the intestinal tract, both of which lead to diarrhea.
- **Side effect of antibiotics or other drugs.** The overgrowth of certain strains of intestinal flora that are not affected by antibiotics is believed to cause diarrhea. These flora digest formula, producing excess gas and acid and resulting in diarrhea. Antibiotic-associated diarrhea may also be related to a superinfection with *Clostridium difficile* or *Staphylococcus aureus*. Medications that may produce diarrhea include antiarrhythmic drugs (quinidine, propranolol), aminophylline, digitalis, potassium supplements, phosphorus supplements, and cimetidine. Investigate possible alternatives; administer antidiarrheals as ordered.

CLIENT GOALS

The client will:

Attain/maintain "healthy" body weight.
Receive ___ calories in ___ mL/day of ___ (product used), as ordered.
Be free of any signs or symptoms of diarrhea or other side effects.
Maintain adequate fluid status.

NURSING INTERVENTIONS

Nutrition Therapy

Implement appropriate interventions for diarrhea based on probable cause.
Reduce rate of administration to highest level tolerated by patient. After 8 to 12 hours, advance feeding slowly and observe tolerance. Gradually attain desired rate as ordered.
Provide supplemental water as needed, based on input and output records and serum sodium concentration, blood urea nitrogen, hematocrit, and urine specific gravity.
Encourage oral intake, if appropriate.

Client Teaching

Instruct the client:

On the importance of tube feedings when oral intake is inadequate or impossible
On the signs and symptoms of intolerance of tube feeding and to alert the nurse if any problems arise
Not to adjust the flow rate unless otherwise instructed

When home enteral nutrition is indicated, discharge teaching should encompass formula preparation, administration, and monitoring, as well as the rationales and interventions for tube feeding complications (Box 15–2).

BOX 15.2

Client Teaching for Home Enteral Nutrition

Provide verbal and written instructions to the client and family on the following:

Formula preparation, including

- Handwashing techniques
- How to mix and prepare, if applicable
- How to store the formula and for how long

Enteral administration, including

- Proper procedure for intubation, if applicable
- How to check for proper tube position
- How to fill and hang the administration bag
- How to check for residuals
- The feeding schedule, with the volume and rate specified
- Correct body positioning during and after feedings
- Which medications to administer through the tube

Oral care, incuding

- Whether and what the client can eat by mouth
- Oral hygiene procedure

Insertion site care, including

- How the skin should look
- How to care for it

Tube care, including

- The name of the tube
- The measurement of the length of feeding tube outside the body
- How to flush the tube
- How to connect the feeding tube, how to cap/clamp the tube

Equipment care, including

- How to use an enteral pump, if indicated
- How to clean the pump
- Maintenance of alarms/batteries

Problem solving, including how to manage

- Diarrhea, constipation, nausea
- Tube malposition and breakage
- A clogged tube
- Mechanical problems with the pump

How frequently to collect the following data:

- Intake and output
- Weight
- Temperature and pulse
- Gastric residuals
- Urine glucose and acetone
- Signs and symptoms to report, such as increased breathing rate, fever, decreased urine output, altered level of consciousness, change in bowel function

Emergency phone numbers, including

- Home care agency/nursing agency
- When to call the physician

How to dispose of equipment

Evaluation

The client:

Attains/maintains "healthy" body weight
Receives ___ calories in ___ mL/day of ___ (product used), as ordered
Is free of signs and symptoms of diarrhea and other side effects
Maintains normal fluid status

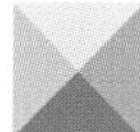

Parenteral Nutrition

Parenteral nutrition delivers nutrients directly into the bloodstream, thereby bypassing the gastrointestinal tract. Parenteral nutrition is used when a patient physically or psychologically cannot consume enough nutrients orally or enterally, or when alteration in gastrointestinal function precludes oral and enteral feedings. The usual fluid volume given to adults over a 24-hour period is 1.5 to 3 L.

COMPOSITION

Parenteral nutrition solutions include dextrose, amino acids, lipid emulsion, electrolytes, vitamins, and trace elements in sterile water. The actual composition of the parenteral solution depends on the site of infusion and the patient's fluid and nutrient requirements. Because there are standard concentrations of protein, carbohydrate, and fat in standard volumes, individualization of parenteral solutions is somewhat limited.

Carbohydrate

The carbohydrate in parenteral solutions is dextrase (a form of glucose that contains water), which provides 3.4 cal/g, not 4.0 cal/g like glucose. Glucose ranges from 10% in peripheral solutions to final concentrations of about 25% in total parenteral solutions. Glucose may be restricted in ventilator-dependent patients because the oxidation of glucose produces more carbon dioxide than does oxidation of fat.

Protein

Protein is provided as a mixture of essential and nonessential amino acids ranging in initial concentration from 5% to 15% of the solution. The quantity of amino acids provided depends on the patient's estimated requirements and hepatic and renal function.

Fat

Lipid emulsions, made from safflower and soybean oil with egg phospholipid as an emulsifier, are isotonic, provide a significant source of calories, and can correct or prevent fatty acid deficiency. They are available in 10% and 20% concentrations, supply 1.1 and 2 cal/mL respectively, and come in 250- and 500-mL volumes. The usual dosage of fat is 0.5 to 1 g/kg/day to supply up to 30% of total calories. Intravenous fat may be provided daily if calorie needs are high, or it may be given several times per week for the purpose of preventing essential fatty acid deficiency. Intravenous fat is contraindicated for patients with severe liver disease, some types of hyperlipidemia, or severe egg allergies. It is used cautiously in patients with atherosclerosis, moderate liver disease, blood coagulation disorders, pancreatitis, or certain types of lung disorders.

Electrolytes, Vitamins, and Trace Elements

The quantity of electrolytes provided is based on the patient's blood chemistry values and physical assessment findings. The electrolyte content can potentially be adjusted three times per day when a 1-L bag is administered over 8 hours. However, total nutrient admixture (TNA) bags may hold a 24-hour quantity of total parenteral nutrition (TPN) solution, which limits flexibility in changing the composition but reduces the risk of contamination.

A standard multivitamin preparation may be added to the TPN solution. Although it is now recognized that minerals and trace elements are a necessary component of TPN to prevent deficiency symptoms, exact parenteral requirements for many of them are not known.

Medications

Medications are sometimes added to intravenous solutions by the pharmacist or infused into them through a separate port. Patients receiving TPN may have insulin ordered to help control serum glucose; this intervention is often necessary because of the high glucose concentration of the solution. Heparin may be added to reduce fibrin buildup on the catheter tip. In general, medications should not be added to TPN solutions because of the potential incompatibilities of the medication and nutrients in the solution.

TYPES OF PARENTERAL NUTRITION

Depending on the patient's nutritional requirements and anticipated length of need, parenteral nutrition is either administered peripherally (PPN) or centrally (TPN). The basic difference between the two types is the concentration of the solutions infused. Solutions infused into peripheral veins must be isotonic (ie, they must have low concentrations of dextrose and amino acids) to prevent phlebitis and increased risk of thrombus formation.

The need to maintain isotonic concentrations of dextrose and amino acids while avoiding fluid overload limits the caloric and nutritional value of PPN. Hypertonic solutions provide more dextrose and/or protein, but they must be delivered centrally in a large-diameter vein so that they can be quickly diluted. TPN is used when nutritional requirements are high and anticipated length of need is relatively long.

Peripheral Parenteral Nutrition

PPN delivers complete but limited nutrition. The final concentration of the solution cannot exceed 10% dextrose and 5% amino acids; vitamins, electrolytes, and trace elements are added. Lipid emulsion may be used to supplement calories, depending on the patient's tolerance.

Three liters of this 10% dextrose and 5% amino acid solution provides only 1620 calories:

10% dextrose = 100 g/L		5% amino acids = 50 g/L
×3 L		×3 L
300 g dextrose		150 g amino acids
×3.4 cal/g		×4 cal/g
1020 cal dextrose	+	600 cal protein = 1620 total calories
To increase calories, one 500-mL bottle of a 20% fat solution may be ordered:		500 mL × 2 cal/mL = 1000 cal fat
		2620 total calories

PPN provides temporary nutritional support. It is best suited for patients who need short-term nutritional support (7–10 days) but do not require more than 2000 to 2500 cal/day. It may also be used for patients with a postsurgical ileus or an anastomotic leak, or for patients who require nutritional support but are unable to use TPN because of limited accessibility to a central vein. Sometimes PPN is used to supplement an oral diet or tube feeding, or as a transition from TPN to an enteral intake.

PPN is not adequate for patients who have increased nutritional requirements or who need more than 2500 cal/day, and it is contraindicated in patients with abnormal lipid metabolism (eg, elevated serum triglycerides) or poor peripheral veins.

Central Vein Total Parenteral Nutrition

TPN infuses hypertonic nutritional solutions through an indwelling central venous catheter (CVC) with the tip placed in the superior vena cava. It provides more concentrated nutrition in an equal volume of fluid.

A typical order for TPN may specify 3 L of solution daily with a final concentration of 25% dextrose and 3.5% amino acids. An additional 250 mL of 20% lipid is ordered.

25% dextrose = 250 g dextrose/L		3.5% amino acids = 35 g/L
×3 L		×3 L
750 g dextrose		105 g amino acids
×3.4 cal/g		×4 cal/g
2550 cal dextrose	+	420 cal protein = 2970 total calories
For the additional 250 mL of a 20% lipid emulsion added to the infusion:		250 mL × 2.0 cal/mL = 500 lipid cal
		3470 total cal

TPN is used to provide complete, long-term nutritional support for patients who cannot or will not consume an adequate oral or enteral intake. Possible indications for TPN include:

- Severe malnutrition; weight loss of 10% or more
- Gastrointestinal abnormalities: obstruction, peritonitis, impaired digestion and absorption, enterocutaneous fistulas, chronic vomiting, chronic diarrhea, prolonged paralytic ileus, radiation enteritis, extensive small bowel resection, severe acute pancreatitis
- Need for supplementation of inadequate oral intake in patients who are being treated aggressively for cancer
- After surgery or trauma, especially that involving extensive burns, multiple fractures, or sepsis
- Acute liver and renal failure when amino acid requirements are altered
- Acquired immunodeficiency syndrome (AIDS)
- Bone marrow transplantation

Because TPN is expensive, requires constant monitoring, and has potential infectious, metabolic, and mechanical complications (Box 15–3), it should be used only when an enteral intake is inadequate or contraindicated and when prolonged nutritional support is needed. Likewise, TPN should be discontinued as soon as possible. Gradual weaning to enteral nutrition or oral feedings is required to prevent metabolic complications and nutritional inadequacies. TPN is never an emergency procedure and is always accompanied by potential risks.

Cyclic TPN infuses a constant rate of solution for 8 to 12 hours/day. Cyclic TPN is suited for patients receiving TPN at home and when TPN is needed to support an inadequate oral intake. Cyclic TPN allows serum glucose and insulin levels to drop during the periods when TPN is not infused, thus promoting fat and glycogen mobilization and a more normal intake. When it is given during the night, cyclic TPN frees the patient to participate in normal activities during the day.

During the switch from continuous to cyclic TPN, the infusion time should be gradually decreased by several hours each day, as ordered, and assessment should be ongoing for signs of glucose intolerance and fluid overload (shortness of breath, crackles, pedal and sacral edema, weight gain of more than 1 kg/d). To give the pancreas time to adjust to the decreasing glucose load, the infusion rate should be tapered near the end of each

BOX 15.3

Potential Complications of Total Parenteral Nutrition

Infection and Sepsis Related to

Catheter contamination during insertion
Long-term indwelling catheter
Catheter seeding from bloodborne or distant infection
Contaminated solution

Metabolic Complications

Dehydration; hypovolemia
Hyperglycemia
Rebound hypoglycemia
Hyperosmolar, hyperglycemic, non-ketotic coma
Azotemia
Electrolyte disturbances
- Hypocalcemia
- Hypophosphatemia, hyperphosphatemia
- Hypokalemia
- Hypomagnesemia

High serum ammonia levels
Deficiencies of
- Essential fatty acids
- Trace elements

Altered acid–base balance
Elevated liver enzymes

Mechanical Complications Related to Catheterization

Catheter misplacement
Hemothorax (blood in the chest)
Pneumothorax (air or gas in the chest)
Hydrothorax (fluid in the chest)
Hemomediastinum (blood in the mediastinal spaces)
Subcutaneous emphysema
Hematoma
Arterial puncture
Myocardial perforation
Catheter embolism
Cardiac dysrhythmia
Air embolism
Endocarditis
Nerve damage at the insertion site
Laceration of lymphatic duct
Chylothorax
Lymphatic fistula
Thrombosis

cycle: reduce the rate by one half during the last hour of infusion to prevent rebound hypoglycemia.

ADMINISTRATION

Before parenteral nutrition begins, the nurse should review the patient's weight, BMI, nutritional status, diagnosis, and current laboratory data. The patient's educational needs should also be assessed.

Maintain strict aseptic procedures in all techniques to reduce the risk of infection.

Initially, the infusion is started slowly (ie, 1 L in the first 24 hours) to give the body time to adapt to the high concentration of glucose and the hyperosmolality of the solution. Continuous drip by pump infusion is needed to maintain a slow, constant flow rate. After the first 24 hours, the rate of delivery is gradually increased by 1 L/day until the optimal volume is achieved.

Because rapid changes in the infusion rate can cause severe hyperglycemia or hypoglycemia and the potential for coma, convulsions, or death, rate changes must be made incrementally. If the rate of delivery falls behind or speeds up, the drip rate should be adjusted to the correct hourly rate only; no attempts should be made to "catch up" to the ordered volume.

NURSING MANAGEMENT

Once parenteral nutrition solutions are prepared, they must be used immediately or refrigerated. It is recommended that solutions be removed from the refrigerator 1 hour before infusion, because they must reach approximately room temperature before they are hung. Once hung, the solution must be infused or discarded within 24 hours.

Inspect the solution for **"cracking,"** which appears as a layer of fat on top or oily globules in the solution. This sometimes occurs in TNA mixtures if the calcium or phosphorus content is relatively high or if salt-poor albumin has been added. A "cracked" solution cannot be infused; notify the pharmacy and the physician, who may need to adjust the original TPN order to eliminate or reduce the offending component.

Monitor the flow rate to avoid complications and ensure adequate intake. Solutions that are infused too rapidly can cause hyperosmolar diuresis, leading to seizures, coma, and even death; solutions that are administered too slowly prevent an optimal nutritional intake.

Observe for side effects of parenteral nutrition: weight gain greater than 1 kg/day (indicative of fluid overload), elevated temperature or sepsis, high blood glucose levels, shortness of breath; tightness of chest, anemia, nausea and vomiting, jaundice, allergy to protein content of the solutions, pneumothorax, or cardiac arrhythmias.

Exact requirements for vitamins, minerals, and trace elements given parenterally are not known. Close monitoring of laboratory data and clinical signs is necessary to prevent the development of nutrient deficiencies or toxicities.

Some patients may feel hungry while receiving TPN and should be allowed to eat, if possible. If oral intake is contraindicated, give mouth care.

Begin weaning the client from TPN to an enteral or oral intake as soon as possible to reduce the risk of bacterial translocation and sepsis. Patients must be weaned off TPN gradually to prevent rebound hypoglycemia. TPN can be discontinued when enteral intake (an oral diet, tube feeding, or combination of the two) provides at least 60% of estimated calorie requirements.

Patients who have permanently nonfunctional gastrointestinal tracts may require TPN indefinitely. For home TPN to be successful, clients and their families must be physically and emotionally prepared. Intensive counseling should focus on preparation and administration of the solution, catheter and equipment care, and assessment skills, as well as the psychological impact of permanent TPN.

Client and Family Teaching

Instruct the client:

- On the importance of TPN when oral or enteral intake is inadequate or impossible
- To alert the nurse if any problems arise
- Not to adjust the flow rate unless otherwise instructed

When home TPN is indicated, discharge teaching should encompass aseptic preparation and administration techniques, criteria to monitor signs and symptoms of system failure, when to call the doctor, when to call the dietitian, and when to call the pharmacist.

Encourage the client to discuss anxiety, anger, or adaptation to TPN and oral deprivation.

Questions You May Hear

Is it good practice to color tube feedings? Some facilities color tube feedings with food dye so that pulmonary secretions can be monitored for aspirated formula. Although this practice can help *detect* aspirate, it does *not protect* against aspiration. In addition, blue food coloring causes a false-positive result on a Hematest for occult blood, and red or orange food coloring added to the formula makes the stool look bloody. A better approach for testing pulmonary secretions for aspiration is to use a glucose dipstick. Unless they are bloody, pulmonary secretions normally do not contain glucose, whereas enteral formulas do.

My patient claims he can taste his tube feeding. Can he? Except for patients who experience gastric reflux, patients cannot truly taste a tube feeding. However, the appearance and aroma of the formula may influence the patient's acceptance and perception of palatability. If the formula's appearance is offensive, cover the feeding reservoir or remove it from the patient's field of vision, if possible.

KEY CONCEPTS

- Hospital food is intended to prevent nutrient deficiencies, not prevent chronic disease. Regular diets may not be consistent with *Dietary Guidelines for Americans*, which recommends limiting intakes of fat, saturated fat, cholesterol, and sodium.
- Oral diets may be modified in their consistency, or in their concentration of certain nutrients or dietary components, depending on the needs of the individual patient. Combination diets (eg, a low-sodium, soft diet) are often ordered.
- Patients with altered appetites or increased needs may benefit from supplements given with or between meals. A variety of supplements are available (clear liquid, milk-based, routine, modified routine, puddings, and bars); they vary in nutritional composition, cost, and taste.
- Enteral nutrition commonly means tube feedings. Tube feedings are preferred to parenteral nutrition whenever the gastrointestinal tract is at least partially functional, accessible, and safe to use. Tube feedings may be delivered through transnasal tubes or through ostomy sites to the gastrointestinal tract.
- The choice of tube feeding method depends on the patient's digestive and absorptive capacity, where the feeding is to be infused, the size of the feeding tube, and the patient's nutritional needs, present and past medical history, and tolerance.

- Standard tube feeding formulas require normal digestion; they contain intact molecules of protein, carbohydrate, and fat. Intact formulas come in several varieties: high-protein, high-calorie, fiber-added, and disease-specific.
- Hydrolyzed formulas are made from partially or totally predigested nutrients; they are higher in cost and osmolality and usually are not well accepted orally. Specially defined formulas are available for specific metabolic disorders (eg, renal failure, hepatic failure).
- Continuous drip infusion with a pump is the preferred method for delivering tube feedings to critically ill patients and should be used whenever feedings are infused into the jejunum. Intermittent feedings may be preferable for long-term tube feeding and home enteral nutrition because they more closely resemble a normal intake and allow the client freedom between feedings. Bolus feedings are not recommended.
- Diarrhea is a frequent complication of tube feedings that may be caused by bacterial contamination, a feeding rate that is too rapid, giving too much volume of formula, hyperosmolar formula, misplacement of the feeding tube, hypoalbuminemia, or antibiotic therapy.
- Parenteral nutrition delivers nutrients by vein when the gastrointestinal tract is non-functional or when oral or enteral intake is inadequate to meet the patient's needs. Amino acids, dextrose, lipid emulsions, electrolytes, multivitamins, and trace elements may be given by vein.
- PPN must be near-isotonic to avoid collapsing small-diameter veins. CVC infusions are hypertonic and are quickly diluted by the rapid blood flow.
- Because parenteral nutrition has numerous potential metabolic, infectious, and mechanical complications, it should be used only when necessary and discontinued as soon as feasible.

Focus on Critical Thinking

Mrs. Tanner is a 72-year-old woman who experienced a stroke 5 days ago. She does not have a significant medical history and was adequately nourished before the stroke. She is unable to eat because of impaired swallowing. The doctor is hopeful that she will regain her swallowing ability over the next few weeks. Yesterday Mrs. Tanner started being fed via continuous drip through a nasogastric tube. The doctor has ordered a routine intact formula that provides 1.06 cal/mL and 34 g of protein per 1000 mL; she is receiving 75 mL of the formula per hour. The dietitian estimates that Mrs. Tanner needs 1800 cal and approximately 60 g of protein each day.

Is this the best approach and type of feeding for Mrs. Tanner?

Calculate the total volume and amount of calories, protein, and fluid Mrs. Tanner is receiving from the nasogastric feeding. Is she meeting her needs? How much additional fluid does she need? Is she getting enough additional fluid through routine flushes of the tube?

The doctor changes the order to give the formula intermittently over 24 hours.

Develop a schedule for feeding Mrs. Tanner. How many 240-mL cans of formula does she need?

What steps should you take to reduce Mrs. Tanner's risk of aspiration?

Mrs. Tanner becomes constipated. What are the possible causes and what can be done to alleviate her constipation?

ANSWER KEY

1. **FALSE** Hospital menus are intended to prevent deficiency disease, not prevent chronic disease, and they often fail to meet the recommendations of the *Dietary Guidelines for Americans*.
2. **TRUE** Full liquid diets can be carefully planned or supplemented to approximate the nutritional value of a regular or high-calorie, high-protein diet. Therefore they are suitable for long-term use.
3. **TRUE** Modular products, either singly or in combination, can increase the nutrient density of enteral formulas.
4. **TRUE** In general, the more digested a protein is in a formula, the greater the osmolality.
5. **FALSE** Although the terms *fiber* and *residue* are often used interchangeably, they are not synonymous. Fiber refers to carbohydrates that are not digested in the gastrointestinal tract. Residue is composed of fiber along with undigested food, intestinal secretions, bacterial cell bodies, and cells from the intestinal lining.
6. **TRUE** The individual's capability of absorbing and digesting food is a primary consideration when choosing a tube feeding method for a patient.
7. **TRUE** PPN cannot supply more than 2000 to 2500 cal/day, because hypertonic concentrations of dextrose and amino acids cannot be infused through peripheral veins.
8. **TRUE** Tolerance of intermittent feedings is optimized by infusing the formula at room temperature by slow gravity drip or by pump over a 20- to 30-minute period.
9. **TRUE** Diarrhea may be averted by initiating hypertonic formulas at a slower rate or strength.
10. **FALSE** Coloring tube formulas with food dye may help detect aspirate, but it does not prevent aspiration.

REFERENCES

American Dietetic Association. (1994). Position of the American Dietetic Association: Nutrition monitoring of the home parenteral and enteral patient. *Journal of the American Dietetic Association 94*, 664–666.

American Dietetic Association. (1996). *Manual of clinical nutrition* (5th ed.). Chicago: American Dietetic Association.

American Dietetic Association. (1997). Position of the American Dietetic Association: The role of registered dietitians in enteral and parenteral nutrition support. *Journal of the American Dietetic Association 97*, 302–304.

American Dietetic Association & Morrison Health Care, Inc. (1997). *Medical nutrition therapy across the continuum of care: Supplement 1*. Chicago: American Dietetic Association.

Chima, C., Barco, K., Dewitt, M., Maeda, M., Teran, J., & Mullen, K. (1997). Relationship of nutritional status to length of stay, hospital cost, and discharge status of patients hospitalized in the medicine service. *Journal of the American Dietetic Association 97*, 975–978.

Gallagher-Allred, C., Voss, A., Finn, S., & McCamish, M. (1996). Malnutrition and clinical outcomes: The case for medical nutrition therapy. *Journal of the American Dietetic Association* 96, 361–366.

Lau, C., & Gregoire, M. (1998). Quality ratings of a hospital foodservice department by inpatients and postdischarge patients. *Journal of the American Dietetic Association* 98, 1303–1307.

Singer, A., Werther, K., & Nestle, M. (1998). Improvements are needed in hospital diets to meet dietary guidelines for health promotion and disease prevention. *Journal of the American Dietetic Association* 98, 639–641.

Skipper, A., Bohac, C., & Gregoire, M. (1999). Knowing brand name affects patient preferences for enteral supplements. *Journal of the American Dietetic Association* 99, 91–92.

Traviss, K., & Barr, S. (1997). Rethinking postoperative diets for short-stay orthopedic surgery patients. *Journal of the American Dietetic Association* 97, 971–974.

Whitney, E., Cataldo, C., & Rolfes, S. (1998). *Understanding normal and clinical nutrition* (5th ed.). Belmont, CA: Wadsworth.

CHAPTER 16

Protein-Calorie Malnutrition and Physiologic Stress

TRUE	FALSE	Check your knowledge of protein-calorie malnutrition and physiologic stress.
⬭	⬭	1 Metabolism slows during starvation.
⬭	⬭	2 Metabolism slows during severe stress.
⬭	⬭	3 Acute protein deficiency can develop in a matter of weeks when there is stress and intake is inadequate.
⬭	⬭	4 Rapid, aggressive refeeding in patients who are chronically malnourished can cause a potentially fatal complication known as refeeding syndrome.
⬭	⬭	5 The risk in refeeding patients with acute protein deficiency is providing too much protein.
⬭	⬭	6 Malnutrition interferes with the body's ability to adapt to stress.
⬭	⬭	7 A signal that the adaptive phase of the stress response is beginning is a drop in serum glucose levels.
⬭	⬭	8 After trauma, the intestines regain motility quicker than the stomach.
⬭	⬭	9 Providing nutrition orally or enterally promotes blood flow to the intestines and may help preserve intestinal cell function and translocation of gastrointestinal bacteria.
⬭	⬭	10 Extensive burns increase protein and calorie needs more than any other stress.

Upon completion of this chapter, you will be able to

- Describe how the body adapts to starvation.
- Name the two major types of protein-calorie malnutrition (PCM) and the signs and symptoms of each.

- Explain the nutritional interventions for each type of PCM and why the risks associated with refeeding differ between the types.
- Discuss how the metabolic changes that occur after the stress response differ from those of starvation.
- Calculate a person's calorie requirements using the Harris-Benedict formula adjusted for activity and injury.
- Describe the roles of the following nutrients in wound healing and recovery: protein, calories, vitamin C, and zinc.
- Lists ways to increase intake of protein and calories.
- Discuss nutritional considerations for thermal injuries and chronic obstructive pulmonary disease (COPD).

Introduction

Stress is any threat to an individual's emotional or physical well-being. *Physiological stress*, a normal part of everyday living, includes events such as marriage, divorce, moving to a new house, and even going on a vacation. *Pathologic stress* is stress caused by disease or injury or even malnutrition. Severe stressors (eg, trauma, extensive surgery, major burns, severe infection) produce a rapid and predictable stress response as the body seeks to reestablish homeostasis.

The intensity of the stress response depends on the severity of the stress, the number of stressors, and the individual's ability to adapt to stress. For instance, the stress of minor surgery in a well-nourished patient may have little impact, whereas patients who are burdened with severe stress and who develop malnutrition may lack the nutrient reserves needed for adaptation to occur. The result may be multisystem organ failure and death.

This chapter reviews the stress of starvation and compares it to the body's metabolic response to severe stress. The effect of severe stress on nutritional status and requirements is discussed. Also presented are additional nutritional considerations of certain hypermetabolic conditions, namely surgery, thermal injuries, and COPD.

The Stress of Starvation

Starvation may be self-imposed (eg, an adolescent girl fasting to lose weight) or involuntary, occurring secondary to the inability to consume any or enough calories and protein. Regardless of the cause, the body adapts to starvation in an attempt to survive.

In simple starvation (ie, starvation not complicated by other stressors), the initial response is to break down glycogen and protein to provide glucose, the body's preferred fuel. The loss of protein tissue slows metabolism, so that energy requirements decrease. Within a matter of days, the body adapts to starvation by using ketones (from fat breakdown) for the majority of its fuel. At this point, the body needs only a minimal amount of glucose to fuel the brain cells which are unable to switch from use of glucose to ketones. Protein is still broken down to supply amino acids for gluconeogenesis, but the catabolism continues at a much slower rate. The ability to use ketones as a major energy source, combined with the decrease in energy requirements, is an adaptive response aimed at prolonging survival.

PROTEIN-CALORIE MALNUTRITION

Although PCM is a major health concern in developing countries, it is rare in the United States except among the elderly, fad dieters, and, ironically, hospitalized patients. Consequences of PCM include weakness, apathy, increased risk of infection, poor drug tolerance, and poor wound healing. The two major types of PCM are **marasmus,** a normal adaptive response to chronic energy deficiency (starvation), and **kwashiorkor,** an acute protein deficiency that occurs when the body cannot adapt to starvation because of a superimposed illness or infection. Such maladaptation may account for the clinical and biochemical differences between kwashiorkor and marasmus.

Kwashiorkor

Patients with kwashiorkor appear well nourished or overnourished because of edema, but they have depleted visceral proteins owing to acute inadequate protein intake and stress. Weight for height is often normal, but the serum albumin concentration is less than 3.0 g/dL, and transferrin, total lymphocyte count, blood urea nitrogen, and creatinine levels are low. The patient may have pitting edema and changes in skin and hair pigments. Protein depletion leads to fatty infiltration of the liver and increased susceptibility to infection. Diarrhea and malabsorption develop because of a decrease in the number and function of intestinal cells. Numerous nutrient deficiencies occur secondary to malabsorption. Wound healing is impaired, and skin breakdown may occur. Kwashiorkor may develop in as little as 2 weeks.

The primary focus of treating kwashiorkor is to correct the protein deficiency. Initially, feeding 2.5 to 3.0 g of protein per kilogram of body weight is recommended, with calories equal to 0.8 to 1.0 basal energy expenditure (BEE) (see later discussion). Enteral or parenteral nutrition may be necessary depending on the patient's medical status. Calories are gradually increased as tolerated.

Marasmus

Unlike kwashiorkor, marasmus is a chronic condition that develops over a period of months to years as the result of a low calorie intake. Patients with marasmus look chronically starved with little no subcutaneous fat. They are lethargic and weak. Anthropometric measurements (eg, weight, triceps skinfold) are low, yet albumin, transferrin, and muscle mass may all be within normal limits. Protein tissues are preserved because adaptation to the chronically low calorie intake has occurred.

Initial treatment for marasmus may consist of intravenous or oral glucose followed by liquids. When solids are introduced, calories should be limited to 25 to 30 cal/kg to avoid overfeeding. After 1 week, calories are increased as tolerated to approximately 35 cal/kg. Multivitamins and mineral supplements may be necessary to correct nutrient deficiencies. If enteral nutrition is used, it should be infused by the continuous drip method.

Mixed Marasmic Kwashiorkor

Mixed marasmic kwashiorkor develops in chronically starved or malnourished patients who experience stress (eg, surgery, trauma). They appear cachectic, unless they have edema that masks their wasted appearance. Anthropometric measurements are depleted, as are somatic and visceral proteins. The severe loss of body protein hinders the patient's ability to withstand stress, so catabolic illness becomes life-threatening. Mixed marasmic kwashiorkor usually develops within a matter of weeks. It is important to determine which type of malnutrition predominates—marasmus or kwashiorkor—because the treatment and treatment risks differ for each. The risk in feeding kwashiorkor patients is underfeeding, or not meeting their needs. The risk in feeding starving patients with lowered metabolism is overfeeding.

REFEEDING SYNDROME

Although on the surface it would seem that the best approach to treating starving patients is to quickly give them as much protein and calories as possible, this is not the case. In fact, that approach may cause **refeeding syndrome,** a potentially fatal complication of rapid and aggressive refeeding of malnourished patients. Although refeeding syndrome is more common and develops more quickly with parenteral than with enteral nutrition, it can occur in any semistarved patient who is refed too aggressively.

Depleted patients who have adapted to starvation are at risk of being metabolically overwhelmed by the introduction of excess protein and calories. Rapid changes in thyroid and endocrine function cause increases in oxygen consumption, cardiac output, and energy expenditure. Excessive insulin secretion produces rapid uptake of glucose by cells. Phosphorus also rushes into cells. In fact, a major manifestation of refeeding syndrome is hypophosphatemia, which may cause anorexia, bone pain, dizziness, muscle weakness, respiratory failure, and cardiac decompensation. Other potential problems of rapid refeeding include alterations in sodium balance possibly leading to congestive heart failure; hypokalemia and arrhythmias as potassium shifts into cells; hypomagnesemia, which can lead to cardiac depression, arrhythmias, tetany, and seizures; fluid intolerance leading to fluid retention and weight gain; and thiamine deficiency due to increased carbohydrate metabolism.

To prevent refeeding syndrome, nutrients (especially carbohydrates) must be introduced slowly during the first week to allow the body time to readapt from fasting to feeding. It is essential that laboratory data, particularly serum phosphorus, magnesium, and potassium levels, be monitored closely so that abnormalities can be swiftly identified and corrected. Weight gain should be less than 1 kg/week; gains higher than this are indicative of fluid retention. After the first week, the intake of calories, fluid, and sodium may be safely liberalized because metabolic adaptations should have occurred.

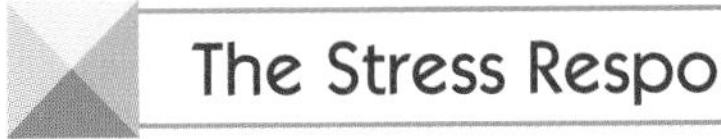

The Stress Response

The **stress response** is a complex series of hormonal and metabolic changes that occur to enable the body to adapt to stressors. Its two major phases are the *ebb phase* and *flow phase*. Hormonal and metabolic characteristics of these phases are listed in Table 16–1.

EBB PHASE

The "ebb" or shock phase occurs during the first 12 to 24 hours after trauma. Blood pressure, cardiac output, body temperature, and oxygen consumption fall. Increased levels of catecholamines and glucagon promote the breakdown of glycogen (glycogenolysis) and increase glucose synthesis from amino acids (gluconeogenesis), resulting in hyperglycemia. Insulin levels are lowered. Lethargy occurs and digestion slows. The immediate goals are to restore tissue perfusion, maintain adequate oxygenation, and stop hemorrhage. Usually within 36 to 48 hours after the injury, the ebb phase is replaced by the flow phase.

FLOW PHASE

The "flow" phase, or acute phase, is the period in which the body mobilizes nutrients to meet the high metabolic demands of stress. Increased levels of glucocorticoids, catecholamines, and glucagon, the so-called *stress hormones*, cause marked hypermetabolism (increased energy expenditure), hypercatabolism (protein breakdown), and persistent hyperglycemia despite normal or increased serum insulin levels. Urinary losses of potassium and nitrogen increase, and sodium and fluid are retained. Decreased gastrointestinal

TABLE 16.1 ***Metabolic and Hormonal Changes Characteristic of the Ebb and Flow Phases of Stress***

Changes	Ebb Phase	Flow Phase
Hormonal	Decreased insulin	Normal or increased insulin
	Increased catecholamines	Increased catecholamines
	Increased glucagon	Increased glucagon
		Increased aldosterone
		Increased antidiuretic hormone
Metabolic	Hyperglycemia	Hyperglycemia, insulin insensitivity
	Decreased O_2 consumption	Hypermetabolism (increased O_2 consumption)
	Decreased blood pressure	Increased tissue catabolism
	Decreased cardiac output	Increased cardiac output
	Decreased body temperature	Increased body temperature
	Decreased renal output	Increased urinary nitrogen losses
		Muscle use of branched-chain amino acids for energy
		Sodium and fluid retention
		Increased fat oxidation

motility can result in anorexia, distention, nausea, vomiting, or constipation. The loss of protein and fat tissue may be significant as the body breaks down its own reserves to meet increased energy needs. An adequate nutritional intake may help to minimize the effects of hypermetabolism and catabolism; however, the ability to eat may be impaired or precluded, necessitating the use of enteral or parenteral nutritional support.

Protein catabolism peaks 7 days after the initial stress response. During this *adaptive phase,* stress hormone levels subside, serum glucose levels decline, and metabolism returns to normal. Nitrogen balance is gradually achieved. Successful adaptation leads to recovery.

If adaptation fails, the body eventually becomes unable to respond to the stress, resulting in *exhaustion* and possibly death.

Effect of Stress on Nutritional Status

Major stress has a profound impact on nutritional status; the greater the stress, the greater the impact. Unlike starvation, to which the body adapts by lowering its metabolic rate and switching from glucose to predominately ketones for energy, severe stress increases metabolism and catabolism for an extended period. Instead of preserving energy and body protein, this accelerates losses of both. During the adaptive period, the body is literally breaking itself down to wage the war against the stressor.

The overwhelming concern is the catabolism of body proteins. Because the body does not "store" extra protein, the increased demand for protein is met by breaking down lean body mass to release amino acids. From them the body makes:

- Glucose to meet increased energy needs. Because the body does not convert predominately to ketones for fuel, the need for glucose is high. Although only certain amino acids can be converted to glucose, whole proteins must be broken down to release those glucogenic amino acids. Alanine and glutamine, which are synthesized in the body from branched-chain amino acids (BCAAs), are important amino acids used in glucose synthesis.
- Stress hormones, which are protein molecules
- Immune factors needed to fight infection
- Collagen, the protein matrix needed to repair damaged tissue and bone

Without adequate protein, the body loses its ability to adapt. Failure to adapt leads to exhaustion and ultimately to death.

People with marasmus lack the nutritional reserves to respond to severe or prolonged stress. Yet because they have adapted to starvation, their lean body mass is relatively preserved and they are generally able to withstand mild to moderate stress with adequate nutritional support. By comparison, severe or prolonged stress combined with inadequate intake can cause acute malnutrition (kwashiorkor) in a previously healthy person who has not had the "benefit" of already adapting to starvation. Meeting the needs of a patient with acute malnutrition related to stress is extremely difficult.

POTENTIAL COMPLICATIONS

Without effective nutritional intervention, the problems of PCM and stress are exacerbated. Malnutrition robs the body of the reserves needed to support a normal stress response; stress aggravates malnutrition. A worsening nutritional status impairs the patient's ability to adapt and recover and increases the risk of complications such as skin breakdown, infections, and poor drug tolerance.

- **Skin breakdown.** Decubitus ulcers (pressure sores) are areas where skin and underlying tissues break down because of constant pressure and a lack of oxygen and nutrients. Immobility compounds the risk of pressure sores brought about by severe stress and malnutrition. The areas most susceptible to pressure sores are the bony or cartilaginous prominences of the hip, sacrum, elbow, and heels. Pressure ulcers are painful and increase the risk for infection. Pressure ulcers increase requirements for protein, vitamin C, and zinc to promote healing.
- **Infections.** Systemically, PCM negatively affects immune system functioning by impairing the effectiveness of phagocytes, reducing the number and function of T lymphocytes, and decreasing the production of antibodies. Locally, PCM impairs the gastrointestinal tract's important role in protecting the body from infectious agents. For instance, PCM decreases the number and function of intestinal border cells, which normally form a protective barrier to prevent the translocation of infectious substances from the bowel to the bloodstream. Researchers speculate that translocation of gut bacteria may be a major factor in the development of sepsis and multiple organ failure.
- **Poor drug tolerance.** Malnutrition can affect the way the body responds to drugs. For instance, patients with malabsorption related to the decreased number and function of intestinal cells may not adequately absorb drugs. A low serum albumin concentration, indicative of protein malnutrition, means that drugs that normally bind to albumin for transport through the blood take longer to be delivered. These drugs also remain in circulation longer because transport to the liver or kidneys for detoxification is delayed.

NUTRITION THERAPY FOR SEVERELY STRESSED PATIENTS

The immediate poststress objective is to simply keep the patient alive. Life support and intensive monitoring may be required. Intravenous fluids and electrolytes are given. Aggressive nutritional support during the initial period is contraindicated because it increases metabolic demands on the body.

Nutrition therapy begins when the serum glucose level drops, indicating adaptation has occurred. Initially the goal of nutritional interventions is to minimize losses and prevent acute malnutrition. Until a normal metabolic rate is restored, it is unlikely that interventions will be able to stop or reverse the drain on nutritional status. After a normal metabolic rate has been restored, nutrition therapy promotes a positive nitrogen balance (protein anabolism) and weight gain. Table 16–2 summarizes nutrients important for wound healing and recovery.

Regardless of the method or standards used to estimate calorie and nutrient requirements, they are still, at best, *estimates* not *exact requirements*. Estimates often need to be adjusted upward or downward based on the patient's response. This is an example of how the science of nutrition is applied as an art.

Calories

It is important to provide enough calories to promote recovery, yet not too many calories to overwhelm an already stressed system. An excess of calories increases metabolism, oxygen consumption, and carbon dioxide production. This compounds the burden already placed on the heart and lungs to regulate blood gases. And as mentioned previously, too many calories tax endocrine and thyroid function and may precipitate dangerous shifts in serum phosphorus and other electrolytes.

One method of estimating calorie requirements is the Harris-Benedict equation, which calculates the basic energy needs and adjusts for stress and activity factors:

Step 1: Calculate basal energy expenditure (calories per day) from the actual body weight in kilograms, the height in centimeters, and the age in years.

Men: BEE = 66 + (13.7 × weight in kg) + (5 × height in cm) – (6.8 × age in y)

Women: BEE = 655 + (9.6 × weight in kg) + (1.7 × height in cm) – (4.7 × age in y)

Step 2: Multiply BEE by the appropriate activity factor:

Confined to bed	1.0–1.2
Out of bed, light activity	1.3
Light activity	1.5 for women
	1.6 for men
Moderate activity	1.6 for women
	1.7 for men
Heavy activity	1.9 for women
	2.1 for men

Step 3: Multiply the activity-adjusted BEE by the appropriate injury factor:

Minor surgery, mild infection	1.0–1.2
Major surgery	1.1–1.2
Moderate infection	1.2–1.4
Skeletal trauma	1.2–1.35
Severe infection	1.4–1.8
Burns (20%–40% of body surface area)	1.5–1.85
Burns (>40% of body surface area)	1.85–1.95

Example: A 20-year-old woman who is 5 feet 5 inches (165 cm) tall and weighs 132 pounds (60 kg) is out of bed with minor surgery.

Step 1: BEE = 655 + (9.6 × 60) + (1.7 × 165) – (4.7 × 20) = 1417

Step 2: 1417 × 1.3 = 1842

Step 3: 1842 × 1.0 = 1842

The client's estimated energy requirement is 1842 cal/d.

TABLE 16.2 ***Nutrients Important for Wound Healing and Recovery***

Nutrient	Rationale for Increased Need	Possible Deficiency Outcome
Protein	To replace the lean body mass lost during the catabolic phase after stress To restore blood volume and plasma proteins lost during exudates, bleeding from the wound, and possible hemorrhage To replace losses resulting from immobility (increased excretion) To meet the increased needs for tissue repair and resistance to infection	Significant weight loss Impaired/delayed wound healing Shock related to decreased blood volume Edema related to decreased serum albumin Diarrhea related to decreased albumin Anemia Increased risk of infection related to decreased antibodies, impaired tissue integrity Decreased lipoprotein synthesis → fatty infiltration of the liver → liver damage Increased mortality
Calories	To replace losses related to lack of oral intake and hypermetabolism during catabolic phase after stress To spare protein To restore normal weight	Signs and symptoms of protein deficiency due to use of protein to meet energy requirements Extensive weight loss
Water	To replace fluid lost through vomiting, hemorrhage, exudates, fever, drainage, diuresis To maintain homeostasis	Signs, symptoms, and complications of dehydration, such as poor skin turgor, dry mucous membranes, oliguria, anuria, weight loss, increased pulse rate, decreased central venous pressure
Vitamin C	Important for capillary formation, tissue synthesis, and wound healing through collagen formation Needed for antibody formation	Impaired/delayed wound healing related to impaired collagen formation and increased capillary fragility and permeability Increased risk of infection related to decreased antibodies
Thiamine, niacin, riboflavin	Requirements increase with increased metabolic rate	Decreased enzymes available for energy metabolism
Folic acid, vitamin B_{12}	Needed for cell proliferation and therefore tissue synthesis Important for maturation of red blood cells. Impaired folic acid synthesis related to some antibiotics; impaired vitamin B_{12} absorption related to some antibiotics	Decreased or arrested cell division Megaloblastic anemia
Vitamin A	Important for tissue synthesis, wound healing, and immune function Enhances resistance to infection	Impaired/delayed wound healing related to decreased collagen synthesis; impaired immune function Increased risk of infection

(continued)

TABLE 16.2 ***Nutrients Important for Wound Healing and Recovery (continued)***

Nutrient	Rationale for Increased Need	Possible Deficiency Outcome
Vitamin K	Important for normal blood clotting Impaired intestinal synthesis related to antibiotics	Prolonged prothrombin time
Iron	To replace iron lost through blood loss	Signs, symptoms, and complications of iron deficiency anemia, such as fatigue, weakness, pallor, anorexia, dizziness, headaches, stomatitis, glossitis, cardiovascular and respiratory changes, possible cardiac failure
Zinc	Needed for protein synthesis and wound healing Needed for normal lymphocyte and phagocyte response	Impaired/delayed wound healing Impaired immune response

There are disadvantages to using the Harris-Benedict equation. In some patients, this formula has been shown to overestimate actual energy expenditure; in others, calorie needs are underestimated. From a practical standpoint, the equation is time-consuming and complex.

An alternative method for estimating calorie needs consists of simply multiplying the patient's weight in kilograms by specified calorie level. This is the approach most often given in this text because it is simpler to use and yields similar results to the Harris-Benedict approach. As a reference point, the following values are used to estimate total calorie needs (calories per kilogram of body weight) for *healthy* people:

Weight Range	Sedentary	Moderately Active	Active
Overweight	20–25	30	35
Normal weight	30	35	40
Underweight	30	40	45–50

The factors for stress in this simpler method are:

Mild stress	35
Moderate stress	45
Severe burns	40–60

For the 60-kg woman with mild stress in the example, this method calculates total calorie needs as 60 kg × 35 cal/kg = 2100 cal, a difference of only 258 calories from the value determined by the Harris-Benedict method.

Protein

An adequate protein intake is essential to minimize and correct body protein catabolism and help maintain normal immune functioning. Because the body meets its energy requirements first, dietary protein is used for anabolism only if adequate nonprotein calories (carbohydrate and fat) are available to meet the body's energy needs. Generally, protein requirements (in grams per kilogram body weight) range as follows:

Normal	0.8
Fever, fracture, infection, wound healing	1.5–2.0
Protein repletion, trauma	1.5–2.0
Burns	1.5–3.0

Besides the total quantity of protein provided, the specific types of amino acids given may influence stress response and recovery. For instance, arginine and glutamine, two nonessential amino acids, may become conditionally essential during periods of stress. Arginine helps minimize protein losses, improve wound healing, and stimulate the immune system. Glutamine helps maintain the integrity and function of intestinal cells and therefore may help prevent translocation of gastrointestinal bacteria. Other studies suggest that supplementing intake with BCAAs (leucine, isoleucine, and valine) may minimize protein losses. There is not enough evidence to make recommendations about the quantities or percentages of specific amino acids that may be optimal during stress.

Fluid

During periods of stress, fluid requirements are highly individualized according to losses that occur through exudates, hemorrhage, emesis, diuresis, diarrhea, and fever. To accurately assess fluid requirements and status, the fluid intake and output, blood pressure, heart rate, respiratory rate, and body temperature are carefully monitored. Care should be taken to avoid overhydration; decreased renal output is a frequent complication of stress.

Micronutrients

Vitamin, mineral, and electrolyte requirements during stress are unclear and undefined. Because of their role in tissue healing and immune function, supplements of the B-complex vitamins, zinc, vitamin A, and vitamin C may be appropriate.

Type of Feeding

Oral and enteral nutrition are the preferred routes if the gastrointestinal tract is functional, because they carry lower risks and help prevent the translocation of gut bacteria. However, an initial response to severe stress is reduced blood flow to the gastrointestinal tract, which slows motility and precludes oral intake. Lack of use of the gastrointestinal tract causes the problems of reduced gastrointestinal blood flow and slower motility to become worse. Even when oral nutrients are provided, they may not be well absorbed because of the loss of gastrointestinal cells and secretions secondary to protein depletion caused by stress or malnutrition. The actual type of nutrition provided (oral, enteral, or parenteral) depends on the location and extent of the injury. Well-nourished patients who experience mild to moderate stress are given intravenous fluid and electrolytes until gut motility returns to normal, usually within a few days. The normal diet progression, from clear liquids to full liquids to a soft diet and then a regular diet, advances as tolerated. Supplements and small, frequent feedings help to maximize intake. Box 16–1 lists methods by which protein and calories can be added to the diet.

BOX 16.1

Ways to Add Protein and Calories to the Diet

To increase protein and calories

- Add skim milk powder to milk to make double-strength milk; chill well before serving.
- Use double-strength milk on hot or cold cereals and in scrambled eggs, soups, gravies, casseroles, milk shakes, and milk-based desserts.
- Substitute whole milk or evaporated milk for water in recipes.
- Add grated cheese to soups, casseroles, vegetable dishes, rice, and noodles.
- Use peanut butter as a spread on slices of apple, banana, pear, crackers, or waffles; use as a filling for celery.
- Add finely chopped, hard-cooked eggs to sauces, soups, and casseroles.
- Choose desserts made with eggs or milk, such as sponge cake, angel food cake, custard, and puddings.
- Dip meat, poultry, and fish in eggs or milk and coat with bread or cereal crumbs before baking, broiling, or pan frying.
- Use yogurt as a topping for fruit, plain cakes, or other desserts; use in gravies and dips.

To increase calories

- Mix cream cheese with butter and spread on hot bread and rolls.
- Whenever possible, add butter to hot foods: breads, pancakes, waffles, soups, vegetables, potatoes, cooked cereal, rice, and pasta.
- Substitute mayonnaise for salad dressing in salads, eggs, casseroles, and sandwiches.
- Add dried fruit, nuts, or granola to desserts and cereal.
- Use whipped cream on pies, fruit, pudding, gelatin, ice cream, and other desserts and in coffee, tea, and hot chocolate.
- Use marshmallows in hot chocolate, on fruit, and in desserts.
- Top baked potatoes, vegetables, and fruits with sour cream.
- Snack frequently on nuts, dried fruit, candy, buttered popcorn, cheese, granola, and ice cream.
- Use honey on toast, cereal, and fruit and in coffee and tea.

Malnourished or severely stressed patients may be given enteral or parenteral nutrition. Because motility returns to the intestines much sooner than to the stomach, intestinal feedings can be initiated much sooner than feedings into the stomach and are associated with improved clinical outcomes. For instance, surgeons frequently insert a needle-catheter jejunostomy tube during surgery in patients who are malnourished, hypermetabolic, or not expected to resume oral intake within a few days after surgery. This allows the patient to benefit from feedings several hours after surgery instead of waiting 24 to 48 hours for stomach motility to resume. In severely stressed patients, infusion feedings into the intestine within 36 hours after stress stimulate blood flow to the intestine, which may help preserve intestinal function, promote adaptation, minimize hypermetabolism, and prevent translocation. Stress formulas enriched with BCAAs may be appropriate for patients receiving enteral nutritional support. Because of the increased risk of infectious, metabolic, and mechanical complications, parenteral nutrition is used only when necessary and is discontinued as soon as possible.

Nutrition Therapy for Certain Stress Conditions

The preceding sections on malnutrition and stress pertain to a number of conditions, including extensive surgery and burns. Yet surgery and burns have additional considerations with nutritional implications, which are presented here. Additional considerations for COPD are also included, because it is a condition that is frequently compounded by malnutrition.

SURGERY

Ideally, patients should have an optimal nutritional status before surgery to enable them to withstand the stress of surgery and the short-term starvation that follows. However, surgical patients are often malnourished as a result of disease-related symptoms experienced before surgery, such as anorexia, nausea, vomiting, fever, malabsorption, and blood loss. To optimize the chance for a successful surgical outcome, malnourished patients and those at risk for malnutrition should be identified and given preoperative nutritional support, which may range from a high-calorie, high-protein diet to enteral or parenteral nutrition.

Patients are restricted to nothing by mouth (NPO) for at least 8 hours before surgery to avoid aspiration related to anesthesia. To minimize fecal residue and postoperative distention after intestinal surgery, a low-residue, residue-free (see Chapter 17), or hydrolyzed formula diet may be used for 2 to 3 days before surgery.

Oral intake is resumed after bowel sounds return, usually 24 to 48 hours after surgery. The traditional diet progression is from clear liquids to full liquids and then to a soft or regular diet as tolerated. However, short-stay patients may benefit physically and psychologically from a more rapid diet progression.

Usually a high-protein, high-calorie diet is appropriate, with a liberal intake of nutrients important for wound healing. Actual needs depend on the extent of surgery and the patient's nutritional status.

BURNS

Extensive burns are the most severe form of stress that a person can experience. Hormonal responses and extensive evaporative water losses may increase metabolism by 100% above normal (hypermetabolism). The patient is hypercatabolic. Large quantities of fluid, electrolytes, protein, and other nutrients leach through the burned area. Nutritional support may be complicated by fluid and electrolyte imbalances, paralytic ileus, anorexia, pain, infection or other complications, emotional trauma, and medical-surgical procedures. Weight loss and malnutrition lead to increased morbidity and mortality unless aggressive nutritional support is initiated as soon as possible after fluid resuscitation. Weight loss of 40% to 50% may be fatal. Sepsis is the most common cause of death among burn victims, followed by pneumonia. Risk factors for complications in burned patients appear in Box 16–2.

Fluid requirements in the immediate postburn ebb phase range from 3 to 5 L daily; up to 10 L/day may be needed for extensive burns. Immediate use of intravenous fluids helps prevent gastric distention and paralytic ileus.

The high incidence of impaired immunocompetence and protein depletion among burned patients makes aggressive nutritional support vital to decrease the risk of infectious complications. Primary goals during the flow period, which begins 48 to 72 hours after the burn, are to maintain fluid and electrolyte balance and to minimize the loss of lean body tissue and body weight. Oral intake should begin as soon as fluid resuscitation is completed and paralytic ileus is resolved, usually at about the third postburn day. If bowel sounds have not returned by the fourth postburn day, peripheral or central vein parenteral nutrition should be given. Although it is easier to meet calorie needs than protein needs, patients should be able to achieve neutral balances of both by the seventh postburn day. Goals of this secondary feeding period are to replace nutritional losses and promote wound healing.

Periodic adjustments in intake are made according to the patient's progress. Nutritional requirements increase with the development of complications and lessen as wound healing progresses. General needs are as follows:

BOX 16.2

Risk Factors for Complications in Burn Patients

Burn surface area greater than 20%
Poor nutritional status before burn
Preburn illness or disease
Morbid obesity
History of substance abuse
Associated injuries
Pulmonary, circulatory, infectious, metabolic, or gastrointestinal complications
Weight loss of more than 10% of preburn weight while hospitalized
Low serum transferrin and anergy (impaired immunocompetence), which are strongly correlated with a high risk of infectious complications

- **Protein** needs increase to 1.5 to 3 g/kg, approximately two to four times greater than the Recommended Dietary Allowance (RDA).
- **Calorie** needs increase by 40 to 60 cal/kg—30% to 100% above normal. Calorie requirements may also be calculated by using the Harris-Benedict equation, accounting for activity and stress factors. Although the metabolic rate peaks at about the tenth postburn day, metabolism (and, therefore, the calorie requirement) remains high for several weeks or longer, depending on the extent of the burn. The distribution of calories should be approximately 25% protein, 50% carbohydrate, and 25% fat.
- **High fluid.** Water losses may be 10 to 12 times greater than normal in the first few postburn weeks. Encourage consumption of fruit juices high in potassium and vitamin C.
- **Vitamin and mineral supplementation.** There are no set guidelines for vitamin and mineral supplementation for burned patients. Some nutrient needs increase directly to promote wound healing (eg, vitamin C, zinc) or indirectly in proportion to the increased calorie intake (eg, thiamine, riboflavin, niacin). Multivitamin and mineral supplements or megadoses of certain nutrients may be prescribed at the physician's discretion, depending on the patient's previous nutritional status.

To promote maximum intake:

- Work with the client and family to solicit food preferences. Young children may regress in their eating behaviors; adults may prefer foods that they associate with recovery as children (eg, chicken soup).
- Encourage the family to bring food from home.
- Discourage the intake of empty-calorie food and beverages.
- Provide small, frequent meals; assist as needed.
- Provide emotional support and allow the patient to verbalize feelings.
- If possible, schedule debridement and other medical and surgical procedures at times when they are least likely to interfere with meals.
- Provide pain medication as needed before meals.

Supplemental or complete enteral or parenteral nutrition may be necessary for patients with:

- Extremely high calorie and protein requirements (who cannot consume enough food orally to meet their needs)
- Inability to swallow because of facial or neck burns
- Adynamic ileus
- Bleeding related to Curling's ulcer (who need total parenteral nutrition)
- Anorexia related to fear, pain, altered body image, and frequent medical or surgical procedures (nutritional requirements are highest when appetite is poorest)

Total parenteral nutrition should be used with extreme caution because of the increased risks for infection and sepsis.

Decreased weight bearing during immobility results in increased bone resorption and a negative calcium imbalance, regardless of calcium intake. Encourage ambulation to minimize calcium and nitrogen excretion and to improve appetite and outlook. Once weight-bearing activity resumes, the calcium requirement increases to replace calcium that has been lost from bone.

RESPIRATORY STRESS: CHRONIC OBSTRUCTIVE PULMONARY DISEASE

As many as half of hospitalized patients with emphysema have PCM, even if they are not critically ill. Weight loss and malnutrition in these patients is multifactorial and may be related to one or more of the following:

- Increased energy expenditure related to labored breathing
- Early satiety related to flattening of the diaphragm
- Abdominal bloating related to swallowed air
- Peptic ulcer disease secondary to steroid therapy
- Dyspnea while eating
- Anorexia related to fatigue
- Anorexia related to excess mucus
- Anorexia related to decreased peristalsis and digestion secondary to inadequate oxygen to gastrointestinal cells

A downhill spiral often occurs: A reduced respiratory rate reduces blood flow to the gastrointestinal tract, thereby decreasing nutrient absorption and increasing the risk of malnutrition. Conversely, malnutrition weakens respiratory muscles, reduces respiratory rate, and exacerbates existing respiratory impairments.

Improving weight in underweight patients improves muscle strength, endurance, and exercise tolerance, even though it cannot increase expiration volume and may not influence life expectancy. To correct malnutrition, calorie requirements are estimated by multiplying the BEE by a factor of 1.5 to 1.7. For depleted patients, provide 1.2 to 1.5 g of protein per kilogram body weight. Overweight patients should be encouraged to lose weight to improve breathing.

The metabolism of carbohydrates, proteins, and fats yields carbon dioxide and water. The term **respiratory quotient** (RQ) refers to the ratio of carbon dioxide produced to oxygen consumed; the more carbon dioxide produced, the greater the burden on the lungs to exhale carbon dioxide. Because the RQ is higher for carbohydrates than for either proteins or fats, it may be beneficial to limit carbohydrate intake in patients who require ventilator support. Instead of the normal calorie distribution of 50% to 60% carbohydrate, 20% to 30% fat, and 15% to 20% protein, it may be appropriate to limit carbohydrate intake to 25% to 30% of calories and increase fat intake to 50% to 55% of total calories. Low-carbohydrate, high-fat enteral products that are designed for use in patients with pulmonary disease are available. It is not thoroughly understood whether lowering carbohydrate and increasing fat consumption provides the same benefits in ambulatory patients eating an oral diet.

A soft diet may be appropriate for patients who have difficulty chewing and swallowing related to shortness of breath. Fatigued patients may need assistance with cutting food, opening containers, and so forth. Breathing exercises should be avoided for at least 1 hour before and after eating.

Limiting "empty" liquids with meals (eg, coffee, tea, water, carbonated beverages) and providing small, frequent, nutritionally dense feedings help maximize intake and reduce gastric distention and pressure on the diaphragm. Gassy foods should be avoided unless they are well tolerated. Consider "feedings" of high-calorie, high-protein eggnogs, shakes, and commercial supplements.

Unless it is contraindicated, a high fluid intake is needed to help thin mucus secretions; fever also increases fluid requirements. Usually, 1 mL fluid per calorie consumed is adequate.

To avoid straining at stool, a high-fiber diet is recommended; this includes bran cereals, whole grains, prunes, fruits, and vegetables. Fiber intake should be increased gradually to avoid excessive gas, distention, and diarrhea.

Supplements of B-complex vitamins (for increased energy metabolism) and vitamins A and C (for healing and tissue repair) may be appropriate.

Additional diet modifications may be necessary, depending on the patient's drug therapy.

DRUG ALERT

Drugs Commonly Used to Treat COPD

Theophylline (a bronchodilator) commonly causes anorexia. A high-carbohydrate, low-protein diet slows the metabolism of theophylline, thereby increasing the risk of side effects, including dizziness, flushing, and headache. A sudden increase in protein intake may decrease the duration of theophylline action. Caffeine in any form also slows the rate of theophylline elimination; concurrent use of caffeine increases the risk for insomnia and cardiac arrhythmias.

Albuterol (a bronchodilator) may cause hyperglycemia in diabetics.

Prednisone (an antiinflammatory glucocorticoid) stimulates appetite and therefore may cause weight gain. Hyperglycemia may occur in diabetics and nondiabetics. Prednisone promotes sodium retention, potassium excretion, loss of calcium from the bones, and gastrointestinal upset.

NURSING PROCESS

Mr. Rameriz is a 74-year-old, frail man admitted to the hospital with multiple, non–life-threatening injuries resulting from a car accident. He weighs 128 pounds and is 5 feet tall.

Assessment

Obtain clinical data:

Current body mass index (BMI); recent weight history

Medical history, including hyperlipidemia, hypertension, cardiovascular disease, renal impairments, diabetes, gastrointestinal complaints
Extent of injuries; significance of gastrointestinal trauma, if appropriate
Hemodynamic status; signs and symptoms of hemorrhaging
Altered fluid and electrolyte balance, particularly sodium and fluid accumulation. Rapid weight gain of more than 1 kg per day indicates fluid retention.
Altered neurologic status (eg, confusion, disorientation); ability to eat, ability to self-feed
Altered gastrointestinal function, such as hypoactive bowel sounds, distention, complaints of nausea, anorexia
Abnormal laboratory values, especially albumin, transferrin, glucose, and electrolytes. After the initial stress response and peak period of catabolism subside, monitor albumin, transferrin, total lymphocyte count, and creatinine height index to assess protein status. Low serum transferrin and anergy are strongly correlated with the development of wound infection.
Diminished renal output; measure intake and output
Clinical signs of malnutrition, such as pitting edema, easily pluckable hair, changes in hair or skin pigment, wasted appearance
Medications that affect nutrition, such as lipid-lowering medications, cardiac drugs, antihypertensives

Interview the patient to assess:

Understanding of normal weight and perception of why he is undernourished
Usual 24-hour intake, including portion sizes, frequency and pattern of eating, food intolerances, adequacy of protein intake, and adequacy of calorie intake
Cultural, religious, and ethnic influences on eating habits
Psychosocial and economic issues, such whether finances, loneliness, or isolation negatively affect food intake. Determine who does food shopping and preparation and whether the client is a candidate for the Meals on Wheels program.
Use of vitamins, minerals, and nutritional supplements: what, how much, and why they are taken
Use of alcohol, nicotine, and caffeine

Nursing Diagnosis

Altered Nutrition: Less Than Body Requirements, related to low calorie intake and increased requirements related to injuries.

Planning and Implementation

CLIENT GOALS

The client will:

Maintain normal fluid and electrolyte balance
Avoid complications of malnutrition, stress, and refeeding syndrome

Initially, by:
- Consuming adequate calories to prevent weight loss
- Consuming adequate protein to prevent protein losses

When oral diet is advanced and tolerated, by:
- Consuming adequate calories to promote weight gain
- Consuming adequate protein to achieve positive nitrogen balance, restore lean body mass, and experience adequate healing and recovery

Describe the principles and rationale of diet management, as appropriate, and implement the recommended dietary interventions

NURSING INTERVENTIONS

Nutrition Therapy

Initially, give intravenous fluid and electrolytes as ordered to maintain hydration until oral intake is resumed.

When oral intake resumes, provide calories based on the BEE adjusted for activity and injury and adequate protein based on the extent of injury. Gradually increase intake as tolerated to avoid refeeding syndrome.

Adjust fluid intake according to need, based on intake and output and physical findings.

Provide small, frequent feedings as tolerated to maximize intake.

Client Teaching

Instruct the client:

On the importance of protein and calories in promoting wound healing and recovery and overall health

On the eating plan essentials, including:
- How to increase calories and protein in the diet (Box 16-1)
- Eating small, frequent meals if anorexia or nausea occurs

Evaluation

The client:

Maintains normal fluid and electrolyte balance

Avoids complications of malnutrition, stress, and refeeding syndrome

Initially, by:
- Consuming adequate calories to prevent weight loss
- Consuming adequate protein to prevent protein losses

When the oral diet is advanced and tolerated, by:
- Consuming adequate calories to promote weight gain
- Consuming adequate protein to achieve positive nitrogen balance, restore lean body mass, and experience adequate healing and recovery

Describes the principles and rationale of diet management, as appropriate, and implements the recommended dietary interventions

Questions You May Hear

Are omega-6 fatty acids (predominate in plant oils) bad for the immune system? In amounts that exceed the requirement for essential fatty acids, omega-6 fatty acids may impair immune system functioning. Because of this, large amounts of omega-6 fatty acids, which are typically found in intravenous lipid emulsions and enteral formulas, may not be appropriate for patients who are severely stressed. Researchers are trying to determine whether omega-3 fatty acids, commonly referred to as "fish oils," are a better source of fat calories for stressed patients.

How do enteral formulas designed for stress differ from routine formulas? Stress formulas tend to be high in protein and calories and may contain higher than normal amounts of certain nutrients, such as vitamin C, the B-complex vitamins, vitamin E, copper, and zinc. Some stress formulas are also fortified with arginine and/or glutamine, omega-3 fatty acids, and nucleotides (components of DNA), all of which may boost immune system functioning. Although the specialized formulas are more expensive than routine formulas, they may help reduce overall costs by reducing the incidence of infections and the length of hospital stays.

KEY CONCEPTS

- The body adapts to starvation (chronically low calorie intake) by lowering its metabolic rate and relying on ketones (fat) as its primary fuel. These adaptations preserve lean body mass and thus prolong survival.
- Acute protein deficiency (kwashiorkor) results from an inadequate intake with superimposed stress. It develops within a matter of weeks, and although the patient may look adequately nourished, visceral and somatic proteins are depleted.
- Chronic PCM (marasmus) results from an inadequate intake consumed over a period of months to years. Adaptation occurs, so that body proteins are preserved. The patient looks emaciated.
- The concern in feeding patients with kwashiorkor is not giving them enough protein. With marasmus, the risk is feeding the patient too rapidly and too aggressively, which can precipitate a potentially fatal refeeding syndrome.
- The impact of stress on nutritional status and requirements depends on the severity of the stress, the number of stressors, and the individual's ability to adapt to stress.
- The release of stress hormones during the ebb phase after injury causes an increase in serum glucose and decreases in oxygen consumption, blood pressure, cardiac output, body temperature, and renal output. Nutritional intervention during this period is usually contraindicated.
- Hypermetabolism and increased catabolism occur during the flow phase. Nutritional support begins when serum glucose levels fall and the adaptive phase begins usually within 2 to 5 days after stress. Adequate calories and protein are needed to minimize weight loss and catabolism.
- Patients who are well nourished before surgery have a lower incidence of infections and experience fewer complications than malnourished patients. If time allows, nutritional deficits should be corrected before surgery. Healing increases the requirements for calories, protein, vitamin C, and zinc.

- Extensive burns are the most severe form of stress that a person can experience. Calorie requirements may increase by 100%, and protein needs may increase to more than three times the normal RDA. Nutritional support may be complicated by paralytic ileus, stress ulcers, anorexia, pain, multisystem organ failure, and the consequences of medical-surgical treatments.
- Patients with COPD are often underweight and malnourished. Shortness of breath can make eating difficult, and decreased oxygenation of the gastrointestinal cells can impair peristalsis and digestion. Conversely, poor nutrition impairs respiratory status.
- Nutrition-dense, easy-to-consume foods are preferred for patients with chronic respiratory disorders. Patients with hypercapnia and those receiving ventilator support may benefit from a restricted carbohydrate intake. Carbohydrates produce more carbon dioxide when they are metabolized than do either proteins or fats, so they create a greater burden on the lungs.

Focus on Critical Thinking

Mr. Stevens is 45-years-old. He is 5 feet 11 inches tall, weighs 160 pounds, and was brought to the emergency room after being struck by a car while jogging. It was quickly determined that Mr. Stevens had a ruptured spleen, a broken femur, a broken jaw, and two cracked ribs. He underwent surgery to remove his spleen, set his leg, and wire his jaw; his course in the intensive care unit was typical of post-trauma clients. By the third post-trauma day, Mr. Stevens still had a paralytic ileus, and parenteral nutrition was started.

Calculate Mr. Stevens' calorie and protein requirements. Explain why parenteral nutrition was or was not the best method of feeding to initiate. When would it be appropriate to discontinue parenteral nutrition? What method of feeding would you then recommend? When Mr. Stevens is able to tolerate oral feedings, what type of diet would you recommend? Devise an appropriate diet that would provide adequate calories and protein in a form Mr. Stevens could consume.

ANSWER KEY

1. **TRUE** The body adapts to starvation in an attempt to survive. Loss of protein tissue slows the metabolism.
2. **FALSE** In an attempt to adapt to severe stress, the body mobilizes nutrients to counteract the high metabolic demands of the stress.
3. **TRUE** Kwashiorkor is an acute protein deficiency that occurs when the body cannot adapt to starvation because of a superimposed illness or infection. It can develop in as little as 2 weeks.
4. **TRUE** People who have adapted to starvation are at risk of becoming metabolically overwhelmed by the sudden introduction of excessive protein and calories, a condition called refeeding syndrome.
5. **FALSE** The risk involved in feeding patients with kwashiorkor is underfeeding, or not meeting their protein needs.

6. **TRUE** Well-nourished surgical patients have a lower incidence of infections and experience fewer complications than malnourished surgical patients.
7. **TRUE** The adaptive phase begins as stress hormone levels subside, serum glucose levels decline, and metabolism returns to normal.
8. **TRUE** After trauma, motility returns to the intestines much sooner than to the stomach.
9. **TRUE** Oral and enteral routes are preferred if the gastrointestinal tract is functional. Since intestinal blood flow is reduced in response to severe stress, using the gastrointestinal tract increases the blood flow, to help prevent translocation of gut bacteria.
10. **TRUE** Extensive burns are the most severe form of stress. Calorie requirements may increase 100%, and protein requirements may increase threefold.

REFERENCES

Chicago Dietetic Association & South Suburban Dietetic Association. (1996). *Manual of clinical dietetics* (5th ed.). Chicago: American Dietetic Association.

Escott-Stump, S. (1998). *Nutrition and diagnosis-related care* (4th ed.). Baltimore: Williams & Wilkins.

Timby, B., Scherer, J., & Smith, S. (1999). *Introductory medical-surgical nursing* (7th ed.). Philadelphia: Lippincott.

Whitney, E., Cataldo, C., & Rolfes, S. (1998). *Understanding normal and clinical nutrition* (5th ed.). Belmont, CA: Wadsworth Publishing Company.

CHAPTER 17

Nutrition for Patients With Gastrointestinal Disorders

TRUE	FALSE	Check your knowledge of nutrition for patients with gastrointestinal disorders.
		1 People who have nausea should limit liquids with meals.
		2 Carbonated beverages may contribute to diarrhea.
		3 Thin liquids, such as clear juices and clear broths, are usually the easiest items for patients with swallowing disorders to swallow.
		4 People with reflux and heartburn should be encouraged to switch from regular coffee to decaffeinated coffee.
		5 People with gastritis or ulcers should eat a bedtime snack to reduce the risk of nocturnal pain.
		6 Steatorrhea is treated with a low-residue diet.
		7 Simple sugars contribute to diarrhea in patients with dumping syndrome.
		8 Patients with celiac disease need a gluten-free diet even when they are asymptomatic.
		9 The nutrient most problematic for people with chronic pancreatitis is fat.
		10 The nutrient most problematic for people with end-stage liver disease is fat.

Upon completion of this chapter, you will be able to

- Discuss nutritional management of the following conditions: anorexia, nausea and vomiting, diarrhea, constipation, dysphagia, gastroesophageal reflux disease, peptic ulcers, dumping syndrome, malabsorption syndromes, diverticular disease, liver disease, pancreatitis, and gallbladder disease.
- Discuss the characteristics and indications for the following therapeutic diets: low-residue, high-fiber, dysphagia, gluten-free, low-fat, and lactose-restricted.

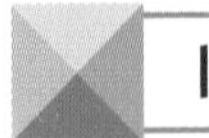

Introduction

Nutrition therapy is a major component in the management of digestive system disorders. It is the foundation of treatment for some disorders; for others, it alleviates symptoms rather than altering the disease. Nutrition therapy is frequently needed to restore nutritional status that has been compromised by dysfunction or disease.

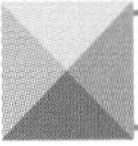

Assessment of Gastrointestinal Status

Before the optimal nutrition therapy can be planned, a nutrition-focused assessment of gastrointestinal status is indicated. Criteria to consider include historical data, physical findings, and laboratory data.

HISTORICAL DATA

- Is the patient underweight, overweight, or obese? Has the patient recently experienced unintentional weight loss? If so, how much and over what time period? Does the patient correlate the weight loss with gastrointestinal symptoms?
- Is the patient following a special diet? Has the patient's appetite changed? Has the patient changed his or her usual intake in response to symptoms? What foods does the patient avoid? What foods does the patient prefer? Does the patient use alcohol or caffeine?
- Is the patient active?
- What gastrointestinal signs or symptoms does the patient experience (eg, reflux, indigestion, nausea, vomiting, diarrhea, constipation, bloating, cramping)? How frequently do symptoms occur? Does the patient know what brings about symptoms? What does the patient do to relieve symptoms? Has there been a change in bowel habits?
- Does the patient use tobacco or recreational drugs? What over-the-counter or prescribed medications does the patient take? What nutritional supplements does the patient use and for what purpose?
- Is the patient willing to change his or her eating habits?

PHYSICAL FINDINGS

- Can the patient chew, swallow, and taste?
- Is the patient's oral and dental health adequate?
- Does the patient look ill?
- Does the patient have ascites or edema?

LABORATORY DATA

- What laboratory values are abnormal?
- Are sodium and potassium levels depleted or increased, indicative of fluid imbalances?
- Are the hemoglobin and hematocrit values low, indicative of blood loss?
- Is the serum albumin concentration low because of protein malnutrition?

Common Gastrointestinal Problems

Anorexia, nausea and vomiting, diarrhea, and constipation are common symptoms experienced by most people from time to time. Among the "well" population, these problems may simply be related to eating unusual or excessive amounts of specific foods or types of food. These problems may be more severe or long-lasting when they occur as symptoms of underlying gastrointestinal disorders, as a result of viral or bacterial infection, or secondary to drug therapy or medical treatment.

ANOREXIA

Anorexia is defined as the lack of appetite. It differs from anorexia nervosa, a psychological condition that is characterized by the denial of appetite. Anorexia is a common symptom for numerous physical conditions, not just gastrointestinal problems, and is a side effect of certain drugs. Emotional issues, such as fear, anxiety, and depression, frequently cause anorexia.

The aim of nutrition therapy is to stimulate the appetite and attain or maintain adequate nutritional intake. The following interventions may help maximize intake:

- Serve food attractively and season according to individual taste. If decreased ability to taste is contributing to anorexia, enhance food flavors with tart seasonings (eg, orange juice, lemonade, vinegar, lemon juice) or strong seasonings (eg, basil, oregano, rosemary, tarragon, mint).
- If possible, schedule procedures and medications at a time when they are least likely to interfere with appetite.
- Control pain, nausea, or depression with medications, as ordered.
- Provide small, frequent meals.
- Provide liquid supplements between meals. These supplements can significantly improve protein and calorie intake and usually are well accepted. In addition, liquids tend to leave the stomach quickly and therefore are less likely to interfere with meals.
- Limit fat intake if fat is contributing to early satiety. High-fat foods include fried foods; fatty meats and luncheon meats; whole milk and milk products; butter, margarine, and oils; and rich desserts.
- Solicit food preferences and allow food from home, if possible.

- Provide encouragement and a pleasant eating environment. Advise the patient to stay calm at mealtimes and not to hurry through eating.

NAUSEA AND VOMITING

Nausea and vomiting may be related to a decrease in gastric acid secretion, a decrease in digestive enzyme activity, a decrease in gastrointestinal motility, gastric irritation, or acidosis. Other causes include bacterial and viral infection; increased intracranial pressure; equilibrium imbalance; liver, pancreatic, and gallbladder disorders; and pyloric or intestinal obstruction. Drugs and certain medical treatments may also contribute to nausea. Prolonged nausea and vomiting can lead to weight loss; vomiting can cause metabolic alkalosis related to the loss of gastric hydrochloric acid.

Food is withheld until nausea or vomiting subsides. Clear liquids are used for fluid and electrolytes, if tolerated. Some patients may need intravenous fluid and electrolytes if vomiting is severe or prolonged. Clear liquids are eventually replaced by full liquids, then by diet as tolerated. Small, frequent meals of readily digested carbohydrates (eg, dry toast, crackers, plain rolls, pretzels, angel food cake, oatmeal, soft and bland fruit) are best tolerated. Other interventions include the following:

- Solicit food preferences and observe individual food intolerances.
- Elevate the head of the bed.
- Encourage the patient to eat slowly and not to eat if he or she feels nauseated.
- Promote good oral hygiene with mouthwash and ice chips.
- Limit liquids with meals, because they can cause a full, bloated feeling. Encourage a liberal fluid intake between meals with whatever liquids the patient can tolerate, such as clear soup, juice, gelatin, ginger ale, and Popsicles.
- Serve foods at room temperature or chilled; hot foods may contribute to nausea.
- Avoid high-fat and spicy foods if they contribute to nausea. These include fried foods, fatty meats and luncheon meats, whole milk and milk products, butter, margarine, oils, and rich desserts.

DIARRHEA

Diarrhea can cause large losses of potassium, sodium, and fluid, and it also reduces the time that is available for the absorption of all other nutrients. Severe or chronic diarrhea can lead to nutritional complications, including weight loss, hypoproteinemia, metabolic acidosis, and nutrient deficiencies related to decreased transit time.

Common causes of diarrhea include emotional or physical stress; gastrointestinal disorders and malabsorption syndromes (eg, lactose intolerance); metabolic and endocrine disorders; surgical bowel intervention; bacterial, viral, and parasitic infections; and certain drug therapies (Box 17–1). Nutritionally, food allergies and the use of tube feedings may cause diarrhea. Also, coffee or caffeine stimulates peristalsis in some people. Stool frequency may increase from an excessive intake of high-fiber foods or foods with

BOX 17.1

Drugs That Commonly Cause Diarrhea

Allopurinol
Alprazolam
Many antibiotics
Many antineoplastics
Atenolol
Carbamazepine
Chlorpropamide
Cisapride
Clofibrate
Clomipramine HCl
Colchicine
Colestipol
Cyclosporine
Cyproheptadine HCl
Digitalis
Disopyramide phosphate
Doxazosin mesylate
Enalapril maleate
Epoetin alfa
Ethosuximide
Famciclovir
Fluoxetine HCl
Flurazepam HCl
Furosemide
Glipizide
Haloperidol
Ibuprofen
Interferon
Ketorolac tromethamine
Lisinopril
Lovastatin
Methyldopa
Metoclopramide HCl
Metoprolol tartrate
Milk of magnesia
Naproxen
Niacin
Nifedipine
Omeprazole
Paroxetine
Pentoxifylline
Phosphorus supplements
Potassium supplements
Pravastatin sodium
Prazosin HCl
Ramipril
Risperidone
Sertraline HCl
Simvastatin
Sodium phosphate
Spironolactone
Sulfasalazine
Tacrine
Temazepam
Tolbutamide
Topiramate
Zafirlukast
Zolpidem tartrate

laxative properties, such as bran, whole-grain breads and cereals, raw vegetables, fresh fruits, and prunes or prune juice.

Nutrition therapy varies with the severity and duration of diarrhea. Acute diarrhea lasting 24 to 48 hours usually requires no nutrition intervention other than encouraging a liberal fluid intake to replace losses. For chronic diarrhea, food is withheld for 24 to 48 hours and intravenous fluid and electrolytes are given to maintain hydration. After 1 to 2 days of clear liquids, the diet progresses to a low-residue diet as tolerated (Box 17–2), to reduce stool bulk and slow gastrointestinal transit time. Small, frequent meals are better tolerated than three large meals. High-potassium foods are encouraged to replace losses. These include bananas, canned apricots and peaches, apricot nectar, tomato juice, fish, potatoes, and meat.

Until diarrhea completely subsides, it may be prudent to restrict the following:

- Milk and milk products, because lactose intolerance may be contributing to diarrhea.
- Very hot or very cold food and beverages, because they stimulate peristalsis.
- Coffee, strong tea, some sodas, and chocolate, because they contain caffeine.
- Carbonated beverages, because their electrolyte content is low and their osmolality is high, which can promote osmotic diarrhea.

(text continues on page 502)

BOX 17.2

Low-Residue Diet (Low-Fiber Diet)

Characteristics

This diet restricts fiber and residue to reduce the frequency and volume of fecal output and to slow transit time.

Indications

- Bowel inflammation, as seen in the acute stages of diverticulitis, ulcerative colitis, and regional enteritis
- Esophageal and intestinal stenosis
- Preparation for bowel surgery

Contraindications

- Irritable colon
- Diverticulosis

Guidelines to Achieve a Low-Residue Diet

You may eat the following foods:

- Meats: eggs; ground or well-cooked tender meat, fish, and poultry
- Dairy: up to 2 cups of milk per day; mild cheeses
- Fruits: juices without pulp, except prune juice; canned fruit; ripe bananas
- Vegetables: vegetable juices without pulp; lettuce if tolerated; most well-cooked vegetables without seeds; potatoes without skins
- Breads and cereals: only white bread and refined bread and cereal products; rolls, biscuits, muffins, pancakes, plain pastries; crackers, bagels; melba toast, waffles, refined cereals such as Cream of Wheat, Cream of Rice, and puffed rice; pasta, white rice
- Miscellaneous: plain desserts made with allowed foods, such as fruit ices, plain cakes, puddings (rice, bread, plain), and cookies without nuts or coconut; sherbet, ice cream (no nuts or coconut); gelatin; candy such as butterscotch, jelly beans, marshmallows, plain hard candy; honey, molasses, sugar

Avoid the following foods:

- Protein: tough meats, dried peas and beans, nuts, seeds, lentils, peanut butter
- Dairy: more than 2 cups of milk per day
- Fruits: all other raw, cooked, or dried fruits; prune juice
- Vegetables: most raw vegetables and vegetables with seeds; sauerkraut, peas, corn
- Breads and cereals: breads made with whole-grain flour, bran, seeds, nuts, coconut, or dried fruit; corn bread, graham crackers, oatmeal; whole-grain, bran, or granola cereal; cereals containing seeds, nuts, coconut, or dried fruit

(continued)

BOX 17.2

Low-Residue Diet (Low-Fiber Diet) (continued)

- Miscellaneous: nuts, coconut, anything made with nuts or coconut, olives, pickles, seeds, popcorn

Sample Menu

Breakfast

Strained orange juice
Cream of Rice
Poached egg
White toast with butter and jelly
½ cup milk
Coffee/tea
Salt/pepper/sugar

Lunch

Tomato juice
Sandwich made with white bread, ham, and mayonnaise
Canned peach halves
Sponge cake
½ cup milk
Coffee/tea
Salt/pepper/sugar

Dinner

Roast chicken
White rice
Gelatin made with ripe bananas
½ cup milk
Cooked carrots
Italian bread with butter
Coffee/tea
Salt/pepper/sugar

Snack

Saltine crackers
½ cup milk

Potential Problems	Recommended Interventions
Deficiencies of calcium, caused by the limited allowance of milk and dairy products Deficiencies of iron, because many adults refuse to eat ground meats (the best source of iron in the diet), and other sources of iron, such as dried fruits and many iron-fortified cereals, are prohibited Deficiencies of vitamins, because few kinds of vegetables are allowed on a low-residue diet and those that are allowed may be vitamin poor because the processing used to remove fiber also removes vitamins	Provide supplements as needed. Encourage as varied an intake as possible, and liberalize the diet as soon as possible.

(continued)

BOX 17.2

Low-Residue Diet (Low-Fiber Diet) (continued)

Potential Problems	Recommended Interventions
Inadequate calorie intake related to the highly restrictive nature of the diet. Also, many adults refuse to eat strained food because it resembles baby food.	Honor special requests for allowed foods, if possible. Liberalize the diet as soon as possible.
Constipation related to the low fiber content of the diet: Insufficient fiber intake causes a decrease in stool bulk and slowing of intestinal transit time.	Liberalize the diet to allow more fiber.
Persistent diarrhea related to poor tolerance of even the small amounts of fiber contained in a low-residue diet. Tolerance of fiber varies among patients and conditions.	Further reduce the residue content of the diet by eliminating all fruits and vegetables, except strained fruit juice.

Patient Teaching

Instruct the patient that:

- Fiber is a component of plants and therefore is found in fruits, vegetables, grains, and nuts.
- "Low residue" means "low fiber" plus avoiding or limiting foods that increase residue and stool weight: prune juice, meat and shellfish with tough connective tissue, and milk or milk products.
- Reducing residue intake slows the passage of food through the bowel.
- The diet will probably be short-term.
- Food preparation techniques to reduce residue include removing skins, seeds, and membranes of fruits and vegetables that are high in fiber and cooking allowed vegetables until they are very tender.

- Foods that may contribute to cramping, such as gassy vegetables (broccoli, cauliflower, cabbage, brussels sprouts, onions, legumes), melons, spicy foods, and excessive sweets.

Patients with intractable diarrhea that does not respond to traditional medical and nutrition therapy may need bowel rest (*total parenteral nutrition*, or TPN).

CONSTIPATION

Constipation, defined as the difficult or infrequent passage of stools that may be hard and dry, can occur secondary to irregular bowel habits, psychogenic factors, lack of activity, chronic laxative use, inadequate intake of fluid and fiber, metabolic and endocrine disorders, and bowel abnormalities (eg, tumors, hernias, strictures, diverticular disease, irritable colon). Certain drug therapies cause constipation (Box 17–3). Contrary to popular belief, daily bowel movements are not necessary, provided the stools are not hard and dry.

Usually, a high-fiber diet is used to alleviate constipation. American adults consume approximately 12 to 18 g of fiber per day, about half the recommended intake of 20 to 35 g/day suggested by leading health organizations. A high-fiber diet is rich in both soluble and insoluble fiber, even though only insoluble fiber has been credited with increasing stool bulk and stimulating peristalsis. It is achieved by substituting high-fiber foods for refined, low-fiber foods (Box 17–4). Fiber intake is increased gradually to avoid symptoms of intolerance, such as increased intestinal gas production, cramping, and diarrhea. Individuals vary in the amount of fiber they need to alleviate constipation and in how well they tolerate fiber. In addition:

- Increase fluid to at least 8 to 10 glasses daily. To help stimulate peristalsis, encourage the patient to drink hot coffee, tea, or lemon water after waking.
- Discourage the use of fiber "pills," which can cause constipation or even intestinal blockages, especially when taken in large amounts and with inadequate fluid. Likewise, over-the-counter laxatives and stool softeners should be used only if recommended by the physician.
- Increasing fat intake may help in some cases. Fat stimulates bile secretion, which draws water into the gastrointestinal tract (because of high salt content), to produce softer stools and stimulate peristalsis.
- Encourage the intake of prunes and prune juice, which have laxative effects.
- Encourage regular aerobic exercise, which promotes muscle tone and stimulates bowel activity.

BOX 17.3

Drugs That Frequently Cause Constipation

Aluminum hydroxide	Diclofenac	Naproxen
Amantadine	Dicyclomine HCl	Nifedipine
Aminophylline	Disopyramide phosphate	Paroxetine
Aventyl	Famotidine	Phenytoin
Basaljel	Haloperidol	Prazosin HCl
Benztropine	Ibuprofen	Ramipril
Chlorpromazine HCl	Iron supplements	Sucralfate
Cholestryamine	Kayexalate	Theophylline
Clonidine	Lovastatin	Thioridazine HCl
Clonidine HCl	Meperidine HCl	Tolbutamide
Clozapine	Methyldopa	Vicodin
Codeine	Metoprolol tartrate	Vincristine sulfate
Colestipol	Morphine	Zolpidem tartrate

BOX 17.4

High-Fiber Diet

Characteristics

- A high-fiber diet is a regular diet that substitutes high-fiber foods for foods low in fiber. Fiber intake should come from eating a wide variety of plant foods, rather than from fiber supplements.
- Unprocessed bran may be added as tolerated. At least eight 8-oz glasses of fluid are recommended daily.
- This diet is used to alleviate constipation (a function of insoluble fiber) and to help lower serum cholesterol levels and improve glucose tolerance in diabetes (a function of soluble fiber).

Indications

- For the prevention or treatment of diverticular disease, constipation, irritable bowel syndrome, hypercholesterolemia, and diabetes mellitus
- May aid weight reduction; may help protect against colon cancer

Contraindications

- Intestinal inflammation or stenosis

Guidelines to Achieve a High-Fiber Diet

- Eat 6–11 servings from the bread and cereal group daily. Breads and cereals with adequate fiber provide 2–5 g of fiber per serving. High-fiber cereals provide 7–11 g of fiber per serving.
- Eat 1 serving of dried peas or beans daily.
- Eat 2–4 servings of fruit per day. Apples, nectarines, oranges, peaches, bananas, pears, and berries are high in fiber. Eat fruit with the skin on whenever possible.
- Eat 3–5 servings of vegetables per day. Cooked asparagus, green beans, broccoli, cabbage, carrots, cauliflower, greens, raw broccoli, tomatoes, celery, and zucchini are good choices.

Sample Menu

Breakfast

Prune juice
Milk
Whole wheat toast with butter
Orange
Bran cereal
Coffee/tea
Salt/pepper/sugar

(continued)

BOX 17.4

High-Fiber Diet (continued)

Lunch

Split pea soup
Julienne salad made with cheese, egg, lettuce, tomato, carrots, and other vegetables as desired
Salad dressing
Whole wheat crackers
Apple
Milk
Coffee/tea
Salt/pepper/sugar

Dinner

Roast chicken
Brown rice
Buttered peas
Coleslaw
Bran muffin with butter
Fresh strawberries
Coffee/tea
Salt/pepper/sugar

Snack

Oatmeal raisin cookies
Milk

Potential Problems	Recommended Interventions
Flatus, distention, cramping, and osmotic diarrhea related to increasing the fiber content of the diet too much or too quickly	Initiate a high-fiber diet slowly to develop the patient's tolerance. If symptoms of intolerance persist, reduce the fiber content to the maximum amount tolerated by the patient.
Possible malabsorption of calcium, zinc, and iron, from increased gastrointestinal motility (which allows less time for absorption to occur) or from binding of these minerals with fiber to form compounds that the body cannot absorb	Actual fiber-induced deficiencies are unlikely because the body adapts to a high-fiber diet. However, foods rich in calcium, zinc, and iron should be encouraged.

Patient Teaching

Instruct the patient that:

- A high-fiber diet increases stool bulk and speeds the passage of food through the intestines.
- Fiber intake may be increased by making subtle changes in eating and cooking habits, such as eating more fresh fruits and vegetables, especially with the skin on.
- Switching to high-fiber breads and cereals can significantly increase fiber intake. The first ingredient on the label should be "whole wheat," not just "wheat."

(continued)

BOX 17.4

High-Fiber Diet (continued)

- A variety of foods high in fiber should be eaten; numerous forms of fiber exist, and each performs a different action in the body (see Chapter 2).
- A meatless main dish made with legumes should be eaten once a week.
- Fresh or dried fruit should be eaten for dessert or snack.
- Although nuts and seeds are high in fiber, they are also high in fat and should be used sparingly.
- Coarse, unprocessed wheat bran is most effective as a laxative and usually is cheaper than fresh fruits and vegetables. It can be incorporated into the diet by mixing it with juice or milk; by adding it to muffins, quick breads, casseroles, and meat loaves before baking; or by sprinkling it over cereal, applesauce, eggs, or other foods.
- Bran should be added to the diet slowly (up to 3 tbsp/day) to decrease the likelihood of developing flatus and distention.
- Certain foods (in addition to being high in fiber) have laxative effects: prunes and prune juice, figs, and dates.
- At least eight 8-oz glasses of fluid should be consumed daily.

NURSING PROCESS

Ms. Scott is a 79-year-old, frail woman who has been hospitalized for a stroke (*cerebrovascular accident*, or CVA) for 6 days. Her physical impairments have gradually improved, but she continues to have difficulty swallowing and left-sided weakness. Upon discharge from the hospital she was admitted to a nursing home, where a speech therapist performed a swallowing evaluation. The results indicated that Ms. Scott should be given semisolid foods until her ability to swallow improves. The patient's usual body mass index (BMI) is 19.6. Her current BMI is 18.2.

Assessment

The following clinical data were obtained:

- Underweight according to BMI with recent weight loss
- Status post-CVA with dysphagia
- Increased serum sodium, blood urea nitrogen (BUN), and serum osmolality indicate dehydration
- Intake and output records indicate poor oral fluid intake

Interviews with patient and nursing staff revealed:

- Patient is fearful of eating and drinking because of frequent choking episodes in the hospital when given liquids
- Patient is anxious about her weight loss

Nursing Diagnosis

Altered Nutrition, Less Than Body Requirements, related to impaired swallowing secondary to CVA.

Planning and Implementation

CLIENT GOALS

The client will:

Swallow food and liquids without aspirating
Return to a regular diet
Consume adequate fluid to correct dehydration
Consume adequate calories and protein to increase BMI to 19.6

NURSING INTERVENTIONS

Give mouth care immediately before mealtime to enhance the sense of taste.
Provide a semisolid diet as ordered.
Position the patient in an upright position and tilt her head forward to facilitate swallowing.
Feed small amounts at a time, and place the food on the right side of the mouth.
Provide encouragement during mealtime.
Offer the patient pudding, custard, and yogurt between meals.
Provide thickened liquids between meals.
Monitor:

- Intake and output, as well as laboratory values for dehydration
- Swallowing ability, episodes of choking
- For signs and symptoms of aspiration
- Weight and BMI

Evaluation

The client:

Swallows food and liquids without aspirating
Returns to a regular diet
Consumes adequate fluid to correct dehydration
Consumes adequate calories and protein; increases body mass index to 19.6

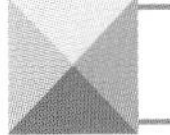

Disorders of the Esophagus

DYSPHAGIA

Dysphagia is an alteration in the ability to swallow. It can have a profound impact on intake and nutritional status, and it greatly increases the risk of aspiration and its complications of bacterial pneumonia, bronchial obstruction, and chemical pneumonitis. Many conditions cause swallowing impairments. Mechanical causes include obstruction, inflammation, edema, and surgery of the throat. Neurologic causes include amyotrophic lateral sclerosis (ALS), myasthenia gravis, cerebrovascular accident, traumatic brain injury, cerebral palsy, Parkinson's disease, and multiple sclerosis. Refer patients with actual or potential swallowing impairments to the speech pathology department for a thorough swallowing assessment.

Pathophysiology

Swallowing is a complex series of events characterized by four distinct phases.

The *oral preparatory phase* takes place in the mouth, where food (bolus) is chewed in preparation for swallowing. Obviously, liquids need little preparation compared with meat and raw vegetables. Patients who have difficulty with this phase may "pocket" food in the cheek, lose food from the lips, or be unable to move food toward the back of the mouth.

In the *oral phase*, the bolus is pushed steadily backward toward the pharynx, which opens to receive the bolus. Impairments in the tongue's muscles or nerves interfere with the oral phase and can cause coughing or choking before the patient swallows. Liquids, because they are difficult to control, are especially problematic.

The *pharyngeal phase* follows. As the food reaches the opening of the pharynx, the swallowing reflex is triggered and the food moves toward and into the esophagus. Food remaining in the throat, prolonged chewing, nasal regurgitation, coughing, choking during or after swallowing, and hoarseness after swallowing are all signs of problems with this phase.

The *esophageal phase* completes the process of swallowing. Peristaltic movements carry the bolus through the esophagus into the stomach. Neurologically impaired patients have less difficulty with this phase than with the other phases. However, obstruction and reduced esophageal peristalsis are concerns. Problems with this phase are less amenable to intervention than problems with the other three phases.

Nutrition Therapy

Crucial strategies in nutrition therapy for dysphagia are modifying the texture of the diet, to enable the patient to control chewing and movement of food, and decreasing the risk of aspiration (Table 17–1). Semisolid or medium-consistency foods, such as pudding, custards, scrambled eggs, yogurt, cooked cereals, and thickened liquids, are easiest to swallow and usually safest. As the patient's ability to swallow improves, the variety of food textures may be increased. For instance, patients who master swallowing thick liquids may be introduced to soft foods, such as mashed potatoes, plain custards, and smooth cooked cereals. Keep in mind the textures of foods for patients with dysphagia.

- Sticky foods, such as peanut butter, white bread, milk, chocolate, ice cream, and bananas can be mucus-forming.
- Melted butter, gravy, and jelly help to moisten foods.

TABLE 17-1 *Dysphagia Diets*

Level*	Description	Examples
Thick liquids	Blended or puréed liquids that are not solid, lumpy, or grainy	Applesauce; smooth, creamed soups; liquids thickened to pudding-like texture
Soft foods and thick liquids	Able to run off a spoon slowly	Pancakes soaked in syrup; plain custards; plain yogurts; mashed potatoes
Semisolid foods, thick liquids, and carbonated beverages	Gelatinous or sticky, but not crumbly	Smooth, cooked cereals; fruit nectars; eggnog; liquids thickened to pudding-like or nectar consistency
Solid foods and thick liquids	Firm, but not tough	Soft fruit; poached eggs; pasta; puréed entrée mixes; soufflés; liquids thickened to nectar or honey consistency
Regular food and beverages	Firm, chewy, crispy, but not hard (eg, no raw vegetables)	Diced meat; soft-cooked vegetables; casseroles; toast; soft cookies; liquids thickened as necessary

*Based on results of a modified barium swallow, the speech pathologist and physician determine which level is most appropriate for the patient.

To stimulate the swallowing reflex, food and beverages should be served at optimum temperature—either hot or cold—rather than tepid or at room temperature. Tepid foods can be difficult to locate in the mouth and may increase the risk of choking.

Proper feeding techniques are especially important:

- Serve small, frequent meals to help maximize intake.
- Encourage dysphagic patients to rest before mealtime. Postpone meals if the patient is fatigued.
- Give mouth care immediately before meals to enhance the sense of taste.
- Instruct the patient to think of a specific food to stimulate salivation. A lemon slice, lemon hard candy, or dill pickles may also help trigger salivation. Moderately flavored foods also help stimulate salivation.
- Reduce or eliminate distractions at mealtime so that the patient can focus his or her attention on swallowing. Limit disruptions, if possible, and do not rush the patient; allow at least 30 minutes for eating.
- Place the patient in an upright or high Fowler's position. If the patient has one-sided facial weakness, place the food on the other side of the mouth. Tilt the head forward to facilitate swallowing.
- Use adaptive eating devices, such as built-up utensils and mugs with spouts, if indicated. Syringes should never be used to force liquids into the patient's mouth,

because this can trigger choking or aspiration. Unless otherwise directed, do not allow the patient to use a straw.
- Encourage small bites and thorough chewing.
- Consider tube feedings if the patient is unable to consume an adequate oral diet.

Alcohol interferes with effective swallowing and reduces cough and gag reflexes.

HIATAL HERNIA AND GASTROESOPHAGEAL REFLUX DISEASE

Hiatal hernia and gastroesophageal reflux disease (GERD) produce "indigestion" and "heartburn," a burning type pain caused by the backflow of acidic gastric juices onto the lower esophageal mucosa. The pain may radiate to the neck and throat. It worsens when the person lies down, bends over after eating, or wears tight-fitting clothing. Some people experience regurgitation, and over time hiatal hernia and esophagitis can lead to dysphagia and esophageal ulcerations and bleeding.

Pathophysiology

People frequently blame spicy foods for their symptoms, even though other causes are more likely. Recurrent GERD is often related to reduced lower esophageal sphincter (LES) pressure, which means that the sphincter at the end of the esophagus fails to stay closed, allowing acidic gastric juice to splash into the esophagus. Several substances are known to reduce LES pressure, especially fat and caffeine. Also, eating a large volume of food distends the stomach, increasing intra-abdominal pressure and the likelihood of reflux. Delayed gastric emptying is another contributing factor.

Nutrition Therapy

Nutrition therapy is the cornerstone of treatment for hiatal hernia and GERD. Symptoms are geatly relieved or avoided by:

- Losing weight (if overweight), because weight loss decreases intra-abdominal pressure
- Avoiding items that decrease LES pressure, namely alcohol, caffeine, chocolate, decaffeinated coffee and tea, high-fat foods, peppermint and spearmint oils, and cigarette smoke

Advise the patient to sleep with the head of the bed elevated, and to adapt his or her eating habits. Small, frequent meals are better tolerated than three large meals. Foods that irritate a sensitive esophagus should be avoided if not tolerated by the individual. These foods include citrus fruits and juices, tomatoes and tomato products, carbonated beverages, pepper, spices, and very hot or very cold foods. People who avoid citrus juices because of their acidity should be encouraged to eat other sources of vitamin C, such as broccoli, brussels sprouts, strawberries, cantaloupe, greens, and raw cabbage. In addition, patients should avoid:

- Liquids immediately before and after meals, to help prevent gastric distention
- Coffee (regular and decaffeinated) and pepper, which stimulate gastric acid secretion
- Bending over or rigorous exercise after eating
- Lying down within 3 hours after eating
- Tight-fitting clothing

DRUG ALERT

Drugs That Lead to Decreased LES Pressure and Increased Risk of GERD

Anticholinergics (atropine, Bentyl, Librax)
Beta-blockers
Calcium channel blockers (Isoptin)
Prednisone
Valium (Diazepam)
Oral contraceptives
Theophylline

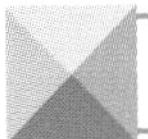

Disorders of the Stomach

PEPTIC ULCERS

Peptic ulcer, characterized by erosion of the mucosal layer of the stomach (gastric ulcer) or duodenum (duodenal ulcer), is caused by an excess secretion of, or decreased mucosal resistance to, hydrochloric acid. Peptic ulcers are classified as either gastric or duodenal.

Pathophysiology

Eighty percent to 90% of patients with peptic ulcers have the *Helicobacter pylori* organism in their stomach. The bacterium appears to secrete an enzyme that may deplete gastric mucus, making the mucosal layer more susceptible to erosion. Another cause is stress ulcers, which occur secondary to severe physiologic stress, such as cardiac or respiratory arrest, severe burns, or trauma. The stress response causes decreased gastric blood flow and vasoconstriction, which impairs the mucosal cells' ability to secrete mucus. The mucosal lining becomes more vulnerable to erosion without adequate mucus to act as a protective barrier.

Typically, duodenal ulcers produce dull, burning, or piercing pain when the stomach is empty (usually 1 to 4 hours after eating), whereas gastric ulcer pain may be worsened by intake of food. Heartburn, nausea, vomiting, and melena are possible. Scarring and obstruction can occur. The course of duodenal ulcers usually alternates between periods of exacerbation and remission, with occurrences more frequent in spring and fall. Cigarette smoking, genetics, and use of nonsteroidal antiinflammatory drugs have been identified as risk factors for ulcers; the effects of alcohol, caffeine, diet, and psychological stress are controversial.

Without proper treatment, ulcers can lead to hemorrhage, perforation, pyloric obstruction, and intractable ulcers. Various drug therapies (Box 17–5), bed rest (to reduce environmental stress), and nutrition therapy are used as treatment. Complications may be treated surgically if medical treatment fails. Gastric ulcers are more likely than duodenal ulcers to recur, and they have a higher incidence of undergoing malignant changes.

GASTRITIS

Gastritis is an inflammation of the gastric mucosa. Acute gastritis is a temporary irritation, usually self-limiting, that is caused by the ingestion of infectious or corrosive substances (eg, aspirin), food poisoning, acute alcoholism, and uremia. Symptoms vary with the source of the irritation and range from mild (heartburn) to severe (vomiting, bleeding, hematemesis).

BOX 17.5

Drugs Used to Treat Peptic Ulcers

- Antacids: Antacids interfere with iron absorption and may cause iron deficiency anemia. They produce other side effects, depending on their composition: magnesium leads to diarrhea, aluminum to constipation, calcium to hypercalcemia, and sodium to fluid retention (sodium-containing antacids are contraindicated for patients who require low-sodium diets).
- Anticholinergics
- Receptor antagonists: Histamine H_2 blockers are commonly used in the treatment of peptic ulcers. Cimetidine (Tagamet) decreases gastric secretion, which reduces the absorption of iron, folic acid, and vitamin B_{12}; hyperglycemia and diarrhea may occur. Ranitidine (Zantac) usually produces fewer side effects and interactions than cimetidine, but it may cause abdominal discomfort, constipation or diarrhea, and decreased absorption of vitamin B_{12} with long-term use.
- Antisecretory agents: The antisecretory drug omeprazole (Prilosec) can cause dry mouth and anorexia.
- Antispasmodics
- Antimotility drugs
- Sedatives
- Tranquilizers
- Bismuth and amoxicillin (if *H. pylori* is present)

Pathophysiology

Chronic gastritis is marked by progressive and irreversible atrophy of the gastric mucosa, which can lead to achlorhydria (lack of hydrochloric acid in the stomach) and pernicious anemia. The exact cause of chronic gastritis is unknown, but it may be related to overeating, stress, coffee and alcohol consumption, cigarette smoking, or chronic uremia. Symptoms include nausea, vomiting, stomach pain, malaise, anorexia, headache, hematemesis, and hiccupping. Perforation, hemorrhage, and pyloric obstruction related to scar tissue formation may occur. Gastritis is treated by eliminating the offender and controlling symptoms (ie, vomiting, pain, blood loss) through drugs and diet. Surgery may be needed to treat complications.

Nutrition Therapy for Peptic Ulcers and Gastritis

The objectives of nutrition therapy for both peptic ulcers and gastritis are to decrease gastric acid secretion, eliminate gastric irritants, and promote healing. During an attack of acute gastritis, food is withheld and intravenous fluids are provided until symptoms subside. Thereafter, the diet is liberalized according to individual tolerance.

Traditional bland diets have been replaced by a more liberal approach that centers on eliminating individual intolerances. Individual tolerance determines the use of spicy food. Beneficial eating strategies include eating in a relaxed environment and chewing food thoroughly. The following foods are known to irritate gastric mucosa and should be avoided:

- Alcohol (if the patient refuses to give up alcohol, it should be consumed with meals or immediately after eating)
- Caffeine
- Decaffeinated coffee and tea
- Pepper
- Peppermint and spearmint oils

Educate the patient about lifestyle changes:

- Encourage the patient to attain and maintain "healthy" weight. Weight loss is experienced by many patients with ulcers or chronic gastritis.
- Patients should avoid eating before going to bed to prevent acid stimulation during sleep.
- Rigorous activity immediately before or after eating should be avoided.
- Cigarettes should be avoided.

Ensure that the patient is aware of altered nutrition needs:

- Encourage protein and vitamin C intake to facilitate healing.
- Encourage iron supplements, if indicated. Iron deficiency anemia may result from blood loss and poor iron absorption related to antacid therapy or achlorhydria.
- Vitamin B_{12} status should be evaluated every few years, because chronic gastritis can impair the secretion of intrinsic factor and result in pernicious anemia.

- Be aware of the potential side effects and nutritional problems associated with antacid therapy (see previous discussion in the section on Hiatal Hernia).

DUMPING SYNDROME

Dumping syndrome is a complication of gastric surgeries in which the pyloric sphincter is removed, bypassed, or disrupted. Nutritional problems and weight loss occur until the patient's body adapts to the altered pyloric sphincter. Weight loss after gastric surgery is caused by many factors: diarrhea, steatorrhea, a voluntary restriction of food intake to avoid symptoms, early satiety, and a restrictive diet.

Pathophysiology

When the pyloric sphincter is disabled, undigested food is quickly dumped from the stomach into the small intestine. Even when the duodenum is left intact, the food moves quickly into the jejunum because of the duodenum's short length. When the duodenum is bypassed, digestive activity that normally occurs there is also bypassed.

As food is then digested in the jejunum, the osmolarity of the intestinal contents increases rapidly, and extracellular fluid shifts from circulating blood into the intestine to dilute the high particle concentration. This rapid decrease in circulating blood volume causes weakness, dizziness, and a rapid heartbeat. The large volume of hypertonic fluid in the jejunum causes distention, cramping, pain, and diarrhea. The decreased exposure to enzymes and bile, along with the rapid transit time, contribute to protein and fat maldigestion.

Reduced gastric acid secretion may lead to bacterial overgrowth in the stomach or small intestine, causing the malabsorption of fat, fat-soluble vitamins, folate, vitamin B_{12}, and calcium.

A secondary reaction, called reactive hypoglycemia, occurs 2 to 3 hours later. The rapid absorption of carbohydrate causes a rapid rise in blood glucose levels. The body compensates by oversecreting insulin, which causes a rapid drop in blood glucose levels and symptoms of dizziness, fainting, nausea, and sweating.

Nutrition Therapy

Advise the patient regarding strategies to manage dumping syndrome:

- Eat five to six or more small meals daily, because the holding capacity of the stomach is reduced (Box 17–6).
- Eliminate simple sugars, because they are quickly digested and form a hyperosmolar solution in the jejunum that attracts water. Avoid sugar, gelatin, cookies, soft drinks, and other high-sugar items.

BOX 17.6

Guidelines for Maintaining an Anti-Dumping Diet

You may eat the following foods:

- Grains and starchy vegetables: up to 5 servings daily of plain breads, crackers, rolls, unsweetened cereal, rice, pasta, corn, lima beans, parsnips, peas, potatoes, sweet potatoes, pumpkins, yams, winter squash
- Vegetables: unlimited amounts of cabbage, Chinese cabbage, celery, cucumbers, lettuce, parsley, radishes, watercress
- Up to two ½-cup servings, as tolerated, of asparagus, bean sprouts, beets, broccoli, carrots, cauliflower, eggplant, green pepper, greens, mushrooms, okra, onions, rhubarb, sauerkraut, summer squash, tomatoes, turnips, zucchini
- Fruit: up to 3 servings daily of unsweetened fruit and fruit juices
- Milk and milk products: initially withheld and gradually introduced as tolerated
- Meat and meat alternatives: all allowed
- Fats: all allowed
- Beverages: coffee, tea, artificially sweetened beverages

You should avoid the following foods:

- Sweetened cereals; cereals containing dried fruit
- Creamed vegetables
- Dried fruit, sweetened fruit, sweetened fruit juices
- Milk and milk products (initially)
- Alcohol, milk-based beverages, fruit drinks and ades
- Cakes, cookies, ice cream, sherbet, gelatin, honey, jam, jelly, syrup, sugar

Sample Menu

Breakfast

1 soft-cooked egg
1 slice white toast with butter
1 hour later: 6 oz pineapple juice

Midmorning snack

Firm banana
Butter crackers

Lunch

½ cup cottage cheese with two unsweetened, canned peach halves
Dinner roll with butter
1 hour later: 8 oz artificially sweetened ginger ale

(continued)

BOX 17.6

Guidelines for Maintaining an Anti-Dumping Diet (continued)

Midafternoon snack

1 oz cheddar cheese
4 saltine crackers

Dinner

2 oz baked chicken
½ cup white rice with butter
½ cup cooked carrots with butter
1 hour later: hot tea

Bedtime snack

½ plain bagel with cream cheese

- Include some fat and protein at each feeding because they are digested more slowly than carbohydrates and do not increase osmolarity as readily.
- Adjust total calorie intake to attain and maintain weight.
- Avoid fluids with meals and 1 hour before or after eating.
- Lie down for 20 to 30 minutes after eating to delay gastric emptying time. (Patients who have reflux should not lie down.)
- Eat foods high in pectin (eg, apple) and guar gum (eg, oats), which may help slow transit time. Milk is restricted or eliminated based on tolerance. (Lactose intolerance is common.) Lactose-reduced milk may not be well tolerated, because its lactose has been broken down to glucose and galactose, simple sugars that may promote dumping.

Eventually the diet can be liberalized to include limited amounts of concentrated sweets, larger meal sizes, and some liquid with meals as the remaining portion of the stomach or duodenum hypertrophies to hold more food and allow for more normal digestion.

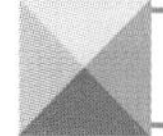

Disorders of the Intestines

MALABSORPTION SYNDROME

A major clinical manifestation of many intestinal disorders is malabsorption syndrome, which is characterized by *steatorrhea* (fatty diarrhea that produces loose, foamy, and foul-smelling stools), weight loss, muscle wasting, abdominal cramps, and distention. Numerous secondary nutrient deficiencies and metabolic disturbances are related to failure of the intestinal mucosa to adequately absorb nutrients (Table 17–2).

TABLE 17-2 ***Secondary Nutrient Deficiencies and Metabolic Disturbances of Malabsorption Syndrome***

Nutrient	Problems Caused by Malabsorption of Nutrients
Potassium	Muscle weakness
Protein	Hypoalbuminemia, edema, muscle weakness, increased risk of infection, poor wound healing
Iron, folic acid, vitamin B_{12}	Anemia, fatigue, pallor, weakness, palpitations, anorexia, indigestion, sore mouth
Vitamin K	Purpura and easy bleeding
Vitamin A	Roughening of the skin, impaired night vision, increased risk of infections
Calcium, magnesium, vitamin D	Osteomalacia and bone pain
Calcium, magnesium	Tetany
B-Complex vitamins	Stomatitis, cheilosis, glossitis, and dermatitis
Lactose	Cramping, distention, flatus, and diarrhea after milk ingestion
Bile salt	Cholesterol gallstone formation (cholesterol from cholesterol-saturated bile may precipitate out into gallstones)
Oxalate (increased absorption)	Increased risk of kidney stone formation

A complication of malabsorption syndrome is an increased risk of oxalate kidney stone formation.

Pathophysiology

Oxalate normally binds with some of the calcium in the intestinal tract and is excreted in the feces. During malabsorption, calcium binds with fatty acids instead of oxalate, resulting in increased oxalate absorption. The body rids itself of excess oxalate by excreting it in the urine. A high concentration of oxalate in the urine increases the risk of developing oxalate kidney stones.

Other factors that may contribute to malnutrition include blood loss, drug therapy, surgical intervention, and impaired intake, which may be related to restrictive diets, fear of eating, decreased pleasure from eating, or depression. The task of restoring nutritional status without aggravating the bowel in an anorexic patient is difficult and frustrating for both the health care team and the patient.

Nutrition Therapy

The goal of nutrition therapy is to control steatorrhea, promote normal bowel elimination, restore optimal nutritional status, prevent complications, and promote healing, when applicable. Regardless of the underlying disorder, the diet should always be individualized as much as possible to correspond with the patient's likes, dislikes, and intolerances. Small, frequent meals are indicated to maximize intake. Patients who are apprehensive about eating need emotional support and encouragement. If the patient is malnourished, nasojejunal tube feeding of a hydrolyzed formula diet or TPN may be used until oral intake is resumed (see Chapter 15). Oral intake should progress to a nutrient-rich diet as soon as possible.

Controlling Steatorrhea

Fat maldigestion occurs from impaired bile salt reabsorption when steatorrhea is present. Fat intake should be reduced to 35 to 45 g or less as tolerated (Box 17–7). If necessary, use medium-chain triglycerides (MCT) oil to increase calorie intake (see Chapter 4). MCT oil should be added to the diet gradually to avoid nausea, vomiting, abdominal pain, and distention. The palatability of MCT oil can be improved by substituting it for regular oils in salad dressings and in cooking and baking.

BOX 17.7

Low-Fat Diet

Characteristics

This diet limits the total amount of fat to reduce symptoms of steatorrhea and pain in patients who are intolerant of fat. Foods are baked, broiled, or boiled instead of fried or prepared with added fat. Visible fats on meats are trimmed and poultry skin is removed, preferably before cooking. Allowed fats can be used as seasonings or in cooking.

A 50-g fat diet allows:

- 6 oz of lean meat or meat substitutes
- Three to five fat equivalents per day
- Moderate portions of all other low-fat and fat-free items

A 25-g fat diet allows:

- 4 oz of lean meat or meat substitutes
- One fat equivalent per day
- Moderate portions of all other low-fat and fat-free items

Indications for Use

Malabsorption syndromes: acquired immunodeficiency syndrome, celiac disease, chronic pancreatitis, Crohn's disease, radiation enteritis, short-bowel syndrome, GERD, type 1 hyperlipoproteinemia (25–35 mg fat)

Contraindications

None

(continued)

BOX 17.7

Low-Fat Diet (continued)

Guidelines to Achieve a Low-Fat Diet

You may eat the following foods:

- Meats: lean meat, fish, and skinless poultry; egg whites and low-fat egg substitutes as desired
- Dairy products: 2 or more servings/day of skim milk, skim-milk cheeses, yogurt, and puddings
- Fruits and vegetables: all fruits and vegetables prepared without added fat, except avocado
- Bread and cereals: plain cereals, pasta, macaroni, rice, whole-grain or enriched breads; plain corn or flour tortillas; bagels
- Miscellaneous: sherbet, fruit ices, gelatin, angel food cake, vanilla wafers, graham crackers, nonfat ice cream and frozen yogurt; fruit whips with gelatin; fat-free or skim-milk soups, soft drinks, honey, sugar, seasonings as desired
- Fats: each of the following constitutes one serving:
  - 1 tsp butter, margarine, shortening, oil, or mayonnaise
  - 1 tbsp diet margarine, diet mayonnaise, or reduced-calorie cream salad dressing
  - 1 strip crisp bacon
  - 1 tbsp heavy cream
  - 2 tsp regular creamy salad dressing
  - 2 tsp peanut butter
  - 2 tsp light cream
  - 6 small nuts
  - 10 olives

You should avoid the following foods:

- Meats: fried, fatty, or heavily marbled meats; sausage, lunch meat, spareribs, frankfurters, salt pork, tuna and salmon packed in oil; egg yolks; duck, goose
- Dairy products: 1%, 2%, and whole milk; whole-milk cheeses and yogurt; ice cream
- Fruits and vegetables: any buttered, au gratin, creamed, or fried vegetables; potato chips; chow mein noodles
- Breads and cereals: products made with added fat, such as biscuits, muffins, pancakes, doughnuts, waffles, and sweet rolls; breads made with eggs, cheese, or added fat; buttered popcorn; granola-type cereals; popovers; snack crackers with added fat; snack chips; stuffing
- Miscellaneous: cream sauces, gravy; desserts, candy, and anything made with chocolate or nuts; cakes, cookies, pies, pastries

Sample Menu

Breakfast

Orange juice	Toast with 1 tsp margarine and jelly
Oatmeal	Coffee/tea
Skim milk	Salt/pepper/sugar

(continued)

BOX 17.7

Low-Fat Diet (continued)

Lunch

Sandwich: whole-wheat bread, 2 oz skinless chicken breast, lettuce, and 1 tbsp mayonnaise
Tossed salad with fat-free dressing
Fruit cocktail
Skim milk
Coffee/tea
Salt/pepper/sugar

Dinner

3 oz broiled fish
Baked potato with fat-free sour cream
Steamed broccoli
Carrot and celery sticks
Dinner roll with 1 tsp butter
Sherbet
Fresh strawberries
Skim milk
Coffee/tea
Salt/pepper/sugar

Snack

Unbuttered popcorn
Fruit juice

Potential Problems	Recommended Interventions
Noncompliance related to decreased palatability and satiety from the reduction in fat intake	Encourage the patient to eat a variety of foods and to use nonfat and fat-free versions of familiar foods. Encourage the use of butter-flavored sprinkles and sprays to season hot vegetables and potatoes.
Persistent symptoms of steatorrhea or pain after eating related to fat intolerance	Decrease fat content by eliminating fat equivalents and limiting the amount of low-fat meat allowed.
Inadequate intake of iron related to the limited allowance of meat (red meat is the best source of iron in the diet)	Monitor hemoglobin and hematocrit; recommend iron supplements as needed. Encourage a liberal intake of high-iron foods, such as fortified cereals and grains and dried peas and beans. Advise the patient to consume a rich source of vitamin C at each meal to maximize iron absorption.

Patient Teaching

Ensure the patient understands that:

- The total amount of dietary fat must be reduced, regardless of the source.

(continued)

BOX 17.7

Low-Fat Diet (continued)

- Sources of fat may be visible (eg, butter, margarine, shortening, fat on meat, salad dressings) or invisible (eg, marbled meat, whole milk and whole-milk products, egg yolks, nuts).
- Substitutions can be made to individualize the diet.
- Oil-packed tuna and salmon may be used if thoroughly rinsed.
- Fat-free salad dressings may be used as desired.
- Tips for reducing fat content when eating out:
  a. Choose juice instead of soup as an appetizer.
  b. Use lemon, vinegar, low-calorie dressing (if available), or fresh ground pepper on salad, or request that the dressing be brought on the side.
  c. Order plain baked or broiled foods.
  d. Avoid warm bread and rolls, which absorb more butter than those at room temperature.
  e. Order fresh fruit, gelatin, or sherbet for dessert.
  f. Request milk for coffee or tea in place of cream and nondairy creamers.

Food preparation techniques to reduce fat content:

- Trim fat from meat and remove skin from chicken before cooking.
- Place meats to be baked or roasted on a rack to allow the fat to drain.
- Bake, broil, steam, or sauté foods in a vegetable cooking spray or allowed fats.
- Cook with bouillon, lemon, vinegar, wine, herbs, and spices instead of adding fat.
- Make fat-free soup stock by preparing the stock a day ahead and refrigerating it overnight. The fat will harden and can easily be removed from the surface. Make fat-free gravies by this method also.
- Purchase "select" grade meats, because they are lower in fat than "choice" and "prime" grades.

Promoting Normal Bowel Elimination

Because the enzyme activity of lactase may be temporarily impaired during malabsorption syndromes, it is prudent to restrict dietary lactose (milk sugar) even when a lactase deficiency has not been objectively diagnosed. Lactase activity may return to normal after malabsorption has been resolved. Reduce lactose to the maximum amount tolerated by the individual as indicated (see later discussion).

Restoring Optimal Nutritional Status

Patients with significant weight loss need a high-calorie, high-protein diet to restore nutritional status. However, it is difficult to meet protein and calorie needs with a low-residue diet, especially if the patient is lactose intolerant. If commercial formulas are used to supplement intake, be sure to consider osmolality, residue content, and lactose content. Patient acceptance may improve by serving the formula over ice, enhanced with commercial flavor packets, or incorporating it into appropriate recipes.

Multivitamin, mineral, and water-miscible supplements of fat-soluble vitamins are needed, not only to replenish losses, but also to facilitate healing via the metabolism of a high-calorie, high-protein diet.

Increase fluid intake to compensate for increased fluid output (eg, diarrhea, fistula drainage, blood loss).

Preventing Complications

To decrease the risk of oxalate kidney stone formation, avoid the following high-oxalate items: dark green leafy vegetables, sweet potatoes, summer squash, rhubarb, beets, nuts, peanut butter, chocolate, instant tea and coffee, grits, wheat bran, strawberries, baked beans with tomato sauce, and tofu.

Promoting Healing

Patients with increased requirements for healing (eg, regional enteritis, ulcerative colitis, postsurgical patients) may need 2000 to 3500 cal/day, and 1.0 to 1.5 g protein per kilogram.

Other diet modifications for malabsorptive disorders depend on the underlying disorder and the presenting symptoms.

LACTOSE INTOLERANCE

Lactase is the enzyme responsible for digestion of lactose into its component simple sugars, glucose and galactose. For the majority of the world's population, especially Asians, Native Americans, Africans, Hispanics, and people from the Mediterranean, lactase in adults is reduced to only 5% to 10% of the peak levels that occur in infancy.

Pathophysiology

Without adequate lactase, lactose passes through the small intestine undigested. Short-chain fatty acids and gases are produced in the colon by the fermentation of lactose. Abdominal discomfort and flatulence are common symptoms, and diarrhea occurs occasionally. For most people, symptoms do not occur at doses less than 4 to 12 g of lactose (eg, ¼ to 1 cup of milk) or when lactose is consumed as part of a meal. The lactose in the milk used to make cheese and yogurt is removed during manufacturing, so these items are usually well tolerated, as is acidophilus milk. For "well" people with primary lactose intolerance, simply knowing individual limits (eg, 8 ounces of milk with dinner is tolerated, but 8 ounces of milk between meals is not) is enough to prevent symptoms. Individual tolerance varies considerably.

A more problematic lactose intolerance occurs secondary to gastrointestinal disorders that alter the integrity and function of intestinal villi cells, where lactase is secreted. For instance, people with inflammatory bowel disease lose lactase activity when the disease is active, and sometimes for a prolonged period afterward. The loss of lactase also occurs secondary to malnutrition, because the rapidly growing intestinal cells that produce lactase are reduced in number and function. Secondary lactose intolerance tends to be more severe than primary lactose intolerance. Distention, cramps, flatus, and diarrhea occur within 15 to 30 minutes after lactose ingestion, because undigested lactose increases the osmolality of the intestinal contents, resulting in a large fluid shift into the intestines to dilute the particle concentration.

Nutrition Therapy

Nutrition therapy for lactose intolerance is to reduce lactose to the maximum amount tolerated by the individual. For "well" people, this may simply mean consuming lactose-reduced milk with food. For patients with gastrointestinal disorders, a lactose-restricted diet is indicated at least until the gastrointestinal disorder is resolved, and sometimes for a prolonged period thereafter (Box 17–8). Because lactose is used as an ingredient in many foods and drugs, it is difficult to eliminate lactose from the diet.

BOX 17.8

Teaching Patients With Primary or Secondary Lactose Intolerance

Teach the patient to limit lactose (milk sugar) to the level tolerated. Tolerated levels vary among individuals.

The following foods contain high amounts of lactose:

- Milk: whole, 2%, 1%, skim, evaporated, nonfat dry milk, milk solids
- Cream; sour cream
- All cheese, except aged natural cheeses
- Creamed soups and sauces
- Specialty or flavored instant coffee blends made with creamer
- Cocoa and most chocolate beverages
- Ice cream, sherbet, ice milk, custard
- Puddings, commercial desserts and mixes

Teach the patient to read labels to identify sources of lactose. Products that have milk, butter, margarine, dry milk solids, or whey listed as ingredients contain some lactose. Examples are:

- Breads and cereals, such as Total, Special K, and Cocoa Krispies
- Cookies, cakes, pastries, commercial fruit pie fillings, sherbet

(continued)

BOX 17.8

Teaching Patients With Primary or Secondary Lactose Intolerance (continued)

- Cold cuts and hot dogs
- Creamed or breaded meats and vegetables
- Gravy, dried soups, dips, salad dressings
- Commercial French fries, instant potatoes, mashed potatoes
- Butterscotch, caramels, chocolate candy, molasses, peppermints, toffee, chewing gum
- Cordials and liqueurs
- Maraschino cherries
- Powdered soft drinks, powdered coffee creamer
- Some dietetic and diabetic foods
- Sugar substitutes (Sweet 'N Low and Equal tablets)
- Monosodium glutamate (MSG)
- Some vitamin and mineral preparations

Other foods with small amounts of lactose include:

- Liver, sweetbreads
- Acidophilus milk

Lactate, lactalbumin, and calcium compounds are lactic acid salts and are lactose free. Kosher foods labeled *pareve* are made without milk. Nondairy creamer is also lactose free and may be used in beverages, on cereal, and in cooking, if desired. Acidophilus milk or Lactaid milk may be tolerated. The lactose in Lactaid has been converted into other absorbable sugars. Lactaid is available in supermarkets and can be used as a beverage or in cooking.

Make sure the patient is aware of the risk for calcium deficiency related to reduction or elimination of milk and dairy products from the diet. Encourage the intake of calcium from nondairy sources, such as green leafy vegetables, dates, prunes, canned sardines and salmon with bones, egg yolks, whole grains, nuts, dried peas and beans, and calcium-fortified orange juice. Provide calcium supplements as needed.

Encourage the patient to drink small amounts of milk as part of a meal, as tolerated. Some amount of milk may be tolerated by those with acquired lactose intolerance, especially if it is consumed slowly, at room temperature, and with food. Yogurt and hard cheeses are usually well tolerated. Sometimes chocolate milk is tolerated because of its higher sucrose content and slower emptying rate from the stomach.

INFLAMMATORY BOWEL DISEASE

Regional enteritis (Crohn's disease) and ulcerative colitis are chronic, inflammatory bowel diseases that produce similar symptoms during periods of exacerbation: diarrhea with possible melena, nausea, vomiting, weight loss, crampy abdominal pain, fever, fatigue, and anorexia.

Pathophysiology

Maldigestion and malabsorption of nutrients may occur from the disease, from surgery to treat the disease, or from medications. As a result, nutritional status is often poor. Patients may avoid specific foods or food types based on experience of pain or diarrhea related to eating. Misconceptions and restrictive diets further limit choices. Malnutrition and anemia are common. Other potential complications with nutritional implications include fistulas and abscesses, hemorrhages, bowel perforations, intestinal obstructions, and dehydration. Inflammatory bowel diseases are characterized by alternating periods of exacerbation and remission.

Nutrition Therapy

The focus of nutrition therapy for acute inflammatory bowel disease is to correct deficiencies by providing nutrients in a form the patient can tolerate. Supplements may be indicated. In the acute stage, an elemental tube feeding, possibly one fortified with glutamine, may be indicated to minimize fecal volume. TPN is used for patients who need complete bowel rest or who are unable to meet their nutritional requirements through an oral diet or tube feeding. Other patients are fed orally.

High amounts of protein and calories are needed to promote healing and restore weight, but patients whose fat digestion and absorption are impaired usually need to restrict lactose and fat. Supplemental vitamins and minerals are also needed.

Patients are often reluctant to eat, because they associate eating with pain and diarrhea. Encourage the patient to eat; discuss the role of nutrition as part of treatment and recovery. Small, frequent meals are better tolerated than three large meals. Symptoms may be improved by avoiding sugar alcohols and caffeine. Omega-3 fatty acids, commonly known as "fish oils," may mitigate the inflammatory response. Avoid iced and carbonated beverages, because they may stimulate peristalsis. During remission, a well-balanced diet based on individual tolerance is recommended. The need for special diets varies among patients.

- A low-residue diet may be needed if the patient has a partial bowel obstruction.
- Sometimes wheat and gluten intolerances occur.
- Lactose and fiber tolerance vary among individuals.

DRUG ALERT

Corticosteroids and Sulfasalazine

Corticosteroids can cause calcium and potassium depletion, sodium retention, and glucose intolerance. Monitor potassium and sodium status. Encourage intake of potassium-rich and calcium-rich foods. Limit sodium if edema or hypertension develops. Monitor serum glucose; long-term use of corticosteroids may necessitate the use of a diabetic diet.

Sulfasalazine interferes with the metabolism and physiologic function of folic acid, leading to folic acid deficiency anemia. Crystalluria and renal stone formation may also occur. Other common side effects include anorexia, nausea, and gastrointestinal upset. Provide folic acid supplements as needed. Encourage a high fluid intake to prevent renal stones. Give with food or milk.

NURSING PROCESS

Mr. Wittmeyer is a 22-year-old man who is admitted to the hospital for suspected Crohn's disease. His chief complaints are crampy abdominal pain, diarrhea, weight loss, fatigue, and anorexia. He has lost 15 pounds since his symptoms began 2 weeks ago. He is prescribed intravenous fluids, sulfasalazine, prednisone, an antidiarrheal medication, and a diet as tolerated.

Assessment

The following clinical data were obtained:

Recent weight loss of 15 pounds; BMI at 19
Admitted with Crohn's disease; no previous history
Low albumin, hemoglobin, hematocrit showing improvement
Increased serum sodium, BUN, and serum osmolality indicate dehydration

Interview with the patient revealed:

Patient is fearful of eating because he relates eating to pain and diarrhea; has been relying mostly on cola for nourishment
Patient complains of fatigue and anorexia
Before admission the patient consumed an unrestricted diet with irregular meal schedules and a high intake of milk.

Nursing Diagnosis

Altered Nutrition, Less Than Body Requirements, related to malabsorption secondary to Crohn's disease.

Planning and Implementation

CLIENT GOALS

The client will:

Experience improvement in symptoms (diarrhea, abdominal pain, fatigue, anorexia)
Restore normal fluid balance
Consume adequate calories and protein to restore normal weight
Describe the principles and rationale of nutrition therapy for Crohn's disease and implement the appropriate interventions

NURSING INTERVENTIONS

Nursing Therapy

Provide a low-fat, lactose-restricted diet
Provide lactose-free commercial supplements between meals to enhance protein and calorie intake
Encourage high fluid intake, especially of fluids high in potassium, such as tomato juice, apricot nectar, and orange juice
Monitor:

- Intake and output, as well as fluid and electrolyte status
- Appetite
- Tolerance to fat (may need to reduce fat level)
- Diarrhea (if patient does not tolerate an oral diet, determine whether an elemental diet or TPN is appropriate)
- Weight changes and BMI

Client Teaching

Instruct the client:

On the purpose and rationale of a low-fat, lactose-restricted diet. Advise the patient that he may be able to tolerate milk after the disease goes into remission.
On the importance of consuming adequate protein, calories, and fluid to promote healing and recovery
To maximize intake by eating small, frequent meals
To avoid colas and other sources of caffeine, because they stimulate peristalsis
To eliminate individual intolerances
To chew food thoroughly and avoid swallowing air
On the importance of consuming adequate fluid while taking sulfasalazine
That prednisone should improve his appetite but may cause fluid retention and gastrointestinal upset
To communicate any side effects he experiences from the medications

Evaluation

The client:

Experiences improvement in symptoms (diarrhea, abdominal pain, fatigue, anorexia)

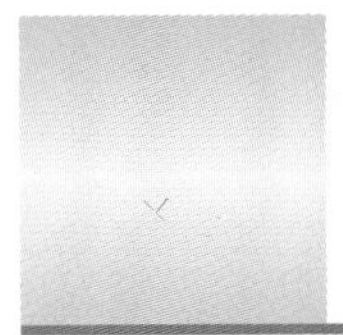

Attains normal fluid balance
Consumes adequate calories and protein to restore normal weight
Describes the principles and rationale of nutrition therapy for Crohn's disease and implements the appropriate interventions

CELIAC DISEASE (GLUTEN-INDUCED ENTEROPATHY, NONTROPICAL SPRUE)

People with celiac disease are hypersensitive to gliadin, the protein component of gluten. Although the exact cause is unknown, immune and hereditary factors are believed to play a role in the development of celiac disease.

Pathophysiology

For patients with celiac disease, eating foods that contain gliadin (eg, wheat, oats, rye, barley) causes the intestinal villi to become flattened and atrophied, resulting in a decreased absorptive surface and loss of disaccharidases. Many nutrients are malabsorbed, including fat, protein, carbohydrate, fat-soluble vitamins, iron, calcium, magnesium, zinc, and some water-soluble vitamins.

The severity of weight loss, muscle wasting, fatigue, and malnutrition varies among individuals. Many patients with celiac disease eat gliadin occasionally or in normal amounts and do not complain of symptoms. Yet even without symptoms, the intestinal mucosa is abnormal in most patients and the risk of cancer is increased. Therefore, the long-term effects of eating even small amounts of gliadin are harmful even in asymptomatic patients.

Nutrition Therapy

The cornerstone of management of celiac disease is to completely and permanently eliminate gluten from the diet. A gluten-free diet (Box 17–9) allows the villi to return toward normal, usually within a few weeks, although complete regeneration may never occur. Lactose intolerance secondary to celiac disease may be temporary or permanent.

Gluten is found in wheat, oats, rye, and barley—grains that form the foundation of a healthy diet in most cultures. A gluten-free diet requires a major lifestyle change, so compliance is often a major problem. Gluten-free products (eg, breads, pastry) made with rice, corn, or potato flour have different textures and tastes than "normal" products and are not well accepted. They are also expensive. Even patients who are willing to comply have difficulty following the diet because of the pervasiveness of gluten in prepared foods and medications and confusion over identifying sources of gluten on food labels. The diet is very restrictive, requires conscientious label reading, and is difficult to adhere to while eating out.

(*text continues on page 533*)

BOX 17.9

Gluten-Free Diet

Characteristics

This is a general diet that eliminates gliadin, a protein fraction of gluten found in wheat, rye, oats, and barley.

Indications

It is used to prevent intestinal villi changes, steatorrhea, and other symptoms characteristic of gluten-sensitive enteropathy, which is also known as celiac disease, celiac sprue, or nontropical sprue. This diet is also used for dermatitis herpetiformis.

Contraindications

None

Guidelines to Achieve a Gluten-Free Diet

You may eat the following foods:

- Beverages: carbonated drinks, cocoa, coffee, tea, fruit juice, milk, decaffeinated coffee containing no wheat flour, soy milk, wine, rum, vodka derived from grapes or potatoes
- Breads and cereals: products made with arrowroot, cornstarch, cornmeal, potato, rice, soybean, and gluten-free wheat starch flours; pure rice, sago, and tapioca; gluten-free macaroni products; corn bread, muffins, and pone made without wheat flour; corn or rice cereals such as cornflakes, Cream of Rice, hominy, puffed rice, rice flakes, Rice Krispies; grits; rice cakes and wafers; pure corn tortillas; popcorn
- Desserts: cakes, cookies, pastries, and other baked products made with allowed flours; custard, gelatin, homemade cornstarch, tapioca, and rice puddings; ice cream and sherbet prepared without gluten stabilizers
- Fats: butter, corn oil, homemade salad dressings, pure mayonnaise made with allowed vinegar, margarine, other pure vegetable oils
- Fruits: all fruit and fruit juices
- Meat and meat substitutes: all meats, poultry, fish, and shellfish; eggs; dried peas and beans; nuts; peanut butter; aged cheese; soybean and other meat substitutes; tofu; cold cuts, hot dogs, and sausage without fillers.
- Soups: broth, bouillon, clear soups, cream soups thickened with allowed flours
- Vegetables: all plain, fresh, frozen, or canned vegetables except those listed as excluded
- Miscellaneous: pepper; pickles; popcorn; potato chips; sugars and syrups, honey, jelly, jam; hard candy, plain chocolate; pure cocoa; molasses; cider, white, and rice vinegars

(continued)

BOX 17.9

Gluten-Free Diet (continued)

The following foods should be avoided:

- Beverages: ale, beer, instant coffee containing wheat, Postum, Ovaltine and other cereal beverages, malted milk, instant milk drinks, hot cocoa mixes; nondairy cream substitutes; some herbal teas with barley or barley malt; alcoholic beverages distilled from cereal grains, such as gin, whiskey, vodka, beer, ale, malt liquor; some root beers
- Breads and cereals: all products made from wheat, rye, oats, barley, buckwheat, durum, or graham, including the following items:

All commercial yeast and quick-bread mixes
All-purpose flour
Baking powder biscuits
Bran
Bread crumbs
Bread flour
Bulgur
Crackers and cracker crumbs
Farina
Graham flour
Kasha
Macaroni
Malt and malt flavoring
Matzoh
Millet
Noodles
Pancakes
Pastry flour
Pretzels
Quinoa
Rye flour
Self-rising flour
Semolina
Spelt
Teff
Vermicelli
Waffles
Whole or cracked wheat flours
Wheat germ
Zwieback

- Cooked or ready-to-eat cereals containing malt, bran, rye, wheat, oats, barley, wheat germ, buckwheat, bulgur, millet, kasha, quinoa, spelt, teff, cereals made with low-gluten flours
- Desserts: cakes, cookies, pastries, and other baked products made with flours not allowed; prepared mixes, prepared pudding thickened with wheat flour; ice cream cones; ice creams with gluten stabilizers; commercial pie fillings
- Fats: commercial salad dressings that contain gluten stabilizers; homemade salad dressings thickened with flour
- Fruit: any thickened fruits
- Soups: all soups thickened with wheat products or containing barley, noodles, or other wheat, rye, or oat products in any form; bouillon and bouillon cubes with hydrolyzed vegetable protein (HVP)
- Meats prepared with wheat, rye, oats, or barley, or gluten stabilizers or fillers, such as some hot dogs, cold cuts, sandwich spreads, sausages, and canned meats; canned pork and beans; turkey basted or injected with HVP or texturized vegetable protein (TVP); breaded fish or meats; tuna canned with HVP

(continued)

BOX 17.9

Gluten-Free Diet (continued)

- Sweets: all others not listed previously
- Vegetables: any creamed or breaded vegetables, unless allowed ingredients are used; canned baked beans; commercially prepared vegetables with cream sauce or cheese sauce
- Miscellaneous: Because the following ingredients may contain gluten, check with the manufacturer before using products containing them:

  Emulsifiers
  Flavorings
  HVP
  Ketchup, chili sauce, mustard, bottled meat sauces, horseradish, steak sauce
  Modified starch and modified food starch
  Some dry seasoning mixes
  Distilled white vinegar
  Stabilizers
  Sauces and gravies with gluten sources
  Some chewing gum
  Some chip dips
  Soy sauce, soy sauce solids
  Vegetable gum
  Vegetable protein or TVP

Additional Considerations

- Patients may be discouraged and overwhelmed when faced with a lifelong restricted diet. Provide support, encouragement, and thorough diet instructions.
- The patient may be temporarily or permanently lactose-intolerant and may require a lactose-restricted diet.
- A celiac crisis may be precipitated by emotional stress.

Potential Problems	Recommended Interventions
Difficulty obtaining a variety of allowed foods from grocery stores related to the highly restrictive nature of the diet.	Encourage the patient to use as many "normal" items as possible, such as corn cereals, grits, rice, and rice cereals. They are easy to obtain and less expensive than special products. Encourage the patient to shop in health-food stores to obtain hard-to-find items such as potato and soybean flours.

Patient Teaching

Instruct the patient on the importance of adhering to the diet, even when no symptoms are present. "Cheating" on the diet can damage intestinal villi, even if no symptoms develop. To eliminate all wheat, oat, rye, and barley flours and products permanently, the patient should:

(continued)

BOX 17.9

Gluten-Free Diet (continued)

- Read labels to identify less obvious sources of wheat, rye, oats, and barley used as extenders and fillers. Patients should check with the manufacturer *before* using products of questionable composition.
- Use corn, potato, rice, arrowroot, and soybean flours and their products.
- Use the following as thickening agents: arrowroot starch, cornstarch, tapioca starch, rice starch, sweet rice flour.

The patient should eat an otherwise normal, well-balanced diet adequate in nutrients and calories and should avoid milk and other sources of lactose if not tolerated. Weight gain may be slowly achieved.

Provide the patient with the following aids:

- A detailed list of foods allowed and not allowed
- Information regarding support groups
- Gluten-free recipes

The following companies offer gluten-free products:

Dietary Specialties, Inc.
PO Box 227
Rochester, NY 14601
To order: 800-544-0099
For information and a price list: 716-263-2787

Ener-G Foods, Inc.
PO Box 84487
5960 1st Ave South
Seattle, WA 98124-5787
800-331-5222 (outside Washington)
900-325-9877 (in state)

Encourage the patient to contact support groups, such as:

The Gluten Intolerance Group of North America
PO Box 23053
Seattle, WA 98102-0353
206-325-6980

Celiac Sprue Assoc./United States of America, Inc.
PO Box 31700
Omaha, NE 68131-0700
402-558-0600

Celiac Disease Foundation
PO Box 1265
Studio City, CA 91614-0265
213-558-4085

ILEOSTOMIES AND COLOSTOMIES

Ileostomies and colostomies are surgical openings (stomas) to the surface of the abdomen performed after part or all of the colon, anus, and rectum is removed, usually for treatment of severe inflammatory bowel disease, intestinal lesions, obstructions, or colon cancer.

Pathophysiology

Potential nutritional problems arise because large amounts of fluid, sodium, and potassium are normally absorbed in the colon. The less colon that remains, the greater the potential for nutritional problems. That is why ileostomies, where the stoma extends from the ileum, create more problems than colostomies, in which some of the colon is retained. In addition to fluid and electrolyte losses, ileostomies cause a decrease in fat, bile acid, and vitamin B_{12} absorption. Effluent from an ileostomy is liquidy, and fluid and electrolyte losses are considerable. Effluent through a colostomy varies from liquid to formed stools, depending on the length of colon that remains. Over time, adaptation occurs.

Nutrition Therapy

Nutrition therapy for ileostomies and colostomies is based on the individual's tolerance and fluid and electrolyte status. A high fluid intake (8 to 10 cups daily) is recommended to replenish losses. A high fluid intake is especially important for ileostomy patients to maintain a normal urine output and minimize the risk of renal calculi.

Weight loss related to diarrhea or a fear of eating is common. Encourage a high-calorie, high-protein diet to promote healing, replenish losses, and restore normal weight. Encourage patients to verbalize their fears. Many patients inaccurately assume that a high fluid intake contributes to diarrhea. Reassure the patient that excess fluid is excreted through the kidneys, not the stoma.

Counsel the patient on the importance of eating to attain or maintain wellness and teach the patient strategies to help control symptoms:

- Advise the patient regarding what foods cause gas, what foods are likely to cause stomal blockage, what foods help thicken the stool, what foods produce odor, and what foods act as natural intestinal deodorizers (Box 17–10).
- Encourage the patient to eat meals on a schedule to help promote a regular bowel pattern. A small evening meal helps reduce nighttime stool output.
- Teach the patient to chew food thoroughly, because improperly chewed food can cause a stomal blockage.

A patient with an ileostomy or colostomy may need supplemental nutrients:

- Because vitamin B_{12} is normally absorbed in the distal ileum, anemia related to vitamin B_{12} malabsorption can occur in patients with ileostomies, necessitating lifelong parenteral injections of vitamin B_{12}.
- Additional salt may be needed for patients with ileostomies.

BOX 17.10

Foods That Cause Side Effects

Foods That May Cause Gas

Apples	Cream sauces	Milk
Asparagus	Cucumber	Molasses
Barley	Dried peas and beans	Nuts
Beer	Eggplant	Onions
Bran	Eggs	Prunes
Broccoli	Figs	Radishes
Brussels sprouts	Fish	Raisins
Cabbage	Fried food	Sorbitol
Carbonated beverages	Garlic	Soybeans
Cauliflower	Honey	Wheat
Celery	Kohlrabi	Yeast
Chinese vegetables	Mannitol	
Coconut	Melon	

Foods That May Cause Stomal Blockage

Cabbage	Green peppers	Pineapple
Celery	Lettuce	Popcorn
Coconut	Nuts	Seeds
Corn	Olives	Skins and seeds from fruits and vegetables
Cucumbers	Peas	
Dried fruit	Pickles	

Foods That Thicken Stools

Applesauce	Cheese	Starchy foods
Bananas	Creamy peanut butter	
Breads	Pasta	

Foods That Produce Odor

Asparagus	Garlic	Onions
Eggs	Green pepper	Radish
Fish	Mustard	Spicy foods

Foods That Are Natural Intestinal Deodorizers

Buttermilk	Parsley
Cranberry juice	Yogurt

The patient may experience depression and anxiety related to altered body image, altered body function, and dietary restrictions. Provide emotional support and allow the patient and family to verbalize their feelings. Advise the patient that with time a more normal diet is possible as adaptation occurs. Foods not tolerated initially can be reintroduced in a few months.

SHORT-BOWEL SYNDROME

Short-bowel syndrome is a complex condition resulting from extensive surgical resection of the intestinal tract, usually because of inflammatory bowel disease, cancer, or obstruction. Complications include malabsorption, maldigestion, dehydration, malnutrition, and metabolic abnormalities related to a decrease in the absorptive area of the intestine when more than 50% of the bowel has been removed.

Pathophysiology

The actual problems experienced and their severity depend on the amount and location of resected and remaining bowel and whether the ileocecal valve was resected. For instance, patients with 150 cm or more of remaining small intestine do not develop short-bowel syndrome, whereas resections of more than 70% of the bowel cause permanent and severe impairments in absorption and metabolic function. Another important factor in the occurrence of symptoms is the amount of time that has elapsed since the resection. Symptoms improve during the first 1 to 2 years after surgery as adaptation takes place.

Short-bowel syndrome is characterized by three postsurgical phases. The first phase lasts for 7 to 10 days after surgery. During this phase, patients experience large fluid and electrolyte losses related to massive diarrhea. The second phase occurs 1 to 3 months after surgery and is the phase during which the majority of adaptation occurs. Diarrhea stabilizes, and a positive fluid and electrolyte balance can be achieved with an oral intake. Fat malabsorption continues, and deficiencies of calcium and magnesium may become apparent. Some patients reach the third phase of complete adaptation, in which nutritional requirements are met through an oral diet.

Nutrition Therapy

Nutrition therapy for short-bowel syndrome is highly individualized depending on the patient's tolerance. Usually, TPN is used as the primary source of nutrition during the first two phases. During the third phase, enteral nutrition is gradually introduced to stimulate the gastrointestinal tract. The complete transition to an oral diet usually occurs when diarrhea is controlled and tolerance to oral feedings improves. Tolerance is enhanced by restricting fat, lactose, fiber, oxalates, and concentrated sweets. Calorie needs may be one and a half to two times above normal in patients who have had 50% or more of their bowel removed. General guidelines to slow the passage of food through the gastrointestinal tract and help reduce diarrhea are to:

- Eat six to eight small meals daily.
- Avoid liquids 1 hour before and after each meal.
- Avoid caffeine (coffee, tea, chocolate) and alcohol for the first year after surgery; then use sparingly.
- Reduce fat to a minimum, with a goal of less than 8 g per meal if eating six meals per day. It is necessary to read labels to identify hidden sources of fat. MCT oil, in doses of 15 mL three to four times a day, may be used to supply additional calories.
- Use yogurt and aged cheeses, which do not contain lactose and should be well tolerated. Limit lactose to small amounts.
- Avoid foods and medications that contain mannitol and sorbitol (sugar alcohols), because they have a laxative effect.
- Dilute fruit juices and soft drinks to 50% strength by adding water. This lowers their osmolality.
- Avoid acidic foods, such as tomato products and citrus juices, if they cause heartburn.
- Avoid concentrated sweets, because they are hyperosmotic and may promote diarrhea.

After a baseline diet is tolerated, restricted categories are reintroduced one at a time. Categories of restricted items should be attempted at 6-month intervals during the first 2 years after surgery. Patients who are unable to adapt need TPN permanently.

DIVERTICULAR DISEASE

Diverticula are pouches that protrude outward from the muscular wall of the intestine, usually in the sigmoid colon, that characterize an asymptomatic condition known as diverticulosis. Diverticula are caused by increased pressure within the intestinal lumen, which may be related to chronic constipation and long-term low-fiber diets. Studies suggest that the incidence of symptomatic diverticular disease is increased by diets that are low in total dietary fiber and high in total fat or red meat.

Pathophysiology

Diverticulitis occurs when fecal matter gets trapped in the diverticula, causing inflammation and infection. Symptoms include cramping, alternating periods of diarrhea and constipation, flatus, abdominal distention, and low-grade fever. Complications include occult blood loss and acute rectal bleeding leading to iron deficiency anemia; abscesses and bowel perforation leading to peritonitis; fistula formation causing bowel obstruction; and bacterial overgrowth (in small bowel diverticula) that leads to malabsorption of fat and vitamin B_{12}.

Nutrition Therapy

High-fiber diets appear to decrease the incidence of diverticular disease by producing soft, bulky stools that are easily passed, resulting in decreased pressure within the colon and shortened transit time. However, once the diverticula develop, a high-fiber diet cannot make them disappear. Foods with husks and seeds, such as nuts, popcorn, cucumbers, okra, strawberries, raspberries, tomatoes, and corn, should be avoided because they can become trapped in diverticula and cause inflammation.

A high-fiber diet as tolerated (Box 17-4) is recommended to prevent and treat diverticulosis. However, a low-residue diet may be used during an acute phase of diverticulitis, or when complications of intestinal bleeding, perforation, or abscess exist. Patients who are treated with a low-residue diet in the hospital may be reluctant to switch to a high-fiber diet on discharge. Diet compliance depends on the patient's understanding of the rationale and benefits of a high-fiber diet for long-term prevention and treatment of diverticulosis and prevention of diverticulitis.

Disorders of the Liver

The liver is a highly active organ that is involved in the metabolism of almost all nutrients. After absorption, almost all nutrients are transported to the liver, where they are "processed" before being distributed to other tissues. The liver synthesizes plasma proteins, blood clotting factors, and nonessential amino acids and forms urea from the nitrogenous wastes of protein. Triglycerides, phospholipids, and cholesterol are synthesized in the liver. Glucose is synthesized (*gluconeogenesis*), and glycogen is formed, stored, and broken down, as needed. Vitamins and minerals are metabolized, and many are stored in the liver. Finally, the liver is vital for detoxifying drugs, alcohol, ammonia, and other poisonous substances.

Liver damage can have profound and devastating effects on the metabolism of almost all nutrients. Liver damage can range from mild and reversible (eg, fatty liver) to severe and terminal (eg, hepatic coma).

HEPATITIS AND CIRRHOSIS

Hepatitis is an inflammation of the liver that is caused by viral infections (types A, B, C, D, and E), alcohol abuse, and hepatotoxic chemicals such as chloroform and carbon tetrachloride. Liver cell damage that occurs from hepatitis is reversible with proper rest and nutrition. The term **cirrhosis** encompasses all forms of end-stage liver disease that are characterized by extensive loss of liver cells, fibrosis, and fatty infiltration of the liver.

Pathophysiology

Early symptoms of hepatitis include anorexia, nausea and vomiting, fever, fatigue, headache, and weight loss. Later, dark-colored urine, jaundice, liver tenderness, and possibly liver enlargement may develop.

In cirrhosis, liver function is seriously impaired as liver cells are replaced by functionless scar tissue. Normal blood circulation through the liver also is disrupted. During the early stages of cirrhosis, fever, anorexia, weight loss, and fatigue may be evident. Impaired glucose tolerance is common. Later, portal hypertension, dyspepsia, diarrhea or constipation, jaundice, esophageal varices, hemorrhoids, ascites, edema, bleeding tendencies, anemia, hepatomegaly, and splenomegaly may develop. Cirrhosis can progress to terminal hepatic coma.

Nutrition Therapy

The objectives of nutrition therapy for hepatitis and cirrhosis are to avoid or minimize permanent liver damage, promote liver cell regeneration, restore optimal nutritional status, and alleviate symptoms. For patients with cirrhosis, nutrition therapy may help avoid complications of ascites, esophageal varices, and hepatic coma. However, depending on the extent of liver damage, regeneration may not be possible.

The importance of optimal nutrition in the management of liver disorders cannot be overestimated. Adequate protein and calories are paramount: protein is needed for liver cell regeneration and calories are used to spare protein. However, if liver damage is extensive, a high protein intake may overburden the liver and precipitate a hepatic coma. Ironically, too little protein has the same effect, because protein tissue is degraded to meet normal requirements. In the later stages of cirrhosis, there is a fine line between enough protein and too much protein. In addition, it may be difficult to provide adequate calories if the patient experiences steatorrhea or an intolerance to fat.

Nutrition therapy guidelines are as follows:

- Increase protein to 1.0 to 2.0 g protein/kg, emphasizing sources of high biologic value: milk, meat, and eggs. If hepatic coma is impending, decrease protein to the maximum amount tolerated by the individual.
- Increase calories to 3000 to 4000/day to spare protein and meet energy needs, allowing a liberal carbohydrate intake of 300 to 400 g but moderate amounts of fat. Restrict fat intake if steatorrhea develops.
- Eliminate alcohol.
- Limit sodium if ascites is present. Allowances are determined by the accumulation of fluid as measured by sudden weight gain and range from 1000 to 2000 mg (see Chapter 18). High-protein foods are also relatively high in sodium. Low-sodium milk is an option; however, it is unpalatable and most patients find its taste offensive.
- If sodium restriction alone does not effectively control ascites, fluid intake is limited to 1000 to 2000 mL/day as tolerated. Amounts are liberalized as liver function improves. Some patients need a high fluid intake to replace losses caused by fever and vomiting. Patients with severe anorexia, nausea, or vomiting may need enteral or parenteral nutritional support.
- Multivitamin and mineral supplements, especially the B vitamins, vitamin C, and vitamin K, may be necessary to compensate for alterations in metabolism. Impaired liver function increases the risk of vitamin A toxicity; therefore, excess amounts of this vitamin should be avoided. Zinc supplements may help improve appetite.
- Provide small, frequent meals. Malnourished, anorexic patients have difficulty consuming an adequate diet, and nausea may worsen as the day progresses. High-calorie, high-protein liquid nourishments may be better tolerated than traditional meals. Solicit individual food preferences and work closely with the family. A

texture-modified diet (ie, soft, low-residue, or full liquid) may be needed if a regular diet irritates the esophageal mucosa. Spices, pepper, caffeine, and coarse foods may also irritate esophageal varices. Withhold food if esophageal varices bleed.

HEPATIC ENCEPHALOPATHY, FAILURE, OR COMA

Hepatic failure is common in critical illnesses. **Hepatic encephalopathy** refers to the central nervous system (CNS) manifestations of advanced liver disease; it is characterized by mental disturbance or loss of consciousness. Symptoms of impaired memory and concentration, slow response time, drowsiness, irritability, flapping tremor, and fecal odor of the breath may progress to terminal coma.

Pathophysiology

The exact cause of hepatic encephalopathy is not known; however, increased serum ammonia levels may be at least partially responsible. Ammonia is a CNS toxin that is produced by the action of gastrointestinal flora on protein (dietary sources, products of muscle catabolism, and protein from gastrointestinal blood loss). Because the malfunctioning liver cannot convert ammonia to urea, serum ammonia levels increase. The drug lactulose is used to draw blood ammonia into the colon so that it can be excreted in the feces. Because the degree of increased ammonia in the blood does not correlate with the degree of coma, other nitrogen-containing substances may be involved in the development of hepatic encephalopathy.

Blood amino acid patterns are altered in hepatic coma. The concentration of aromatic amino acids increases because the liver is not able to break them down. Higher than normal insulin levels increase the uptake of branched-chain amino acids into muscle cells, so that blood concentrations of these amino acids decrease. The increased ratio of aromatic amino acids to branch-chained amino acids interferes with the formation of certain neurotransmitters (dopamine and norepinephrine) and causes the formation of substances that may contribute to hepatic coma.

Nutrition Therapy

The goals of nutrition therapy are to help preserve liver function, control symptoms, and prevent coma. Texture modification may be necessary to prevent damage to esophageal varices. A soft, puréed, or liquid diet may facilitate swallowing. The amount of protein, sodium, and fluid allowed is adjusted according to the patient's symptoms.

Protein

Manipulation of dietary protein is critical. Providing protein in excess of what the liver can handle increases serum ammonia levels and worsens CNS symptoms. The same results occur from too little protein; a protein intake that is inadequate to meet the body's needs stimulates body protein catabolism, which, in effect, is like eating too much protein. Some studies suggest that low protein intake may be independently associated with worsening of hepatic encephalopathy.

Optimal protein allowance is derived by observation of clinical symptoms and serum ammonia levels. Patients showing signs of impending coma may be restricted to 40 to 60 g of protein from food daily, with additional amounts supplied by enteral formulas specially designed for hepatic failure (eg, formulas with altered amino acid patterns). Protein allowance for patients with coma may initially be 0 g and progressed by 10 g/day as tolerated. Vegetable and dairy proteins may be better tolerated than meat proteins because they contain fewer aromatic amino acids and more branched-chain amino acids. The protein content of the diet is adjusted frequently according to the patient's mental symptoms. Restrict foods that are sources of preformed ammonia or that contain amino acids that readily convert to ammonia: cheese, chicken, ground beef, ham, salami, buttermilk, gelatin, Idaho potatoes, onions, and peanut butter.

Sodium and Fluid

Sodium and fluid are restricted to alleviate the fluid accumulation of ascites. Sodium restrictions may be severe (250 mg/day) to moderate (up to 2000 mg/day). Fluid allowance ranges from 1500 to 2000 mL/day. Intakes of sodium and fluid are liberalized as the patient improves.

Calories

Calorie requirements are increased to 35 to 45 cal/g to prevent tissue breakdown and promote protein sparing. Fat should supply 25% to 30% of total calories.

To increase calorie intake without increasing protein, use the following supplements:

- Butter or margarine on potatoes, bread, vegetables, rice, cereal
- Honey, sugar, on toast or cereal; glucose in coffee or fruit juice
- Hard candy and jelly
- Modular carbohydrate supplements (see Chapter 15)

Patients with steatorrhea need to limit dietary fat and use MCT oil for additional calories.

Enteral and Parenteral Nutrition

Patients who are unable to consume adequate food or formula orally need enteral or parenteral nutrition. Enteral and parenteral formulas designed for patients with liver failure have fewer aromatic amino acids and more branch-chained amino acids than normal formulas do.

LIVER TRANSPLANTATION

Liver transplantation is a treatment option for patients with severe and irreversible liver failure. Patients awaiting a transplant usually have long-standing malnutrition, which increases the risk of complications and death after transplantation. Whenever possible, nu-

BOX 17.11

Low-Bacteria Diet

A low-bacteria diet eliminates the following foods:

- Undercooked meats
- All cheese and cheese products, including cottage cheese
- Unpasteurized milk and milk products
- All raw vegetables, including vegetable garnishes
- Fresh fruit with peels that are eaten, such as grapes, cherries, and berries

All other foods are allowed, including fresh fruit that is peeled and rinsed, such as apples, oranges, bananas, pears, melon, pineapple, peaches, nectarines, and kiwi.

trient deficiencies and imbalances are corrected before the transplantation to promote a positive outcome. Patients waiting for a liver transplant may be given a low-bacteria diet to decrease the risk of infection (Box 17–11).

TPN has traditionally been used to deliver nutrition after the surgery. However, intestinal tube feedings may be equally as effective, and they offer protection against gastrointestinal atrophy and bacterial translocation. Immunosuppressant drugs used to prevent rejection can complicate feeding by causing nausea, vomiting, diarrhea, and mouth sores. Nutrition guidelines when an oral intake resumes are as follows:

- Provide 1.3 to 2.0 g protein per kilogram body weight initially.
- Increase calories to 35 to 45 cal/kg. MCT oil may be needed for fat intolerance.
- Limit simple sugars if blood glucose levels are elevated.
- Adjust sodium and potassium intake according to the patient's profile. Sodium allowances range from 2 to 4 g. Patients taking cyclosporine may develop high blood potassium levels.
- Provide supplements of calcium, magnesium, and zinc, which may help alleviate muscle cramping or impaired sense of taste.
- After the initial hypermetabolic period, the patient's calorie and protein needs return toward normal. However long-term complications, such as excessive weight gain, hypertension, and diabetes, may require nutrition therapy.

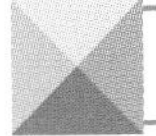

Disorders of the Pancreas

PANCREATITIS

Inflammation of the pancreas, known as **pancreatitis,** causes the retention of pancreatic enzymes, leading to autodigestion of the pancreas. Symptoms of both acute and chronic pancreatitis include severe abdominal pain, nausea, vomiting, distention, fever, and jaundice. Hyperglycemia, steatorrhea, weight loss, and malnutrition may develop as chronic manifestations.

Acute Pancreatitis

Acute pancreatitis may develop from unknown causes, alcoholism, biliary tract disease, pancreatic cancer; after gastric or biliary tract surgery; or secondary to mumps or a bacterial infection. Chronic pancreatitis, characterized by scarring and tissue calcification, is most often caused by alcohol abuse, although it is also associated with gallstones, hyperparathyroidism, and hyperlipidemia.

Nutrition Therapy

Acute pancreatitis is treated by reducing pancreatic stimulation. The patient is ordered to have nothing by mouth (NPO), and a nasogastric tube is inserted to suction gastric contents. Appropriate measures are taken to correct fluid and electrolyte imbalance, to control pain, and to treat or prevent symptoms. If the patient is malnourished, a nasojejunal tube feeding (feeding into the jejunum does not stimulate pancreatic secretions) or TPN may be used until oral intake is resumed. As bowel sounds return, serum amylase levels fall, and as pain subsides, clear liquids are given. This is progressed to a low-fat diet and then a regular diet as tolerated. Small, frequent meals may be better tolerated initially, because they help reduce the amount of pancreatic stimulation at each meal.

Acute pancreatitis that is not resolved or recurs frequently can permanently damage pancreatic cells, leading to chronic pancreatitis. The goals of nutrition therapy for chronic pancreatitis are to reduce steatorrhea, to minimize pain, and to avoid acute attacks. Because the pancreas normally secretes enzymes in amounts that exceed physiologic need, a decrease in pancreatic enzyme secretion does not necessarily mean that digestion is significantly impaired. However, extensive pancreatic damage does impair digestion, especially fat digestion. When maldigestion occurs, fat is limited to the maximum amount that the patient can tolerate without causing steatorrhea or pain, usually 50 g/day or less. Liberal quantities of protein and carbohydrates are recommended to replace calorie and nutrient losses. Patients whose insulin secretion is impaired may need a diabetic diet to help control hyperglycemia. It is prudent to eliminate individual intolerances and gastric acid stimulants (ie, alcohol, regular and decaffeinated coffee, caffeine, and pepper). Supplements of vitamin C and the B-complex vitamins, as well as water-miscible forms of the fat-soluble vitamins, may be necessary. If pancreatic enzyme replacements are prescribed, they must be taken with every meal and snack.

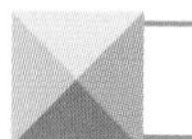

Gallbladder Disorders

CHOLELITHIASIS AND CHOLECYSTITIS

Abdominal pain, nausea and vomiting, jaundice, fever, fat intolerance, and flatulence are symptoms of **cholecystitis,** an inflammation of the gallbladder.

Pathophysiology

Cholecystitis can be caused by the presence of gallstones (*cholelithiasis*) that obstruct the cystic duct, by trauma, or by previous surgery. Cystic duct obstruction can lead to abscess, necrosis, perforation, and peritonitis.

Nutrition Therapy

The role of nutrition therapy in the treatment of cholecystitis is to minimize gallbladder stimulation. During an acute attack of cholecystitis, food is withheld and the patient is maintained on intravenous fluids and electrolytes. After 12 to 24 hours, a clear liquid diet may be offered and then progressed to a regular diet as tolerated.

Low-fat diets (20–60 g/day of fat) are frequently used in the management of gallbladder disease, based on the rationale that limiting fat intake reduces stimulation to the gallbladder and minimizes pain. Although some patients' symptoms are aggravated by fat, fat intolerance, according to some studies, is no more common among patients with gallbladder disease than it is among the general population. Some physicians recommend a low-fat diet for 4 to 6 weeks; others believe that no diet modification is necessary.

Diet modification, therefore, should be individualized. Individual intolerances should be eliminated. Foods that are most likely to cause problems are highly seasoned foods, coffee, eggs, broccoli, cauliflower, brussels sprouts, cabbage, onions, legumes, and melons. Coffee, both regular and decaffeinated, has been shown to induce significant increases in plasma cholecystokinin, the hormone released in the upper small bowel that stimulates gallbladder contraction. It is recommended that patients with symptomatic gallstones avoid coffee.

Fat-soluble vitamin deficiencies may develop as a result of impaired bile secretion, making supplementation with water-soluble forms of vitamins A, D, E, and K necessary.

Promote gradual weight loss, if the patient is overweight. Rapid weight loss favors the development of gallstones and should be avoided.

KEY CONCEPTS

- Nutrition therapy for gastrointestinal disorders is usually aimed at minimizing or preventing symptoms. For some gastrointestinal disorders, nutrition therapy is the cornerstone of treatment.
- Small, frequent meals may help maximize intake in patients who are anorexic, and avoidance of high-fat foods may lessen the feeling of fullness.
- After nausea and vomiting subside, low-fat carbohydrate foods, such as crackers, toast, oatmeal, and bland fruit, usually are well tolerated. Patients should avoid liquids with meals, because they can promote the feeling of fullness.
- A low-residue diet is used to reduce the frequency and volume of fecal output and to slow transit time. It is a short-term diet used for diarrhea, diverticulitis, and malabsorption syndromes, and in preparation for bowel surgery.

- A high-fiber diet increases stool bulk and stimulates peristalsis; it is therefore effective against constipation. Fiber intake should be increased gradually to prevent gas, distention, and diarrhea.
- Semisolid foods, such as pudding, yogurt, and cooked cereals, are usually the easiest and safest foods for people with dysphagia. Thin liquids and sticky foods should be avoided.
- Nutrition therapy strategies for GERD and hiatal hernia include losing weight if overweight, eliminating individual intolerances, and avoiding the following items that reduce LES pressure: alcohol, caffeine, chocolate, fatty foods, peppermint and spearmint flavors, and cigarette smoke.
- Patients with ulcers or gastritis should avoid foods that stimulate gastric acid secretion, such as pepper, chili powder, alcohol, caffeine, and all coffee.
- Nutrition therapy for dumping syndrome consists of eating small, frequent meals; eating protein and fat at each meal; and avoiding concentrated sugars. Lactose may have to be restricted, and liquids should be consumed 1 hour before or after eating instead of with meals.
- Depending on their severity and chronicity, malabsorption syndromes can cause numerous nutritional problems. When steatorrhea occurs, fat is reduced to the maximum amount tolerated. MCT oil may be used to increase calorie intake when fat digestion is impaired.
- Lactose intolerance is common in much of the world's adult population; tolerance varies considerably among individuals. Some people tolerate milk with food, and others tolerate only lactose-reduced milk. Lactose intolerance that occurs secondary to intestinal disorders is usually more symptomatic than acquired lactose intolerance and requires a more restrictive intake.
- During exacerbation of inflammatory bowel diseases, patients need increased amounts of calories and protein and may not tolerate fiber and lactose. Patients are often reluctant to eat, fearing that food will cause pain and diarrhea. Some patients require enteral or parenteral nutrition for bowel rest. During remission, the diet is liberalized as tolerated.
- A gluten-free diet prevents intestinal villi changes, steatorrhea, and other symptoms in patients with celiac disease. All forms and sources of wheat, oats, rye, and barley must be permanently eliminated from the diet, even in patients who are asymptomatic. A gluten-free diet requires major lifestyle changes and is difficult to follow.
- Fluid and electrolytes are of primary concern for patients with ileostomies and colostomies. Low-residue foods may help reduce stoma discharge and irritation. Additional calories and protein are needed to promote healing.
- Short-bowel syndrome occurs in patients who have had more than 50% of the small intestine removed. Maldigestion and malabsorption may lead to malnutrition. TPN is usually used until adaptation begins. Needs for calories and protein increase. Tolerance to fat, lactose, and fiber is impaired.
- A high-fiber diet may prevent diverticulosis and diverticulitis. During acute diverticulitis, however, patients may be given a low-residue diet to reduce bowel stimulation. Patients are often confused about the apparent inconsistency in nutrition therapy.

- Adequate calories and protein promote liver cell regeneration in patients with hepatitis and cirrhosis. In the advanced stages of cirrhosis, a high-protein diet—or a protein intake that is too low—can precipitate a hepatic coma.
- People who have undergone liver transplantation have high protein and calorie needs. Glucose intolerance may occur, and sodium and potassium intakes may be restricted depending on the individual's profile. Immunosuppressant drugs may interfere with intake and appetite.
- Chronic pancreatitis is treated with a low-fat diet. Patients who develop glucose intolerance may benefit from a diabetic diet.
- Patients with symptomatic gallstones should avoid coffee (regular and decaffeinated) and eliminate individual intolerances. Overweight patients are encouraged to lose weight gradually.

Focus on Critical Thinking

Mrs. Templeton is 45-years-old, weighs 153 pounds, and is 5 feet 1 inch tall. Recently, she has been complaining about heartburn that radiates to her throat and regurgitation. She notes that the pain is particularly bothersome when she eats before going to bed. Her doctor has diagnosed hiatal hernia with GERD. She avoids all citrus products because they are "too acidic" but has not made any other dietary changes related to her diagnosis.

In questioning Mrs. Templeton about her usual dietary habits, on which foods would you specifically focus?

Why is it important to find out how frequently and at what times Mrs. Templeton eats?

What would be the most effective dietary intervention for her?

What other advice would you give Mrs. Templeton to help relieve her symptoms?

What nutrient may be deficient in her diet because she avoids all citrus products?

What foods would you recommend she consume to avoid a deficiency of that nutrient?

ANSWER KEY

1. **TRUE** Avoid consuming liquids with meals, because they can cause a full, bloated feeling. Encourage a liberal fluid intake between meals with whatever liquids the client tolerates, such as clear soup, juice, gelatin, ginger ale, and Popsicles.
2. **TRUE** Carbonated beverages can contribute to diarrhea because their electrolyte content is low and their osmolality is high, possibly leading to osmotic diarrhea.
3. **FALSE** Semisolid or medium-consistency foods, such as pudding, custards, scrambled eggs, yogurt, cooked cereals, and thickened liquids, are easiest to swallow and usually safest.
4. **FALSE** All coffee, both regular and decaffeinated, stimulates gastric acid secretion.
5. **FALSE** Patients should avoid eating before going to bed to prevent acid stimulation during sleep.

6. **FALSE** A low-fat diet is indicated for patients with steatorrhea: fat intake should be reduced to 35 to 45 g or less as tolerated.
7. **TRUE** Simple sugars are quickly digested and form a hyperosmolar solution in the jejunum that attracts water.
8. **TRUE** For a patient with celiac disease, the long-term effects of eating even small amounts of gliadin are harmful, even when patients are asymptomatic.
9. **TRUE** Extensive pancreatic damage impairs digestion, especially fat digestion.
10. **FALSE** In the advanced stages of cirrhosis, a high-protein diet—or protein intake that is too low—can precipitate a hepatic coma.

REFERENCES

Beyer, P. (1998). Gastrointestinal disorders: Roles of nutrition and the dietetics practitioner. *Journal of the American Dietetic Association*, 98, 272–277.

Chartrand, L., Russo, P., Duhaime, A., & Seidman, E. (1997). Wheat starch intolerance in patients with celiac disease. *Journal of the American Dietetic Association*, 97, 612–618.

Chicago Dietetic Association and the South Suburban Dietetic Association. (1992). *Manual of clinical dietetics* (4th ed.). Chicago: The American Dietetic Association.

Dehkordi, N., & Warren, A. (1995). Lactose malabsorption as influenced by chocolate milk, skim milk, sucrose, whole milk, and lactic cultures. *Journal of the American Dietetic Association*, 95, 484–486.

Escott-Stump, S. (1997). *Nutrition and diagnosis-related care* (4th ed.). Baltimore: Williams & Wilkins.

Lykins, T., & Stockwell, J. (1998). Comprehensive modified diet simplifies nutrition management of adults with short-bowel syndrome. *Journal of the American Dietetic Association*, 98, 309–315.

Roche-Dudek, M., & Roche-Klemma, K. (1998). *Drug-nutrition resource: Part of the drug-nutrient intervention system* (3rd ed). Riverside, IL: Roche Dietitians, LLC.

Timby, B., Scherer, J., & Smith, N. (1999). *Introductory medical-surgical nursing* (7th ed.). Philadelphia: Lippincott Williams & Wilkins.

CHAPTER 18

Nutrition for Patients With Cardiovascular Disorders

TRUE	FALSE	Check your knowledge of nutrition for patients with cardiovascular disorders.
		1 Restricting saturated fat and cholesterol intake is the only dietary intervention likely to reduce the risk of coronary heart disease (CHD).
		2 Canola, olive, and peanut oils are rich in monounsaturated fats.
		3 The levels of vitamin E used in studies to reduce the risk of heart disease can easily be obtained through food.
		4 Increasing soluble fiber intake helps lower total and low-density lipoprotein cholesterol (LDL-C) without lowering high-density lipoprotein cholesterol (HDL-C).
		5 A high homocysteine level often is related to an inadequate intake of folic acid.
		6 People who don't drink alcohol should be encouraged to do so to lower their risk of heart disease.
		7 People who do not eat fish should take fish-oil supplements to lower their risk of heart disease.
		8 Very-low-fat diets may have the undesirable effect of lowering "good" cholesterol.
		9 Weight loss lowers high blood pressure.
		10 Unlike the Food Guide Pyramid, the Dietary Approaches to Stop Hypertension (DASH) diet has a "Nuts, Seeds, and Dried Peas and Beans" food group.

Upon completion of this chapter, you will be able to

- List risk factors for CHD.
- Discuss the significance of LDL-C and HDL-C and nutritional interventions to improve each.
- Describe the characteristics of the Step One and Step Two diets.
- Describe other nutritional interventions aimed at decreasing CHD risk.
- List questions you would ask to determine how closely a patient's diet resembles the Step One diet.
- Discuss the characteristics of the DASH diet.
- Describe other lifestyle modifications that are effective in the prevention and treatment of hypertension.
- Describe teaching points for low-sodium diets.

Introduction

Atherosclerotic CHD is the leading cause of death in the United States and other Western countries. A decrease in cigarette smoking and changes in eating habits, as well as improvements in health care, are credited with reducing the incidence of CHD mortality by approximately 40% over the last 40 years. Several intervention trials have shown that treating CHD risk factors, such as high blood pressure and high LDL-C, decreases fatal and nonfatal cardiovascular events.

This chapter discusses the role of diet in the prevention and treatment of cardiovascular disorders, including CHD, hypertension, and congestive heart failure (CHF). The Step One and Step Two diets are explained, as is the DASH diet.

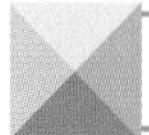

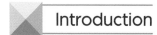

Atherosclerosis and Coronary Heart Disease

Atherosclerosis, a common and severe form of arteriosclerosis, is characterized by the formation of plaques along the smooth inner walls of arteries, which results in progressive narrowing. Studies show that the process of atherosclerosis begins early in life.

PATHOGENESIS OF ATHEROSCLEROSIS

The process of atherosclerosis begins asymptomatically with the development of fatty streaks on the lining of the arterial wall. It is believed that these fatty streaks result from chronic minimal injury to the arterial endothelium, especially at points where the force of blood flow is greatest, such as where the artery bends. Other factors that may injure the artery lining are chemicals from tobacco, high blood pressure, high glucose and cholesterol levels, and infection.

The fatty streaks enlarge and harden through a complex series of events. LDL particles enter the artery wall, where they are oxidized. Macrophages take up oxidized LDL particles, causing the cells to become larger and harder. Interplay among other factors, such as monocytes, platelets, and abnormal blood clotting, promotes the progression of fatty streaks to **plaques**.

Plaques are composed mostly of fats, cholesterol, calcium, other blood components, and connective tissue. They eventually cause artery walls to lose their elasticity and become narrowed, resulting in restricted blood flow and increased blood pressure. When blood flow is impaired, damage to organs and tissues that are "serviced" by those arteries can occur. The increase in blood pressure further damages artery walls, making them more susceptible to plaque formation. Thus, the progression of atherosclerosis is self-perpetuating (Fig. 18–1).

The three sites most often affected by atherosclerosis are the legs (peripheral vascular disease and increased risk of gangrene), the brain (cerebral vascular accident [CVA]), and the coronary arteries (CHD). Although angina may be a symptom of blocked coronary arteries, most people are asymptomatic until three-fourths of a coronary artery is occluded.

COMPLICATIONS

In rare instances, plaques grow to fully occlude an artery. An aneurysm is another potential complication arising from increased pressure that causes the artery to weaken and balloon. A ruptured aneurysm in a major artery can lead to massive bleeding and death. The most likely complication from atherosclerosis is clot formation. Platelets interpret plaque formation as an injury and respond in normal fashion by stimulating clot formation. Once they have been formed, clots may enlarge and remain stationary (thrombus) until they completely block off the blood supply to tissues fed by that artery (thrombosis).

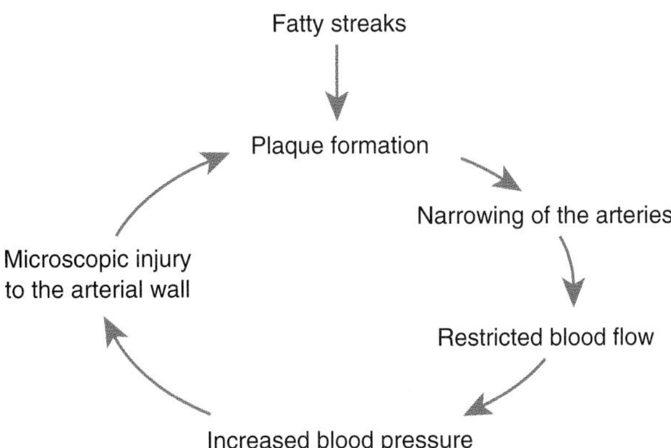

FIGURE 18-1 Perpetuating progression of atherosclerosis.

Slow tissue death occurs, and scar tissue forms. Thrombosis can occur in coronary arteries (coronary thrombosis) or in arteries that nourish the brain (cerebral thrombosis). A clot can break off from the thrombus (embolus) and travel until it gets stuck in a narrowed artery (embolism). The surrounding tissue is then deprived of oxygen and suddenly dies. This can lead to the death of heart tissue (heart attack) or brain tissue (stroke).

RISK FACTORS

CHD is a multifactorial disease. Most risk factors are modifiable, some are not. Risk factors can be grouped according to how certain it is that their management will reduce the risk of CHD. With the exception of smoking and exercise, all the selected risk factors presented here have nutritional implications.

Category I Risk Factors

Management of these risk factors has been *proven* to reduce the risk of heart disease.

Cigarette Smoking

Compelling evidence shows that cigarette smoking increases the risk of CHD. Smoking promotes endothelial damage, increases heart rate, increases blood pressure, lowers HDLC, and promotes thrombus formation. The risk of CHD improves with smoking cessation.

High-Saturated-Fat, High-Cholesterol Diet

It is well documented that saturated fats raise serum cholesterol, particularly LDLC, the "bad" type of cholesterol. In fact, reducing saturated fat and cholesterol intake is the foundation of nutrition therapy for the prevention and treatment of CHD. Yet, as a review of the remaining risk factors shows, the complex process of CHD is more than simply the result of excess serum cholesterol. The belief that a high-fat diet leads to a high serum cholesterol level, which in turn leads to CHD, is an oversimplified but frequently held view. Opponents to this hypothesis raise several thought-provoking questions:

- Why is it that people who eat high-fat diets do not always have elevated cholesterol levels?
- Why do many people with low or normal serum cholesterol levels have CHD, but most of those with increased serum cholesterol levels do not have CHD?
- Why does death from cardiovascular disease occur in people with minimal atherosclerosis?
- Conversely, why do so many people with extensive atherosclerosis exhibit no apparent clinical problems?

These questions underscore the fact that, although much has been learned about CHD, much has yet to be determined. Restricting saturated fat and cholesterol intake is prudent for almost all Americans older than 2 years of age, but it is not the only dietary intervention likely to reduce the risk of CHD. Other components of nutrition therapy help reduce CHD risk by different mechanisms, such as reducing the oxidation of LDL-C, decreasing the propensity of blood to clot, and altering platelet aggregation. Some of the other dietary substances that affect risk include omega-3 fatty acids, soluble fibers, folic acid, and antioxidant vitamins.

Elevated Total Cholesterol

Total serum cholesterol is a measure of all cholesterol: HDL-C + LDL-C + very-low-density lipoprotein (VLDL) cholesterol (VLDL-C). It is influenced by many variables, including genetics, diet, various diseases, activity, certain drugs, and age. High levels of total cholesterol are associated with an increased risk of CHD. Desirable, borderline, and high levels of total cholesterol and LDL-C are listed in Table 18–1.

Because it is widely available and relatively inexpensive, the total cholesterol measurement is commonly used as a screening tool to estimate a person's risk of CHD. It is closely correlated with the concentration of LDL-C, because LDL-C constitutes the largest percentage of total cholesterol. Total cholesterol is composed of approximately:

- 20% to 30% HDL-C, the "good" cholesterol that acts as a scavenger to take cholesterol out of the serum and transport it to the liver, where it is either recycled or excreted in the bile. The HDL value is inversely related to CHD risk.
- 10% to 15% VLDL-C, which is a precursor of LDL. VLDLs are composed mostly of triglycerides. VLDL remnants appear to be atherogenic.
- 60% to 70% LDL-C, the "bad" cholesterol that transports cholesterol out of the liver to the cells.

However, the total cholesterol measurement does not reveal the amount of "good" and "bad" cholesterol contributing to the total cholesterol number. Because the level of LDL-C more accurately reflects CHD risk than does total cholesterol, anyone who meets any of the following criteria should have a lipoprotein analysis done to determine their LDL-C:

- A total cholesterol level greater than 240 mg/dL

TABLE 18.1 ***Classification of Total Serum Cholesterol and Low-Density Lipoprotein Cholesterol***

Classification	Total Serum Cholesterol	LDLC
Desirable	<200 mg/dL	<130 mg/dL
Borderline—high risk	200–239 mg/dL	130–159 mg/dL
High	≥240 mg/dL	≥160 mg/dL

Public Health Service, United States Department of Health and Human Services, National Institutes of Health: National Cholesterol Education Program. (1993). *Second report of the expert panel on detection, evaluation, and treatment of high blood cholesterol in adults*. (NIH Publication No. 93-3095). Washington, DC: Government Printing Office.

- A total cholesterol level of 200 to 239 mg/dL with two or more other risk factors for CHD
- An HDL-C level of 35 mg/dL or less

Elevated Low-Density Lipoprotein Cholesterol

Comprehensive data show that LDL-C is associated with the development of atherosclerosis. Conversely, lowering total cholesterol and LDL-C reduces CHD risk, and it may even help prevent recurrent myocardial infarction and death in people who have already had a heart attack. High levels of LDL-C are related to obesity and excessive intakes of saturated fat, total fat, and cholesterol. LDL-C is reduced by losing weight if overweight, modifying the type and amount of fat consumed, and increasing soluble fiber intake.

Hypertension

Hypertension is an independent risk factor for heart disease and stroke. Conversely, normalizing blood pressure reduces mortality and morbidity. Nutrition therapy is the cornerstone of the nonpharmacologic approach to managing hypertension.

Category II Risk Factors

Management of these risk factors is *likely* to reduce the risk of heart disease.

Diabetes

Diabetes clearly increases the risk of CHD. Diabetics, especially type 2 diabetics, characteristically have metabolic abnormalities associated with increased CHD risk, such as high triglycerides, low HDL-C, small LDL particles, hypertension, and upper body obesity.

Physical Inactivity

Regular aerobic exercise reduces the risk of CHD by lowering blood pressure, lowering triglyceride levels, increasing HDL-C, promoting weight management, and improving insulin sensitivity. Exercise may also decrease platelet aggregation and promote electrical stability in the heart.

Low High-Density Lipoprotein Cholesterol

A low level of HDL-C and an increased ratio of total (or LDL-C) to HDL-C is an independent risk factor for CHD. Low HDL-C levels are associated with cigarette smoking, obesity, and postmenopausal status. Exercise, smoking cessation, weight loss if overweight, and moderate alcohol consumption increase HDL-C levels.

Obesity

Obesity is associated with hypertension, physical inactivity, glucose intolerance, low HDL-C, and increased triglycerides. Even though it is not certain that reducing body fat decreases coronary events, losing excess body weight improves blood pressure, blood lipid profiles, insulin sensitivity, and other CHD risk factors.

Category III Risk Factors

Management of these risk factors *may* reduce the risk of heart disease.

Elevated Triglycerides

When considered alone, elevated triglycerides appear to increase the risk of CHD. However, after adjustment for other risk factors, especially HDL-C, the significance of high triglyceride levels becomes less clear. It may be that high triglyceride levels are not responsible for an increased risk but rather are a marker for other metabolic abnormalities that do increase risk. For instance, high triglycerides are associated with obesity, diabetes, hypertension, low HDL-C, and small, dense LDL particles. Triglyceride levels decline with weight loss, increased physical activity, and reduced alcohol intake.

Elevated Homocysteine

A high blood level of the amino acid homocysteine has been identified as an independent risk factor for CHD, cerebrovascular disease, peripheral vascular disease, and venous thromboembolism. Although the process by which high homocysteine levels cause atherosclerosis is not completely known, an increase in smooth muscle cell growth, arterial damage, and an increased propensity for clot formation are among the suspected mechanisms. High homocysteine levels can occur from a deficiency of folic acid, vitamin B_{12}, and/or vitamin B_6, but a deficiency of folic acid is more likely to cause increased homocysteine levels than deficiencies of the other two vitamins. Researchers speculate that some people have high homocysteine levels because they are born with an inefficient form of an enzyme that normally enables folic acid to interact with homocysteine. Other potential causes of high homocysteine include chronic renal failure, hypothyroidism, and malignancies.

The optimal doses of folic acid may be within the range of 650 to 1000 μg/day. The average American intake of folic acid is approximately 200 μg/day. Rich sources of folic acid are fortified breads and cereals, leafy green vegetables, organ meats, milk, eggs, wheat germ, and dried peas and beans. Even though it is not yet proven that reducing elevated homocysteine levels reduces the risk of atherosclerosis, it is prudent and safe for American adults to increase their intake of folate-rich foods and to consider taking a daily multivitamin containing 400 μg of folic acid.

Oxidation and Antioxidants

Many studies indicate that vitamin E, as well as other antioxidants, make LDL-C resistant to oxidation. By preventing the oxidation of LDL-C, vitamin E may play a key role in the prevention of cardiovascular disease. Another benefit of large doses of vitamin E (200–400 IU) is that platelets are less likely to adhere to arterial walls. Studies show that among supplement users, the greatest reduction in CHD risk occurs at daily intakes of 100 IU to 249 IU for more than 2 years. The National Cholesterol Education Program (NCEP) claims that there is not enough evidence to recommend that people take vitamin E supplements, but it is impossible to get 100 IU of vitamin E through food alone.

Until all the results are in, it may be prudent, safe, inexpensive, easy, and effective to take 100 IU of vitamin E daily. The only potential drawback is that large doses of vitamin E (>400 IU/day) may increase the risk of hemorrhagic stroke.

Alcohol Intake

Moderate alcohol consumption (one to two drinks per day) is associated with a reduced risk of CHD, possibly because it raises HDL-C and reduces platelet aggregation. However, studies show an increased risk of breast cancer among women who consume one alcoholic drink daily. Heavier alcohol consumption increases the risk of alcoholic liver disease, hypertension, and accidental death. In some people, alcohol raises triglyceride levels. Because of the potential risks of using alcohol, many health professionals are reluctant to encourage people who do not drink to do so as a means of reducing their risk of CHD.

Category IV Risk Factors

These risk factors are not amenable to change: advancing age, male gender, and family history of premature heart disease.

ASSESSMENT OF ATHEROSCLEROSIS AND CORONARY HEART DISEASE

Before the optimal nutrition therapy can be planned, a nutrition-focused assessment is indicated.

Historical Data

- Does the patient's body mass index (BMI) indicate that the patient is obese? Is the patient's weight stable?
- What is the patient's blood pressure?
- Is the patient's usual intake adequate? Is the food budget adequate?
- Is the patient following a special diet?
- Does the patient use low-fat or low-sodium products?
- Does the patient read food labels?
- Does the patient shop for and cook food?
- Does the patient frequently eat out?
- What cultural, religious, or ethnic influences affect the patient's food choices?
- Is the patient willing to change his or her eating habits?
- Can the patient identify foods he or she is not willing to give up?
- Does the patient have food allergies or intolerances?
- Does the patient use alcohol or caffeine?
- Does the patient use tobacco or recreational drugs?
- What nutritional supplements does the patient use and for what purpose (Box 18–1)?

- What is the patient's understanding about the relationship between diet and heart disease?
- Does the patient have medical conditions that benefit from nutrition therapy, such as diabetes and hypertension?

BOX 18.1

Nutritional Supplements Used to Prevent or Treat Cardiovascular Problems

Green tea extract: A high intake of green tea (>10 cups/day) is significantly associated with lower levels of LDL-C and triglycerides and an increase in HDL-C. Green tea also contains antioxidants that may help prevent the oxidation of LDL-C. Even though it has not been proven that green tea effectively helps prevent atherosclerosis, it is safe to use and has the potential to be beneficial. Green tea extract capsules that are standardized are purported to be equivalent to 4 cups of green tea.

Red yeast: The dietary supplement Cholestin is made from red yeast and rice. Its active ingredient is lovastatin, the same active ingredient found in the drug Mevacor. Like Mevacor, red yeast interferes with the liver's ability to synthesize cholesterol. It produces the same therapeutic benefits as lovastatin and also the same side effects, namely gastritis, abdominal discomfort, and increased liver enzyme levels. People who use red yeast are actually self-medicating, a potentially dangerous practice that may circumvent physician-supervised treatment based on the patient's overall CHD risk and actual lipid profile.

Soluble fiber: Fiber supplements may significantly reduce LDL-C in people with hypercholesterolemia, depending on the type of fiber contained in the supplement. One such supplement is Metamucil, the over-the-counter product approved for sale only as a laxative. Six studies have demonstrated that about 3 tsp of regular flavor Metamucil taken daily for 1.5 to 4 mo lowers LDL-C by 6% to 26% in people with an average initial total cholesterol of 250 mg/dL. As with any source of fiber, an adequate fluid intake is essential. A potential drawback is that some people are allergic to psyllium, the fiber in Metamucil. Possible symptoms of psyllium allergy include wheezing, chest tightness, rashes, and, in rare instances, anaphylactic shock.

Chromium: Although chromium supplements are advertised to help reduce cholesterol levels, studies have failed to show any beneficial effects.

Hawthorn: An extract of the dried leaves and blossoms of hawthorn is widely used in Europe to treat CHF in its early stages. It reportedly improves the pumping capacity of the heart and reduces susceptibility to cardiac angina by reducing vascular resistance peripherally and in the heart. Hawthorn has a very low incidence of side effects and is considered safe. Even though hawthorn has potential as an important drug for patients with mild CHF, self-treatment of heart disorders is not recommended.

- What over-the-counter or prescribed medications does the patient take?
- Does the patient have a "type A" (easily excitable) personality or admit to a stressful lifestyle?
- Is there a family history of premature heart disease?
- Does the patient exercise regularly? If so, how frequently and at what intensity?

Physical Findings

- Assess for ascites or edema.
- Assess for xanthomas.
- Determine whether the patient has an "apple" (excess weight around waist or upper body) or a "pear" (excess weight around hips and thighs) shape.

Laboratory Data

- Obtain the patient's total cholesterol, LDL-C, and HDL-C values.
- Note abnormal triglycerides.
- Note an elevated blood glucose concentration.
- Note any other abnormal laboratory values.

PREVENTION AND TREATMENT OF ATHEROSCLEROSIS

Correcting abnormal blood lipid levels (*dyslipidemia*) is the primary goal of strategies aimed at preventing and treating atherosclerosis. The five general categories of dyslipidemias differ in the types of lipoproteins that are abnormal (Table 18–2). However, the nonpharmacologic interventions recommended for all types of dyslipidemias are remarkably similar. Smoking cessation and an increase in physical activity are the non-nutritional strategies. The nutrition interventions are presented below.

Step One and Step Two Diets

Although the term "diet" is used to describe the nutritional recommendations put forth by the NCEP to treat high blood cholesterol levels, diet really is a misnomer. What is needed are lifestyle modifications that include changes in eating habits, not a "diet" with short-term and restrictive implications. Changes in eating habits are more likely to be long-lasting when the changes are individualized and occur gradually and sequentially over time.

The **Step One diet** is consistent with the dietary recommendations for the general public suggested in the *Dietary Guidelines for Americans* and by the American Heart Association to reduce the risk of chronic diseases. It is also the initial therapy for people with high blood cholesterol levels who have not already changed their eating habits. Many people can comply with this diet by making only moderate changes in their dietary habits. If the goals of the Step One diet are not accomplished after 3 months of good

TABLE 18.2 ***Dyslipidemias***

Lipid Abnormality	Clinical Management
Elevated LDL-C (most common lipid abnormality)	Lifestyle modifications including Step One and Step Two diets, weight loss (if overweight), regular physical activity, and increased intake of soluble fiber Hydroxymethylglutaryl Coenzyme A (HMG-CoA) reductase inhibitors (the most commonly used class of drug) Hormone replacement therapy (an option for postmenopausal women)
Elevated VLDL-C and triglycerides	Control of contributing factors, including obesity, poorly controlled diabetes, excessive alcohol intake, and inactivity Omega-3 fatty acids to lower triglycerides Gemfibrozil (the drug of choice to lower triglycerides); niacin
Low HDL-C (with or without elevated triglycerides)	Weight loss and increased physical activity to increase HDL-C (most effective when triglycerides are elevated) Strategies to lower LDL-C (to improve the ratio of LDL-C to HDL-C) Gemfibrozil or niacin to raise HDL-C or improve the ratio of LDL-C to HDL-C
Combined dyslipidemias (high LDL-C, low HDL-C, high triglycerides)	Lifestyle modifications as listed for elevated LDL-C (initial intervention) Combinations of drugs to lower LDL-C and triglycerides and to increase HDL-C
Chylomicronemia (chylomicra and hypertriglyceridemia in fasting state)	Low- to very-low-fat diet; cholesterol restriction Control of contributing factors, including obesity, poorly controlled diabetes, excessive alcohol intake, and inactivity Omega-3 fatty acids Drug therapies, including gemfibrozil, niacin, and progestins (for women)

compliance, the person may need to progress to the **Step Two diet,** which more severely limits saturated fat and cholesterol. Examples of foods to include and avoid for both the Step One and Step Two diets appear in Table 18–3. Sample menus for the Step One and Step Two diets are provided in Box 18–2.

Typically, LDL-C is reduced 3% to 10% by the Step One diet and 5% to 15% by the Step Two diet in free-living subjects. Similar results for total cholesterol and LDL-C have been reported for large intervention trials. For every 1% drop in serum cholesterol, the risk of CHD decreases by 2%. Although dietary changes can lower serum cholesterol levels, dietary changes are not guaranteed to prevent atherosclerosis. Despite the uncertainty, most experts agree that the majority of Americans older than 2 years of age have the potential to benefit from a low-fat, low-saturated-fat, low-cholesterol diet with

TABLE 18.3 *Examples of Foods to Choose or Decrease for the Step One and Step Two Diets**

Food Group	Choose	Decrease
Lean Meat, Poultry, and Fish ≤5–6 oz/day	Beef, pork, lamb—lean cuts well trimmed before cooking	Beef, pork, lamb—regular ground beef, fatty cuts, spareribs, organ meats
	Poultry without skin	Poultry with skin, fried chicken
	Fish, shellfish	Fried fish, fried shellfish
	Processed meat—prepared from lean meat (eg, lean ham, lean frankfurters, lean meat with soy protein or carrageenan)	Regular luncheon meat (eg, bologna, salami, sausage, frankfurters)
Eggs ≤4 yolks per week, Step One ≤2 yolks per week, Step Two	Egg whites (two whites may be substituted for one whole egg in recipes), cholesterol-free egg substitute	Egg yolks (if >4/wk on Step One or if >2/wk on Step Two); includes eggs used in cooking and baking
Low-Fat Dairy Products 2–3 servings per day	Milk—skim or 1% fat (fluid, powdered, evaporated) buttermilk	Whole milk (fluid, evaporated, condensed), 2%-fat milk (low-fat milk), imitation milk
	Yogurt—nonfat or low-fat yogurt or yogurt beverages	Whole-milk yogurt, whole-milk yogurt beverages
	Cheese—low-fat natural or processed cheese	Regular cheeses (American, blue, Brie, cheddar, Colby, Edam, Monterey Jack, whole-milk mozzarella, Parmesan, Swiss), cream cheese, Neufchatel cheese
	Low-fat or nonfat varieties (eg, cottage cheese—low-fat, nonfat, or dry curd with 0 to 2% fat)	Cottage cheese (4% fat)
	Frozen dairy dessert—ice milk, frozen yogurt (low fat or nonfat)	Ice cream
	Low-fat coffee creamer Low-fat or nonfat sour cream	Cream, half & half, whipping cream, nondairy creamer, whipped topping, sour cream
Fats and Oils ≤6–8 tsp/day	Unsaturated oils—safflower, sunflower, corn, soybean, cottonseed, canola, olive, peanut	Coconut oil, palm kernel oil, palm oil
	Margarine—made from unsaturated oils listed above, light or diet margarine, especially soft or liquid forms	Butter, lard, shortening, bacon fat, hard margarine
	Salad dressings—made with unsaturated oils listed above, low fat or fat free	Dressings made with egg yolk, cheese, sour cream, whole milk
	Seeds and nuts—peanut butter, other nut butters	Coconut
	Cocoa powder	Milk chocolate
Breads and Cereals ≥6 servings per day	Breads—whole-grain bread, English muffins, bagels, buns, corn or flour tortillas	Bread in which eggs, fat, or butter is a major ingredient; croissants

(continued)

TABLE 18.3 ***Examples of Foods to Choose or Decrease for the Step One and Step Two Diets* (continued)***

Food Group	Choose	Decrease
	Cereals—oat, wheat, corn, multigrain	Most granolas
	Pasta	
	Rice	
	Dry beans and peas	
	Crackers, low-fat—animal-type, graham, soda crackers, bread sticks, melba toast	High-fat crackers
	Homemade baked goods using unsaturated oil, skim or 1% milk, and egg substitute—quick breads, biscuits, corn bread muffins, bran muffins, pancakes, waffles	Commercial baked pastries, muffins, biscuits
Soups	Reduced- or low-fat reduced-sodium varieties (eg, chicken or beef noodle, minestrone, tomato, vegetable, potato, reduced-fat soups made with skim milk)	Soup containing whole milk, cream, meat, fat, poultry fat, or poultry skin
Vegetables 3–5 servings per day	Fresh, frozen, or canned, without added fat or sauce	Vegetables fried or prepared with butter, cheese, or cream sauce
Fruits 2–4 servings per day	Fruit—fresh, frozen, canned, or dried Fruit juice—fresh, frozen, or canned	Fried fruit or fruit served with butter or cream sauce
Sweets and Modified Fat Desserts	Beverages—fruit-flavored drinks, lemonade, fruit punch	
	Sweets—sugar, syrup, honey, jam, preserves, candy made without fat (candy corn, gumdrops, hard candy), fruit-flavored gelatin	Candy made with milk chocolate, coconut oil, palm kernel oil, palm oil
	Frozen desserts—low-fat and nonfat yogurt, ice milk, sherbet, sorbet, fruit ice, Popsicles	Ice cream and frozen treats made with ice cream
	Cookies, cake, pie, pudding—prepared with egg whites, egg substitute, skim milk or 1% milk, and unsaturated oil or margarine; gingersnaps; fig and other fruit bar cookies, fat-free cookies; angel food cake	Commercial baked pies, cakes, doughnuts, high-fat cookies, cream pies

*Careful selection of processed foods is necessary to stay within the sodium <2400 mg guideline.

Public Health Service, United States Department of Health and Human Services, National Institutes of Health. (1993). *National Cholesterol education program: Second report of the expert panel on detection, evaluation, and treatment of high blood cholesterol in adults*, (NIH Publication No. 93-3095). Washington, DC: Government Printing Office.

BOX 18.2

Step One and Step Two Diet Menus (Traditional American Cuisine: Males 25–49 Years of Age)

Step One Sample Menus

Breakfast

Bagel, plain (1 medium)
  Cream Cheese, low fat (2 tsp)
Cereal, shredded wheat (1½ cups)
Banana (1 small)
Milk, **1%** (1 cup)
Orange juice (¾ cup)
Coffee (1 cup)
  Milk, **1%** (1 oz)

Lunch

Minestrone soup, canned, low sodium (1 cup)
Roast beef sandwich
  Whole wheat bread (2 slices)
  *Lean roast beef, unseasoned (**3 oz**)
  American cheese, low-fat and low sodium (¾ oz)
  Lettuce (1 leaf)
  Tomato (3 slices)
  Mayonnaise, low fat and low sodium (2 tsp)
Fruit and cottage cheese salad
  Cottage cheese, **2%** and low sodium (½ cup)
  Peaches, canned in juice (½ cup)
Apple juice, unsweetened (1 cup)

Dinner

***Salmon** (3 oz)
  Vegetable oil (1 tsp)
Baked potato (1 medium)
  Margarine (2 tsp)
*Green beans (½ cup), seasoned with margarine (½ tsp)

Step Two Sample Menus

Breakfast

Bagel, plain (1 medium)
  Margarine (2 tsp)
  Jelly (2 tsp)
Cereal, shredded wheat (1½ cups)
Banana (1 small)
Milk, **skim** (1 cup)
Orange juice (¾ cup)
Coffee (1 cup)
  Milk **skim** (1 oz)

Lunch

Minestrone soup, canned, low sodium (1½ cups)
Roast beef sandwich
  Whole wheat bread (2 slices)
  *Lean roast beef, unseasoned (**2 oz**)
  American cheese, low-fat and low sodium (¾ oz)
  Lettuce (1 leaf)
  Tomato (3 slices)
  Margarine (2 tsp)
Fruit and cottage cheese salad
  Cottage cheese, **1%** and low sodium (½ cup)
  Peaches, canned in juice (½ cup)
Apple juice, unsweetened (1 cup)

Dinner

***Flounder** (3 oz)
  Vegetable oil (1 tsp)
*Baked potato (1 medium)
  Margarine (2 tsp)
Green beans (½ cup), seasoned with margarine (½ tsp)

(continued)

BOX 18.2

Step One and Step Two Diet Menus (Traditional American Cuisine: Males 25-49 Years of Age) (continued)

Step One		Step Two	
*Carrots (½ cup), seasoned with margarine (½ tsp)		Carrots (½ cup), seasoned with margarine (½ tsp)	
White dinner rolls (1 medium)		White dinner roll (1 medium)	
Margarine (1 tsp)		Margarine (1 tsp)	
Ice milk (1 cup)		**Frozen yogurt** (1 cup)	
Iced tea, unsweetened (1 cup)		Iced tea, unsweetened (1 cup)	
Snack		**Snack**	
Popcorn (3 cups)		*Popcorn (3 cups)	
Margarine (1 T)		Margarine (1 T)	
Analysis		**Analysis**	
Calories	2518	Calories	2533
Total fat, % kcals:	29	Total fat, % kcals:	28
Saturated fatty acids, % kcals:	8.6	Saturated fatty acids, % kcals:	6.6
Cholesterol, mg:	181	Cholesterol, mg:	150
Protein, % kcals:	18	Protein, % kcals:	17
Total carbohydrate, % kcals:	53	Total carbohydrate, % kcals:	55
Simple carbohydrate, % carbohydrate:	36	Simple carbohydrate, % carbohydrate:	36
Complex carbohydrate, % carbohydrate:	64	Complex carbohydrate, % carbohydrate:	64
*Sodium, mg:	1821	*Sodium, mg:	1803
100% RDA met for all nutrients except: Zinc 90%		100% RDA met for all nutrients except: Zinc 90%	

Boldface food items represent differences between the Step One and Step Two Diets. See companion menu.

*No salt is added in recipe preparation or as seasoning. All margarine is low sodium.

calorie intake appropriate for "healthy" weight. Possible exceptions include high-risk elderly people and pregnant women.

The characteristics of the Step One and Step Two diets appear in Table 18–4. Although these diets refer to "percentage of total calories" and "milligrams" of cholesterol, such terms are meaningless to the general public. Overall, emphasizing portion sizes, portions per day, and specific eating strategies is much more effective and less intimidating than discussing specific nutrient and caloric composition of the diet.

Total Fat

Total fat intake is limited to 30% or less of total calories on both the Step One and Step Two diets. A high fat intake increases blood cholesterol levels and increases the risk of

TABLE 18.4 *Characteristics of the NCEP Step One and Step Two Diets*

Nutrient	Step One Diet	Step Two Diet
Total fat (% of calories)	≤30	≤30
Saturated fat	8–10	<7
Polyunsaturated fat	≤10	≤10
Monounsaturated fat	≤15	≤15
Carbohydrate (% of calories)	55	55
Protein (% of calories)	~15	~15
Cholesterol (mg/d)	<300	<200
Total calories	For desirable weight	For desirable weight

obesity. High-fat diets, regardless of the type of fat they contain, may also promote the formation of blood clots. Currently, the average American consumes 34% of total calories from fat. It is estimated that less than 20% of the population meets the recommendations for total fat and saturated fat intake. Most people know that fat is found in meat, butter, oil, and fried foods, but they may be unaware of "hidden" fat in pies, cakes, cookies, cheese, salty snacks, and nuts.

Some experts recommend that fat intake be more severely limited so that greater improvements in cholesterol levels and weight can be achieved. For instance, Dean Ornish's program limits fat to 10% of total calories, and the Pritikin program is designed with fewer than 10% of total calories from fat. When the amount of fat in the diet is reduced and no other changes in intake are made, weight loss is promoted. However, when fat is drastically reduced or when carbohydrate calories replace the decrease in fat calories, the result may be an undesirable decrease in HDL-C. This outcome may be particularly problematic for diabetics. For them, a fat intake greater than 30% of total calories that comes from a higher intake of monounsaturated fats may be more desirable; an example is the Mediterranean Diet, which is credited with the low rate of chronic disease and increased longevity seen in people living in the Mediterranean area (Box 18–3).

Saturated Fat

Saturated fat intake is limited on both the Step One and Step Two diets. Saturated fat is the dietary component most consistently linked to high LDL-C levels. It is limited to 8% to 10% of total calories on the Step One diet and to less than 7% of total calories on the Step Two diet. Currently the average American consumes 12% of calories from saturated fat.

The majority of saturated fat in the typical American diet comes from animal fats, such as meats, cheese, egg yolks, ice cream, cream, whole and 2% milk, butter, lard, suet, salt pork, and bacon drippings. Coconut oil, palm oil, and palm kernel oil are high in saturated fat, but their overall contribution to the diet is relatively small.

To reduce saturated fat intake, lean cuts of meat are emphasized and visible fat is removed. Skinless chicken and fish are frequently used in place of red meats, and occasional meatless meals are recommended. Egg yolks are limited to four or fewer per week,

BOX 18.3

The Mediterranean Diet

The traditional Mediterranean Diet is associated with low rates of chronic disease and a high adult life expectancy. This diet may be most beneficial for people who have high triglycerides, low HDL-C, or type 2 diabetes and for those who find it difficult to follow a low-fat diet.

Mediterranean Diet characteristics:

- This is a plant-based diet that relies heavily on fruit, vegetables, grains, beans, nuts, and seeds.
- An emphasis is placed on minimally processed foods.
- Olive oil is the principal fat; it is used in place of, not in addition to, other fats and oils, such as butter and margarine.
- 35% or less of calories are from fat; saturated fat is limited to 7–8% of total calories.
- Dairy products, fish, and poultry are eaten in low to moderate amounts.
- Red meat is used sparingly (eg, 12–16 oz/mo); 0–4 eggs are eaten weekly.
- Low to moderate amounts of red wine are consumed daily, with meals.
- Regular physical activity promotes healthy weight and fitness.

and organ meats are used sparingly. Reduced-fat or fat-free cheese, ice cream, dressings, and spreads are used in place of full-fat varieties.

Polyunsaturated Fats

Polyunsaturated fats should contribute up to 10% of total calories on the Step One and Step Two diets. Polyunsaturated fats (corn, sunflower, safflower, and soybean oil) currently provide about 7% of total calories in the average American diet, which is an acceptable level. When used in place of saturated fats, polyunsaturated fats tend to lower blood levels of both LDL-C (a positive outcome) and HDL-C (a negative outcome). In addition, there are concerns about the long-term safety of a diet high in polyunsaturated fats. Therefore is it recommended that the polyunsaturated fat intake remain at its current level, and that intake not exceed 10% of total calories.

Trans-fatty acids are created during the process of hydrogenation, in which a vegetable oil is converted to a more solid (more saturated) fat through the addition of hydrogen molecules. The prefix "*trans*" refers to the type of configuration around the fatty acid's double bond (Fig. 18–2). Although small quantities of *trans*-fatty acids occur naturally in meat and dairy products, the majority of *trans*-fats in the typical American diet come from partially hydrogenated fats and foods containing those fats. *Trans*-fats are unsaturated (they contain double bonds), but they act like saturated fats in the body, raising LDL-C and possibly lowering HDL-C. The *trans*-fat content of commercially prepared baked goods and fried foods varies among brands. *Trans*-fat content is currently not specified on the food label, but proposed changes in labeling regulations that will require

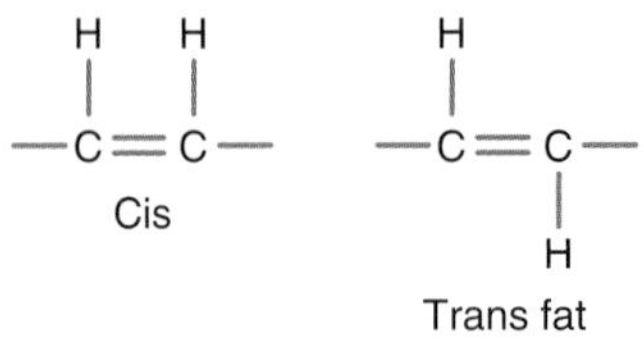

FIGURE 18-2 Structure of a *trans*-fatty acid.

their disclosure, are being considered. In the meantime, consumers can reduce *trans*-fat intake by choosing soft margarine in place of firm margarine whenever possible.

Monounsaturated Fats

Monounsaturated fats contribute up to 15% of total calories on the Step One and Step Two diets. Monounsaturated fats, including those predominant in olive oil, canola oil, peanut oil, nuts, seeds, and avocado, tend to lower LDL-C when they replace saturated fat in the diet. At high intakes, monounsaturated fats decrease LDL-C and increase HDL-C. This benefit occurs only with higher total fat and high monounsaturated fat intakes (Box 18-3).

Currently, Americans consume 14% to 16% of their total calories from monounsaturated fats. However, much of it is contained in foods containing animal fats, which are also high in saturated fats. A decrease in animal fat intake means that a larger proportion of monounsaturated fats can come from olive oil, canola oil, and peanut oil. Although these oils are low in saturated fat, they are still calorically dense and can cause weight gain if used in excess.

Carbohydrates

Carbohydrates should contribute 55% or more of total calories on the Step One and Step Two diets. A liberal intake of complex carbohydrates is recommended because they are generally low in fat and because whole-grain choices are rich in fiber, vitamins, minerals, and phytochemicals.

Protein

Protein should contribute approximately 15% of total calories on the Step One and Step Two diets. This level is neither restricted nor elevated. Low-saturated-fat sources of protein are recommended, such as lean meats, poultry, fish, egg whites, skim milk, and dried peas and beans.

Cholesterol

Cholesterol is limited on the Step One and Step Two diets. Dietary cholesterol is restricted because it enhances the serum cholesterol–raising effect of saturated fat. Cholesterol is limited to less than 300 mg/day on the Step One diet and to less than 200 mg/day on the Step Two diet. Cholesterol is produced by the body, so dietary intake is not essential. Cholesterol is found only in animal products. It is found in both muscle and fat, so removing the fat from meat does not fully remove the cholesterol. Also, low-fat animal products are not necessarily low in cholesterol (eg, shrimp). The richest sources of cholesterol are organ meats and egg yolks. Fruits, vegetables, grains, cereals, nuts, legumes, and egg whites are cholesterol free.

Calories

On the Step One and Step Two diets, calories to achieve and maintain desirable weight are determined on an individual basis according to the person's body weight and activity patterns.

Loss of Excess Weight

In overweight people, weight loss lowers triglycerides and VLDL-C and raises HDL-C. Changes in LDL-C are usually smaller but favorable. It is estimated that an 11-pound weight loss causes a decrease of approximately 10 mg/dL in total cholesterol, 40% of which is in LDL-C. People with upper body obesity may benefit even more from weight loss.

Increase in Soluble Fiber Intake

High-fiber diets, especially those rich in soluble fiber, lower total cholesterol and LDL-C without lowering HDL-C. On average, adding 6 to 12 g of soluble fiber to a Step One or Step Two diet lowers LDL-C by 5% to 15%. Reductions in LDL-C are even greater when fiber is added to a high-saturated-fat, high-cholesterol diet. Therefore, a high fiber intake may provide a cushion against deteriorating compliance, which often occurs over time.

Excellent sources of soluble fiber include oats and dried peas and beans. To achieve a high fiber intake, the following foods are recommended daily: 3 servings of fruit, 3 servings of vegetables, 6 or more servings of whole-grain products, and 1 serving of dried peas or beans. Ideas for adding fiber to the diet include:

- Eat plant foods in their natural state, such as unpeeled raw vegetables, unpeeled fresh fruit, and unrefined grains (eg, whole-grain breads, whole-grain cereals, whole-grain pasta, brown rice).
- Use pulverized oats or oat bran in cooking and baking, such as in casseroles, as a breading for poultry or fish, in salmon patties, or to thicken sauces.
- Use whole oats in casseroles and quick breads.
- Eat dried peas or beans as a complete or partial meat substitute. Beans can be used in salads, casseroles, and soups or as a side dish.

"FUNCTIONAL FOODS" TO REDUCE THE RISK OF CORONARY HEART DISEASE

Functional foods are defined as nutritious foods with health-promoting properties. The following functional foods may reduce the risk of CHD.

Fish Oils and Fish-Oil Supplements

Omega-3 (n-3) fatty acids, commonly referred to as "fish oils," are most abundant in herring, sardines, Atlantic salmon, bluefish, halibut, sockeye salmon, mackerel, and striped bass. Much smaller amounts are found in green leafy vegetables, nuts, canola oil, flaxseed, soybean oils, and tofu.

In therapeutic doses (3 g or more), n-3 fatty acids lower triglycerides and VLDL-C and usually raise HDL-C. Their effect on LDL-C is variable and may not be favorable. However, n-3 fatty acids may reduce the risk of dying from heart disease by other mechanisms, perhaps by decreasing platelet aggregation, slowing the proliferation of smooth muscle cells in the artery wall, or increasing resistance to cardiac arrhythmia. Although increased consumption of fatty fish is prudent and safe, the use of fish-oil supplements has not been proven effective or safe and is not recommended by the American Medical Association. A sensible recommendation is to eat fish, especially fatty fish, once a week.

Soy Products

The mechanisms by which soy products lower LDL-C when used in place of other proteins are not completely understood. Proposed theories are that soy protein impairs cholesterol absorption or bile acid reabsorption; that it alters cholesterol metabolism; or that its phytoestrogens bind to estrogen receptors and produce effects similar to those of estrogen (namely, a decrease in LDL-C, an increase in HDL-C, and changes in vasomotor tone and arterial wall function).

Sources of soy protein include soymilk, tofu, isolated and textured soy protein supplements, and meat analogues. Although no long-term, large, multicenter clinical studies have investigated the effectiveness and safety of soy protein, it appears that patients with high cholesterol levels benefit from adding low-fat sources of soy protein to their usual intake.

Garlic

Most evidence indicates that garlic probably reduces the risk of CHD. Increased garlic intake is related to decreased LDL-C and triglyceride levels, decreased platelet aggregation, and improved blood pressure. However, studies frequently yield conflicting results owing to lack of consistency in the preparations used (eg, form of garlic used, concentration of active ingredients), in the amount consumed, and in the length of treatment. It is not known how much and what types of garlic are most effective nor what types of patients may benefit most. Until more is known, it is prudent to eat a variety of foods, including those containing garlic. Garlic supplements have no known side effects except for the presence of odor in some people.

PROMOTION OF THE "EATING STYLE" CONCEPT

In theory, nutrition therapy can prevent or reverse atherosclerosis and CHD in most people. In practice, the science of nutrition does not always live up to its expectations. The gap is often blamed on lack of knowledge, social pressures to eat, and the unappetizing taste of healthy foods. Moreover, the "diet" advocated differs from the predominant lifestyle of American culture. Giving clients a "diet" most likely means that they will change their eating habits to match the ideal as closely as possible, follow this plan for as long as they can, "fall off" the diet, and then dismiss it as impractical or unachievable. Clearly, the concept of "diet" must evolve into that of "eating style." A person cannot "fall off" an eating style. An eating style simply reflects where the person is in the evolution of usual intake to healthy intake. The following ideas can help the client move toward a healthier eating style.

Determine How Closely the Patient's Usual Intake Resembles the Step One Diet

There is no absolute way to achieve the nutrition therapy strategies listed in this chapter. For some people, minor changes in intake are sufficient, such as switching from 2% to skim milk or reducing daily meat intake to 5 oz. Some people prefer to implement a vegetarian diet, and others may opt to try the Mediterranean Diet. Instead of making general recommendations that may or may not apply to the individual, it is wise to determine how closely the client's usual intake resembles the Step One diet and then make specific suggestions for change that are relevant for the individual. Figure 18–3 is a dietary assessment questionnaire that can be used to evaluate a client's usual intake according to the Step One and Step Two diet recommendations. Another method is to ask the client:

- What kind, how often, and how much meat do you normally eat?
- How many eggs do you eat weekly?
- What types of fats do you use (eg, butter, solid margarine, soft margarine, vegetable oils)?
- How much fat do you use and on what food items?
- Which method of food preparation do you use most often (eg, baking, roasting, frying, sautéing)?
- How often and in what amounts do you consume convenience foods, fast foods, commercially prepared baked goods, and snack items?
- How many meals do you eat outside of the home each week?
- Do you use fat-reduced or fat-free items, such as margarine, cheese, ice cream, and salad dressings? How often?
- What type of milk do you use?
- What type and how often do you eat high-fiber or whole-grain breads and cereals?
- How many daily servings of fruits and vegetables do you eat?
- How often do you consume dried peas and beans?
- Is your eating pattern to "graze" or to eat fewer than three meals daily?
- Which high-fat foods must you have?

Offer Appropriate Intervention Strategies

In general, people who choose foods consistent with one of the commonly used fat-reduction strategies also make other conscious food choices that result in a more healthful diet. Conversely, people who do not implement specific fat-reduction strategies tend

Name ______________________ Date ____________

MEDFICTS: Dietary Assessment Questionaire
(Meats, Eggs, Dairy, Fried foods, In baked goods, Convenience foods, Table fats, Snacks)

Directions: For each food category for both Group 1 and Group 2 listings: Please check a box in the "Weekly Consumption" column and in the "Serving Size" column. If patient rarely or never eats the food listed, please check only the "Weekly Consumption" box.

FOOD CATEGORY	WEEKLY CONSUMPTION			SERVING SIZE			SCORE
	Rarely/ Never	3 or less serv/wk	4 or more serv/wk	Small	Average	Large	For office use
M Meats • Average amount per day: 6 oz (equal in size to 2 decks of playing cards) • Base your estimate on the food you consume the most of							
Group 1 — **Beef:** Ribs, Steak, Chuck blade, Brisket, Ground beef, Meatloaf, Corned beef; **Processed meats:** Regular hamburger, Fast food hamburger, Bacon, Lunchmeat, Sausage, Hot dogs, Knockwurst; **Pork & others:** Pork shoulder, Pork chops, roast, Pork ribs, Ground pork, Regular ham, Lamb steaks, ribs, chops, Organ meats, Poultry with skin	☐	☐ 3 pts	☐ 7 pts	x ☐ 1 pts	☐ 2 pts	☐ 3 pts	= ____
Group 2 — **Lean Cuts of Beef:** Sirloin tip, Flank steak, Round steak, Rump roast, Chuck arm roast; **Low-fat Processed Meats:** Low-fat lunchmeat, Low-fat hot dogs, Canadian bacon; **Poultry, Fish, Meat:** Poultry without skin, Fish, seafood, Lamb flank, leg-shank, sirloin, roast, Lean ham cured and fresh, Pork loin chops, tenderloin, Veal chops, cutlets, roast, Venison	☐	☐	☐	☐	☐	☐+ 6 pts	= ____
E Eggs • Weekly consumption is expressed as times/week				How many eggs do you eat each time?			
Group 1 — Whole eggs, yolks	☐	☐ 3 pts	☐ 7 pts	x ≤1 1 pts	2 2 pts	≥3 3 pts	= ____
Group 2 — Egg whites, egg substitutes (1/2 cup = 2 eggs)	☐	☐	☐	≤1	2	≥3	
D Dairy							
Milk • Average serving: 1 cup							
Group 1 — Whole milk, 2% milk, 2% buttermilk, yogurt (whole milk)	☐	☐ 3 pts	☐ 7 pts	x ☐ 1 pts	☐ 2 pts	☐ 3 pts	= ____
Group 2 — Skim milk, 1% milk, skim milk-buttermilk, yogurt (nonfat & low-fat)	☐	☐	☐	☐	☐	☐	
Cheese • Average serving: 1 oz.							
Group 1 — Cream cheese, cheddar, Monterey jack, Colby, Swiss, American processed, blue cheese; Regular cottage cheese and ricotta (1/2 cup)	☐	☐ 3 pts	☐ 7 pts	x ☐ 1 pts	☐ 2 pts	☐ 3 pts	= ____
Group 2 — Low-fat & fat-free cheeses, skim-mild mozzarella; String cheese; Low-fat & fat-free cottage cheese, and skim-milk ricotta (1/2 C)	☐	☐	☐	☐	☐	☐	
Frozen Desserts • Average serving: 1/2 cup							
Group 1 — Ice cream, milk shakes	☐	☐ 3 pts	☐ 7 pts	x ☐ 1 pts	☐ 2 pts	☐ 3 pts	= ____
Group 2 — Ice milk, frozen yogurt	☐	☐	☐	☐	☐	☐	

+ Score 6 points if this box is checked

Comments ______________________________________ Total ______

FIGURE 18-3 MEDFICTS: Dietary Assessment Questionnaire. (Source: National Cholesterol Education Program (1993). *Second report of the expert panel on detection, evaluation, and treatment of high blood cholesterol in adults* (Adult Treatment Panel II). Bethesda: USDHHS, Public Health Service, National Institutes of Health, NIH Publication No. 933095.)

FOOD CATEGORY	WEEKLY CONSUMPTION			SERVING SIZE			SCORE
	Rarely/ Never	3 or less serv/wk	4 or more serv/wk	Small	Average	Large	For office use
F Fried Foods • Average serving: see below							
Group 1 French fries, fried vegetables: (1/2 cup) *Fried chicken, fish, and meat: (3 oz.) *check meat category also	☐	☐ 3 pts	☐ 7 pts	x ☐ 1 pts	☐ 2 pts	☐ 3 pts	= ______
Group 2 Vegetables, - not deep fried Meat, poultry, or fish - prepared by baking, broiling, grilling poaching, roasting, stewing	☐	☐	☐	☐	☐	☐	
I In Baked Goods • Average serving: 1 serving							
Group 1 Doughnuts, biscuits, butter rolls, muffins, croissants, sweet rolls, danish, cakes, pies, coffee cakes, cookies	☐	☐ 3 pts	☐ 7 pts	x ☐ 1 pts	☐ 2 pts	☐ 3 pts	= ______
Group 2 Fruit bars, low-fat cookies/cakes/pastries, angel food cake, homemade baked goods with vegetable oils	☐	☐	☐	☐	☐	☐	
C Convenience Foods • Average serving: see below							
Group 1 Canned, packaged, or frozen dinners; e.g., pizza (1 slice), Macaroni & cheese (about 1 cup), pot pie (1), cream soups (1 cup)	☐	☐ 3 pts	☐ 7 pts	x ☐ 1 pts	☐ 2 pts	☐ 3 pts	= ______
Group 2 Diet/reduced calorie or reduced-fat dinners (1 dinner)	☐	☐	☐	☐	☐	☐	
T Table Fats • Average serving: see below							
Group 1 Butter, stick margarine: 1 pat Regular salad dressing or mayonnaise, sour cream: 1-2 Tbsp	☐	☐ 3 pts	☐ 7 pts	x ☐ 1 pts	☐ 2 pts	☐ 3 pts	= ______
Group 2 Diet and tub margarine, low-fat & fat-free salad dressings Low-fat & fat-free mayonnaise	☐	☐	☐	☐	☐	☐	
S Snacks • Average serving: see below							
Group 1 Chips (potato, corn, taco), cheese puffs, snack mix, nuts, Regular crackers, regular popcorn, Candy (milk chocolate, caramel, coconut)	☐	☐ 3 pts	☐ 7 pts	x ☐ 1 pts	☐ 2 pts	☐ 3 pts	= ______
Group 2 Air-popped or low-fat popcorn, low-fat crackers, hard candy, licorice, fruit rolls, bread sticks, pretzels, fat-free chips, fruit	☐	☐	☐	☐	☐	☐	

Directions for scoring:
Multiply weekly consumption points (3 or 7) by serving size points (1, 2, 3) for Group 1 foods only except for a large serving of Group 2 meats

Example: ☐ 3 pts ☑ 7 pts ☐ 1 pts ☐ 2 pts ☑ 3 pts

3 x 7 = 21 points

Add score on page 1 and page 2 to get Final Score

Key
40 - 70 -Step I Diet
less than 40 -Step II Diet

☐ = Foods high in fat, saturated fat, and/or cholesterol

Total ______

Score from page 1 + ______

Final Score ______

Comments ________________________________

(Note frequent use of foods high in fat or saturated fat, e.g. coffee creamer, whipped toping)

FIGURE 18-3 (continued)

to have higher intakes of calories, total fat, saturated fat, and cholesterol and less favorable vitamin and mineral profiles than people who use fat-reduction strategies. The commonly used fat-reduction strategies are to:

- Use skim milk instead of other types of milk.
- Use lean meats in place of high-fat meats.
- Use reduced-fat or nonfat products in place of full-fat products.

Offer interventions strategies that are appropriate for the client's cultural food practices (Box 18–4).

BOX 18.4

Cultural Considerations

For all cultural groups, emphasize the positive aspects of their eating styles and suggest modifications to lower the fat and sodium content of traditional foods.

African-American Tradition

Traditional soul foods tend to be high in fat, cholesterol, and sodium. On the positive side, there is a heavy emphasis on vegetables and complex carbohydrates.

Changes in cooking techniques can improve fat, cholesterol, and sodium content, such as:

- Using nonstick skillets sprayed with cooking spray when pan-frying eggs, fish, and vegetables
- Using small amounts of liquid smoke flavoring in place of bacon, salt pork, or ham
- Using more seasonings, such as onion, garlic, and pepper, in place of some of the salt
- Substituting fat-free mayonnaise for regular mayonnaise in biscuits
- Using turkey ham or turkey sausage in place of bacon
- Using "lite" or sugar-free syrups
- Using egg substitutes or egg whites in pancakes and biscuits

Mexican-American Tradition

The traditional diet is primarily vegetarian, with a heavy emphasis on fruits, vegetables, rice, and dried peas and beans. Processed foods are used infrequently.

Cooking techniques rely on frying and stewing with liberal amounts of oil or lard. High-fat meats and lard are commonly used.

Chinese-American Tradition

Traditional Chinese cooking relies heavily on vegetables and rice, with plants providing the majority of calories. Meat is used more as a condiment than an entree. Cooking techniques tend to preserve nutrients. Sauces add little fat.

(continued)

BOX 18.4

Cultural Considerations (continued)

Sodium intake is high related to heavy use of soy sauce, MSG, and salted pickles.

Native-American/Alaska Native Traditions

Widely diverse eating styles make useful generalizations difficult.

In general:

- Encourage traditional cooking methods, such as baking, roasting, boiling, and broiling.
- Encourage the use of traditional meats, such as fish, deer, and caribou.
- Remove fat from canned meats.
- Use vegetable oil for frying instead of lard or shortening.

Jewish Tradition

Many traditional foods are high in sodium, such as *kosher* meats (salt is used in the koshering process), herring, lox, pickles, canned chicken broth or soups, and delicatessen meats (eg, corned beef, pickled tongue, pastrami).

Pareve (neutral) nondairy creamers are often used as a dairy substitute at meat meals, but they are high in fat. Encourage light and fat-free versions.

Encourage methods to lower fat in traditional recipes, such as:

- Baking instead of frying potato pancakes
- Limiting the amount of schmaltz (chicken fat) used in cooking
- Using reduced-fat or fat-free cream cheese on bagels
- Using low-fat or nonfat cottage cheese, sour cream, and yogurt in kugels and blintzes

Make the Patient an Active Participant

Encourage individual goal setting and self-monitoring. People who record their total intake for one or more days are more aware of eating and food choices. The written account provides an objective tool for identifying areas that need improvement.

Keep the Message Positive

The consumption of fruits and vegetables should be encouraged, not only for their low-fat content, but also because they are rich sources of fiber, vitamins, minerals, and other substances that may eventually be determined to lower CHD risk. Emphasize all the delicious foods the patient should eat, not those he or she should not eat. Take the "Do" approach:

- Do eat up to four egg yolks per week for the Step One diet or up to two per week for the Step Two diet, including those used in food preparation.
- Do eat up to 5 to 6 ounces of meat per day, emphasizing skinless poultry; lean, well-trimmed cuts of beef, pork, and lamb; and fish, shellfish, and processed meats made from lean meat.
- Do use canola, olive, and peanut oils for baking and sautéing.
- Do use soft, liquid, or spray margarine.
- Do choose skim milk and skim-milk products.
- Do fill up on a variety of fruits, vegetables, and whole grains.
- Do enjoy low-fat desserts, such as low-fat and nonfat yogurt, ice milk, sherbet, sorbet, fruit ice, Popsicles, angel food cake, fig bars, gingersnaps, and other low-fat cakes and cookies.

Teach Behavior Skills

Behavioral skills to address include label reading, low-fat cooking techniques, and how to choose a healthy meal when eating out.

Label Reading

Specific definitions of "free," "very low," "low," "reduced," and "less" for fat, saturated fat, cholesterol, and sodium appear in Chapter 8. Basically, the patient needs to know that these descriptions are valid and believable and are useful when comparing different varieties and brands of similar items.

Food Preparation Ideas

Tips for meal planning and cooking are as follows:

- Eat occasional meatless meals.
- Trim fat from meat before cooking; chicken can be cooked with the skin on, but the skin should be removed before eating.
- Use meat more as a condiment than as the main entree. For example, when preparing casseroles, reduce the meat by half and double the complex carbohydrate (rice, potato, pasta).
- Place meats to be baked or roasted on a rack to allow the fat to drain.
- Bake, broil, steam, or sauté foods in vegetable cooking spray or allowed oils.
- Prepare foods from "scratch" instead of purchasing convenience foods and mixes, which tend to be high in saturated fat.
- Use allowed oils to season cooked vegetables and in the preparation of salad dressings, marinades, and barbecue sauces.
- Reduce fat by one half or more in casserole and quick-bread recipes.
- Substitute low-fat items for high-fat items whenever possible. For instance,

In place of . . .	Try:
Whole milk	Skim milk
Light cream	Equal portions of 1% milk and evaporated skim milk
Heavy cream	Equal portions of half-and-half and evaporated skim milk
1 oz baking chocolate	3 tbsp cocoa
Fudge sauce	Chocolate sauce
Whipped cream	Whipped chilled evaporated skim milk or reduced-fat whipped toppings
Sour cream	Low-fat or nonfat sour cream or plain yogurt
Mayonnaise	Reduced-fat or nonfat mayonnaise
Mayonnaise on a sandwich	Fat-free salad dressings (eg, ranch) or mustard, salsa, or fruit chutney
Butter, margarine	one-third less than called for
Oil (in baking)	half oil, half applesauce
1 whole egg	2 egg whites
Regular cheese (ricotta, cream, hard)	Low-fat or nonfat cheeses
Sausage	Ground skinless turkey breast
Bacon, salt pork, or ham	Canadian bacon or 1 tbsp canola oil plus ¼ tsp liquid hickory smoke flavoring

- Make fat-free soup stock by preparing the stock a day ahead and refrigerating it overnight. The fat will harden and can be removed easily from the surface. Also, make fat-free gravies, thickened with cornstarch, by this method.
- Use herbs and spices, lemon juice, and flavored vinegars to flavor foods without fat.
- Use these low-fat snack ideas: low-fat yogurt, fresh fruits and vegetables, dried fruit, unbuttered popcorn, unsalted pretzels, bread sticks, melba toast, frozen juice bars, low-fat crackers.

Tips for Eating Out

Eating out is a growing American cultural trend. It is estimated that on any typical day, half of American adults eat at least one meal outside the home. Meals ordered out tend to be higher in calories, fat, and sodium than home-cooked meals, partly because portion sizes are bigger. Conversely, the fiber and calcium content of restaurant meals is usually less. Adding to the problem is that eating out often gives the diner an excuse to not follow the "diet."

Tips to eat wisely while eating out include:

- **Balance the restaurant meal with better choices the rest of the day.** If the restaurant meal is too large or high in fat, eat less the rest of the day and focus on plant foods.
- **Make wise choices.** Forgo the appetizer, or order two and call it a meal. Split a dessert. Focus on these low-fat choices:
  - Clear broth, vegetable soup, and shrimp cocktail appetizers

- Salad with dressing served "on the side" (dip the fork in the dressing before loading the greens on the fork)
- Meats that are broiled, baked, grilled, or stir-fried
- Sauces and gravies "on the side"
- Vegetables without sauces or breading
- Scrambled egg substitutes
- Burgers with mustard, ketchup, lettuce, tomato, and onions instead of "special sauce"

- **Watch the portion size.** Split a large entree in half, ask for a doggie bag, and enjoy the other half at another meal. Order regular size, not "super" size.
- **Adjust the attitude.** If eating out is an everyday occurrence, the attitude needs to switch from an "excuse to indulge" to an "excuse to not prepare and clean up while maintaining a healthy intake."

Recognize the Value of Ongoing Counseling and Follow-up

Whether one-on-one or group counseling, ongoing contact is necessary to provide nutrition education, teach behavior skills, and promote lifestyle modifications.

PHARMACOLOGIC THERAPIES

People who fail to achieve desired results with nutrition therapy alone are candidates for drug therapy.

Hydroxymethylglutaryl Coenzyme A Reductase Inhibitors

Hydroxymethylglutaryl coenzyme A (HMG-CoA) reductase inhibitors (statins: lovastatin, pravastatin, simvastatin) are the most commonly prescribed drugs to lower cholesterol. They are highly effective at lowering LDLC and are well tolerated. Because they are more effective at lowering LDLC when taken in the evening than in the morning, the U.S. Food and Drug Administration (FDA) recommends that lovastatin be taken with the evening meal, pravastatin at bedtime, and simvastatin in the evening. Side effects are most often gastrointestinal and may include dyspepsia, flatus, constipation, and abdominal pain or cramps.

Bile Acid Sequestrants

Bile acid sequestrants (cholestyramine, colestipol) lower LDLC by reducing bile acid reabsorption. They are powders that must be mixed with water or fruit juice; they are usually taken once or twice a day with meals. Because they are not absorbed from the gastrointestinal tract, they do not produce systemic toxicity. Decreased absorption of the fat-soluble vitamins and folic acid has been reported with prolonged high doses. Gastrointestinal side effects (cramping, constipation, bloating, nausea, and flatulence) may interfere with compliance. A psyllium bulking laxative (eg, Metamucil) may be used to ease gastrointestinal symptoms and enhance the decrease in LDL-C.

Fibric Acid Derivatives

Only one drug in this class, Lopid, has been approved for use in the United States. It is most useful for treating high triglyceride levels, with or without increased LDL-C or low HDL-C levels. Lopid is generally well tolerated.

Niacin

Niacin (nicotinic acid) lowers serum LDL-C and triglyceride levels and raises HDL-C levels. Nicotinamide, which is also frequently referred to as niacin, has no effect on serum lipids and cannot be used as a substitute for nicotinic acid. Nicotinic acid has frequent side effects, including flushing, which may be minimized by gradually increasing the dose, taking the drug with meals, avoiding hot liquids near the dosing time, and taking an aspirin 30 minutes before the drug. Nausea, dyspepsia, flatulence, vomiting, diarrhea, and activation of peptic ulcer may also occur. Liver toxicity and gout occur rarely. High doses of niacin should not be used by diabetics, because niacin can promote insulin resistance and induce or worsen hyperglycemia.

Estrogen and Estrogen-Progestin Replacement

The decrease in circulating estrogen related to menopause is associated with an increase in LDL-C and a decrease in HDL-C. Oral estrogen replacement therapy lowers LDL-C and raises HDL-C and triglycerides. The addition of progestin decreases the risk of estrogen-related uterine cancer but blunts the positive effects on HDL-C. Common side effects include changes in appetite, edema, and diarrhea.

NURSING PROCESS

Mr. Sanders is a 56-year-old man who recently learned during his routine physical that he has high levels of total cholesterol, LDL-C, and triglycerides. His HDL-C is low and his weight is normal. The doctor simply told him to avoid alcohol, exercise, and "watch your diet," but he doesn't know what that means. He comes to you, the corporate nurse, to interpret the doctor's advice.

Assessment

Obtain clinical data:

Current weight, height, BMI
Blood pressure

Medical history and comorbidities, including diabetes, hypertension, myocardial infarction, alcohol abuse, other CHD risk factors
Abnormal laboratory values, especially cholesterol, LDL-C, HDL-C, triglycerides, and glucose
Medications that affect nutrition, such as diuretics, antihypertensives, antidiabetics, lipid-lowering medications

Interview client to assess:

Understanding of the relationship between "diet" and blood cholesterol levels
Motivation to change eating style; previous attempts to modify intake
Usual 24-hour intake, including portion sizes, frequency and pattern of eating, method of food preparation, intake of foods high in fat and saturated fat, intake of foods high in soluble fiber
How often meals are eaten out; what and where he eats out
Cultural, religious, and ethnic influences on eating habits
Use of vitamins, minerals, and nutritional supplements: what, how much, and why taken
Psychosocial issues, such as living situation and cooking facilities
Usual activity patterns
Use of alcohol, tobacco, and nicotine

Nursing Diagnosis

Health-Seeking Behaviors, as evidenced by the lack of knowledge of a heart-healthy diet and a desire to learn.

Planning and Implementation

CLIENT GOALS

The client will:

Experience a decrease in total cholesterol and LDL-C to the desired level or below (Table 18–1)
Experience an increase HDL-C
Explain the principles and rationale of nutrition therapy for hypercholesterolemia
Implement appropriate dietary and lifestyle changes
Consume a varied and nutritious diet
Name foods that are high in saturated fats, polyunsaturated fats, monounsaturated fats, cholesterol, and soluble fiber

NURSING INTERVENTIONS

Nutrition Therapy

Initiate the Step One diet
Restrict alcohol
Increase soluble fiber intake

Client Teaching

Instruct the client:

On the role of the Step One eating plan in managing hypercholesterolemia
On eating plan essentials, including:

- Eating up to four egg yolks per week on the Step One diet, including those used in food preparation.
- Eating up to 5 to 6 ounces of meat per day, emphasizing skinless poultry; lean, well-trimmed cuts of beef, pork, and lamb; and fish, shellfish, and processed meats made from lean meat
- Using canola, olive, and peanut oils for baking and sautéing
- Eating nuts and seeds in moderation
- Using soft, liquid, or spray margarine
- Choosing skim milk and skim-milk products
- Filling up on a variety of fruits, vegetables, and whole grains
- Enjoying low-fat desserts, such as low-fat and nonfat yogurt, ice milk, sherbet, sorbet, fruit ice, Popsicles, angel food cake, fig bars, gingersnaps, and other low-fat cakes and cookies
- Increasing soluble fiber intake, such as eating more oats and dried peas and beans; drinking at least eight 8-ounce glasses of fluid daily
- Eating at least 1 serving of a fatty fish per week, if desired
- Avoiding alcohol as advised by the physician

On behavioral matters, including:

- How to read labels
- How to order in a restaurant
- The importance of trying new recipes to acclimate to the changes in taste and texture of low-fat dishes
- The importance of regular physical activity
- Consulting his physician about the use of supplemental vitamin E, multivitamins containing folic acid, and fish-oil supplements

Resources for additional information:

American Heart Association
National Center
7272 Greenville Ave
Dallas, TX 75231-4596
800-AHD-USA-1
www.amhrt.org

National Heart, Lung, and Blood Institute (NHLBI) Information Center
PO Box 30105
Bethesda, MD 20824-0105
301-251-1222
www.nhlbi.nih.gov

Evaluation

The client:

Experiences a decrease in total cholesterol and LDL-C to the desired level or below
Experiences an increase in HDL-C

- Explains the principles and rationale of nutrition therapy for hypercholesterolemia
- Implements appropriate dietary and lifestyle changes
- Consumes a varied and nutritious diet
- Names foods that are high in saturated fats, polyunsaturated fats, monounsaturated fats, cholesterol, and soluble fiber

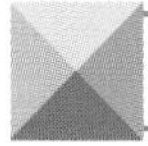

Myocardial Infarction

DESCRIPTION

A **myocardial infarction** (MI) involves the destruction of heart tissue in areas of the heart that are deprived of blood and oxygen. An MI can occur as a result of atherosclerosis, arterial occlusion from embolus or thrombus, or myocardial hypertrophy caused by CHF and hypertension, or it may occur secondary to a temporary reduction in blood flow to the heart related to shock, gastrointestinal bleeding, severe dehydration, or hypotension. MI is the most frequent cause of death in North America.

Treatment of an acute MI seeks to alleviate symptoms and prevent further damage with continual assessment and monitoring, complete rest, sedation, narcotics, oxygen, and intravenous fluids. The diet is modified to prevent diet-induced arrhythmias and to reduce cardiac workload. After the acute phase has passed, treatment focuses on rehabilitation and education of the patient and the family. Nutrition therapy is aimed at reducing the diet-responsive risk factors, such as hypercholesterolemia, obesity, diabetes mellitus, and hypertension.

NUTRITION THERAPY

Initially, patients who experience an MI may be given a liquid diet for approximately 24 hours. The diet is progressed to a regular diet as tolerated. Small, frequent meals are better tolerated than large meals, which can increase myocardial oxygen demand by increasing visceral blood flow. In addition:

- Gassy foods are avoided, but fiber intake should be adequate to prevent constipation.
- Temperature extremes are avoided because they may produce cardiac arrhythmias.
- Caffeine is eliminated because it is a stimulant.

The discharge diet is based on the patient's weight, serum lipid levels, risk factors, and medical condition. A Step One or Step Two diet (Table 18–3) is used, with calories adjusted for healthy weight. Soluble fiber is emphasized. A sodium-restricted diet is usually prescribed to treat or prevent hypertension, edema, or CHF. The physician may prescribe supplemental vitamin E and folic acid. Ongoing patient education is extremely important to promote lifestyle change.

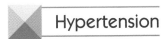

Hypertension

DESCRIPTION

Hypertension is a symptom, not a disease, that is arbitrarily defined as sustained elevated blood pressure greater than or equal to 140/90 mm Hg. It is estimated that hypertension affects one of every four Americans, although only one third of these cases may actually be diagnosed.

Fewer than 5% of cases of hypertension occur secondary to medical problems. In these cases, eliminating the underlying disorder cures the secondary hypertension. In at least 95% of cases, hypertension occurs from unknown causes and is classified as essential, primary, or idiopathic hypertension. *Essential hypertension* is more common among

DRUG ALERT
Antihypertensive Drugs

Potassium-wasting diuretics (thiazide and related agents, loop diuretics) can cause constipation, diarrhea, nausea, vomiting, gastrointestinal upset, dry mouth, increased thirst, anorexia, and fluid and electrolyte imbalances. Modify the diet to alleviate unpleasant gastrointestinal side effects, if possible. Often, patients who require an increased potassium intake are told to "eat a banana and drink orange juice every day," without any further explanation. Instruct the patient on the many other sources of potassium, especially those that are low in sodium (see text and Box 18-6). Advise the client to avoid natural licorice, which tends to cause potassium depletion and sodium retention.

Potassium supplements can lead to nausea, vomiting, gastrointestinal discomfort, and diarrhea and can produce hyperkalemia when used with salt substitutes that contain potassium. Monitor serum potassium levels and observe for signs of hyperkalemia. Advise against the use of potassium-containing salt substitutes.

Because the absorption of **beta-adrenergic blocking agents** (propranolol, metoprolol, atenolol) is enhanced by food, clients should be advised to take them with food.

Elderly patients who are receiving high doses of **captopril** may experience loss of taste.

Some **calcium channel blockers,** such as diltiazem (Cardizem, Dilacor) should be taken on an empty stomach, because foods that contain fat may decrease their absorption.

African-Americans than Caucasians and occurs more frequently among men than women until late middle age. In the United States and other developed countries, the prevalence of hypertension rises progressively with aging, but biologic changes are not the only factor. Age-related increases in blood pressure appear to be related to certain environmental factors, namely a high salt intake, obesity, physical inactivity, excessive alcohol consumption, and an inadequate intake of potassium and perhaps other minerals. Essential hypertension cannot be cured, but it may be prevented in large numbers of people through lifestyle changes.

Because nutrition therapy and other lifestyle changes have the potential to be completely effective, produce no adverse side effects, and may preclude the need for drug therapy, it is the focus of primary prevention and the initial treatment of choice for all patients with hypertension. If the patient fails to achieve desired goals, drug therapy (eg, diuretics, vasodilators, adrenergic blocking agents) may be added to nutrition therapy.

NUTRITION THERAPY

For years, the nonpharmacologic approach to preventing and treating high blood pressure has centered on four lifestyle modifications: reduce salt (sodium) intake, lose excess weight, increase physical activity, and limit alcohol intake to two drinks per day. The same approaches are outlined in the *Dietary Guidelines for Americans*, with additional advice to eat a liberal intake of fruits and vegetables because they provide potassium.

As the result of the DASH clinical study (Dietary Approaches to Stop Hypertension), the DASH diet has been added to the list of lifestyle modifications that prevent or treat hypertension. Although it had long been suspected that higher intakes of some minerals (eg, potassium, magnesium, calcium) lower blood pressure, results of studies using these nutrients in pill form were inconsistent. The DASH study set out to test whether eating whole "real" foods, rather than individual nutrients, would lower blood pressure as a result of some combination of nutrients, interactions among individual nutrients, or other food factors. The results clearly showed that eating the right foods can lower blood pressure to the same extent as taking blood pressure medication. The drop in blood pressure occurred within 2 weeks after starting the DASH diet. And, this is the same diet that may reduce the risk of cancer, heart disease, and diabetes.

The DASH diet is low in saturated fat, total fat, and cholesterol, like the Step One and Step Two diets. What is different about the DASH diet is that generally provides about two to three times the amounts of potassium, magnesium, and calcium most Americans typically consume and it is high in fiber (Table 18–5). This difference is achieved by increasing the intake of fruit, vegetables, and low-fat dairy products. Unlike the Food Guide Pyramid, the DASH diet has a separate food group entitled "Nuts, Seeds, and Dried Peas and Beans," from which 4 to 5 servings per week are recommended. A general characteristic is to center meals around plant foods instead of meat.

The DASH diet contains about 3000 mg of sodium, which is higher than the Daily Value for sodium (2400 mg) but slightly lower than the average American intake of 3600

TABLE 18.5 *Characteristics of the DASH Diet and the Typical American Diet*

Nutrient	DASH Diet	Average American Diet
Total fat (% of calories)	27	34
Saturated fat	6	12
Polyunsaturated fat	8	7
Monounsaturated fat	13	14–16
Carbohydrate (% of calories)	55	48
Protein (% of calories)	18	15
Cholesterol (mg/d)	150	300+
Fiber (g/d)	31	12–18
Potassium (mg/d)	4700	2220–3450
Magnesium (mg/d)	500	238–320
Calcium (mg/d)	1240	750
Sodium (mg/d)	3000	4000

to 4000 mg. The next phase of the study, called DASH2, is examining the relationship between blood pressure, eating patterns, and a reduced sodium intake. Table 18-6 shows the daily recommended servings and serving sizes for a 2000-cal DASH diet. Tips for implementing the DASH diet are as follows:

- To increase fruit and vegetable intake to 8 servings per day, try to eat 2 servings of either fruits or vegetables at each meal plus 1 serving of each for a snack. Choose vegetables that are fresh, frozen, or canned without salt. Edible skins and seeds of fruits and vegetables should be eaten to increase fiber and micronutrient intake.
- To increase dairy foods to 3 servings per day, try to consume 1 serving of a low-fat dairy food at each meal, or replace carbonated beverages with 1% or skim milk.
- Choose whole-grain foods, which are especially rich in B vitamins, fiber, and minerals.
- Use the Percent Daily Value (%DV) on food labels to compare products.
- Use fresh, frozen, canned, or dried fruits to satisfy a "sweet tooth."

In addition to the DASH diet, the following lifestyle modifications are recommended to prevent or treat high blood pressure:

- **Stop smoking.** Smoking raises blood pressure and is a strong risk factor for CHD.
- **Lose weight, if overweight.** Body weight is one of the strongest determinants of blood pressure. Losing weight lowers blood pressure, even if ideal weight is not attained and regardless of the degree of overweight. Weight loss may also reduce or eliminate the need for medication and thus the potential for toxicity and unpleasant side effects associated with drug therapy. Because weight control has the potential to control hypertension effectively for a large number of people, it is vital for primary prevention and treatment.

TABLE 18.6 *The DASH Diet*

The DASH eating plan shown here is based on 2000 cal/d. The number of daily servings in a food group may vary from those listed depending on your caloric needs.
Use this chart to help you plan your menus or take it with you when you go to the store.

Food Group	Daily Servings (except as noted)	Serving Sizes	Examples and Notes	Significance to the DASH Eating Plan
Grains and grain products	7–8	1 slice bread 1 cup dry cereal* ½ cup cooked rice, pasta, or cereal	Whole wheat bread, English muffin, pita bread, bagel, cereals, grits, oatmeal, crackers, unsalted pretzels, and popcorn	Major sources of energy and fiber
Vegetables	4–5	1 cup raw leafy vegetable ½ cup cooked vegetable 6 oz vegetable juice	Tomatoes, potatoes, carrots, green peas, squash, broccoli, turnip greens, collards, kale, spinach, artichokes, green beans, lima beans, sweet potatoes	Rich sources of potassium, magnesium, and fiber
Fruits	4–5	6 oz fruit juice 1 medium fruit ¼ cup dried fruit ½ cup fresh, frozen, or canned fruit	Apricots, bananas, dates, grapes, oranges, orange juice, grapefruit, grapefruit juice, mangoes, melons, peaches, pineapples, prunes, raisins, strawberries, tangerines	Important sources of potassium, magnesium, and fiber
Low-fat or fat-free dairy foods	2–3	8 oz milk 1 cup yogurt 1½ oz cheese	Fat-free (skim) or low-fat (1%) milk, fat-free or low-fat buttermilk, fat-free or low-fat regular or frozen yogurt, low-fat and fat-free cheese	Major sources of calcium and protein
Meats, poultry, and fish	2 or less	3 oz cooked meats, poultry, or fish	Select only lean; trim away visible fats; broil, roast, or boil, instead of frying; remove skin from poultry	Rich sources of protein and magnesium
Nuts, seeds, and dried peas and beans	4–5 per week	⅓ cup or 1½ oz nuts 2 tbsp or ½ oz seeds ½ cup cooked dry beans	Almonds, filberts, mixed nuts, peanuts, walnuts, sunflower seeds, kidney beans, lentils, and peas	Rich sources of energy, magnesium, potassium, protein, and fiber

(continued)

TABLE 18.6 *The DASH Diet (continued)*

The DASH eating plan shown here is based on 2000 cal/d. The number of daily servings in a food group may vary from those listed depending on your caloric needs.
Use this chart to help you plan your menus or take it with you when you go to the store.

Food Group	Daily Servings (except as noted)	Serving Sizes	Examples and Notes	Significance to the DASH Eating Plan
Fats and oils†	2–3	1 tsp soft margarine 1 tbsp low-fat mayonnaise 2 tbsp light salad dressing 1 tsp vegetable oil	Soft margarine, low-fat mayonnaise, light salad dressing, vegetable oils, (eg, olive, corn, canola, safflower)	In addition to fats added to foods, remember to choose foods that contain less fat
Sweets	5 per week	1 tbsp sugar 1 tbsp jelly or jam ½ oz jelly beans 8 oz lemonade	Maple syrup, sugar, jelly, jam, fruit-flavored gelatin, jelly beans, hard candy, fruit punch, sorbet, ices	Sweets should be low in fat

*Serving sizes vary between ½ and 1¼ cups. Check the product's nutrition label.
†Fat content changes serving counts for fats and oils: For example, 1 tbsp of regular salad dressing equals 1 serving; 1 tbsp of a low-fat dressing equals ½ serving; 1 tbsp of a fat-free dressing equals 0 servings.
National Institutes of Health, National Heart, Lung and Blood Institute. *Facts about the DASH Diet.* (NIH Publication No. 98-4082). Bethesda, MD: U.S. Department of Health and Human Services, NIH, NHLBI.

- **Limit alcohol to no more than one to two drinks per day.** Consistent and powerful evidence links alcohol consumption (three or more drinks per day) with hypertension. Clients who drink habitually should be advised to limit their consumption to two drinks per day or less. A "drink" is defined as 4.5 ounces of wine, 12 ounces of beer, or 1.5 ounces of distilled liquor, such as rum, bourbon, whiskey, gin, or vodka.
- **Get at least 30 to 45 minutes of aerobic activity on most days.** Studies show that increasing activity, either alone or as part of a weight loss program, lowers blood pressure. It appears that 30 to 45 minutes of moderate-intensity aerobic exercise may actually be better than a more intense workout. It is recommended that individuals participate in activities such as walking, cycling, dancing, and gardening at least three to five times per week.
- **Reduce sodium intake.** Even though the diet used in the DASH study provided 3000 mg of sodium daily, it is prudent to limit sodium to the Daily Value of 2400 mg (Box 18–5). Some people prefer to use salt substitutes when regular salt is restricted. Salt substitutes may contain potassium in place of sodium, or they may contain a combination of sodium and potassium chloride. Neither type should be used without a physician's permission.

BOX 18.5

Sources of Sodium

The Rule of 7 S's

Soups: canned soups, freeze-dried soup mixes, broth, bouillon (unless salt free)

Sauces: canned gravy, spaghetti sauce, and other cooking sauces; packaged sauce mixes and convenience mixes; ketchup, barbecue sauce, steak sauce

Snacks: processed varieties like corn chips, potato chips, popcorn, pretzels, snack crackers, and salted nuts

Smoked meat and fish: such as bacon, chipped beef, corned beef, cold cuts, ham, hot dogs, sausage, and lox

Sauerkraut: and other foods preserved in brine, such as pickles, pickled beets, pickled sausage, pickled herring, and pickled eggs

Seasonings: horseradish, soy sauce, Worcestershire sauce, meat tenderizer, and monosodium glutamate (MSG)

Sodium-processed cold cuts: bologna, ham, salami, corned beef

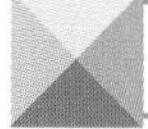

Congestive Heart Failure

DESCRIPTION

CHF is a syndrome that is characterized by the inability of the heart to maintain adequate blood flow through the circulatory system, which leads to decreased blood flow to the kidneys, excessive sodium and fluid retention, peripheral and pulmonary edema, and, finally, an overworked and enlarged heart. The severity of CHF can vary from mild to severe. Although the heart and its circulatory efficiency are principally affected initially, the entire circulation eventually is altered.

The treatment of CHF involves treatment of the underlying cause. Physical and mental rest help to decrease cardiac workload. Digitalis may be used to slow the heart rate and strengthen its beat. Diuretic therapy is used to help rid the body of excess fluid. Oxygen therapy may be necessary. Nutrition therapy is used to reduce sodium and fluid retention and to minimize cardiac workload.

NUTRITION THERAPY

Edema related to CHF can be relieved by reducing sodium intake, because extracellular fluid retention does not occur in the absence of sodium. Permitted sodium intake may vary from 250 to 2000 mg/day, depending on the severity of CHF (Box 18–6). The initial allowance may be progressed as edema subsides. Some clients can tolerate 4000 mg of sodium daily after their condition has stabilized.

(text continues on page 594)

BOX 18.6

Sodium-Restricted Diets

The objective of low-sodium diets is to rid the body of excess sodium and fluid accumulation associated with certain disorders, such as liver disease characterized by edema and ascites, CHF, renal disease characterized by edema and hypertension, and adrenocortical therapy. Low-sodium diets also are used in the treatment, and possible prevention, of hypertension.

Low-sodium diets are contraindicated for clients with sodium-wasting renal diseases, such as pyelonephritis, polycystic renal disease, and bilateral hydronephrosis; in pregnancy; for clients with ileostomies; and for those with myxedema.

The characteristics of low-sodium diets vary according to the level of restriction; 500- and 250-mg sodium diets are unpalatable, extremely difficult to follow, and likely to be inadequate in some nutrients. To promote compliance and to allow greater flexibility, exchange lists featuring the sodium content of high- and low-sodium foods may be used.

Levels of Restriction

3000 mg sodium (130 mEq) per day

- Up to ¼ tsp of salt allowed daily
- Eliminate high-sodium processed foods and beverages

2000 mg (87 mEq) per day

- Eliminate processed and prepared foods and beverages high in sodium
- No salt is allowed in cooking or at the table
- Limit milk and milk products to 16 oz/d

1000 mg (45 mEq) per day

- Follow all of the 2000-mg sodium restrictions
- Use only unsalted butter, margarine, and salad dressings
- Limit regular breads to 2 servings per day; use low-sodium bread, crackers, and other grains

500 mg (22 mEq) per day

- Follow all of the 1000-mg sodium restrictions
- Eliminate vegetables naturally high in sodium: beets, beet greens, carrots, kale, spinach, celery, white turnips, rutabagas, mustard greens, chard, peas, and dandelion greens
- Use only low-sodium bread, no regular bread
- Use distilled water for cooking and drinking
- Eliminate sherbet and flavored gelatin

(continued)

BOX 18.6

Sodium-Restricted Diets (continued)

- Limit meat to 5 oz/d; one egg may be substituted daily for 1 oz of meat
- Limit milk and milk products to 16 oz/d

250 mg (11 mEq) per day

- Follow all of the 500-mg sodium restrictions
- Use low-sodium milk in place of regular milk

Foods Grouped by Sodium Content

Food Group	Foods High in Added Sodium	Foods Naturally High in Sodium	Foods Lower in Sodium
Meats	Real and imitation bacon, cold cuts, chipped or corned beef, frankfurters, smoked meats, sausage, salt pork, canned meats, codfish, canned/salted/smoked fish, kosher meats, frozen and powdered egg substitutes, regular peanut butter	Brain, kidney, clams, crab, lobster, oysters, scallops, shrimp, and other shellfish	Fresh, frozen, or canned low-sodium meat and poultry; eggs; low-sodium cheeses and peanut butter; fresh bass, bluefish, catfish, cod, eel, flounder, halibut, rockfish, salmon, sole, trout, tuna; canned low-sodium tuna and salmon
Dairy products	Buttermilk, regular cheeses and cottage cheese; commercial milk products such as ice cream, malted milk, milk mixes, milk shakes, sherbet		Skim, 2%, whole, evaporated, and low-sodium milk; low-sodium cheeses, low-sodium cottage cheese
Fruits and vegetables	Crystallized or glazed fruit, maraschino cherries, dried fruit with sodium preservatives added; canned	Spinach, celery, beets and beet greens, carrots, artichokes, white turnips, Swiss chard, dandelion	Fresh, frozen without salt, and low-sodium canned vegetables, except those listed; fresh, frozen, canned or dried fruits

(continued)

BOX 18.6

Sodium-Restricted Diets (continued)

Foods Grouped by Sodium Content (continued)

Food Group	Foods High in Added Sodium	Foods Naturally High in Sodium	Foods Lower in Sodium
Fruits and vegetables *(continued)*	vegetables and vegetable juices unless low sodium, sauerkraut, frozen vegetables with added salt	greens, kale, mustard greens	without added sodium
Breads and cereals	Commercial mixes, bread and rolls made from frozen bread dough, graham and all other crackers except low-sodium crackers, instant rice and pasta mixes, commercial casserole mixes, commercial stuffing, instant and quick-cooking cereals, most dry cereals (except puffed rice, puffed wheat, and shredded wheat), self-rising flour, self-rising cornmeal, waffles; quick breads and other baked products containing		Low-sodium breads, crackers, cereals, and cereal products; baked products made without salt, baking powder containing sodium, or baking soda; low-sodium mixes; unsalted cooked cereals, puffed rice, puffed wheat, shredded wheat, barley, cornmeal, cornstarch, unsalted matzo; unsalted macaroni, and rice

(continued)

BOX 18.6

Sodium-Restricted Diets (continued)

Foods Grouped by Sodium Content (continued)

Food Group	Foods High in Added Sodium	Foods Naturally High in Sodium	Foods Lower in Sodium
	salt, baking soda, baking powder, or egg white		
Fats	Salted butter and margarine, regular commercial salad dressings and mayonnaise		Unsalted butter, margarine, salad dressings, and mayonnaise; cooking oils and shortening
Miscellaneous	Regular canned or frozen soups; soup mixes; salted popcorn, nuts, potato chips, and snack foods; instant cocoa mixes; powdered drink mixes, canned fruit drinks; pastries; commercial candies, cakes, cookies, and gelatin desserts		Alcohol; coffee and coffee substitutes, lemonade, tea; salt-free or low-sodium candy, unflavored gelatin, jam, jelly, maple syrup, honey; unsalted nuts and popcorn
Seasonings and condiments	Sea salt, rock salt, and kosher salt; barbecue sauce; bouillon cubes, ketchup; celery salt, seed, and leaves; chili sauce; tartar sauce; garlic salt; horseradish made with salt; meat extracts, sauces, and tenderizers;		Allspice, almond extract, anise seed, basil, bay leaf, low-sodium bouillon, caraway seed, cardamom, low-sodium ketchup, chili powder, chives, cinnamon, cloves, cocoa (1 to 2 tsp), coconut, cumin, curry, dill, fennel, garlic

(continued)

BOX 18.6

Sodium-Restricted Diets (continued)

Foods Grouped by Sodium Content (continued)

Food Group	Foods High in Added Sodium	Foods Naturally High in Sodium	Foods Lower in Sodium
Seasonings and condiments *(continued)*	Kitchen Bouquet, gravy, and sauce mixes; monosodium glutamate (MSG); prepared mustard, olives, onion salt, pickles, relishes; saccharin; soy sauce; teriyaki sauce, sugar substitutes containing sodium; Worcestershire sauce		and garlic powder, ginger, horseradish made without salt, juniper, lemon juice, mace, maple extract, marjoram, low-sodium meat extracts, low-sodium meat tenderizers, mint, mustard (dry and seeds), nutmeg, orange extract, oregano, paprika, parsley, pepper, peppermint extract, poppy seed, poultry seasoning, purslane, rosemary, saffron, sage, salt substitutes (if approved by a physician), savory, sesame seeds, sorrel, sugar, tarragon, thyme, tumeric, vanilla, vinegar, walnut extract, wine

2000-mg Sodium Diet

Breakfast

¼ cup orange juice
¾ cup shredded wheat
2 slices toast
2 tsp margarine

(continued)

BOX 18.6

Sodium-Restricted Diets (continued)

1 tbsp strawberry jam
1 cup 1% milk
Sugar
Coffee/tea
Pepper

Lunch

2 oz sliced chicken breast on 2 slices whole wheat bread with 2 tsp mayonnaise, tomato, and lettuce
Tossed salad with oil and vinegar dressing
Fresh fruit
4 vanilla wafers
1 cup 1% milk
Coffee/tea
Sugar/pepper

Dinner

4 oz broiled halibut
Baked potato
2 tsp margarine
½ cup broccoli
Coleslaw made with oil and vinegar dressing
1 dinner roll
½ cup sherbet
Coffee/tea
Sugar/pepper

Snack

1 cup unsalted popcorn
Apple juice

250-mg Sodium Diet

Breakfast

½ cup orange juice
¾ cup shredded wheat
2 slices low-sodium toast
2 tsp unsalted margarine
1 tbsp strawberry jam
1 cup low-sodium milk

(continued)

BOX 18.6

Sodium-Restricted Diets (continued)

Sugar
Coffee/tea
Pepper

Lunch

2 oz sliced chicken breast on 2 slices low-sodium bread with 2 tsp low-sodium mayonnaise, tomato, and lettuce
Tossed salad with oil and vinegar dressing
Fresh fruit
Fruit ice
Sugar/pepper
Coffee/tea
Apricot nectar

Dinner

4 oz broiled beef patty
Baked potato
2 tsp unsalted margarine
½ cup broccoli
1 slice low-sodium bread
Fresh strawberries
Coffee/tea
Sugar/pepper

Snack

1 cup plain popcorn
Apple juice

Potential Problems	Recommended Interventions
Hyponatremia (nausea, malaise, possible confusion, seizures, and coma) related to a sodium intake that is too low, especially when combined with the use of diuretics. For most people, the risk of hyponatremia is insignificant. However, clients with renal disease and the elderly may not be able to reabsorb enough sodium while following a low-sodium diet.	To allow homeostatic mechanisms time to adapt in the elderly and in clients with renal disease, initiate a low-sodium diet gradually. Observe for signs of sodium deficiency and liberalize the diet if necessary.

(continued)

BOX 18.6

Sodium-Restricted Diets (continued)

Noncompliance, which may be related to the following situations:

Pervasiveness of sodium in the diet. Not all high-sodium foods taste salty.

Preference of salt taste.

Ethnic or religious customs. For instance, Chinese cooking relies heavily on soy sauce and MSG for seasoning. Kosher meats are bathed in a brine solution for 1 hour after slaughter. Although rinsing does remove some of the salt, kosher meats remain high in sodium.

Reliance on convenience products and canned foods, which are high in sodium. This is especially common among the elderly and people living alone.

Reassure the client that, with time, the taste for salt lessens and it becomes easier to follow the diet.

Advise the client that label reading is essential. Foods that supply >480 mg sodium per serving (ie, 20% DV) are high-sodium foods and should be avoided.

Provide thorough and periodic instructions on how to incorporate the diet into the client's lifestyle and budget, information on sources of sodium in food and drugs, and lists of sodium alternatives.

If expense and convenience are a problem, allow the client to continue using regular canned meats and vegetables, if possible. Rinsing canned foods under running water for at least 1 minute removes much of the sodium content.

Encourage support from the client's family and urge them to follow the diet if possible.

Patient Teaching

(Be more or less specific depending on the level of sodium allowed.)

Provide general information:

- Reducing sodium intake will help the body rid itself of excess fluid and help lower high blood pressure.
- Sodium appears in the diet in the form of salt and to some degree in almost all foods and beverages. Most unprocessed, unsalted foods are low in sodium.
- Approximately 15% of sodium intake comes from salt added during cooking and at the table, 75% comes from processed foods, and 10% is from food and water naturally high in sodium.
- Sodium-containing compounds are used extensively as preservatives (sodium propionate, sodium sulfite, and sodium benzoate), leavening agents (sodium bicarbonate, baking soda, and baking powder), and flavor enhancers (eg, salt, MSG) and are found in foods that may not taste salty.

(continued)

BOX 18.6

Sodium-Restricted Diets (continued)

- Many nonprescription drugs (eg, aspirin, cough medicines, laxatives, antacids), toothpastes, tooth powders, and mouthwashes contain large amounts of sodium and should not be used without a physician's approval.
- Salt substitutes replace sodium with potassium or other minerals. "Low-sodium" salt substitutes are not sodium free and may contain half as much sodium as regular table salt. Use neither type without a physician's approval.
- The preference for salt taste eventually will decrease.
- If the client "cheats" by eating a high-sodium meal or snack, compensate by eating less sodium than normally allowed for the rest of the day.

Teach the client how to order off a menu while dining out:

- Request that food not be salted, if possible.
- Choose fruit juice instead of soup for an appetizer.
- Use oil and vinegar or fresh lemon instead of regular salad dressing.
- Order plain meat and vegetables without gravy or sauce.
- Choose plain baked potatoes and season sparingly with sour cream, butter, or pepper.
- Select fresh fruit for dessert. If the client is going to splurge, ice cream or sherbet is a better choice than pie, cake, cookies, or other desserts.
- Avoid fast food restaurant meals, which usually are high in sodium.

Teach the client food preparation techniques to minimize sodium intake:

- Foods made from "scratch" generally have less sodium than processed foods and mixes.
- Experiment with sodium-free seasonings, such as herbs, spices, lemon juice, vinegar, and wine. Fresh ingredients are more flavorful than dried ones.
- Commercial "salt alternatives" are sodium-free blends of herbs and spices that are not intended to taste like salt but to be used as flavor enhancers.
- If permitted by a physician, salt substitutes may be used, although they taste bitter to some people.
- A variety of low-sodium cookbooks are available.

Teach the client how to read labels:

- Salt, MSG, baking soda, and baking powder contain significant amounts of sodium. Other sodium compounds such as sodium nitrite, benzoate of soda, sodium saccharin, and sodium propionate add less sodium to the diet.
- "Sodium free," "low sodium," "very low sodium," and "reduced" or "less" sodium are reliable terms.

(continued)

BOX 18.6

Sodium-Restricted Diets (continued)

- Numerous low- and reduced-sodium products are available: milk, bread and bread products, cereal, crackers, cakes, cookies, pastries, soups and bouillon, canned vegetables, tomato products, meats, entrees, processed meats, hard and soft cheeses, condiments, nuts and peanut butter, butter, margarine, salad dressings, baking powder, and snack foods.
- The difference in taste between some low-sodium products and their high-sodium counterparts is barely noticeable; others taste flat and may need to have herbs or spices added.

In most cases, sodium restriction, used alone or in combination with diuretics (low-sodium diets enhance the sodium-excreting effects of diuretics), effectively reduces fluid volume without the need for fluid restriction. However, fluid restriction may be necessary if edema persists despite a low-sodium diet. Fluid may be limited to 2 L per day or less, depending on the client's response to the sodium restriction.

A diet that is low in calories but otherwise nutritionally adequate is indicated for overweight clients. Attaining ideal or slightly under ideal weight reduces the cardiac workload. In addition:

- Provide five to six small meals per day of nonirritating and non–gas-forming foods to limit gastric distention and pressure on the heart.
- Individualize the diet according to the patient's tolerance. Soft foods reduce the amount of chewing required, an important consideration for fatigued patients.
- Provide adequate potassium, based on the type of diuretic prescribed. A high-potassium diet may be indicated for clients who are taking thiazide (potassium-wasting) diuretics or digitalis (Box 18–7). Spironolactone and triamterene are

BOX 18.7

Sources of Potassium

Fruit: Especially bananas, citrus fruits and their juices, melons, raisins, dried dates, apricots, and avocados

Vegetables: Sweet and white potatoes, tomatoes and tomato products, dried peas and beans, green leafy vegetables, carrots, corn, spinach, winter squash

Whole grains, especially those containing bran

Fresh meat

Milk, yogurt, ice cream, pudding

Potassium-containing salt substitutes: NoSalt, Seasoned NoSalt, Morton Salt Substitute, Morton Lite Salt Mixture, Adolph's Salt Substitute, Adolph's Seasoned Salt, Diamond Crystal, and CoSalt potassium-sparing diuretics that do not warrant the intake or use of additional potassium.

- Initially eliminate caffeine. After the patient's condition has stabilized, coffee intake may be liberalized to 4 or 5 cups/day as tolerated.

Malnutrition among CHF patients, known as *cardiac cachexia,* may occur with poor nutritional intake and long-term use of medication. Nutritional deficiencies can have a severe impact on the heart. Patients with cardiac cachexia need a high-calorie, high-protein, high-nutrient diet within the confines of sodium restriction (1–2 g/day). Caloric and nutrient density is important to maximize intake. Often these patients do not tolerate enteral feedings because of access to the thoracic cavity and decreased blood flow to the gastrointestinal tract.

NURSING PROCESS

Mrs. Gigante is a 79-year-old widow admitted for CHF. She lives alone and, because she prepares her own meals, she relies heavily on convenience foods, such as canned and packaged soups, frozen dinners, canned pasta, and tuna fish sandwiches. She appears thin and has 3+ edema in her lower extremities.

Assessment

Obtain clinical data:

- Current weight, height, BMI
- Blood pressure
- Abdominal girth, presence of edema
- Medical history and comorbidities, including diabetes, hypertension, myocardial infarction, alcohol abuse, and other CHD risk factors
- Abnormal laboratory values, especially cholesterol, lipid profile, triglycerides, blood urea nitrogen, sodium, creatinine, potassium, and glucose
- Medications that affect nutrition, such as diuretics, antihypertensives, antidiabetics, and lipid-lowering medications
- Complaints, including activity intolerance, fatigue, and shortness of breath
- Urine output

Interview client to assess:

- Understanding of the relationship between sodium, fluid accumulation, and symptoms of CHF
- Motivation to change eating style; previous attempts to modify intake
- Usual 24-hour intake, including portion sizes; frequency and pattern of eating; method of food preparation; problems with anorexia or early satiety; intake of foods high in fat and saturated fat, foods high in sodium, and foods high in potassium
- Hydration; input and output

Whether CHF symptoms impair her ability to shop, cook, eat, or perform other activities of daily living

Cultural, religious, and ethnic influences on eating habits

Use of vitamins, minerals, and nutritional supplements: what, how much, and why taken

Psychosocial and economic issues, such as living situation, cooking facilities, financial status, education, and eligibility for the Meals on Wheels program

Use of alcohol, caffeine, and nicotine

Adherence to prescribed drug therapy

Nursing Diagnosis

- Fluid Volume Excess, related to CHF.
- Decreased Cardiac Output, related to CHF.
- Health-Seeking Behaviors, as evidenced by the lack of knowledge of a heart-healthy diet and a desire to learn.

Planning and Implementation

CLIENT GOALS

The client will:

Attain and maintain normal fluid balance

Consume a varied and nutritious diet with adequate calories to attain healthy body weight

Avoid excessive sodium and increase intake of potassium

Avoid cardiac stimulants

NURSING INTERVENTIONS

Nutrition Therapy

Provide a 2-g sodium diet as ordered

Provide five to six small meals to limit gastric distention and pressure on the heart

Monitor input and output for need for fluid restriction

Eliminate caffeine until patient has stabilized

Client Teaching

Instruct the client:

On the roles of sodium, fluid, medication, desirable weight, and smoking in managing CHF

On the availability of the Meals on Wheels program. Explain that Meals on Wheels can provide her with the appropriate diet after discharge to ensure that she gets the proper foods, even on days when she feels short of breath or too tired to cook. (Notify the discharge planner that the client may be a candidate for Meals on Wheels.)

On eating plan essentials, such as:

- Eliminating the use of salt in cooking and at the table
- Using low-sodium canned foods when available
- Avoiding other high-sodium items (Box 18-5)
- Limiting milk intake to 2 cups daily
- Restricting caffeine initially
- Increasing intake of high-potassium foods (Box 18-7)
- Avoiding alcohol
- Adhering to fluid restriction, if appropriate

On behavioral matters, including:

- How to read labels to identify high-sodium foods
- That a gradual reduction in sodium intake may be easier to comply with than an abrupt withdrawal of sodium. Because the preference for salt gradually diminishes when intake is limited, following a low-sodium diet tends to get easier with time.
- Timing of meals and snacks to avoid shortness of breath and fatigue
- Physical activity goals, if applicable and appropriate

Evaluation

The client:

Attains and maintains normal fluid balance
Consumes a varied and nutritious diet with adequate calories to attain healthy body weight; has Meals on Wheels scheduled to provide meals after discharge
Avoids excessive sodium and increases intake of potassium
Avoids cardiac stimulants

Questions You May Hear

Who should have their cholesterol levels measured? The NCEP recommends that total serum cholesterol be measured at least once every 5 years in all adults 20 years of age and older, preferably as part of a total physical examination so that other risks can be identified. Measurements of total serum cholesterol and HDL-C can be used to screen adults who have no symptoms of CHD. Both measurements can be obtained at any time of day in the nonfasting state, because they change little after eating.

Is red wine good for your heart? Cross-cultural and animal studies show greater protection against atherosclerosis for red wine than for other alcoholic beverages. In addition to the beneficial effects of the alcohol in red wine, nonalcoholic components play a role in risk reduction. For instance, red wine is rich in powerful antioxidants and other active substances that are just beginning to be identified. However, populations who drink red wine and have lower rates of heart disease also have different consumption patterns from those of Americans. For them, red wine is more likely to be consumed daily, with meals, and in moderation. Although it appears that red wine offers greater benefits than other forms of alcohol, this has not been proven. The recommendation for red wine is the same for other forms of alcohol: if you don't drink, don't start. If you do drink, consume less than two drinks per day if you're a man, less than one drink per day if you're a woman.

KEY CONCEPTS

- Although diet intervention may not prevent heart disease in individuals, it can reduce the risk of heart disease in Americans.
- Management of these risk factors is proven to reduce the risk of atherosclerosis: cigarette smoking; a high-saturated-fat, high-cholesterol diet; elevated total cholesterol and LDLC concentrations; and hypertension.
- Lifestyle modifications recommended to lower total cholesterol and LDLC include the Step One and Step Two diets (low saturated fat, low cholesterol), loss of excess weight, and increased consumption of soluble fiber.
- The Step One diet is lower in saturated fat, total fat, and cholesterol than the current typical American diet. Calories are adjusted for healthy weight.
- The Step Two diet is recommended when the goals of the Step One diet are not achieved after 3 months of good compliance; it more severely limits saturated fat and cholesterol.
- Changing eating patterns is a lifestyle modification that should be made gradually and sequentially for the greatest chance of long-term success.
- The Mediterranean Diet is higher in fat than the Step One diet (35% of total calories), with the largest percentage of fat coming from olive oil. The plant-based diet, along with daily red wine consumption at meals and regular physical activity, is credited with the low rate of chronic disease and increased longevity seen in people living in the Mediterranean area.
- Functional foods that may help reduce the risk of heart disease include fish oils, soy products, and garlic.
- Determine how closely the patient's diet resembles the Step One diet before recommending changes.
- People who use fat-reduction strategies usually eat less fat and cholesterol and consume more micronutrients than people who do not use a plan when changing their eating habits. The most commonly used strategies are to switch to skim milk, use lean meats in place of fatty meats, and substitute low-fat and nonfat products for regular-fat varieties.
- Nutritional supplements promoted to prevent or treat atherosclerosis include green tea, red yeast, soluble fiber, and chromium. Clients should be cautioned against self-medicating with supplements and herbs, especially supplements that act like drugs.
- Usually a low-sodium diet, used with or without diuretics, can effectively control fluid balance in clients with CHF, without the need for a fluid restriction.
- Nutrition therapy is the cornerstone of primary prevention and treatment of hypertension. The DASH diet, which is similar to a Step One diet but has more fruits, more vegetables, and a food group entitled "Nuts, Seeds, and Dried Peas and Beans," can lower blood pressure as much as drug therapy. Other lifestyle modifications for high blood pressure are to stop smoking, lose excess weight, increase physical activity, drink alcohol only moderately, and avoid a high salt intake.

Focus on Critical Thinking

Mr. Bishop is 56-years-old, weighs 184 pounds, and is 5 feet 9 inches tall. He smokes two packs of cigarettes a day and leads a sedentary lifestyle. He was recently divorced and is now living alone, preparing his own meals occasionally, but mostly eating out or getting takeout foods. The doctor has warned him that his blood pressure is creeping up, with the most recent measurement at 150/95 mm Hg. If Mr. Bishop's blood pressure is not lower at his next office visit, which is scheduled in 3 months, he will have to begin antihypertensive medication. Mr. Bishop has heard that blood pressure medication can have serious side effects, so he says he is determined to get his blood pressure under control. He wonders whether fish-oil pills will help bring down his blood pressure.

List risk factors that may be contributing to Mr. Bishop's elevated blood pressure.

Before recommending that Mr. Bishop change his eating habits, his usual intake needs to be determined, particularly which foods or nutrients are consumed. List three dietary interventions that may benefit Mr. Bishop. Given his present lifestyle, what does Mr. Bishop need to know to implement the appropriate dietary changes? What would you tell him about the use of fish-oil supplements?

ANSWER KEY

1. **FALSE** Restricting saturated fat and cholesterol intake is prudent for almost all Americans older than 2 years of age, but it is not the only dietary intervention likely to reduce the risk of CHD. Other components of nutrition therapy help reduce CHD risk by different mechanisms, such as reducing the oxidation of LDL-C, decreasing the propensity of blood to clot, and altering platelet aggregation. Some of the other dietary substances that affect risk include omega-3 fatty acids, soluble fibers, folic acid, and antioxidant vitamins.
2. **TRUE** Canola, olive, and peanut oils are rich in monounsaturated fats.
3. **FALSE** Studies show that among supplement users, the greatest reduction in CHD risk occurs at daily intakes of 100 to 249 IU vitamin E per day for more than 2 years. It is impossible to get 100 IU of vitamin E through food alone.
4. **TRUE** High-fiber diets, especially those rich in soluble fiber, lower total cholesterol and LDL-C without lowering HDL-C.
5. **TRUE** High homocysteine levels can occur from a deficiency of folic acid, vitamin B_{12}, and/or vitamin B_6.
6. **FALSE** Moderate alcohol consumption (one to two drinks per day) is associated with a reduced risk of CHD. However, because of the potential risks of using alcohol, many health professionals are reluctant to encourage people who do not drink to do so simply to reduce their risk of CHD.
7. **FALSE** The use of fish-oil supplements has not been proven effective or safe and is not recommended by the American Medical Association.
8. **TRUE** When fat is drastically reduced or when carbohydrate calories replace the decrease in fat calories, the result may be an undesirable decrease in HDL-C.
9. **TRUE** Weight loss lowers high blood pressure.

10. TRUE Unlike the Food Guide Pyramid, the DASH diet has a separate food group entitled "Nuts, Seeds, and Dried Peas and Beans," from which 4 to 5 servings per week are recommended.

REFERENCES

Chicago Dietetic Association and The South Suburban Dietetic Association. (1992). *Manual of clinical dietetics* (4th ed.). Chicago: American Dietetic Association.

Connor, S. (1999). The healthy heart: Challenges and opportunities for dietetics professionals in the 21st century. *Journal of the American Dietetic Association*, 99, 164–165.

Ellison, R. (1999). Alcohol and coronary heart disease. *SCAN's pulse: A publication for sports, cardiovascular, and wellness nutritionists*, *18*(1), 1–5.

Escott-Stump, S. (1998). *Nutrition and diagnosis-related care* (4th ed.). Philadelphia: Williams & Wilkins.

Fallest-Strobl, P., Koch, D., Stein, J., & McBride, P. (1997). Homocysteine: A new risk factor for atherosclerosis. [On-line]. *American Family Physician*, *56*(6). Available: www.aafp.org/afp/971015ap/fallest.html. Accessed May 3, 1999.

Joint National Committee on Prevention, Detection, Evaluation, and Treatment of High Blood Pressure. (1997). The sixth report of the Joint National Committee on Prevention, Detection, Evaluation, and Treatment of High Blood Pressure (JNC VI). *Archives of Internal Medicine*, *157*, 2413–2446.

Kris-Etherton, P., & Burns, J. (Eds.). (1998). *Cardiovascular nutrition: Strategies and tools for disease management and prevention*. Chicago: The American Dietetic Association.

Lappalainen, R., Koikkalainen, M., Julkunen, J., Saarinen, T., & Mykkanen, H. (1998). Association of sociodemographic factors with barriers reported by patients receiving nutrition counseling as part of cardiac rehabilitation. *Journal of the American Dietetic Association*, 98, 1026–1029.

Liebman, B. (1997). DASH: A diet for all diseases. *Nutrition Action Health Letter*, *42*(8), 10–13.

Liebman, B. (1998). The soy story. *Nutrition Action Health Letter*, *25*(7), 1,3–7.

Masley, S. (1998). Dietary therapy for preventing and treating coronary artery disease. *American Family Physician* *57*(6), 1299–1313.

National Cholesterol Education Program. (1993). *Second report of the expert panel on detection, evaluation, and treatment of high blood cholesterol in adults (Adult Treatment Panel II)*. (NIH Publication No. 933095). Bethesda, MD: U.S. Department of Health and Human Services, Public Health Service, National Institutes of Health.

National Cholesterol Education Program. (1993). *Report of the expert panel on population strategies for blood cholesterol reduction: Executive Summary*. (NIH Publication No. 933047). Bethesda, MD: U.S. Department of Health and Human Services, Public Health Service, National Institutes of Health, National Heart, Lung, and Blood Institute.

National Institutes of Health, National Heart, Lung, and Blood Institute. (1995). *Facts about the DASH diet*. (NIH Publication No. 98-4082). Bethesda, MD: U.S. Department of Health and Human Services, Public Health Service, NIH, NHLBI.

Nelson, K. (1995). Therapeutic nutrition: An alternative approach to coronary heart disease management. *Nutrition Today*, *30*(3), 114–122.

Peterson, S., Sigman-Grant, M., Eissenstat, B., & Kris-Etherton, P. (1999). Impact of adopting lower-fat food choices on energy and nutrient intakes of American adults. *Journal of the American Dietetic Association*, 99, 177–183.

Robbers, J., & Tyler, V. (1999). *Tyler's herbs of choice: The therapeutic use of phytomedicinals*. Binghamton, NY: Haworth Press, Inc.

Shardt, D. (1997). Cholesterol-lowering supplements. *Nutrition Action Health Letter*, *24*(9), 8–11.

U.S. Department of Agriculture, U.S. Department of Health and Human Services. (2000). Bulletin No. 323. (Home and Garden) *Nutrition and your health: Dietary Guidelines for Americans* (5th ed.).

CHAPTER 19

Nutrition for Patients With Diabetes Mellitus

TRUE	FALSE	Check your knowledge of nutrition for patients with diabetes mellitus.
		1 Nutrition therapy is less important for diabetics taking oral agents than for those treated with nutrition therapy alone.
		2 All diabetics should strive to eat their meals and snacks at approximately the same time every day.
		3 Alcohol is more likely to cause hypoglycemia when consumed without food rather than with food.
		4 Diabetics who are ill should take less insulin when they are not eating their usual amounts of food.
		5 Frequent treatment of hypoglycemia can lead to weight gain.
		6 Type 2 diabetics may benefit from a higher fat intake if that fat is in the form of monounsaturated fat.
		7 Dehydration is often a precipitating factor in hyperglycemic hyperosmolar nonketotic syndrome (HHNS).
		8 All diabetics should be taught how to use exchange lists to plan their meals.
		9 Pregnant diabetics should eat slightly less carbohydrates than normal.
		10 A 10- to 20-pound weight loss may be enough to improve glycemic control in overweight type 2 diabetics, even if reasonable weight is not achieved.

Upon completion of this chapter, you will be able to

- Contrast the pathogenesis of type 1 diabetes with that of type 2 diabetes.
- List goals of nutrition therapy for diabetics.
- Discuss the nutrient recommendations for diabetics.
- Explain why consistent meal timing and composition is important for patients with either types of diabetes.
- Name assessment criteria for diabetics.
- Discuss basic and in-depth teaching strategies for diabetes nutrition therapy.
- Discuss the effect weight loss has on management of type 2 diabetes.

- Discuss diabetes in childhood, in pregnancy, and in older adults.
- Describe the nutrition therapy for functional hypoglycemia.

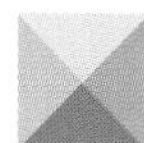

Diabetes Mellitus

Diabetes mellitus is a chronic heterogeneous disorder characterized by elevated blood glucose levels (*hyperglycemia*) related to a relative or absolute deficiency of insulin. Approximately 6% of the American population has diabetes, only half of whom may be diagnosed. The two major types of diabetes are type 1 and type 2. The exact cause is unknown but is believed to be multifactorial for each type.

PATHOGENESIS OF TYPE 1 DIABETES

Type 1 diabetes (formerly known as insulin-dependent diabetes mellitus) accounts for only 5% to 10% of all diabetes cases. Although it can occur at any age, it is most often detected before the age of 30 years in people who are normal or slightly below normal weight. People with type 1 diabetes secrete little or no insulin. It is theorized that, in genetically susceptible people, an autoimmune response triggered by an environmental stress (such as mumps, rubella, Epstein-Barr, or Coxsackie virus infection) damages or destroys beta cells, leaving them unable to produce much or any insulin.

Without insulin, serum glucose levels rise and cells are unable to use glucose for energy. Glucose eventually "spills" over into the urine (glycosuria). To some extent, the body compensates for the lack of usable energy by breaking down protein and fat. Ketone bodies accumulate because the body is not able to completely utilize fat for energy, and ketonuria develops. If left untreated, the accumulation of ketones in the blood lowers serum pH, leading to **diabetic ketoacidosis (DKA)**, a potentially fatal form of metabolic acidosis.

Polyuria and polydipsia, the classic symptoms of diabetes, develop as the body tries to rid itself of excess glucose and ketones. The third hallmark, polyphagia, occurs because the cells are actually starving for energy despite the high glucose levels. Rapid weight loss, muscle wasting, fatigue, weakness, irritability, itchy skin, and poor wound healing may occur.

PATHOGENESIS OF TYPE 2 DIABETES

Approximately 90% to 95% of the diabetic population has type 2 diabetes. Because it is a slowly progressive disease, the number of diagnosed and undiagnosed cases may be equal. It is most often diagnosed after 40 years of age and is most prevalent in minority populations, such as Hispanic-Americans, Native Americans, and African-Americans. The incidence of type 2 diabetes is strongly correlated with obesity (80% to 90% of type 2 diabetics are obese), family history, sedentary lifestyle, and aging.

Unlike type 1, type 2 diabetes is characterized by insulin resistance and hyperinsulinemia. **Insulin resistance** means that skeletal muscle cells and other types of cells are unable to adequately remove glucose from the blood under the action of insulin. The body compensates by secreting higher than normal amounts of insulin (**hyperinsulinemia**) to overcome the effects of insulin resistance. Chronic hyperinsulinemia can lead to a decrease in the number of insulin receptors on the cells and a further reduction in tissue sensitivity to insulin. For instance, it may take 4 to 5 hours instead of the usual 2 hours for blood glucose levels to return to normal after a meal. Eventually and progressively, insulin sensitivity and insulin secretion deteriorate and frank type 2 diabetes develops.

Obesity does not cause hyperglycemia but contributes to insulin resistance, especially among women with upper body obesity. The risk of developing type 2 diabetes increases in proportion to the degree of obesity.

Many people with type 2 diabetes are asymptomatic and do not know they have diabetes until a complication develops. Others display mild classic symptoms or experience drowsiness, fatigue, blurred vision, tingling or numbness of the extremities, or frequent infections. Because insulin is available, ketoacidosis does not develop, even though blood glucose levels are high. A complication that can develop rapidly from severe hyperglycemia is **hyperglycemic hyperosmolar nonketotic syndrome (HHNS)**, or **hyperglycemic hyperosmolar nonketotic coma (HHNC)**. The sudden hyperosmolar state that is triggered by extremely high blood glucose levels (ie, 1000 mg/dL) causes severe dehydration and neurologic dysfunction, including coma.

LONG-TERM COMPLICATIONS

Diabetes significantly increases morbidity and mortality and is the fourth leading cause of death by disease in the United States. The major challenge is to control the progressive microvascular and macrovascular damage that occurs over time, usually 15 to 20 years after diabetes onset. Microvascular injury damages the kidneys (nephropathy), and retina (retinopathy). Macrovascular damage increases the risk of coronary heart disease, peripheral vascular disease, and cerebrovascular accidents. Atherosclerosis is 50% more common among diabetics than in the general population, and the death rate from coronary artery disease is two to three times higher among diabetics compared with age- and sex-matched peers. This increased risk may be partly related to a high incidence of other coronary heart disease risk factors, such as hyperlipidemia, hypertension, and clotting abnormalities. Other complications include neuropathy, which causes gastroparesis (delayed gastric emptying), impaired peripheral circulation, and impotence in men. Impaired wound healing can lead to gangrene and amputation.

Patients develop complications without being aware that the damage is occurring. The presence of higher than normal blood glucose levels for a long period damages the vessels in the eyes, kidneys, and feet. By the time the patient has symptoms of a problem, the damage is done. For this reason, it is important to keep blood glucose levels as near normal as possible. The Diabetes Complication and Control Trial (DCCT) definitively showed that strict blood glucose control delays the onset and slows the progression of long-term complications in type 1 diabetics. The United Kingdom Prospective Diabetes Study (UKPDS) proved that the same is true for people with type 2 diabetes.

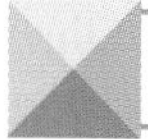

Management of Diabetes

The overall goals of medical therapy for all people with diabetes are to:

- Achieve blood glucose control as near normal as possible.
- Achieve optimal blood lipid levels.
- Provide adequate calories for reasonable weight.
- Prevent, delay, or treat complications.
- Improve overall health through optimal nutrition.

These goals are most effectively met through a combination of exercise, drug therapy, and nutrition therapy. Although the goals are the same for both types of diabetes, the approaches differ somewhat between type 1 and type 2 diabetes.

MANAGEMENT OF TYPE 1 DIABETES

Insulin

All people with type 1 diabetes require exogenous insulin to maintain blood glucose levels. Regardless of the type of diabetes, insulin injections usually are taken two or more times daily to allow adequate glucose control overnight without precipitating daytime hypoglycemia. Ideally, a meal plan that is based on the client's preferred eating pattern serves as the basis for integrating insulin therapy into eating and exercise patterns. However, conventional use of insulin, which limits injections to one or two per day, necessitates that food intake be altered to coincide with insulin action (ie, rapid, short, intermediate, or long-acting preparations). Intensive insulin therapy uses multiple injections or an insulin pump. This allows much greater flexibility in eating and exercise because insulin is adjusted to match the patient's lifestyle. Even with intensive insulin therapy, consistency in food intake and exercise patterns are recommended.

Nutrition Therapy

Nutrition therapy is the cornerstone of treatment for all diabetics, regardless of weight, blood glucose levels, or use of medication. The most recent nutrient recommendations issued by the American Diabetes Association (1994) stress that the diet must be individualized according to assessment data and treatment goals. The nutrient recommendations for diabetes are consistent with intake recommendations to promote health and well-being in the general public. The major difference is that total carbohydrate intake must be consistent from day to day (eg, approximately the same amount of carbohydrate each breakfast, each lunch, each dinner, and each snack).

Nutrient Recommendations

Calories should be adequate to maintain or attain reasonable weight in adults. Most type 1 diabetics are of normal weight and therefore need adequate calories for weight maintenance. Calorie intake should approximate the Recommended Dietary Allowance (RDA) for calories based on the patient's age, sex, and activity patterns. Calorie adjustments are made according to changes in the patient's weight.

Protein should provide 10% to 20% of total calories. This is consistent with the recommendation for protein intake among the general public because there is a lack of evidence to support either higher or lower intakes. Once the glomerular filtration rate (GFR) begins to fall, a reduction in protein intake from 0.8 g/kg (normal RDA) to 0.6 g/kg may help slow the rate of GFR decline. Some evidence suggests that vegetable protein also may help slow the progression of renal disease, allowing for a more liberal protein intake than is usually prescribed to manage nephropathy.

Limit saturated fat to 10% of total calories or less. Saturated fat is limited to less than 10% of total calories to reduce the risk of cardiovascular disease. This recommendation is also consistent with healthy eating suggestions for the general public.

Total fat intake is not specified. There is no recommendation regarding total fat intake except that the percentage of calories from total fat should be based on assessment data and treatment goals. The percentage of calories left after protein, saturated fat, and polyunsaturated fat are accounted for is determined as follows: 10%–20% of calories from protein, plus 10% of calories from saturated fat, plus up to 10% of calories from polyunsaturated fat, equals 30%–40% of total calories accounted for. That leaves 60% to 70% of remaining calories to be divided between carbohydrates and monounsaturated fat. How those calories are actually distributed depends on the individual's weight, lipid levels, and preference. For instance:

- Thirty percent or less of total calories from fat may be appropriate for clients with normal lipid levels and normal weight. The diet would have 10% of total calories from monounsaturated fat and 50% to 60% of calories from carbohydrates. This is the diet recommended for the general population.
- A more drastic reduction in fat may be appropriate for obese clients trying to lose weight. A diet containing 20% or 25% calories from fat may be reasonable. Ideally, the reduction in total fat would come mostly from saturated fat, so that the beneficial effects of monounsaturated fats are retained.
- A Step Two diet (30% fat, 7% saturated fat, 200 mg cholesterol) may be appropriate for people with a high concentration of low-density lipoprotein (LDL) cholesterol (LDL-C).
- Diabetics with a high level of triglycerides may see a greater improvement in their lipid, glucose, and insulin levels by consuming a fat intake higher than

30% (and correspondingly fewer carbohydrate calories), with the increase in fat coming from monounsaturated fat. This eating style is similar to the Mediterranean Diet explained in Chapter 18. However, if triglyceride levels exceed 1000 mg/dL, limiting all types of fat is recommended.

Limit cholesterol to 300 mg or less to decrease the risk of cardiovascular disease. This recommendation is also consistent with suggestions for cholesterol intake among the general population.

The amount of carbohydrate is not specified. Rigid guidelines recommending that up to 60% of calories be taken from carbohydrate (mostly complex carbohydrate) have been replaced by a more flexible approach that is based on the client's usual intake and laboratory data. More emphasis is placed on consistency in the total amount of carbohydrate consumed than on the type of carbohydrate eaten.

Sucrose can be substituted for other carbohydrates, gram for gram, in the context of a healthy diet. Traditional assumptions that sugar causes diabetics' blood glucose levels to rise too high and too quickly no longer hold true. Studies show that substitution of sucrose for starches as part of a meal plan does not impair blood glucose control for either type 1 or type 2 diabetics. Sucrose and sucrose-containing foods are "allowed," but only when substituted for other carbohydrates in the meal plan, not added as "extras." Many long-standing diabetics resist accepting this shift in thinking. Others find the freedom to choose sweetened foods difficult not to abuse. Even though they do not aggravate glycemic control, foods high in sugar are usually nutrient poor and may be high in fat. People with diabetes are advised to consume sucrose judiciously.

Other nutritive sweeteners are similar to sucrose. Fructose and other sweeteners (eg, honey, molasses, corn syrup, dextrose, maltose) do not have any significant advantage or disadvantage over sucrose. Sugar alcohols (sorbitol, mannitol, and xylitol) cause a smaller increase in glucose than sucrose and other carbohydrates do, but they may cause abdominal gas, discomfort, and osmotic diarrhea when consumed in large amounts.

Nonnutritive sweeteners are safe to use. Saccharin, aspartame, and acesulfame-K are approved for use by the U.S. Food and Drug Administration (FDA) and may safely be used by diabetics.

Eat 20 to 35 g of fiber daily, preferably from a wide variety of foods. The recommendations for fiber are the same as for the general population. Although soluble fiber can delay glucose absorption, the effect of fiber on glycemic control is probably insignificant. However, fiber has other benefits, such as increasing the volume of the diet without increasing the calories (a plus for weight management), providing vitamins and minerals, preventing constipation, and reducing serum cholesterol.

Limit sodium intake to less than 3000 mg/day. Because individual sensitivity to sodium differs and is impractical to assess, sodium intake recommendations are the same for diabetics as for the general population: generally no more than 2400 to 3000 mg. For clients with mild to moderate hypertension, sodium intake should not exceed 2400 mg/day.

Moderate use of alcohol in well-controlled diabetics does not affect blood glucose levels. However, alcohol intake should be limited to two or fewer drinks daily.

Alcohol should be consumed with food, not between meals, because it can cause hypoglycemia. In addition, type 1 diabetics should not reduce their food intake to compensate for alcohol calories. Alcohol should be avoided during pregnancy and lactation and by people who have a history of alcohol abuse.

Vitamin and mineral needs of diabetics are not different from those of the general population. Supplements are not necessary if the diet is adequate. Chromium deficiency is associated with high blood glucose levels, but chromium should not be supplemented unless a deficiency is determined. Likewise, magnesium deficiency increases insulin resistance but magnesium repletion should occur only if a deficiency is clearly demonstrated.

Meal Timing

Control of blood glucose improves when meals and snacks are consistent in number, timing, and relative composition every day. A bedtime snack is especially important to prevent hypoglycemia during the night. People with irregular eating schedules and activity patterns need to learn how to adjust their insulin accordingly. This requires that blood glucose be monitored throughout the day. Consistent meal timing is less important, but still recommended, for clients who receive insulin through a pump or by multiple injections.

Exercise

Exercise is an important aspect of treatment for both types of diabetes, regardless of weight status, unless it is contraindicated for other medical reasons. Exercise has not been shown to improve glycemic control among people with type 1 diabetes, but it imparts other important benefits, such as improving cardiovascular fitness, promoting bone strength, and enhancing the sense of well-being. Important considerations regarding exercise for type 1 diabetes include:

- Achieve metabolic control before exercise. When diabetes is poorly controlled, exercise may worsen hyperglycemia; without adequate insulin, the muscle cannot adequately use glucose, so the liver compensates by producing or releasing stored glucose. Exercise should be avoided if the fasting glucose level exceeds 250 mg/dL and ketosis is present, or if the glucose level is higher than 300 mg/dL regardless of whether ketones are present.
- Monitor blood glucose before and after exercise to determine when changes in food and insulin are necessary. Because exercise lowers the blood glucose level, the optimal time for insulin-dependent diabetics to exercise is within 2 hours after eating; exercise beyond that time is more likely to cause hypoglycemia. Clients should test their blood glucose level before exercising and eat a carbohydrate snack if the level is lower than 100 mg/dL. After exercise, the risk of hypoglycemia continues for up to 24 to 36 hours, because exercise increases insulin sensitivity in muscle.
- Consume adequate additional carbohydrates during and after exercise to prevent hypoglycemia. Although no additional food is needed for light exercise of short

duration, type 1 diabetics may need 10 to 15 g of extra carbohydrate (ie, approximately 1 serving of fruit or starch) for each hour of moderate exercise such as hunting or golfing, and 20 to 30 g of extra carbohydrate (2 servings of fruit or starch) for each hour of vigorous exercise such as digging or playing basketball.

- Be aware that exercise is not without risk, especially in patients with certain diabetic complications. For instance, people with extensive retinopathy are at increased risk of retinal hemorrhage or detachment during certain types of strenuous exercise. Exercise may result in foot injury in patients who have decreased feeling related to peripheral neuropathy.

Managing Acute Complications

Clients who effectively manage their blood glucose levels avoid acute complications. Managing blood glucose levels means that food intake, activity patterns, blood glucose readings, and insulin doses are monitored and adjusted as needed to keep fasting and postprandial glucose levels within acceptable ranges. Clients receiving intensive insulin therapy (three to four insulin doses daily by injections or insulin pump) test their blood glucose levels about four times each day and have their glycosylated hemoglobin level evaluated monthly. Clients receiving standard insulin therapy (insulin once or twice daily) check their blood glucose levels one or two times each day and have their glycosylated hemoglobin level checked three or four times per year. Accurate records identify where adjustments need to be made in insulin or food intake to avoid acute complications of hyperglycemia and hypoglycemia.

Routine Hyperglycemia

Persistent hyperglycemia detected through routine monitoring means that there is an imbalance among food, insulin, and activity. Strategies to correct hyperglycemia that occurs at a particular time of day include reducing carbohydrate content of the previous meal, eliminating or reducing the size of the previous snack, changing the time of the previous meal or snack, increasing activity in the hours before the hyperglycemia is detected, adjusting the previous insulin dose, or a combination of these strategies. The actual intervention used depends on the client's needs, lifestyle, and preferences.

Hyperglycemia Related to Acute Illness

Acute illnesses, even mild ones such as a cold or flu, can significantly raise blood glucose levels. Unless otherwise instructed by the physician, clients should maintain their normal medication schedule, monitoring their blood glucose levels and testing their urine for ketones every 3 to 4 hours. Clients should eat the usual amount of carbohydrate, divided into smaller meals and snacks if necessary. Clients whose blood glucose levels are higher than 250 mg/dL do not need to consume all of their usual carbohydrate intake. If a normal diet is not tolerated, clients should rely on liquids to prevent hypoglycemia and to replenish losses that may occur from vomiting or diarrhea. Generally, 15 g of carbohydrate (ie, one starch, fruit, milk, or other carbohydrate exchange) should be eaten every half-hour, and 1½ cups of fluid should be taken every hour. Each of the following has approximately 15 g of carbohydrate and may be acceptable during illness: 6 ounces regular ginger ale, ½ cup ice cream, ½ cup apple juice, 1 frozen juice bar, ¼ cup sherbet, ½ cup regular gelatin, ½ cup orange juice, 1 cup creamed soup.

Diabetic Ketoacidosis

DKA is a life-threatening medical emergency that requires treatment with insulin, fluids, and electrolytes. An absolute lack of insulin causes severe hyperglycemia and an overproduction of keto acids, which may lead to acidosis. The causes are failure to take any insulin or the correct insulin; excess hormones due to stress related to infection, trauma, or surgery; and insulin deficiency due to excessive counterregulatory hormones produced by the body in response to infection, injury, depression, or anxiety. DKA can be prevented by self-monitoring blood glucose and urine ketones, consuming adequate fluid, controlling vomiting, and taking extra insulin.

Hypoglycemia

Hypoglycemia is often referred to as *insulin reaction*. It occurs from taking too much insulin (or sulfonylureas, but less frequently), inadequate food intake, delayed or skipped meals, extra physical activity, or consumption of alcohol without food. Clients should be advised to carry a readily absorbable source of carbohydrate with them at all times to treat hypoglycemia. Blood glucose levels of 70 mg/dL or less require immediate action.

Treatment for hypoglycemia:

1. Consume 15 g of readily absorbable carbohydrate. This amount should raise blood glucose levels by 50 to 100 mg/dL in 15 to 30 minutes. Any of the following will work:

   4 to 6 ounces or regular soft drink
   4 ounces of orange juice
   2 or 3 glucose tablets (5 g each)
   1 tablespoon of honey
   1 tablespoon of brown sugar
   4 or 5 Life Savers
   5 or 6 large jelly beans

2. Retest blood glucose in 15 minutes. If glucose is at or below 50 to 80 mg/dL, consume another 15 g of carbohydrate.
3. Retest blood glucose in 15 minutes. If glucose is within normal range (80–120 mg/dL) and it is still 1 hour or longer until the next meal or snack, consume another 15 g of carbohydrate.
4. Retest blood glucose and monitor symptoms.

Frequent treatment of hypoglycemia can lead to weight gain. Frequent bouts of hypoglycemia mean that the care plan needs to be revised or the client needs to be counseled to ensure better adherence.

Patients with long-standing diabetes may develop hypoglycemic unawareness. This occurs because the body no longer signals hypoglycemia. Consistent monitoring of blood glucose is especially important for people who are not cognizant of hypoglycemic symptoms.

MANAGEMENT OF TYPE 2 DIABETES

The goal of therapy for type 2 diabetes is to control blood glucose levels to a preprandial range of 80 to 120 mg/dL and a bedtime range of 100 to 140 mg/dL. An additional goal is to maintain glycosylated hemoglobin at less than 7%. These goals are aimed at reducing long-term complications.

The classic hallmarks of type 2 diabetes, insulin resistance and hyperinsulinemia, are part of a group of symptoms that characterize **insulin resistance syndrome,** also known as **syndrome X.** Other features of syndrome X are abnormal blood lipid levels, obesity, hypertension, and cardiovascular disease, all of which contribute to morbidity in type 2 diabetes. Ironically, optimal control of blood glucose levels often leads to weight gain, which leads to hyperglycemia and ultimately to greater insulin resistance. Conversely, weight loss in type 2 diabetics improves insulin resistance and glucose tolerance. Even though nutrition therapy and exercise are capable of controlling glucose levels for the majority of type 2 diabetics, most clients require medication because of poor compliance with nutrition and exercise regimens.

Nutrition Therapy

Nutrition therapy goals are to provide a nutritionally adequate meal plan that achieves and maintains reasonable weight, results in normal blood cholesterol levels, and controls blood glucose levels. Meal spacing is an important aspect to prevent large swings in the blood glucose concentration. Except for the differences noted in this section, nutrient recommendations are the same for type 1 and type 2 diabetics.

Weight Loss

Weight loss has traditionally been the focus of nutritional intervention for type 2 diabetics. Clinical symptoms may be immediately improved by a low-calorie diet, and even a mild to moderate weight loss (eg, 10–20 pounds) can lower blood glucose levels and help reverse insulin resistance. Other potential benefits of weight loss include an improvement in blood lipid levels and lowered blood pressure. Even though long-term weight loss is seldom achieved, overweight clients should be encouraged to lose weight.

There is no one proven strategy that can be uniformly recommended to promote weight loss in all clients. For instance, a modest calorie restriction (250–500 fewer calories than usual daily intake) that allows for a gradual loss of ½ to 1 pound/week is recommended but may not be accepted by all patients. Some people prefer to follow a low-fat diet (ie, 20% of total calories); this may be an effective alternative to produce weight loss and improve blood glucose and lipid levels. For others, very-low-calorie diets may be used to improve blood glucose and lipid levels, even though the weight loss they promote is rarely maintained. Clients who are resistant to weight loss by traditional dietary, exercise, and behavioral modification methods may be candidates for gastric surgery or drug therapy. Data on the long-term safety and efficacy of surgery and drug therapy are unavailable.

Nutrient Recommendations

Studies suggest that the most beneficial distribution of carbohydrate and fat calories for people with type 2 diabetes may be 40% carbohydrate and 45% fat, with 10% of calories from saturated fat, 10% from polyunsaturated fat, and 25% from monounsaturated fat. This distribution, similar to the Mediterranean Diet, results in lower blood glucose and insulin levels after meals, lowers daylong triglyceride levels, and may improve high-density lipoprotein (HDL) cholesterol (HDL-C) levels.

Meal Spacing

Meal spacing should also be a consideration for type 2 diabetics. Eating meals 4 to 5 hours apart allows postprandial glucose levels to return to baseline. Type 2 diabetics may maintain appropriate blood glucose levels and maximize drug effectiveness by eating meals of approximately the same composition at approximately the same time every day.

Alcohol

Because alcohol provides empty calories, it should be avoided by people who are trying to lose weight. Others who should avoid alcohol are people with high triglyceride levels, pregnant or lactating women, and people with a history of alcohol abuse. Type 2 diabetics who choose to use alcohol should substitute alcohol for fat calories (eg, substitute 1 alcoholic beverage for 2 fat exchanges).

Exercise

Exercise offers substantial benefits for people with type 2 diabetes. Regular exercise improves blood glucose control independent of weight loss. It also reduces insulin resistance, improves blood lipid levels, improves blood pressure, and enhances sense of well-being and quality of life. Exercise helps maintain long-term weight reduction. It is recommended that type 2 diabetics exercise at least 3 days/week for 20 to 45 minutes at 50% to 70% of maximal heart rate. Like type 1 diabetics, type 2 diabetics who are treated with oral hypoglycemic agents or insulin may experience exercise-induced hypoglycemia. Clients should be encouraged to monitor their blood glucose levels, exercise within 2 hours after eating, and stop activity if signs and symptoms of hypoglycemia develop.

Drug Therapy

Drug therapy is used to help manage type 2 diabetes when exercise and nutrition therapy fail to achieve glycemic control. Drugs are used in addition to, not in place of, diet and exercise. Drug therapy begins with oral agents. Thirty percent to 40% of type 2 diabetics eventually use insulin to help control their blood glucose levels. Paradoxically, sulfonylureas and insulin tend to promote weight gain, which leads to greater insulin resistance. Newer drugs make weight stabilization achievable.

Oral Agents

The type of drug prescribed depends on the patient's fasting and postprandial glucose levels, body weight, and response to therapy. Because each class of oral agents works by a different mechanism to help reduce blood glucose levels, combinations of oral agents are often prescribed. They vary in duration of action, dose response, and side effects. Sometimes, after a few months or years of use, a previously effective drug will fail to work.

Sulfonylureas stimulate pancreatic beta cells to produce more insulin. Because insulin is increased, weight gain, hypoglycemia, and hyperinsulinemia are risks. Sulfonylureas may be used as monotherapy or in combination with other drugs. Brand names in this class include Diabinese, Amaryl, Glucotrol, DiaBeta, Micronase, Tolinase, and Orinase. Although they all have a similar effect on blood glucose levels, they differ in their side effects and in how often they need to be taken.

The biguanide metformin (brand name Glucophage) is the only drug in this class marketed in the United States. It works by suppressing the liver's release of glucose by increasing the sensitivity of liver cells to the action of insulin. It also increases satiety and reduces food intake. Because insulin levels are not increased, weight gain and hypoglycemia are not a problem when metformin is used alone. When used with a sulfonylurea, the drug combination has the potential to control glucose levels without promoting weight gain and hyperinsulinemia. Diarrhea, a common side effect, is lessened when the drug is taken with food.

Thiazolidinediones increase tissue sensitivity to insulin. They are taken once or twice daily with food. Troglitazone (brand name Rezulin), the first drug in this class approved for use in the United States, was removed from the market in March 2000, at the request of the FDA after confirmed reports of severe liver failure and death related to its use. Two other drugs in this class, rosiglitazone (Avandia) and pioglitazone (Actos), are purported to be less toxic than troglitazone. Regular monitoring of liver function is recommended. Thiazolidinediones may be used alone or in combination with insulin, a sulfonylurea, or metformin.

Alpha-glycosidase inhibitors marketed in the United States are acarbose (Precose) and glyset (Miglitol). They delay the absorption of glucose. They are used with other oral agents or insulin. Because they are taken three times daily at the start of meals, poor compliance is a concern. Gas and diarrhea are common side effects.

Meglitinides (repaglinide, brand name Prandin) works like sulfonylureas to stimulate the release of insulin from pancreatic beta cells. Unlike other oral agents, repaglinide works very quickly. It is taken with each meal or up to 30 minutes before mealtime. Because it is gone from the bloodstream in 3 to 4 hours, it does not raise insulin levels over a long period.

Insulin

Patients who are unable to achieve glycemic control with maximum doses of oral agents allowed may be prescribed insulin. Often the use of oral agents continues so that the exogenous insulin requirement is minimized. Insulin is also frequently used to control glucose levels in hospitalized type 2 diabetics who have hyperglycemia related to infection or illness.

A problem with using insulin to treat type 2 diabetes is that it tends to exacerbate hyperinsulinemia. Exogenous insulin increases the risk of hypoglycemia, stimulates appetite, promotes weight gain, and aggravates insulin resistance, leading to an even greater need for insulin. Despite the potentially negative effects of using insulin, it continues to be used in the treatment of type 2 diabetes when it is the only means to achieve glycemic control.

Managing Acute Complications

Hyperglycemic Hyperosmolar Nonketotic Syndrome

HHNS is a serious condition that develops mostly in older adults and people receiving total parenteral nutrition or peritoneal dialysis. Blood glucose levels are greater than 600 mg/dL and may be as high as 2000 mg/dL. Ketones usually are not elevated. Dehydration is often a precipitating cause, and polyuria is common for weeks or days before HHNS occurs. Normally, adequate fluid intake promotes excretion of some excess glucose, keeping blood levels lower than 500 mg/dL. But when fluid intake is inadequate, especially over a period of weeks, blood glucose levels rise rapidly. Treatment involves replacing fluids and administering insulin. The increased risk of excessive clotting is blamed for the high mortality rate associated with HHNS. Most people who recover have no residual problems controlling their blood glucose levels.

Hypoglycemia

Hypoglycemia in type 2 diabetics can occur in people treated with insulin or, to a lesser extent, in those taking oral hypoglycemics. The treatment is the same as that for hypoglycemia in type 1 diabetics.

THE PROCESS OF LIFESTYLE CHANGE

The diagnosis of diabetes often triggers anxiety, uncertainty, and resentment. Patients often see "diet" as the most difficult part of treatment. Even people with healthy eating styles may need to make changes in their intake to improve glycemic control. Effective nutrition therapy encompasses assessment, establishment of goals, institution of appropriate interventions, and evaluation of outcomes.

Assessment

Nutrition therapy for diabetes is assessment-based. Assessment data not only identify problems but also reveal positive eating and activity habits that should be reinforced. A thorough assessment takes into consideration all medical and lifestyle data.

Anthropometric data. What is the patient's weight status based on body mass index (BMI)? Is the patient's weight stable? What is the patient's blood pressure?

Biochemical data. What are the patient's glucose, glycosylated hemoglobin, cholesterol, LDL-C, HDL-C, and triglyceride levels? Does the patient self-monitor glucose levels?

Clinical data. Does the patient have an "apple" or a "pear" shape?

Dietary data. What is the patient's understanding about the relationship between diet and diabetes? Has the patient been counseled regarding a diabetic diet before, and if so, what was the outcome? Is the patient's usual intake adequate? What is its relative composition (eg, proportion of carbohydrate, protein, and fat)? Does the patient consistently eat at regular times? Does the patient use sugar-free or "dietetic" products? Does the patient frequently eat out? Can the patient identify foods he or she is not willing to give up? Does the patient use alcohol? Does the patient have food allergies or intolerances? Does the patient read food labels? Does the patient shop and cook for food? What nutritional supplements does the patient use and for what purpose? Is the patient willing to change his or her eating habits? What obstacles can the client identify that may hinder dietary adherence? For instance, does the client:

- Overeat to cope with stress and negative emotions?
- Have difficulty resisting temptation when faced with food, food cues, or cravings?
- Feel deprived by nutrition therapy?
- Feel that time pressures and a hectic lifestyle make it difficult to eat right?
- Feel tempted to give up after a relapse?
- Have competing responsibilities and obligations that get in the way of eating right?
- Overeat and make poor food choices when tempted at parties and other social events?
- Lack support from family and friends?

Medical socioeconomic data. Does the patient have physical complaints? Does the patient have other medical conditions that benefit from nutrition therapy, such as hypertension? Does the patient have diabetes complications, such as renal impairment or gastroparesis? Is the patient taking insulin and/or oral agents? Does the patient use tobacco or recreational drugs? Does the patient use any medication that interferes with glucose management (Box 19–1)? Is the patient em-

BOX 19.1

Drugs That Commonly Interfere With Blood Glucose Control

Potentiates Hypoglycemia

Alcohol
Allopurinol (Lopurin)
Anticholinergics, such as dicyclomine (Bentyl)
Beta-adrenergic antagonists, such as atenolol (Tenormin) and metoprolol (Lopressor)
Clofibrate (Novofibrate)
Haloperidol (Haldol)
H_2-receptor antagonists, such as cimetidine (Tagamet) and ranitidine (Zantac)
Monoamine oxidase inhibitors, such as phenelzine sulfate (Nardil)
Salicylates, such as aspirin
Sulfonamides, such as trimethoprim/sulfamethoxazole (TMP/SMX; Bactrim)

Potentiates Hyperglycemia

Corticosteroids, such as prednisone (Deltasone)
Diuretics, such as furosemide (Lasix) and all thiazide diuretics
Epinephrine (Primatene Mist)
Estrogens
Niacin (Vitamin B_3)
Phenothiazines, such as chlorpromazine (Thorazine)
Phenytoin (Dilantin)
Rifampin (Rifadin)
Sympathomimetics, such as theophylline (Theolair, Theobid)

ployed? Is the patient's food budget adequate? What cultural, religious, or ethnic influences affect the patient's food choices? Does the patient exercise regularly? If so, how frequently and at what intensity?

Establishing Goals

Goals provide a gauge upon which success is measured. Therefore goals must be realistic, achievable, and measurable. Goals that are mutually agreed on between the health care team and client give the client more responsibility in "owning" the goal and, therefore, a greater commitment to achieving the goal. Goals may be directed at clinical or metabolic parameters, such as weight, glucose, and lipid levels, or lifestyle changes, such as specific behaviors related to eating, physical activity, or blood glucose monitoring.

The role of the health care team is to negotiate goals that meet the client's needs and capabilities. Questions that may help establish goals include:

- What do you want from nutrition counseling?
- What behaviors do you want to change?
- What changes can you make in your present lifestyle?

- What obstacles may prevent you from making changes?
- What changes are you willing to make right now?
- What changes would be difficult for you to make?

Appropriate Interventions

Goals can best be met by providing information in stages, beginning with basic information and progressing to details as information is not only understood but also assimilated. Some clients may never progress beyond basic information—which is fine, as long as goals are met. The types of teaching and intervention strategies used depends on the client's:

- Ability and willingness to learn
- Level of motivation to change eating habits
- Preferred learning style
- Education level
- Nutrition goals
- Drug therapy (if any)
- Activity level
- Lifestyle—work or school schedule, eating habits, financial factors, and social factors

Basic Information

Basic information includes an overview of nutrition and nutrient requirements and an explanation of both the role of diet in the treatment of diabetes and the importance of meal timing and consistency. Survival skill information, such as how to treat hypoglycemia and sick day management, must also be conveyed. Teaching tools available for providing basic information are *The First Step in Diabetes Meal Planning, Healthy Food Choices*, and single-topic handouts.

THE FIRST STEP IN DIABETES MEAL PLANNING

The First Step in Diabetes Meal Planning, published by the American Dietetic Association and the American Diabetes Association, is a trifold brochure that opens to a poster of the diabetes Food Guide Pyramid. The food groups depicted in this guide are based on the exchange list food groupings, which differ slightly from the standard Food Guide Pyramid. For instance, cheese is found in the Meat group instead of the Milk group, and nuts are located in the Fats, Sweets, and Alcohol category instead of the Meat group. Basic meal planning guidelines are provided, as are tips for changing eating behaviors within each food group and general serving sizes from each group.

This resource is essentially a self-teaching education tool that is often used to begin the nutrition education process until the client can see a dietitian. It may be the only meal planning tool used for clients who need or want only basic and simple nutrition guidance. Because it is written at about a sixth-grade reading level, this tool is easy to understand. A drawback to using this resource is that it does not address control of specific nutrients, such as carbohydrates, fat, or calories.

HEALTHY FOOD CHOICES

Healthy Food Choices, also published by the American Dietetic Association and the American Diabetes Association, is a pamphlet that promotes healthful eating by providing nutrition guidelines and a simplified exchange system that uses the term "choices" instead of "exchanges" and features simplified portion sizes with each group. It offers an overview of nutrition therapy for diabetes within a basic framework. Like the *First Steps* tool, this resource may be used to initiate the diabetes education process or it may be the only tool used for clients who want or need only basic, simple information.

This tool is easy to understand and concise. The primary disadvantage of this tool is that two nutrition education approaches are featured in the pamphlet (nutrition guidelines and the simplified exchange system). Clients for whom one approach is appropriate may be confused if both approaches are introduced at the same time. Assessment should identify the most appropriate approach to teaching nutrition and meal planning.

SINGLE-TOPIC RESOURCES

A variety of single-topic handouts are available from the American Dietetic Association and the American Diabetes Association. Titles include "Eating Out: From Burgers to Burritos," "Portions: How Much Is Enough?," "When You Just Can't Eat," and "Children and Diabetes." The handouts are interactive and allow individualization of the content and teaching process. They can be used alone or as a supplement to other resources.

These single-topic resources allow the educator to focus on the specific information of interest to the client. A major advantage to using these tools is that assessment, goal setting, interventions, and evaluation are integrated into the layout and design of the resource. For instance, each handout begins with a simple section ("What About You?") in which clients answer questions regarding their knowledge and behaviors (assessment). The goal-setting section ("Set Your Sights") enables clients to set behavior goals related to the topic. The section entitled "Here's the Challenge; What's Your Solution?" promotes problem solving using examples of situations the client may face. The disadvantage of using these handouts is that only basic information is provided.

In-Depth Interventions

Some clients progress from basic information to more in-depth information that provides more structure to meal planning and more information on macronutrients and calories to facilitate meal planning. Three in-depth approaches are menu approaches, exchanges lists, and carbohydrate counting.

MENU APPROACH

In the menu approach, the dietitian works with the client to develop a set of menus that reflect the client's nutritional needs and prescription and his or her usual intake pattern and preferences. The menus may specify exactly what, when, and how much the client is to eat at each meal and snack, or they may give the client some food choices. This approach is often used to supplement other teaching aids, and frequently hospital patients save their menus to use as a guide for meal planning after discharge. The menu approach may be used for either type 1 or type 2 diabetics, and it is best suited for people who have relatively routine eating habits, have difficulty making healthy food choices, and want to be told what and how much to eat.

The advantages of the menu approach are that it is simple and the menus are individualized for the client. However, this approach is too restrictive and monotonous for some people, and the menus are not intended to be used indefinitely.

EXCHANGE LISTS

The guide *Exchange Lists for Meal Planning* groups foods into three major categories: Carbohydrates, Meat and Meat Substitutes, and Fats (Table 19–1). Subgroups within each major category form the exchange lists. Portion sizes are specified so that each serving within a list contains approximately the same amount of carbohydrates, protein, fat, and calories (see Appendix 8).

Exchange lists simplify meal planning, eliminate the need for daily calculations, ensure a consistent and nutritionally balanced diet, and add variety. However, the exchange lists may not be appropriate or acceptable for all age, ethnic, and cultural groups, and individual adjustments may be vital for compliance. Characteristics of the exchange lists are as follows:

- The Carbohydrate category contains five exchange lists: starch, fruit, milk, other carbohydrates, and vegetables. With the exception of the vegetables list, all other

TABLE 19.1 ***Exchanges***

Groups/Lists	Carbohydrate (grams)	Protein (grams)	Fat (grams)	Calories
Carbohydrate Group				
Starch	15	3	1 or less	80
Fruit	15	—	—	60
Milk				
Skim	12	8	0–3	90
Low-fat	12	8	5	120
Whole	12	8	8	150
Other carbohydrates	15	varies	varies	varies
Vegetables	5	2	—	25
Meat and Meat Substitute Group				
Very lean	—	7	0–1	35
Lean	—	7	3	55
Medium-fat	—	7	5	75
High-fat	—	7	8	100
Fat Group	—	—	5	45

lists within the carbohydrate group contain approximately the same amount of carbohydrate and can generally be substituted for one another.

- The Meat and meat substitute category is divided into four groups based on fat content. All four groups provide the same amount of protein and no carbohydrates.
- The Fat category supplies only fat. It is divided into three sublists based on the predominate type of fat: monounsaturated fats, polyunsaturated fats, and saturated fats.
- With the exception of the starch, fruit, milk, and other carbohydrates exchanges, items from one list cannot be exchanged for items in a different exchange list (eg, 1 cup of milk can be exchanged for 1 serving of fruit, but not for 1 serving of meat or fat).
- Portion sizes are important; weigh or measure food until portion sizes can be estimated accurately.
- The number of servings allowed from each exchange list depends on the calorie content and composition of the diet and corresponds as closely as possible to the client's preferences and food habits.
- Meal patterns specify the number of servings from each exchange list allowed for each meal and snack (Box 19–2). Glycemic control is improved when exchanges are not "saved" from one meal to use at another, especially for clients who are taking insulin or oral agents.
- Certain foods and beverages are considered "free" because they provide less than 5 g of carbohydrate or less than 20 cal per serving. Some of these items have serving sizes specified; those choices should be limited to 3 servings per day, preferably spread out over the course of the day. Items without a portion size, such as sugar substitutes, may be used as desired.
- A combination foods list gives examples of how mixed dishes can be calculated into a meal plan; components are identified and then classified according to their representative exchange lists. For instance, one-fourth of a 10-inch thin-crust pizza is listed as 2 starch exchanges (the crust), 2 medium-fat meat exchanges (the cheese), and 1 fat exchange (oil in and on the crust).
- Fast foods are also calculated into a meal plan according to their composition. For instance, one medium submarine sandwich is listed as 3 starch exchanges (the roll), 1 vegetable exchange (lettuce, tomato, onion), 2 medium-fat meat exchanges (2 ounces of luncheon meats), and 1 fat exchange (oil or mayonnaise).
- The exchange list approach is best suited to people who want or need structured meal-planning guidance and are able to understand complex details. Some clients progress from using the exchange lists to carbohydrate counting. Major advantages of this approach are the consistency in intake and the emphasis on important nutrition principles, such as limiting and modifying fat and controlling sodium intake. The concept of exchanging may not be understood by all clients.

CARBOHYDRATE COUNTING

Carbohydrate counting is a relatively new meal planning approach that offers an alternative to the use of traditional exchange lists. Resulting from advances in diabetes manage-

BOX 19.2

Sample Meal Plan

Meal Plan for: ______________________ Date: ______________
Dietitian: ______________________ Phone: ______________

	Grams	Percent
Carbohydrate	222	50
Protein	88	20
Fat	59	30
Calories	1771	___

Time	Number of Exchanges/Choices	Menu Ideas	Menu Ideas
8:00	4 Carbohydrate group		
	2 Starch	2 slices wheat toast	2 waffles (2 starch plus 2 fat)
	1 Fruit	½ cup orange juice	½ grapefruit
	1 Milk	1 cup skim milk	1 cup skim milk
	0 Meat group		
	2 Fat group	2 tsp margarine	
		2 tsp low-sugar jelly (free)	2 tbsp sugar-free syrup (free)
Snack			
12:00	4 Carbohydrate group		
	3 Starch	1 cup tomato soup (1 starch) 1 hamburger roll (2 starch)	2 slices bread ½ cup sugar-free low-fat pudding
	1 Fruit	1 small banana	1 cup cantaloupe cubes
	___ Milk		
	✓ Vegetables	1 cup tossed salad	½ cup tomato juice
	3 oz Meat group	3 oz lean hamburger patty (3 med-fat)	3 oz smoked turkey breast
	2 Fat group	2 tbsp salad dressing (2 fat)	2 tsp regular mayonnaise
		1 tbsp ketchup (free)	
6:00	5 Carbohydrate group		
	4 Starch	⅓ cup rice ½ cup sweet potato ½ cup peas 1 plain small dinner roll } 4 starch	1½ cups tuna noodle casserole (3 starch, 3 meat) 1 dinner roll (1 starch)
	1 Fruit	1¼ cup strawberries	1 sliced kiwi fruit
	___ Milk		
	✓ Vegetables	½ cup wax beans	½ cup cooked carrots
	3 oz Meat group	3 oz skinless chicken breast (lean)	
	2 Fat group	2 tsp margarine	2 tsp margarine
Snack	1 cup skim milk 1 starch 1 fat	1 cup skim milk 3 cups microwave popcorn (1 starch plus one fat)	1 cup nonfat yogurt sweetened with aspartame 6 butter-type crackers (1 starch, 1 fat)

ment, carbohydrate counting is based on the premise that a carbohydrate is a carbohydrate is a carbohydrate. Emphasis is on consuming a consistent quantity of total carbohydrate, not restricting the type of carbohydrate, as the main priority in establishing glycemic control. This is because published studies indicate no adverse effect when sucrose is substituted for other carbohydrates within the context of a meal plan.

Although carbohydrate counting has the advantage of focusing on a single nutrient (carbohydrates) rather than all the energy-yielding nutrients, protein and fat cannot be disregarded, especially if weight is a concern. Because of its greater flexibility, this method allows the client to feel more in control and offers the potential for improved glucose control. On the minus side, carbohydrate counting requires clients to keep food records initially and periodically, and they must also record blood glucose levels before and after eating. Weighing and measuring foods may be seen as a disadvantage by some clients. In addition, the goals of weight control and healthful eating may be forgotten or forsaken when the emphasis is placed solely on carbohydrate.

The three levels of carbohydrate counting are outlined in Table 19–2.

Evaluating Outcomes

Evaluation reveals which interventions were effective and which were not. It is a continuous and cyclic process that allows for reassessment of the client, new or refined goals, and new or refined interventions. Evaluation is similar to follow-up.

BEHAVIORAL SKILLS

To manage diabetes effectively, clients need not only declarative knowledge (eg, nutrition facts, such as the fact that milk contains carbohydrates) but also procedural knowledge (eg, how to use those facts to make better choices). Behavioral skills are procedural knowledge.

TABLE 19.2 *Three Levels of Carbohydrate Counting*

Level	Goal	Intended Audience
Level I: Getting Started	Carbohydrate consistency, flexible food choices	Type 1, type 2, gestational diabetics
Level II: Moving On	Adjustment of medication/food/activities based on patterns from client's daily records	Any diabetic (diet only, oral agents, type 1) who has mastered the basics of level I
Level III: Intensive Diabetes Management Using Carbohydrate/Insulin Ratios—Advanced	Adjustment of insulin dose using ratio of carbohydrate/insulin dosage	Clients receiving intensive insulin therapy; clients who have mastered insulin adjustment and supplementation

Tips for Eating Out

Clients eating outside the home need to be mindful of portion sizes and methods of food preparation. At fast food restaurants, regular-size burgers, grilled chicken sandwiches, baked potatoes, and chili are good choices. Ketchup, mustard, relish, lettuce, and tomato should replace "special sauces." At better restaurants:

- Choose tomato juice, unsweetened fruit juice, clear broth, bouillon, consommé, or shrimp cocktail as an appetizer instead of sweetened juices, fried vegetables, or creamed or thick soups.
- Choose fresh vegetable salads and use oil and vinegar or fresh lemon instead of regular salad dressings, or request that the dressing be put on the side. Avoid coleslaw and other salads that have the dressing already added.
- Order plain (without gravy or sauce) roasted, baked, or broiled meat, fish, and poultry instead of fried, sautéed, or breaded entrees. Avoid stews and casseroles. Request a doggie bag if the portion exceeds the meal plan allowance.
- Order steamed, boiled, or broiled vegetables.
- Choose plain, baked, mashed, boiled, or steamed potatoes, rice, or noodles.
- Select fresh fruit for dessert.
- Request a sugar substitute for coffee or tea, if desired.

Tips for Food Preparation

The client's food does not have to be prepared separately from the rest of the family's. Portion sizes are important. Cooking methods that do not add fat, such as baking, broiling, roasting, and boiling, are preferred to frying. Diabetic cookbooks specify portion sizes and nutritional analysis and can add variety to meal planning.

Tips on Food Purchasing and Label Reading

Studies show that women use nutrition information on food labels when deciding what foods to buy. The more confident they are in their ability to read food labels, the greater the chance that they will make appropriate food purchases. Therefore it is important to teach people, especially women, about how to read food labels.

A big area of confusion is the claims on food labels, such as "low fat" and "good source of fiber." Clients need assurance that these claims are defined by labeling laws and are reliable. Another misconception regards the sugar content listed on the Nutrition Facts label. Clients need to know that the value listed includes both natural and added sugars. For instance, milk, which has 12 g of sugar per 8-oz serving, appears to be a "high sugar" food, but the "sugar" is lactose that is present naturally, not added sucrose. Clients also need to know that:

- Fresh, frozen (without sugar), and water-packed canned fruits are preferable, but sweetened canned fruit is acceptable if it is rinsed under running water for at least 1 minute to remove the sugary syrup.

- Sugar goes by many names on the ingredient list, such as high-fructose corn syrup, invert sugar, sorghum, dextrose, and maltose.
- Sugar alcohols, such as sorbitol and xylitol, can cause diarrhea in large amounts.
- Dietetic products are not necessarily calorie-free or specifically intended for diabetics. Foods that are labeled "dietetic" may be made without sugar, without salt, with a particular type of fat, or for special food allergies. Read the ingredient label and check with a diet counselor before adding a dietetic food to the diet—or avoid dietetic foods altogether, because they are expensive and usually do not taste as good as the foods they are intended to replace.
- Ingredients are listed in descending order by weight. Therefore, foods that list sugar near the beginning of the ingredient list may be high in sugar (the exception is when foods contain few ingredients).

LIFE CYCLE CONSIDERATIONS

Diabetes nutrition therapy can influence growth and development in children and adolescents, the outcome of pregnancy, and the quality of life in older adults. Special considerations for each group are presented here.

Children and Adolescents

Complicating the management of diabetes in children and adolescents are their increased nutritional needs related to growth. Compared with adults, children and adolescents have more erratic eating and activity behaviors. Nutrition therapy for children is the same for adults, but children require more frequent adjustments in insulin and food intake to compensate for growth and activity needs. Failure to provide adequate calories and nutrients results in poor growth, as does poor glycemic control and inadequate insulin administration. Conversely, excessive weight gain occurs from excessive calorie intake, overtreatment of hypoglycemia, or excess insulin administration. Other unique features among this life cycle group are as follows:

The stage of growth and development must be assessed. The rate of physical and emotional development varies greatly among children and adolescents. Age-based assumptions may not be reliable or valid. Assessment questions to consider include the following: Is the child responsible for any or all of his or her diabetes management? Does the child feed himself or herself? Does the child's routine and activity expenditure differ on weekdays and on the weekend? What is the child's school schedule? What is the child's social life? Are school lunches eaten? Does the child have food jags or use food to manipulate parents? If the child does not attend school, who is the primary caretaker during the day?

Children with diabetes are still children. They may not care what effect food has on blood glucose, only that it tastes good. Conversely, children are often finicky eaters and are not likely to eat foods simply because they "should."

Social situations involving eating may be more stressful. Peer pressure and not wanting to be different from others can make social occasions a problem for children. Teachers should be aware of the diagnosis of diabetes, know the signs and symptoms of hypoglycemia, and know how to treat it. Parents should have advance warning of school parties so that party foods can be incorporated into the day's food plan. Diabetic children who go on sleepovers should test their blood glucose levels before the party. The host parent should be educated about hypoglycemia and appropriate snacks.

Goals may be less stringent. "Good control" for children and adolescents is defined more liberally than for adults. Higher glucose levels are considered acceptable to prevent hypoglycemia.

Changes occur more frequently. More frequent monitoring and evaluation are needed to adjust for physical, emotional, and social changes.

Their future is longer. Generally, the initial approach is more structured. It is easier to introduce flexibility into a structured plan than to add structure to a flexible plan.

Pregnancy

Pregnancy causes insulin levels to rise, affects insulin resistance, and causes erratic glucose levels. Hypoglycemia is common during the first trimester, and hyperglycemia occurs during the second and third trimesters. Spontaneous abortion and pregnancy-induced hypertension are risks. Women with diabetes tend to have bigger babies (macrosomia), probably as a result of high glucose levels. After about 13 weeks' gestation, babies produce their own insulin: high glucose levels in the mother lead to increased fetal insulin secretion, which acts as a growth hormone to stimulate fat deposition. Hyperglycemia also increases the risk of birth defects, especially during the first few weeks of pregnancy. Other risks to the infant include life-threatening hypoglycemia and respiratory distress syndrome.

Preconception counseling, early prenatal care, and ongoing counseling throughout pregnancy are needed to help maintain glycemic control. Most women need 2000 to 2400 cal of approximately 45% to 50% carbohydrate, 20% protein, and 30% to 35% fat. This percentage of carbohydrates, slightly lower than what is recommended for nonpregnant diabetics, is to help limit the rise in blood glucose between meals. Snacks are important, especially before bedtime. The bedtime snack should provide carbohydrate, protein, and fat to help sustain blood glucose levels throughout the night. Some women may need a snack during the night, such as a glass of milk, to prevent morning hypoglycemia.

Gestational diabetes is diabetes that occurs only during pregnancy and is usually resolved after delivery. However, many women with gestational diabetes develop type 2 diabetes later in life. Women with gestational diabetes should avoid excessive weight gain during pregnancy and should maintain a reasonable weight thereafter. They should establish a regular eating pattern of three meals with two to three snacks, including a bedtime snack; monitor their blood glucose levels as directed; and make healthy food choices. To prevent midmorning hyperglycemia, fruit and fruit juices should be avoided at breakfast.

Diabetes in Later Life

There are unique considerations related to aging that affect glycemic control. First, blood glucose levels rise with age, for reasons that are unclear. Treatment may not be instituted for glucose elevations that are considered "high" in younger populations but may be "normal" for the elderly. Cognitive impairments, such as memory loss, impaired concentration, dementia, and depression, may preclude self-management. Physical impairments may impede exercise. Sensory impairments, such as decreased hearing, poor eyesight, and decreased senses of taste and smell, may complicate teaching and self-management. For instance, older clients who could clinically benefit from insulin may be treated instead with oral agents if poor eyesight or decreased manual dexterity precludes self-injection. Older adults may be at greater nutritional risk for a variety of reasons, including poor dentition, physical impairments that make shopping or cooking difficult, poor appetite related to lack of socialization, and an inadequate food budget. For many, a strict calorie-controlled diet is more harmful than beneficial. Because older adults are more susceptible to severe hypoglycemia, a fasting target level of 120 to 150 mg/dL may be considered appropriate.

To maximize teaching effectiveness in an older adult:

- Keep teaching sessions short.
- Relay only as much information as necessary.
- Go slowly and summarize frequently.
- Minimize distractions.
- Include a spouse or family member.
- Speak clearly; face clients who have a hearing impairment.
- Use appropriate written materials; do not overload the client with information that is nice to know but not essential.
- Ask the clients to write down skills or procedures (eg, insulin injection, home glucose monitoring) in their own words.

DIABETIC DIETS IN THE HOSPITAL

Traditionally, standardized meal plans based on the exchange lists have been used to provide "diabetic" diets to hospitalized diabetics. The physician would order a specific-calorie-level "ADA diet" that was composed of specific percentages of carbohydrate, protein, and fat. Because the ADA (American Diabetes Association) no longer endorses any single meal plan or specified nutrient composition, it is recommended that this term and approach no longer be used.

Also considered obsolete are "no concentrated sweets," "no sugar added," "low sugar," and "liberal diabetic" diets. They do not reflect the diabetes nutrient recommendations and unnecessarily restrict sugar. These diets may give patients the false impression that glycemic control is achieved by limiting sugar.

A suggested alternative to the traditional "ADA diet" is a consistent-carbohydrate meal plan. In this approach, calories are not specified, but carbohydrate intake is consistent; that is, breakfast supplies approximately the same amount of carbohydrate each day, lunch is likewise consistent from day to day, and so is dinner. A typical day's intake from meals and snacks may range from 1500 to 2000 cal, with adjustments made for individual patients as needed. Appropriate modifications in fat intake are made, and consistent timing of meals and snacks is stressed. However, just as there is no longer one diabetic diet, neither is there one correct way to provide nutrition therapy to hospitalized diabetics.

Diabetics are no longer admitted to the hospital for diabetes management and education. Hospital stays are shorter, and patients tend to be sicker. For these reasons, diabetes self-management education, including nutrition therapy counseling, is usually best provided in an outpatient or home setting. In the acute care setting there is neither the time nor the resources to completely teach diabetes management.

Additional recommendations for hospitalized diabetics are as follows:

- Patients given clear or full liquid diets should receive approximately 200 g of carbohydrate per day in equally divided amounts at meals and snacks. Sugar-free liquids should not be used. Adjustments in diabetes medications may be needed to achieve glycemic control.
- Food intake should be progressed as soon as possible after surgery, with the goal of providing adequate carbohydrates and calories.
- Continuous monitoring is needed during catabolic illnesses to ensure that nutritional needs are met and hyperglycemia is prevented. Overfeeding exacerbates hyperglycemia.
- Enteral formulas with standard or lower carbohydrate content may be used for patients with diabetes. Both require glucose monitoring so that adjustments can be made in glucose-lowering medications as needed.

NURSING PROCESS

Mrs. Wilson is a 69-year-old woman referred to a home health agency for a home visit to provide nutrition/diabetes education. When she was diagnosed with diabetes 5 years ago, the doctor told her to avoid sugar and take DiaBeta twice a day. She is 5 feet 2 inches tall and weighs 185 pounds.

Assessment

Obtain clinical data:

Current BMI; recent weight history

Medical history and comorbidities, including hyperlipidemia, hypertension, cardiovascular disease, renal impairments, neuropathy, and gastrointestinal complaints

Abnormal laboratory values, especially fasting blood glucose, glycosylated hemoglobin, total cholesterol, LDL-C, HDL-C, triglycerides, and albumin

Record of blood glucose monitoring

Blood pressure measurement

Medications taken that affect nutrition, such as insulin, other oral agents, lipid-lowering medications, cardiac drugs, antihypertensives, and anticoagulants

Interview the client to assess:

Understanding of the relationship between food, exercise, and blood glucose levels

Ability to understand, attitude toward health and nutrition, and readiness to learn

Motivation to change eating style; how she implemented the "avoid sugar" advice. For instance, did she simply not use sugar in her tea, or did she also know that cakes, cookies, pies, and candy are sources of sugar?

Usual 24-hour intake, including portion sizes, frequency and pattern of eating, method of food preparation, intake of high-fat foods, intake of high-sugar foods, use of salt and salty foods. Determine whether mealtimes are relatively consistent or variable from day to day.

Appropriateness of usual calorie intake and overall nutritional adequacy. Assess types of carbohydrate, protein, and fat usually consumed. Assess usual intake of foods high in fiber, especially soluble fiber, such as oats, oat bran, and dried peas and beans.

Cultural, religious, and ethnic influences on eating habits

Psychosocial and economic issues, such as the living situation, cooking facilities, adequacy of food budget, education, need for food assistance, and level of family and social support

Usual activity patterns; willingness and ability to increase activity

Use of vitamins, minerals, and nutritional supplements: what, how much, and why they are taken

Use of alcohol

Nursing Diagnosis

Altered Health Maintenance, related to the lack of knowledge of diet management of diabetes mellitus.

Planning and Implementation

CLIENT GOALS

The client will:

Short-term:

- State three signs/symptoms of hypoglycemia
- Eat three meals plus a bedtime snack at approximately the same times every day
- Use artificially sweetened soft drinks, and use sugar substitute in her tea
- Use fruit for dessert every day, instead of the usual cake or cookie
- Monitor her blood glucose level daily
- State three emergency foods to use during hypoglycemic episodes
- Walk 10 minutes, three times a day at least 3 days per week

Long-term:

- Lose 10 pounds in 6 months
- Consistently maintain preprandial blood glucose levels less than 120 mg/dL
- Avoid hypoglycemia
- Improve lipid profile
- Prevent or delay chronic complications
- Eat a nutritionally adequate, varied, and balanced diet
- Increase physical activity to 30 minutes daily, five times a week

NURSING INTERVENTIONS

Nutrition Therapy

Introduce *The First Step in Diabetes Meal Planning.* Allow the client to verbalize her feelings and thoughts about diabetes and nutrition therapy.

Client Teaching

Instruct the client:

On the role of nutrition therapy in managing blood glucose levels, including:

- That nutrition therapy is essential and that nutrition is important even when no symptoms are apparent
- That medication is used in addition to nutrition therapy, not as a substitute

On eating plan essentials, including the importance of:

- Eating meals and snacks at regular times every day
- Eating approximately the same amount of food every day
- Reducing portion sizes for gradual weight loss
- Eating enough high-fiber foods, such as oats, oat bran, and dried peas and beans
- Using less fat, sugar, and salt

On behavioral matters, including:

- How to read labels to identify foods that are low in fat and low in saturated fat
- Reducing high-sugar and high-fat foods to help promote weight loss
- Not skipping meals or the bedtime snack
- Physical activity goals

Where to get additional information:

American Diabetes Association
1660 Duke Street
Alexandria, VA 22314
800-232-3472
www.diabetes.org

Evaluation

The client:

Short-term:

- States three signs/symptoms of hypoglycemia

- Eats three meals plus a bedtime snack at approximately the same times every day
- Uses artificially sweetened soft drinks, and uses sugar substitute in her tea
- Uses fruit for dessert every day, instead of the usual cake or cookie
- Monitors her blood glucose level daily
- States three emergency foods to be used during hypoglycemic episodes
- Walks 10 minutes, three times a day, at least three times per week

Long-term:

- Loses 10 pounds in 6 months
- Consistently maintains preprandial blood glucose levels below 120 mg/dL
- Avoids hypoglycemia
- Improves lipid profile
- Prevents chronic complications
- Eats a nutritionally adequate, varied, and balanced diet
- Increases physical activity to 30 minutes daily, five times a week

Functional Hypoglycemia (Hyperinsulinism)

Functional hypoglycemia (hyperinsulinism) is characterized by an excessive insulin secretion in response to carbohydrate-rich foods (blood glucose levels of 40 mg/dL or less). Weakness, hunger, nervousness, trembling, sweating, and faintness may occur 2 to 4 hours after eating. Convulsions and loss of consciousness may occur in severe cases. Approximately 15% of cases result in diabetes mellitus. The goal of nutrition therapy is to avoid stimulating insulin secretion.

NUTRITION THERAPY

Total carbohydrate intake is limited to 100 to 125 g/day and only small amounts of simple sugars are allowed, to avoid excessive insulin secretion. Small, frequent meals, each containing protein and/or fat, help slow the rate of carbohydrate absorption, decrease the rise in blood glucose levels, and reduce insulin secretion. A high fiber intake, especially soluble fiber, may be beneficial. A liberal protein intake is encouraged. Obese clients should be encouraged to lose weight. Alcohol and caffeine are prohibited. The diabetic exchange lists may be used for meal planning. A sample menu appears in the Box 19–3.

Questions You May Hear

What do you do when the client is not motivated? Encourage the client to attend group learning sessions, which tend to be more effective than individualized instruction.

BOX 19.3

Hyperinsulinism Diet

Breakfast

½ banana
½ cup oatmeal
1 slice whole-wheat toast with margarine
½ cup 2% milk
Coffee/tea

Midmorning Snack

1 oz cheddar cheese
6 saltine crackers
½ cup 2% milk

Lunch

Tomato soup
Turkey sandwich
Carrot and celery sticks
1 cup 2% milk
Apple

Midafternoon Snack

Peanuts
Sugar-free carbonated beverage

Dinner

Roast beef
Roasted potatoes
Tossed salad
Winter squash
½ cup 2% milk
½ cup rice pudding

Bedtime Snack

Popcorn
1 cup 2% milk

Enlist family support and involvement and encourage their participation in group sessions. Frequent followup and feedback over an extended period may help.

What do you do when the client claims to have a relentless "sweet tooth"? Assure the client that small amounts of sweet foods are permitted, especially if weight is not a problem. Diabetic cookbooks may help the client incorporate sweet foods into the eating pattern occasionally. Calorie-free foods sweetened with nonnutritive sweeteners (eg, saccharin, aspartame) add sweetness and interest without calories. Encourage the client to try artificially sweetened soft drinks, gelatin, and hard candy.

What do you do when the client is intellectually unable to comprehend the reason for the diet and its strategies? Keep the message simple and decide on a single directive each time you see the client. For instance, food models and pictures may help convey portion sizes.

What do you do when the client is under the impression that taking insulin or oral hypoglycemia agents eliminates the need to follow an eating plan? Instruct the client that nutrition therapy is used regardless of whether medication is used and regardless of the type of medication used.

KEY CONCEPTS

- Type 1 diabetes is characterized by the lack of insulin secretion. It is usually diagnosed before the age of 30 years in people who are of normal or below normal weight.
- Ninety percent to 95% of diabetes cases are type 2 diabetes. It is characterized by hyperinsulinemia and insulin resistance. Hyperglycemia provides constant stimulation for insulin secretion, further aggravating hyperinsulinemia.
- Studies of type 1 diabetics show that tight glycemic control delays or prevents the onset of long-term complications. It is assumed that the same is true for type 2 diabetics.
- Nutrition therapy is the cornerstone of treatment for all diabetics, regardless of weight status, use of medication, blood glucose levels, and presence or absence of symptoms. The goals of nutrition therapy are to achieve optimal blood glucose and lipid levels, attain or maintain reasonable weight, and avoid acute and chronic complications.
- Type 1 diabetics need adequate calories to maintain normal weight; a balanced and varied intake that meets nutritional needs; daily consistency in the number, size, and timing of meals and snacks; and extra carbohydrates for moderate and vigorous exercise, especially if exercise occurs more than 2 hours after eating.
- Exercise for type 1 diabetics may not promote glycemic control, but it affects other cardiovascular risk factors and promotes a sense of well-being.
- Type 1 diabetics who consistently experience hyperglycemia before a meal need to reduce the amount of food eaten at the previous meal or snack, change the time of the previous meal or snack, exercise more, or adjust the insulin dosage.
- Type 1 diabetics need to carry a readily absorbable source of carbohydrate with them to treat hypoglycemia. Glucose tablets, sugar cubes, jelly beans, and Life Savers are options.
- The nutrition therapy for type 2 diabetes is similar to that for type 1, except that a mildly hypocaloric diet is recommended to promote gradual weight loss. Consistent meal timing is encouraged to prevent large swings in blood glucose levels.
- The American Diabetes Association recommends that diabetics limit their saturated fat intake to less than 10% of total calories, polyunsaturated fat ≤10% of total calories and that protein provide 10% to 20% of total calories. The remaining calories are to be divided between carbohydrates and monounsaturated fats, depending on the client's lipid levels, usual dietary pattern, and weight status.
- Sucrose ("sugar") is no longer considered detrimental to glucose control, so long as it is eaten as part of the meal plan and not as an "extra." However, if weight loss is a goal, high-sugar foods should be limited.
- Diets for diabetics are not "one size fits all." Dietary changes should be made sequentially and restrictions kept to a minimum to maximize compliance.
- Clients who want or need only basic nutrition therapy information may benefit from using *The First Step in Diabetes Meal Planning, Healthy Food Choices*, or single-topic resources geared to the client's interests.
- Some clients want in-depth nutrition therapy information. Options for them include the menus, the exchanges lists, and carbohydrate counting.
- Behavioral skills help clients use factual knowledge while making food choices. Clients need to know how to order restaurant food, read food labels, and cook food at home.

- Children and adolescents have a greater variation in their day-to-day calorie needs than do adults because of their nutritional needs for growth and their more erratic activity patterns. Most experts recommend a structured program for children and adolescents.
- Pregnant diabetics need to closely monitor their blood glucose levels and eat three meals and two to three snacks daily. The bedtime snack is especially important to avoid morning hypoglycemia.
- Elderly diabetics may need to be treated more conservatively than younger diabetics because they are more susceptible to severe hypoglycemia, are at greater nutritional risk, and may have physical or sensory impairments that complicate self-management.
- Diabetic diets in the hospital were traditionally identified as "ADA diets". Because there is no one diabetic diet recommended for all people with diabetes, this term should be discontinued.
- People with functional hyperinsulinism should limit their total carbohydrate intake, especially their intake of simple sugars. Small, frequent meals should provide protein and fat along with the carbohydrate to slow its absorption.
- To control symptoms of functional hypoglycemia, clients should eat three meals and two to three snacks daily, limit their total carbohydrate intake (especially their intake of simple sugars), eat protein and/or fat with every meal and snack, increase soluble fiber intake, and avoid alcohol and caffeine.

ANSWER KEY

1. **FALSE** Nutrition therapy is a crucial part of treatment, regardless of use of medication or other factors.
2. **TRUE** Control of blood glucose improves when meals and snacks are consistent in timing every day.
3. **TRUE** Hypoglycemia can be triggered by the consumption of alcohol without food.
4. **FALSE** Unless otherwise instructed, clients should maintain their normal medication schedule and consume the usual amounts of carbohydrate. If a normal diet is not tolerated, certain liquids can provide supplementation (eg, ginger ale, apple juice, gelatin).
5. **TRUE** Frequent treatment of hypoglycemia can lead to weight gain.
6. **TRUE** Some studies suggest that the best distribution of carbohydrates and fats for these patients is 40% carbohydrate and 45% fat, with 25% of total calories from monounsaturated sources.
7. **TRUE** Dehydration is often a precipitating cause of HHNS.
8. **FALSE** Exchange lists may not be appropriate for all types of clients.
9. **TRUE** A slightly lower intake of carbohydrates in pregnancy helps limit the rise in blood glucose between meals.
10. **TRUE** A moderate weight loss can lower blood glucose levels and help reverse insulin resistance.

REFERENCES

American Diabetes Association. (1999). What you need to know about pioglitazone hydrochloride (Actos), a new type 2 oral medication. [On-line]. Available: www.diabetes.org/ada/actos.asp. Accessed August 18, 2000.

American Diabetes Association. (1997). Translation of the diabetes nutrition recommendations for health care institutions: Position statement. *Journal of the American Dietetic Association, 97,* 52–53.

American Diabetes Association, American Dietetic Association. (1995). *Exchange lists for meal planning.* Alexandria, VA: American Diabetes Association; Chicago: American Dietetic Association.

American Diabetes Association. (1995). *101 tips for improving your blood sugar.* Alexandria, VA: Author.

American Dietetic Association. (1994). Nutrition recommendations and principles for people with diabetes mellitus. *Journal of the American Dietetic Association, 94,* 504–506.

Deakins, D. (1994). Teaching elderly patients about diabetes. *American Journal of Nursing, 94,* 39–42.

Diabetes Care and Education, Tinker, L., Heins, J., & Holler, H. (1994). Commentary and translation: 1994 nutrition recommendations for diabetes. *Journal of the American Dietetic Association, 94,* 507–511.

Holler, H., & Pastors, J. (1997). *Diabetes medical nutrition therapy.* Chicago: The American Dietetic Association.

Lipkin, E. (1999). New strategies for the treatment of type 2 diabetes. *Journal of the American Dietetic Association, 99,* 329–324.

Miller, C., Jensen, G., & Achterberg, C. (1999). Evaluation of a food label nutrition intervention for women with type 2 diabetes mellitus. *Journal of the American Dietetic Association, 99,* 323–328.

Monk, A., Barry, B., McClain, K., Weaver, T., Cooper, N., & Franz, M. (1995). Practice guidelines for medical nutrition therapy provided by dietitians for persons with non–insulin-dependent diabetes mellitus. *Journal of the American Dietetic Association, 95,* 999–1006.

Riddle, M. (1999). Oral pharmacologic management of type 2 diabetes. *American Family Physician.* [On-line]. Available: www.aafp.org/afp/991201ap/2613.html. Accessed February 14, 2000.

Schaafer, R., Bohannon, B., Franz, M., Freeman, J., Holms, A., McLaughlin, S., Haas, L., Kruger, D., Lorenz, R., & McMahon, M. (1997). Translation of the diabetes nutrition recommendations for health care institutions: Technical review. *Journal of the American Dietetic Association, 97,* 43–51.

Schlundt, D., Rea, M., Kline, S., & Pichert, J. (1994). Situational obstacles to dietary adherence for adults with diabetes. *Journal of the American Dietetic Association, 94,* 874–879.

Wing, R. (1995). Use of very-low-calorie diets in the treatment of obese persons with non–insulin-dependent diabetes mellitus. *Journal of the American Dietetic Association, 95,* 569–572

CHAPTER 20

Nutrition for Patients With Renal Disorders

TRUE	FALSE	Check your knowledge of nutrition for patients with renal disorders.
		1 People with renal insufficiency are allowed only half of the normal Recommended Dietary Allowance (RDA) for protein.
		2 People with renal insufficiency need a high-calcium diet to compensate for altered calcium metabolism.
		3 People receiving dialysis need more than the RDA for protein.
		4 All people with renal impairments need to limit their sodium intake.
		5 People with chronic renal failure (CRF) tend to have accelerated atherosclerosis and may benefit from eating more monounsaturated fat.
		6 The diet for acute renal failure (ARF) is more clear-cut than that for CRF.
		7 People receiving peritoneal dialysis absorb calories from the dialysate.
		8 People who have gained more than 2 pounds between dialysis treatments have eaten too many calories.
		9 People with calcium oxalate renal stones should restrict their intake of calcium.
		10 The most effective nutritional intervention for renal stones is to increase fluid intake.

Upon completion of this chapter, you will be able to

- Explain the recommendations and rationales for intake of protein, calories, sodium, fluid, potassium, phosphorus, and calcium for people with renal insufficiency.
- Discuss how nutrient recommendations differ after dialysis begins.
- Discuss nutrition therapy for ARF.
- Describe nutritional interventions for renal stones.

Introduction

The kidneys perform many vital endocrine and exocrine functions. They maintain normal blood volume and composition by reabsorbing needed nutrients and excreting wastes through the urine. Urinary excretion is the primary method by which the body rids itself of excess water, nitrogenous wastes (ammonia, urea, uric acid, and creatinine), electrolytes, sulfates, organic acids, toxic substances, and drugs. The kidneys help regulate acid-base balance by secreting hydrogen ions to increase pH and excreting bicarbonate to lower pH. Renin, an enzyme important for blood pressure regulation, is synthesized in the kidneys, as is erythropoietin, a hormone that stimulates the bone marrow to produce red blood cells. Because vitamin D is converted to its active form (1,25-dihydroxycholecalciferol) in the kidneys, they have an important role in maintaining normal metabolism of calcium and phosphorus.

This chapter discusses nutrition therapy for CRF and ARF and provides nutrition guidelines for clients receiving peritoneal dialysis, hemodialysis, or a renal transplant. General nutrition therapy recommendations for other selected renal disorders are summarized in Table 20–1. Nutrition recommendations for preventing and treating kidney stones are presented.

TABLE 20.1 ***General Nutrition Therapy Recommendations for Selected Renal Disorders***

Disorder	Symptoms/Complications	Diet Management
Acute glomerulonephritis: inflammation of the glomeruli. Most often caused by an allergic or autoimmune reaction to a streptococcal infection of the throat; may also result from impetigo or scarlet fever.	Nitrogenous waste retention	Decrease protein to 0.2–0.5 g/kg for clients with uremia. Increase calories to 35 cal/kg to promote protein sparing.
	Oliguria	For oliguria, restrict fluid to 500–700 mL, and restrict potassium and phosphorus as needed.
	Edema, high blood pressure	For edema or high blood pressure, limit sodium to 500–1000 mg.
Nephritis: kidney inflammation that may be acute or chronic. Causes include scarlet fever, flu, and tonsillitis.	Edema, hypertension	Limit sodium to 1–2 g/d.
	Uremia; net protein catabolism	Restrict protein to 0.6–0.7 g/kg; increase calories to 35 cal/kg to promote protein sparing. Determine fluid allowance: urine output + 500 mL. Use of fish oils may decrease loss of renal function.

(continued)

TABLE 20.1 ***General Nutrition Therapy Recommendations for Selected Renal Disorders (continued)***

Disorder	Symptoms/Complications	Diet Management
Nephrotic syndrome: increased capillary permeability in the glomeruli leads to leakage of serum proteins into the urine, causing proteinuria, hypoalbuminemia, massive edema, and altered blood lipid levels (elevated cholesterol, triglycerides, LDL-C, and VLDL-C; decreased HDL-C).	Proteinuria, which leads to protein-calorie malnutrition	Provide RDA for protein (0.8 g/kg). Higher intakes are contraindicated because they increase waste production and may promote deterioration of renal function. Increase calories to 40–60 cal/kg to spare protein.
	Edema	Limit sodium to 2–3 g or less. Initially sodium may be restricted to 250 mg/d to potentiate the effectiveness of diuretics in mobilizing excess interstitial fluid. Fluid restriction is not necessary unless renal failure develops. Supplemental nutrients may be needed, especially of potassium (depending on diuretic use), vitamin D, calcium, zinc, vitamin C, and folacin.
	Accelerated atherosclerosis, which increases the risk of cardiovascular disease, stroke, and further kidney damage	Limit fat, saturated fat, and cholesterol. Lipid-lowering medications may be needed to adequately control blood lipid levels.
Pyelonephritis: bacterial invasion of the kidneys leads to fibrosis, scarring, and dilatation of the tubules and impaired renal function.	Hypertension; however, some people excrete excess sodium and may become sodium depleted	Adjust sodium intake according to symptoms.
	Possible hyperkalemia	Adjust potassium according to laboratory values.
	Possible loss of renal function	Limit protein, accordingly. Cranberry juice may be helpful. Encourage high fluid intake to flush bacteria, unless contraindicated because of decreased urine output.

HDL-C, high-density lipoprotein cholesterol; LDL-C, low-density lipoprotein cholesterol; VLDL-C, very-low-density lipoprotein cholesterol.

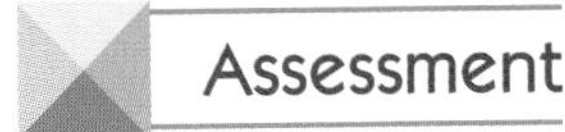

Assessment

Assessment data to consider for renal disorders include:

HISTORICAL DATA

What is the client's weight status according to body mass index (BMI)? Has the client experienced sudden weight gain? What is the client's blood pressure? Has the client's height decreased (indicative of bone disease)?

Is the client following a special diet? Has the client had nutritional counseling before? What is the client's understanding of the relationship between diet and renal disease? Is the client's usual intake adequate? Does the client use low-protein or low-sodium products? Does the client have food allergies or intolerances? Does the client complain of poor appetite or dry mouth? Does the client shop and cook? Does the client read food labels? Is the client willing to change his or her eating habits? What nutritional supplements does the client use and for what purpose?

Does the client have diabetes, hypertension, or heart disease? What over-the-counter or prescribed medications does the client take? What are the client's chief complaints? Is the client's food budget adequate? What cultural, religious, or ethnic influences affect the client's food choices?

PHYSICAL FINDINGS

Does the client have edema? Is the client pale? Is the skin dry and scaly? Do the client's oral mucous membranes bleed? Do the client's breath and body have the odor of urine? Does the client appear to be drowsy or to have decreased mental alertness?

LABORATORY DATA

What are the client's blood urea nitrogen (BUN), creatinine, albumin, lipids, electrolyte, glucose, hemoglobin, hematocrit, phosphorus, and calcium levels? Are there any other abnormal laboratory values? Is urine output normal? Is urine specific gravity normal?

Chronic Renal Failure

CRF is characterized by the slow, progressive loss of renal function related to irreversible nephron deterioration. The clinical course of renal failure can be divided into three phases. **Decreased renal functioning** is an asymptomatic period in which homeostasis is maintained despite a 50% decrease in glomerular filtration rate (GFR). **Renal insuffi-**

ciency occurs when GFR decreases by 75%. Serum creatinine may be eight times greater than normal, the urine becomes more dilute, generalized edema may occur, and mild anemia develops. However, the client is relatively asymptomatic because the remaining nephrons hypertrophy to maintain homeostasis. **Renal failure** occurs when GFR decreases by more than 75%. **End-stage renal disease (ESRD)** occurs when 90% of nephrons are lost; serum creatinine levels steadily increase to about 10 mg/100 mL, overt symptoms develop, and dialysis or kidney transplantation is required.

Renal damage and subsequent loss of renal function profoundly affect metabolism, nutritional requirements, and nutritional status. For instance, fluid, electrolytes, and other compounds in the blood accumulate as urine output decreases. The accumulation of nitrogenous wastes leads to uremia, a toxic systemic syndrome that literally means "urine in the blood." Acidosis occurs because the kidneys are unable to excrete excess acid produced through normal metabolic processes. Conversely, renal damage can impair the kidneys' ability to reabsorb needed nutrients, which are then "wasted" in the urine. Kidney failure impairs gastrointestinal absorption of certain minerals, such as calcium and iron. Impaired synthesis of renin, erythropoietin, and vitamin D can lead to high blood pressure, anemia, and bone demineralization, respectively. Certain peptide hormones, such as insulin, parathyroid hormone, and glucagon, are not adequately inactivated, which contributes to altered metabolism. Accelerated atherosclerosis increases the risk of congestive heart failure and myocardial infarction. Poor intake related to dietary restrictions, anorexia, alterations in taste, nausea, vomiting, stomatitis, depression, or anxiety is common. In addition, nutrients may be lost secondary to drug therapy, dialysis, or renal transplantation.

NUTRITION THERAPY

Nutrition therapy plays a key role in the treatment of renal diseases. Its objectives are to:

1. Lessen renal workload to forestall or prevent further kidney damage.
2. Restore or maintain optimal nutritional status.
3. Avoid the symptoms or complications of uremia.

The optimal interventions that are needed to meet these objectives vary among individuals and according to the nature, severity, and stage of the disease. Generally, diet modifications are made in response to symptoms and laboratory values and, therefore, require frequent monitoring and adjustment. Nutrients affected include protein, calories, sodium, fluid, potassium, phosphorus, calcium, and other vitamins and minerals. Table 20–2 summarizes the nutritional parameters in renal failure discussed here.

Protein

Protein restriction is the cornerstone of nutrition therapy for renal insufficiency.

Studies strongly suggest that reducing protein intake helps preserve nephron function and thus slows renal deterioration. However, a narrow margin of error exists with re-

TABLE 20.2 *Dietary Parameters in Renal Failure*

Energy and Nutrients	Renal Insufficiency (Predialysis)	Hemodialysis	Peritoneal Dialysis	Transplantation
Protein	0.6–0.8 g/kg/d, >50%–60% HBV	1.2–1.4 g/kg/d, >50%–60% HBV	1.2–1.5 g/kg/d, >50%–60% HBV	1.3–1.5 g/kg/d after surgery; 1.0 g/kg/d with chronic, stable renal function
Energy	30–35 cal/kg/d	30–35 kcal/kg/d	25–35 kcal/kg/d, including dialysate energy; 20–25 kcal/kg for weight loss	25–35 kcal/kg/d to maintain desired body weight; limit fat to 30% total energy; <300 mg/d cholesterol
Sodium	2.0–4.0 g/d; variable with disease etiology and urine output	2.0 g/d	2.0–4.0 g/d	2.0–4.0 g/d after surgery; 3.0–4.0 g/d with chronic, stable renal function
Potassium	Not usually restricted	2.0–3.0 g/d	3.0–4.0 g/d	Unrestricted; monitor drug effects
Phosphorus	10–12 mg/g dietary protein	12–15 mg/g dietary protein	12–15 mg/g dietary protein	Unrestriced; monitor
Calcium	1.0–1.5 g/d	1.0–1.5 g/d	1.0–1.5 g/d	1.0–1.5 g/d
Fluid	Unrestricted until urine output decreases	Urine output plus 1000 mL/d	Monitored; most tolerate 2000 mL/d	Unrestricted unless urine output decreases or fluid overload occurs
Vitamins and minerals	Daily RDA of vitamins B, C, and D plus iron and zinc; do not supplement vitamin A or magnesium	Daily RDA except: vitamin C, 60–100 mg/d; vitamin B_6, 5–6 mg/d; folic acid, 0.8–1.0 µg/d; do not supplement vitamin A or magnesium	Daily RDA except: vitamin C, 60–100 mg/d; vitamin B_6, 5–10 mg/d; folic acid, 0.8–1.0 µg/d; do not supplement vitamin A or magnesium	Daily RDA

HBV, protein of high biologic value; RDA, Recommended Dietary Allowance.

Beto, J. (1995). Which diet for which renal failure: Making sense of the options. The American Dietetic Association. Reprinted by permission from the *Journal of the American Dietetic Association*, 95, 898–903.

gard to protein intake. Too much protein increases BUN levels and the symptoms of uremia. Conversely, too little protein results in body protein catabolism (which increases serum potassium and BUN levels) and protein malnutrition, as evidenced by low serum albumin levels. Low serum albumin is a strong predictor of mortality in patients starting dialysis.

The most severe level of protein restriction is for renal insufficiency without dialysis. The recommended daily intake of 0.6 to 0.8 g/kg is at, or slightly below, the normal RDA for protein (0.8 g/kg), yet the diet is viewed as unrealistically restrictive because most Americans habitually consume almost twice this level. Once dialysis is initiated, protein requirements are increased to greater than normal levels to ensure adequacy and to compensate for the loss of serum proteins and amino acids in the dialysate.

It is recommended that at least 60% of total protein intake be from high biologic sources, such as eggs, milk, yogurt, cheese, meat, fish, poultry, and soy. The rationale for using high biologic proteins, which provide adequate amounts of all the essential amino acids, is that they promote reuse of circulating nonessential amino acids for protein synthesis and by doing so minimize urea production.

Calories

Adequate calories are needed to prevent weight loss and body protein catabolism. Taking in too few calories can have the same effect as eating too much protein: BUN levels rise because body proteins are broken down for energy.

Daily consumption of 35 cal/g is recommended for most adults who are not undergoing dialysis. Clients receiving peritoneal dialysis need to decrease their calorie intake to compensate for the calories absorbed from the dialysate (average, 680 cal/day). Likewise, sedentary clients and post-transplantation clients who are taking immunosuppressive steroids may require fewer calories to avoid excess weight gain.

Pure sugars and pure fats are recommended for calories because they do not provide protein, even though they are not considered "nutritious" foods (Box 20–1). However, approximately 50% of CRF clients exhibit glucose intolerance, and many develop hyperlipidemia (increased levels of triglycerides and very-low-density lipoproteins). Emphasis on monounsaturated fats may help minimize cardiovascular risks.

Children with renal failure experience growth failure, which may be permanent if it is not corrected before puberty. Aggressive nutrition therapy is needed to overcome nutrient deficits. Calcium supplements, vitamin D supplements, and phosphate binders may be used to promote calcium uptake by the bones and subsequent bone growth. Human growth hormone may be prescribed for children who are short for their age and may help treat malnutrition in children with renal failure.

Sodium and Fluid

The client's blood pressure, weight, serum electrolyte levels, and urine output determine the amount of sodium and fluid allowed. Most renal diets contain a moderate amount of sodium (2–4 g/day). However, some clients with advanced renal failure are unable to conserve sodium, and a sodium deficit may occur if sodium intake is restricted. If the client does not have edema, hypertension, or signs of heart failure, increasing the sodium intake as tolerated may slightly improve GFR.

BOX 20.1

Sources of Protein-Free Calories and Seasonings

Protein-Free Calories

Beverages*
- Alcoholic
- Carbonated (colas may be restricted due to their relatively high phosphorus content)
- Cranberry juice cocktail
- Fruit drinks and punches
- Kool-Aid
- Lemonade, limeade
- Tang

Candies
- Buttermints
- Candy corn, fondant
- Chewy fruit snacks
- Cotton candy
- Fruit chews, fruit rollups
- Gum
- Gumdrops
- Jelly beans
- Life Savers
- Lollipops
- Marshmallows
- Mints

Desserts
- Fruit ice*
- Juice bar
- Popsicle*
- Sorbet

Fats
- Butter and margarine (unsalted)
- Coconut
- Mayonnaise, oils
- Powdered coffee whitener
- Shortening
- Tartar sauce

Sweeteners
- Corn syrup
- Honey
- Jams
- Jellies

(continued)

BOX 20.1

Sources of Protein-Free Calories and Seasonings (continued)

Sweeteners (continued)
- Maple syrup
- Marmalade
- Sugar: confectioners, white, brown

Protein-Free Seasonings

Flavoring extracts
Herbs
Spices
Vinegar

*As allowed by fluid restriction.

If blood pressure and serum sodium levels are normal and edema does not occur, fluid intake can exceed 24-hour urine output by 500 mL (the amount of fluid lost through skin, lungs, and perspiration) (Box 20–2). Typical fluid allowances range from 500 to 3000 mL/day. The goal is to limit weight gain between hemodialysis treatments to approximately 2 pounds, although much larger gains are common.

Potassium

Most clients with renal insufficiency and those undergoing peritoneal dialysis do not need to restrict their intake of potassium. A moderate potassium restriction of 2 to 3 g/day is recommended for hemodialysis clients with hyperkalemia. Clients who are taking potassium-wasting diuretics and those experiencing severe potassium losses from gastrointestinal fistulas or gastric suctioning may need more potassium to avoid hypokalemia.

Phosphorus and Calcium

Vitamin D deficiency occurs when the kidneys are unable to convert the vitamin to its active form. The metabolism of calcium, phosphorus, and magnesium is altered, resulting in hyperphosphatemia, bone demineralization, bone pain, and possible calcification of the soft tissues (eg, eyes, skin, heart, lungs, blood vessels). Renal osteodystrophy may be prevented by the following measures:

- **Limiting phosphorus intake.** Low-protein diets are usually low in phosphorus and may control hyperphosphatemia effectively. Allowances are often calculated

BOX 20.2

Sources of Fluid

Liquids

Alcoholic beverages
Carbonated beverages
Cereal beverages
Coffee
Cream
Fruit juices, drinks, and punches
Juice and syrup from canned fruit and vegetables
Liquid medications
Milk
Soup, bouillon, consommé, broth
Tea
Vegetable juices
Water

Foods That Liquefy at Room Temperature

Ice (melts to 9/10 initial volume)
Ice cream (melts to 1/2 initial volume)
Ice milk (melts to 1/2 initial volume)
Gelatin
Popsicles
Sherbet

per gram of protein consumed (eg, 12–15 mg phosphorus per gram of protein for clients receiving dialysis). Phosphate binders, such as the calcium salts calcium carbonate and calcium acetate, are used to prevent the absorption of phosphorus from the gastrointestinal tract. Phosphate binders must be taken with meals.

- **Providing vitamin D supplements.** Supplements of the active form of vitamin D (calcitriol) promote calcium absorption to help maintain blood calcium levels and prevent bone disease. Doses are individualized to maintain desirable serum calcium levels (see Drug Alert).
- **Providing calcium supplements.** Supplements are used to increase calcium intake, because foods high in calcium (eg, dairy products) are usually restricted because of their high protein and phosphorus contents (Table 20–3). The amount of calcium absorbed from calcium binders varies among types used.
- **Avoiding aluminum, which may cause encephalopathy and osteodystrophy.** Aluminum may be found in antacids, parenteral nutrition systems, albumin replacements, and dialysate. Dietary sources include canned carbonated beverages, drinking water, and foods cooked in aluminum utensils.

DRUG ALERT

Drugs Used During Chronic Renal Failure

Epoetin alfa (EPO, Epogen) is recombinant human erythropoietin, which stimulates bone marrow production of red blood cells. It is used to treat anemia of chronic renal failure, in which there is an erythropoietin deficiency.

Possible side effects include worsening of hypertension, edema, fatigue, nausea, vomiting, and diarrhea.

Because deficiencies of iron, vitamin B_{12}, and folic acid can cause a poor response to Epogen therapy, it is important to identify and prevent nutritional deficiencies.

Higher hematocrit causes a decrease in phosphorous clearance; an adjustment in dietary phosphorous intake, use of phosphate binders, or both may be indicated.

Calcitriol (Calcijex, Rocaltrol) is the active form of vitamin D. It is used to manage hypocalcemia in patients receiving chronic renal dialysis. Vitamin D raises serum calcium levels and decreases parathyroid hormone levels. The most common side effects are nausea and vomiting. An adequate intake of calcium and fluids is important. The risk of hypermagnesemia is increased when calcitriol is used with magnesium-containing antacids.

Vitamins

Deficiencies of water-soluble vitamins occur frequently in clients with renal failure and may be caused by inadequate intake related to anorexia or dietary restrictions; altered metabolism related to uremia or medications; or increased losses related to dialysis. With few exceptions, supplements of the water-soluble vitamins at RDA levels are recommended for both nondialyzed and dialyzed clients. Amounts greater than the RDA of folic acid and vitamin B_6 are suggested to promote red blood cell production. Because vitamin C increases the risk of oxalate stones, total intake from food and supplements should be less than 100 mg.

Except for vitamin D mentioned previously, supplements of fat-soluble vitamins usually are not necessary. Vitamin A supplementation is contraindicated in clients with ESRD because of reported toxicity.

Trace Minerals

Clients who are undergoing dialysis may develop a deficiency of zinc, which could contribute to anorexia and taste alterations. Supplements are recommended if a zinc deficiency is identified. It is recommended that all other trace elements be routinely removed from the dialysate to prevent toxicities. Dialysate that is contaminated with aluminum has been associated with progressive mental disorders and osteomalacia.

Iron supplements, plus human erythropoietin, are used to treat anemia of CRF. Iron supplements may cause gastrointestinal upset and constipation, and they should not be

TABLE 20.3 *Calcium, Phosphorus, and Protein Content of Selected Foods*

Item	Amount	Calcium (mg)	Phosphorus (mg)	Protein (g)
Bread, Cereal, Rice, and Pasta Group				
White bread	1 slice	27	24	2
Whole wheat bread	1 slice	20	64	3
Long-grain rice	½ cup	10	81	3
Corn tortilla	1 med	44	79	1
Vegetable Group				
Artichoke, boiled	1 med	135	258	10
Cassava, raw	3.5 oz	91	70	3
Kale, frozen, boiled	½ cup	90	18	2
Okra, boiled	½ cup	77	37	2
Spinach, boiled	½ cup	122	50	3
Turnip greens, boiled	½ cup	99	21	1
Fruit Group				
Orange juice, calcium-fortified	¾ cup	200	25	0
Avocado, raw	1 med	33	119	5
Cherimoya, raw	1 med	126	219	7
Mango, raw	1 med	21	23	1
Strawberries, raw	½ cup	10	14	0
Milk, Yogurt, and Cheese Group				
Skim	1 cup	302	247	8
1%	1 cup	300	235	8
2%	1 cup	297	232	8
Whole	1 cup	291	228	8
Goat milk	1 cup	326	270	9
Chocolate milk (with 1% milk)	1 cup	287	256	8
Plain low-fat yogurt with nonfat dry milk	1 cup	415	326	12
Plain whole-milk yogurt	1 cup	274	215	8
Low-fat fruit-flavored yogurt	1 cup	314	247	8
Cheddar	1 oz	214	145	7
Cottage cheese, 1% fat	½ cup	78	170	14
Mozzarella, part skim	1 oz	147	105	7
Ricotta, part skim	½ cup	337	226	14
Swiss	1 oz	272	171	8
Ice cream, vanilla soft serve	½ cup	138	106	4
Meat, Poultry, Fish, Dry Beans, Eggs, and Nuts Group				
Ground beef, broiled	3½ oz	12	191	27
Ham, cured, roasted	3½ oz	6	224	19
Veal, ground, broiled	3½ oz	17	217	24
Beef liver, braised	3½ oz	7	404	24
Chicken breast, roasted	½	13	196	27

(continued)

TABLE 20.3 *Calcium, Phosphorus, and Protein Content of Selected Foods (continued)*

Item	Amount	Calcium (mg)	Phosphorus (mg)	Protein (g)
Meat, Poultry, Fish, Dry Beans, Eggs, and Nuts Group (continued)				
Salmon, chinook	3 oz	24	316	22
Tuna, white, canned	3 oz	12	185	20
Refried beans, canned	½ cup	45	109	7
Great northern beans, canned	½ cup	70	178	10
Egg, poached	1	25	89	6
Almonds, blanched	1 oz	73	150	6
Peanut butter	2 tbsp	13	101	8
Sunflower seeds, dry roasted	1 oz	20	327	6
Fats, Oils, and Sweets				
Sour cream	2 tbsp	28	20	1
Cola	12 oz	11	44	0
Milk chocolate bar	1.55 oz	84	95	3
Orange sherbet	½ cup	52	38	1

taken with calcium supplements. Potential side effects of recombinant human erythropoietin appear in the accompanying Drug Alert.

MEAL PLANNING

Meal planning is simplified by the use of renal exchange lists (referred to as "choices," rather than "exchanges," to eliminate confusion with diabetic exchanges). Allowed foods are grouped into lists based on their protein, sodium, potassium, and phosphorus content; calories are also addressed, and fluids may be considered. Portion sizes are specified so that each serving contains approximately the same amount of protein, sodium, potassium, and phosphorus (Table 20–4). Items within a list may be substituted for each other; substitutions from one list to another are not allowed. An individualized meal pattern specifies the number of choices that are permitted from each list; allowances are based on laboratory data and clinical symptoms and should correspond as closely as possible to the client's food preferences and habits (Box 20–3). The composition, complexity, and number of exchange lists used in the treatment of renal failure vary considerably among institutions.

Despite the use of "choice" lists, adherence to nutrition therapies for chronic renal disease is extremely challenging. The diet is complex; modifications are numerous, extensive, and lifelong; and changes are frequent as the disease progresses. Additional meal planning considerations are as follows:

- Clients with uremia may experience a deterioration of their appetite as the day progresses. Encourage a good breakfast.

TABLE 20.4 *Renal Diet "Choice" Lists*

Choice	Various Serving Sizes	Nutritional Content				
		g Pro	*Calories*	*mg Na*	*mg K*	*mg P*
Milk	½ cup milk 1 cup low-protein milk ½ cup yogurt, ice cream, or light cream	4	120	80	185	110
Nondairy milk substitutes	½ cup	0.5	140	40	80	30
Meat	1 oz meat, fish, poultry 1 egg ¼ cup cottage cheese	7	65	25	100	65
Starch	1 slice bread ½ bagel or hamburger roll ¾ cup most ready-to-eat cereals ⅓ cup pasta, oatmeal ½ cup rice	2	90	80	35	35
Vegetable	Generally ½ cup, prepared or canned without added salt					
Low potassium		1	25	15	50	20
Medium potassium		1	25	15	150	20
High potassium		1	25	15	270	20
Fruit	Generally, ½ cup					
Low potassium		0.5	70	trace	50	15
Moderate potassium		0.5	70	trace	150	15
High potassium		0.5	70	trace	270	15
Fat	1 tsp oil, margarine, butter, mayonnaise 1 tbsp salad dressing, low-calorie mayonnaise, reduced-calorie margarine, powdered coffee whitener	0	45	55	10	5
High-calorie	Varies 1 cup carbonated beverage, lemonade, fruit-flavored drinks; 1 Popsicle, juice bar; 2 fruit rollups, 15 gumdrops; 2 tbsp jam, honey, sugar, or syrup; 5 large marshmallows; ½ slice low-protein bread	Trace	100	15	20	5
Salt	Varies ⅛ tsp salt ⅓ cup bouillon 1½ tbsp ketchup 4 tsp mustard 2 medium green olives 2½ tsp steak sauce 2 tbsp taco sauce	0	0	250	0	0

Pro, protein; Na, sodium; K, potassium; P, phosphorus.

BOX 20.3

Sample Renal Failure Menu: 2075 Calories, 42 g Protein, 1785 mg Sodium, 1810 mg Potassium

Meal	Choices
Breakfast	
½ cup orange juice	1 high-potassium fruit
¾ cup cornflakes with ½ cup nondairy creamer	1 starch, 1 salt
1 poached egg	1 nondairy milk substitute
1 slice toast	1 meat
2 tsp margarine	1 starch
2 tbsp jelly	2 fats
½ cup coffee*	1 high-calorie choice
1 tbsp powdered coffee whitener	1 fat
Lunch	
Sandwich made with:	
1 oz turkey	1 meat
2 slices low-protein bread	2 high-calorie choices
2 teaspoons mayonnaise	2 fats
1 cup lettuce	1 low-potassium vegetable
2 tbsp low-calorie salad dressing	1 fat, 1 salt
1 small apple	1 medium-potassium fruit
2 fruit rollups	1 high-calorie choice
Dinner	
2 oz roast beef	2 meat
2½ tsp steak sauce	1 salt
½ cup unsalted noodles with 2 tsp butter and parsley	1 starch, 2 fat
½ cup carrots	1 medium-potassium vegetable
½ cup beets	1 high-potassium vegetable
½ cup blueberries	1 low-potassium fruit
1 cup ginger ale*	1 high-calorie choice
4 sugar wafers	1 starch
Snacks	
½ cup apple juice*	1 low-potassium fruit
5 large marshmallows	1 high-calorie choice

*As allowed, depending on fluid needs.

- Highly seasoned or strongly flavored foods may be preferred because of changes in the sense of taste attributed to uremia.
- Clients should initially weigh or measure portion sizes and thereafter periodically spot-check portion sizes for accuracy, because either too little or too much protein in the diet can cause BUN levels to increase and uremic symptoms to return.
- Protein allowance should be spread over the whole day instead of saving it all for one meal.
- Low-protein breads, cereals, cookies, gelatin, and pastas are available to help boost calorie intake without sacrificing protein restriction. However, their taste and texture differ from those of the products they are intended to replace, and they are more costly. Because acceptability varies greatly among low-protein products, encourage clients to try a variety.
- Sometimes very-low-protein diets (30 g or less) and supplements of essential amino acids or their keto analogues are used to promote a neutral or positive nitrogen balance, reduce uremic symptoms, and even prevent further kidney damage in people with advanced renal disease. Very-low-protein diets are extremely difficult to follow (Box 20–4).
- An easy way to measure fluid intake is to place a pitcher of water that contains a total daily fluid allowance in the refrigerator. As fluids are consumed, the equivalent amount of water should be discarded from the pitcher.
- To help relieve thirst when fluid intake is restricted, encourage the client to use hard candies, refrigerated water instead of tap water, and Popsicles and ices (as allowed by fluid restriction). Petroleum jelly applied to the lips, frequent mouth rinsing with refrigerated water, and good oral hygiene are encouraged to relieve mouth dryness.

BOX 20.4

Renal Formulas

Amin-Aid (Kendall McGaw): Contains free essential amino acids plus histidine in a high-calorie, low-electrolyte supplement. Does not contain vitamins or minerals. Provides 2.0 cal/mL, 4% of calories from protein.

Suplena (Ross Laboratories): Provides complete and balanced nutrition for nondialyzed renal clients. Low in fluid, protein, phosphorus, magnesium, and electrolytes. Provides 2.0 cal/mL, 6% of calories from protein.

Nephro (Ross Laboratories): Provides complete and balanced nutrition for patients on dialysis with either acute or chronic renal failure. Low in fluid, phosphorus, magnesium, electrolytes, and vitamins A, D, and C. Provides 2.0 cal/mL and moderate amounts of protein (14% of total calories).

Travasorb Renal Diet (Clintec): Contains esssential amino acids in a high-calorie, low-protein, electrolyte-free supplement. Does not contain fat-soluble vitamins. Provides 1.4 cal/mL, 7% of calories from protein.

- Foods that are high in potassium include fruit (especially bananas, citrus fruits and juices, melons, raisins), potatoes, tomatoes, dried peas and beans, whole grains, milk, and fresh meat. The potassium content of vegetables and potatoes can be reduced by cutting them into small pieces, soaking them overnight, and boiling them in fresh water.

PROMOTING ADHERENCE

Studies show that, even though a substantial and significant reduction in protein intake can be observed in clients who are highly motivated and receive individualized dietary counseling, clients have difficulty consistently achieving their prescribed levels of protein. This may be a result of the highly restrictive nature of the diet or because the "choice" listings are imprecise and, in some groups, protein content is underestimated.

Clients who are not satisfied with their diets are not likely to maintain long-term adherence to a modified protein-eating plan. Adherence may be improved if counseling focuses on satisfaction with the diet. Other factors that may improve adherence include the following:

- Greater knowledge and skills, such as how to weigh and measure foods
- Positive messages about what to eat, rather than emphasizing food restrictions, especially protein modification guidelines
- Praise and encouragement, which help maintain motivation and sustain adherence
- More social support. Enlist the support of family and friends.
- Self-perception as successfully adhering to the plan. People who are more confident in their ability to adhere to the eating plan make better choices.
- More frequent self-monitoring of protein intake. This is especially important because the protein allowance may change as the disease progresses.
- More feedback on self-monitoring records and biochemistry data. Correlation of records with laboratory data enables the client to see cause-and-effect, reinforces the importance of nutrition therapy, and opens the door for problem solving.
- More food-tasting experiences, such as sampling new protein-modified products or recipes
- More guidelines for increasing energy; more what-to-eat information, not what-not-to-eat

NURSING PROCESS

Allen Parker is 34-years-old and has had type 1 diabetes for 27 years. He has a history of mild hypertension and mild anemia and complains of sudden weight gain and "swelling." His BUN and creatinine have been steadily increasing over the last several years. During his last appointment, the doctor told Allen to watch his protein intake and avoid salt. His diabetes is fairly well controlled with diet and multiple insulin injections. The doctor has diagnosed renal insufficiency and asked you to talk to Allen about his diet.

Assessment

Obtain clinical data:

- Current height, weight, BMI, recent weight history
- Medical history, including cardiovascular disease, hypertension, diabetes, and history of renal disease
- Abnormal laboratory values, especially BUN, creatinine, lipid levels, glucose, albumin, electrolytes, phosphorus, calcium, hemoglobin, and hematocrit
- Urine specific gravity
- Blood pressure
- Medications that affect nutrition, such as diuretics, insulin, and lipid-lowering medications

Interview client to assess:

- Understanding of the relationship between diet and renal function, specifically the role of protein, calories, sodium, potassium, phosphorus, calcium, and fluid
- Motivation to change eating style; how successful he was at avoiding salt
- Usual 24-hour intake, portion sizes, frequency and pattern of eating. Assess usual quantity and quality of protein consumed and whether most of the protein is of high biologic value (usually animal sources) or of low biologic value (gelatin and plant sources). Assess the use of salt and intake of high-sodium foods: cold cuts, bacon, frankfurters, smoked meats, sausage, canned meats, chipped or corned beef, buttermilk, cheese, crackers, canned soups and vegetables, convenience products, pickles, and condiments. Determine whether a salt substitute is used and, if so, its chemical composition. Assess intake of calories, potassium, calcium, and fluid.
- Cultural, religious, and ethnic influence on eating habits
- Psychosocial and economic issues, such as living situation, cooking facilities, financial status, employment, and education
- Use of vitamins, minerals, and nutritional supplements: what, how much, and why taken
- Use of alcohol and nicotine
- Physical complaints, such as fatigue, taste changes, anorexia, nausea, vomiting, diarrhea, muscular twitches, and muscle cramps

Nursing Diagnosis

Fluid Volume Excess, related to impaired renal function.

Planning and Implementation

CLIENT GOALS

The client will:

Maintain normal urinary output
Achieve and maintain normal blood pressure
Achieve normal or near-normal electrolyte levels
Maintain adequate glucose control
Consume adequate calories to minimize tissue catabolism
Attain and maintain adequate nutritional status
Describe the rationale and principles of nutrition therapy for renal insufficiency and implement the appropriate dietary changes
Practice self-management strategies, especially self-monitoring of protein intake

NURSING INTERVENTIONS

Nutrition Therapy
The doctor has prescribed a 50-g protein, 2-g sodium diet in addition to the patient's normal 2400-cal diabetic diet.

Client Teaching
Instruct the client:

On the role of nutrition therapy in the treatment of renal insufficiency
On eating plan essentials, including:
- Limiting protein, emphasizing high-quality proteins, spreading protein allowance over the whole day
- Consuming adequate calories
- Limiting high-sodium foods, not adding salt during cooking or at the table

On behavioral matters, including:
- How to weigh and measure foods to ensure accurate portion sizes
- To self-monitor protein intake
- To weigh himself at approximately the same time every day, with the same scale, and while wearing the same amount of clothing. Unexpected weight gain or loss should be reported to the physician.
- That renal diet cookbooks are available to increase variety

On attitudinal adjustment. Learn to view the diet as an integral component of treatment and a means of life support. Strict adherence to the diet can improve the quality of life and decrease the workload on the kidneys.
On where to find additional information (Box 20–5)

Evaluation

The client:

Maintains normal urinary output
Achieves and maintains normal blood pressure

BOX 20.5

Where to Get Additional Information

National Kidney Foundation
600 South Federal
Suite 201
Chicago, IL 60605
312-663-3103
www.nkfi.org/

National Institute of Diabetes and Digestive and Kidney Diseases
Building 31, Room 9A04
9000 Rockville Pike
Bethesda, MD 20892
301-496-3583
www.niddk.nih.gov/PG

Achieves normal or near-normal electrolyte levels
Consumes adequate calories to minimize tissue catabolism
Attains and maintains adequate nutritional status
Describes the rationale and principles in nutrition therapy of renal insufficiency and implements the appropriate dietary changes
Practices self-management strategies, especially self-monitoring of protein intake

KIDNEY TRANSPLANTATION

Kidney transplantation is a treatment option for people with ESRD. As with any surgery, the postoperative diet is high in protein and calories to promote healing. Thereafter, nutrition therapy is aimed at reducing the side effects and complications of immunosuppressant drug therapy. General guidelines are as follows:

Provide 1.0 g protein per kilogram body weight and adjust as needed. Higher amounts may be needed to outweigh the catabolic effects of glucocorticoids (negative nitrogen balance, muscle wasting, poor wound healing, stunted growth in children). Conversely, lower amounts are indicated if symptoms of uremia return.
Provide calories to maintain reasonable weight and spare protein. Corticosteroids may contribute to obesity, but other drugs may promote weight loss related to anorexia, nausea, vomiting, and diarrhea.
Limit fat to less than 30% of total calories, because blood lipid levels are often elevated.
Limit sodium to 3 to 4 g/day to help prevent sodium retention and hypertension.
Adjust potassium intake according to diuretic therapy.

DRUG ALERT

Drugs Used After Renal Transplantation

Corticosteroids (eg, prednisone) cause protein catabolism, negative nitrogen balance, glucose intolerance, sodium and fluid retention, potassium excretion, and impaired calcium absorption. Gastrointestinal upset may occur. Possible diet modifications include increasing protein and potassium and limiting sodium. Small, frequent meals may help minimize gastrointestinal distress. A diabetic diet may be indicated for hyperglycemia.

Cyclosporine commonly causes nausea, vomiting, and diarrhea. Other potential side effects include hypertension, hyperlipidemia, and hyperkalemia. Sodium and potassium intakes may be restricted, and because cyclosporine is nephrotoxic, a renal diet may be used.

Immunosuppressants (muromonab-CD3, Orthoclone, antithymocyte globulin) are less toxic than cyclosporine but may cause nausea, vomiting, diarrhea, and anorexia. Fever and stomatitis may occur.

Azathioprine (Imuran) may cause esophageal sores, vomiting, diarrhea, and macrocytic anemia. A liquid or soft diet may be needed.

Temporary or permanent rejection of the transplanted kidney may result in uremia, which may require the resumption of CRF dietary restrictions.

Acute Renal Failure

ARF is characterized by a decrease in renal blood flow, or glomerular or tubular damage, that leads to sudden loss of renal function, with rising blood levels of urea and other nitrogenous wastes (azotemia) and oliguria or anuria. Renal dysfunction can range from mild to severe.

Its clinical course begins with an *oliguric phase* that is characterized by a low urine output of less than 400 to 600 mL/24 hours, which may deteriorate to anuria. Sometimes large amounts of urine are excreted despite loss of renal function and nitrogenous waste retention (this is called **high-output renal failure**). The oliguric phase may last 10 to 20 days or longer.

The *diuretic phase* occurs when the kidneys are unable to conserve water. Large volumes of urine are excreted; losses of fluid, sodium, and potassium are extensive. The diuretic phase usually lasts 14 to 21 days. Today, few clients experience the diuretic phase because dialysis is usually performed earlier, minimizing extracellular fluid accumulation. The *recovery phase* is characterized by a gradual improvement in renal function over a 3- to 12-month period. Rapid improvement may be noted during the first 1 to 2 weeks, followed by a period of slower improvement. Some loss of renal function may be permanent.

Complications of ARF include infection, which is the leading cause of death in these clients. Hyperkalemia may result in cardiac arrest, metabolic acidosis, hypercatabolism, circulatory overload (dyspnea, orthopnea, pulmonary congestion, pulmonary edema), hypertension, hypertensive crisis, convulsions, and neurologic abnormalities. ARF may progress to CRF; at least 5% of clients with acute tubular necrosis require long-term hemodialysis. ARF is fatal in 50% of cases.

The primary focus of treatment is to correct the underlying disorder so as to prevent permanent renal damage. Dialysis is used to keep BUN levels lower than 100 mg/dL and creatinine levels lower than 8 mg/dL. Diuretics and other measures to restore fluid and electrolyte balance are used. Symptomatic anemia is treated with transfusions of packed red blood cells. Nutrition therapy may help to lessen the workload of the kidneys and restore optimal nutritional status.

NUTRITION THERAPY

The optimal diet for clients with ARF is more elusive than the optimal diet for CRF. Although the exact nutritional requirements are not known, it is evident that needs vary among individuals and according to the phase of ARF, and that once dialysis is instituted, diet restrictions are liberalized.

Protein

Controversy exists over whether protein intake should be restricted because of nitrogenous waste retention or increased because of hypercatabolism and infection or sepsis imposed by a major underlying illness. Some clinicians believe that restricting protein helps preserve nephron functioning; others believe that a high-protein diet is necessary to correct for negative nitrogen balance. People not receiving dialysis therapy may be limited to 0.8 g protein per kilogram body weight. As GFR returns to normal or dialysis begins, the protein allowance is increased to promote nitrogen balance and tissue healing. Depending on the type of dialysis used, protein intake may increase to 1.1 to 2.5 g/kg.

Calories

Calorie requirements depend on the rate of catabolism and metabolism and range from 30 to 50 cal/kg. Carbohydrate modules, pure fats, refined sugars, and low-protein starches are used liberally.

Fluid

For both the oliguric and diuretic phases of ARF, fluid intake should equal total fluid output per 24 hours, plus an additional 400 to 500 mL, depending on the client's hydration status. Up to 3 L of fluid may be needed daily to replenish losses after diuresis begins.

Potassium

Life-threatening hyperkalemia that occurs during the oliguric phase of ARF is related to potassium retention and tissue catabolism, which causes potassium to leave the cells and enter the serum. Diets that are low in potassium (2 g/day or less) and exchange resins such as Kayexalate may be used during the oliguric phase to reduce serum potassium levels. Intravenous dextrose and insulin may be given as a temporary measure to lower serum potassium (insulin causes dextrose and potassium to leave the serum and enter the cells). Once diuresis begins, large amounts of potassium are excreted, and potassium supplements may be necessary to avoid hypokalemia.

Sodium

Sodium intake is adjusted according to urine output, serum sodium level, symptoms of sodium imbalance, and concurrent use of dialysis. Sodium intake may be restricted to 500 to 1000 mg/day during the oliguric phase. As with potassium, sodium requirements increase during the diuretic phase to replace increased losses.

METHOD OF FEEDING

Clients who are unable to eat because of critical illness or impaired gastrointestinal function secondary to ARF may need enteral or parenteral nutrition. Special enteral and parenteral renal formulas are low in protein, low in electrolytes, and high in calories. The carbohydrate-dense formulas may contribute to hyperglycemia that occurs with stress and renal failure. Insulin may be used to lower glucose levels. When oral intake resumes, small, frequent meals and assistance with eating may be needed if the client is weak or fatigued.

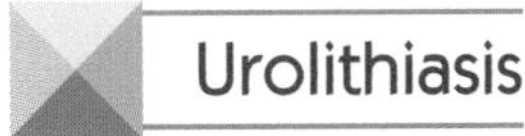

Urolithiasis

DESCRIPTION

The precipitation of insoluble crystals in the urine leads to the formation of stones (**calculi**) that vary in size from sand-like "gravel" to large, branching stones. Although they form most often in the kidney, they can occur anywhere in the urinary system. Usually, stones smaller than 1 cm in diameter are spontaneously voided; larger stones may require removal. Renal stones can lead to infection and obstruction, resulting in renal damage, which may require nephrectomy. Approximately 80% of stones contain calcium, and most of these are composed of calcium oxalate; fewer calcium stones are composed of calcium phosphate or of oxalate and phosphate salts. Approximately 10% of stones are composed of uric acid, and 10% are struvite (magnesium, ammonium, phosphate). Cystine (an amino acid) stones occur only in people with cystinuria, an autosomal recessive disorder.

Urolithiasis may result from low urine volumes, which may occur secondary to ileostomies or arise from certain occupational circumstances that limit fluid intake (eg, in delivery people and salespeople). People living in the southeastern United States (the "stone belt") are at increased risk of stone formation. It has been suggested that the increased risk is related to reduced urine volume secondary to increased perspiration caused by high environmental temperatures or to increased absorption of calcium secondary to vitamin D activation from greater sunlight exposure.

Certain dietary factors are implicated in stone development, namely high intakes of animal protein, sodium, and oxalate, and low intake of calcium. Under debate is whether excluding dietary components of the stone is preventive against future stone formation.

- **Animal protein.** A high intake of animal protein makes the urine more acidic, which promotes calcium excretion and inhibits calcium reabsorption. Animal protein is also the major dietary source of purines, the precursors of uric acid. High levels of urinary uric acid make calcium oxalate less soluble, thereby increasing the risk of calcium stone formation.
- **Sodium.** Because the body rids itself of excess sodium through the urine, the greater the sodium intake, the greater the level of urinary sodium. High urinary sodium increases urinary excretion of calcium and uric acid and increases calcium mobilization from bone. However, limiting sodium intake has not been shown to prevent stone formation.
- **Oxalates.** Certain foods are rich sources of oxalate, including nuts, chocolate, dark green leafy vegetables, rhubarb, beets, okra, tomato sauce, and jams. However, endogenous oxalate production provides more urinary oxalate than dietary intake does. Also, the bioavailability of oxalate from some foods may be impaired. For instance, tea and beer are high in oxalates, but they may actually protect against stone formation. Restricting dietary oxalate intake has been shown to reduce urinary oxalate levels but not to prevent stone formation.
- **Calcium.** Calcium intake from dairy products may be associated with high urinary calcium levels and stone formation. However, an inverse relation between dietary calcium and stone formation has been shown; people with the highest calcium intake had almost half the rate of stones as people with the lowest intake of calcium. Dietary calcium may bind with dietary oxalate in the intestines, forming an insoluble compound that the body cannot absorb. The decrease in urinary oxalate that occurs with increased dietary calcium is proportionally more significant than the rise in urinary calcium levels that occurs.

NUTRITION THERAPY

The most effective nutritional intervention for the treatment and prevention of all renal calculi is to increase fluids and thereby dilute the urine. A high urine output not only helps the client to pass an existing stone, but also decreases the likelihood that another stone will precipitate out of the urine. A daily fluid intake of 2.5 to 3 L is recommended. Fluid intake should increase when perspiration increases, such as with hot weather and exercise. At least 8 to 12 ounces of fluid, preferably water, should be consumed before bedtime, because urine normally becomes more concentrated at night.

Recommendations for clients with hypercalciuria are as follows:

- Increase fluid intake to produce a urine output of at least 2 L/day.
- In clients with hypercalciuria, limit animal protein intake to 8 ounces/day, sodium to 2 g/day, and oxalate to as low as tolerated. These are achievable goals and are potentially beneficial, especially if dietary excesses have been identified. Vitamin B_6 supplements reduce oxalate production by 50% and may help treatment. Megadoses of vitamin C should be avoided by people at risk for oxalate stones, because the body can synthesize oxalate from vitamin C.
- Maintain adequate calcium intake. Restricting calcium intake has not been shown to decrease stone formation and may worsen osteoporosis.

Clients with uric acid stones are urged to limit animal protein and sodium intakes. Drugs are used to alter urinary pH.

Questions You May Hear

Does cranberry juice prevent urinary tract infections? Although conclusive evidence is lacking, it now appears that, if cranberry juice is effective against urinary tract infections, it is because it contains an ingredient that may prevent bacteria from adhering to the lining of the urinary tract, thereby promoting their excretion. However, not all bacteria are sensitive to the juice, and protection lasts only as long as the juice is consumed regularly. Clients who are prone to urinary tract infections and like cranberry juice should be encouraged to consume it regularly, just in case. The only other dietary recommendation for urinary tract infections is to increase fluid intake to flush out bacteria.

KEY CONCEPTS

- Loss of renal function profoundly affects metabolism, nutritional status, and nutritional requirements. The nutrients most affected are protein, calcium, phosphorus, vitamin D, fluid, sodium, and potassium.
- Diet modifications for renal insufficiency are complex, unpalatable, and frequently adjusted according to the client's laboratory values and symptoms.
- Although it has not been proven that protein restriction can slow the decline in renal function, protein restriction remains the cornerstone of dietary treatment for renal insufficiency because it has the potential to lessen renal workload.
- There is a narrow margin of error regarding protein intake: too little protein results in body protein catabolism, which has the same effect as eating too much protein, namely an increase in BUN levels.
- A high-calorie diet is indicated whenever protein intake is restricted to ensure that the protein consumed will be used for specific protein functions, not for energy requirements.
- Usually, clients with renal insufficiency tolerate 2 to 4 g of sodium per day. Potassium usually is not restricted.
- Fluid allowance is based on urine output, plus an additional 400 to 500 mL to account for insensible losses.
- Calcium metabolism is impaired because of faulty vitamin D metabolism secondary to loss of renal function. A high calcium intake from food is not achievable when protein and phosphorus are restricted.

- When dialysis is instituted, dietary restrictions are liberalized; a high protein intake is recommended to compensate for protein lost through the dialysate.
- There is little agreement on the optimal diet for ARF. Protein intake may start at 0.8 g/kg and advance with improvement or dialysis.
- Clients who experience renal transplantation may need to alter their diet to lessen the side effects of drug therapy. Steroids cause hyperglycemia, sodium retention, potassium depletion, loss of calcium from the bones, and gastrointestinal upsets.
- A fluid intake of 2.5 to 3 L/day or more is the most effective nutritional intervention for the prevention of renal calculi.

Focus on Critical Thinking

Michael Murphy is a 42-year-old active male who recently experienced ARF secondary to scleroderma. While he was hospitalized in the intensive care unit, Michael received total parenteral nutrition (TPN) and dialysis and stayed in a coma for 2 weeks. As his condition improved, he was weaned from TPN and resumed an oral diet. The only discharge dietary instructions he recalls are to avoid salt, limit fluid to 1 quart daily, and limit daily meat intake to 6 ounces. Although he has some urine output, he requires hemodialysis three times each week. Doctors hope that he will eventually regain enough renal function so that he can discontinue dialysis.

Michael has lost 22 pounds since he became ill; his present weight of 168 pounds is the least his 6-foot 2-inch frame has ever weighed. He complains of fatigue, anorexia, and being "mentally fuzzy." He forces himself to eat and says that the only thing that tastes good to him is ice cream. He has not been gaining any weight between dialysis treatments. As his outpatient dialysis nurse, you find that he wants to do whatever he can to feel better and maximize his chance of getting off dialysis treatments.

- Is it appropriate that Michael limit his meat intake to 6 ounces daily? How much protein does he require? What other sources of protein might he be eating that would contribute to his daily intake?
- Is not gaining weight between dialysis treatments an appropriate goal? What nutrient may he not be getting enough of?
- What other nutrients may need to be restricted in Michael's diet?
- Explain why he may have symptoms of fatigue, anorexia, and "mental fuzziness."
- Michael thought he could eat as much ice cream as he wanted because it's just "a sweet." What would you tell Michael about ice cream to convince him that it should not be eaten freely?
- Calculate Michael's calorie requirements; list high-calorie foods that he may use to boost his calorie intake. What would you suggest he do to help improve his intake?

ANSWER KEY

1. **FALSE** The recommended protein intake for patients with renal insufficiency is only slightly below the normal Recommended Dietary Allowance.
2. **FALSE** Foods high in calcium (dairy products) are usually restricted because of their high protein and phosphorus content; therefore, calcium supplements are used to increase calcium intake.

3. **TRUE** Once dialysis is initiated, protein requirements are increased to above normal levels to ensure adequacy and to compensate for protein and amino acid losses in the dialysate.
4. **FALSE** Some people with advanced renal failure are unable to conserve sodium, and a sodium deficit may occur if sodium intake is restricted.
5. **TRUE** Accelerated atherosclerosis increases the risk of congestive heart failure and myocardial infarction, and a dietary emphasis on monounsaturated fats may help minimize the cardiovascular risks.
6. **FALSE** Although the diet for CRF is complex, that for ARF is even more so.
7. **TRUE** People on peritoneal dialysis need to decrease their calorie intake to compensate for the calories absorbed from the dialysate.
8. **FALSE** Weight gain between dialysis treatments reflects fluid retention, not excess calorie intake.
9. **FALSE** An inverse relationship between dietary calcium and stone formation has been demonstrated: The rate of stone formation in people with the highest calcium intake was approximately 50% that of people with the lowest calcium intake.
10. **TRUE** The most effective nutrition intervention for the treatment and prevention of all renal calculi is to increase fluids to dilute the urine.

REFERENCES

Beto, J. (1995). Which diet for which renal failure: Making sense of the options. *Journal of the American Dietetic Association, 95*, 898–903.

Coyne, T., Olson, M., Bradham, K., Garcom, M., Gregory, P., & Scherch, L. (1995). Dietary satisfaction correlated with adherence in the Modification of Diet in Renal Disease Study. *Journal of the American Dietetic Association, 95*, 1301–1306.

Curhan, G., Willett, W., Speizer, F., & Stampfer, M. (1998). Beverage use and risk for kidney stones in women. *Annals of Internal Medicine, 128*, 534–540.

Escott Stump, S. (1998). *Nutrition and diagnosis-related care* (4th ed.). Philadelphia: Williams & Wilkins.

Gillis, B., Caggiula, A., Chiavacci, A., Coyne, T., Doroshenko, L., Milas, C., Nowalk, P., & Scherch, L. (1995). Nutrition intervention program of the Modification of Diet in Renal Disease Study: A self-management approach. *Journal of the American Dietetic Association, 91*, 1288–1294.

Goldfarb, D., & Coe, F. (1999). Prevention of recurrent nephrolithiasis. *American Family Physician, 60*, 2269–2276.

Milas, N., Nowalk, M., Akpele, L., Castaldo, L., Coyne, T., Doroshenko, L., Kigawa, L., Korzec-Ramirez, D., Scherch, L., & Snetselaar, L. (1995). Factors associated with adherence to the dietary protein intervention in the Modification of Diet in Renal Disease Study. *Journal of the American Dietetic Association*, 95, 1295–1300.

MDRD Study Group. (1994). Reduction of dietary protein and phosphorus in the Modification of Diet in Renal Disease Feasibility Study. *Journal of the American Dietetic Association, 94*, 986–990.

National Kidney and Urologic Diseases Information Clearinghouse. Growth failure in children with kidney disease. [On-line]. Available: www.niddk.nih.gov/health/kiendy/summary/grwofail/index.htm. Accessed February 13, 2000.

Renal Dietitians Dietetic Practice Group, National Kidney Foundation Council on Renal Nutrition. (1993). *National renal diet: Professional guide*. Chicago: American Dietetic Association.

Sanders, H., Rabb, H., Bittle, P., & Ramirez, G. (1994). Nutritional implications of recombinant human erythropoietin therapy in renal disease. *Journal of the American Dietetic Association, 94*, 1023–1029.

CHAPTER 21

Nutrition for Patients With Cancer or HIV/AIDS

TRUE	FALSE	Check your knowledge of nutrition for patients with cancer or HIV/AIDS.
		1 Nutrition problems are not likely to develop until cancer metastasizes.
		2 Cachexia is responsible for more deaths than cancer itself.
		3 Cachexia is directly related to the amount of calories consumed.
		4 The appetite of clients with anorexia tends to improve as the day progresses.
		5 The risk of nausea may be lessened by not eating 1 to 2 hours before chemotherapy and radiation.
		6 A cheese sandwich may be a better option than hot roast beef for someone with taste alterations.
		7 All clients with cancer need a high-calorie diet.
		8 Weight loss and malnutrition are inevitable consequences of HIV/AIDS.
		9 Clients with HIV/AIDS have problems with appetite and intake similar to those of cancer clients.
		10 Nutritional counseling of clients with HIV/AIDS should include how to avoid foodborne illnesses.

Upon completion of this chapter, you will be able to

- Discuss how cancer and cancer therapies affect nutritional status.
- List criteria to consider when assessing the nutritional status of someone with cancer.
- Describe nutritional interventions to minimize the following side effects: anorexia, nausea and vomiting, taste alterations, and sore mouth.
- Describe the role of nutrition therapy for clients receiving palliative care.
- Discuss how HIV/AIDS affects nutritional status.
- Describe nutrition therapy for clients with HIV/AIDS.

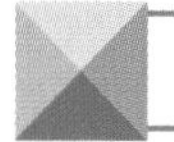

Introduction

This chapter is devoted to cancer and acquired immunodeficiency syndrome (AIDS), two diseases characterized by body wasting and malnutrition. Although nutrition therapy cannot cure either disease, it has the potential to maximize the effectiveness of drug therapy, minimize side effects of the disease and its treatments, and improve overall quality of life.

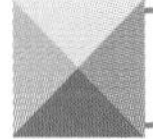

Nutrition and Cancer

The relationships among diet, nutritional status, and cancer are complex and multifaceted. As discussed in Chapter 8, approximately one third of all cancer deaths are related to dietary factors. Some components of food may promote cancer, and others may help prevent cancer promotion. For people who have cancer and are being aggressively treated, nutrition therapy aimed at maintaining nutritional status helps optimize the chance for successful cancer treatment and may decrease morbidity and mortality. Palliative nutritional support for the terminally ill may improve quality of life and enhance the client's sense of well-being.

PATHOGENESIS OF CANCER

Cancer develops when an **initiating event** (eg, repeated or prolonged exposure to carcinogens or radiation) changes the structure of deoxyribonucleic acid (DNA), or the reproductive code, in normal cells. Exactly why this change in normal cell structure occurs is not known. After a latent period of usually 5 to 30 years, a **promoting event** (eg, a favorable hormonal environment) transforms initiated cells into cancer cells that autonomously proliferate, then infiltrate and destroy surrounding tissues. Eventually, cancer cells detach from the tumor mass and migrate, or are transported, to a distant site, where they lodge and grow (**metastasize**) in the new location to form a secondary tumor mass. Left untreated, cancer ends in death.

There is no single etiology of cancer in humans. External causes include chemicals, radiation, and viruses. Internal causes include hormones, immune conditions, and inherited mutations. Many cancers are curable if detected early, and the risk of getting cancer can be greatly reduced by lifestyle changes. Seventy percent to 80% of all cases of cancer may be related to environmental causes, such as smoking, exposure to the sun, and diet, and therefore are potentially preventable.

EFFECT OF CANCER ON NUTRITIONAL STATUS

Cancer and its treatments can have profound and devastating effects on nutritional status, leading to protein-calorie malnutrition, the most common secondary diagnosis in cancer patients. Protein-calorie malnutrition is a major cause of morbidity and mortality.

Moreover, cancer patients identify nutrition problems as the most important factor affecting their sense of well-being, more important than sexuality or continued employment.

Local Effects

Local tumor effects produce many nutritional problems. Most notably, growing tumors of the gastrointestinal tract can cause obstruction, nausea, vomiting, impaired digestion, delayed transit, and malabsorption. Ascites related to ovarian and genitourinary cancers may lead to early satiety, progressive protein malnutrition, and fluid and electrolyte imbalances. Pain related to tumor bulk or location may cause severe anorexia and poor oral intake. Tumors of the central nervous system that cause confusion or somnolence may lead to poor intake related to poor attention. Other potential problems vary with the cancer location (Table 21–1).

Systemic Effects

Cancer causes systemic effects by altering metabolism, and these effects lead to nutritional problems of a pervasive nature. Although metastatic cancers may produce more pronounced changes, even cancers that are limited to one site can produce generalized effects. Metabolic alterations include increased energy expenditure, increased protein catabolism and whole-body protein turnover (reuse of amino acids that are generated by protein metabolism), increased lipolysis, and preferential use of fat as an energy source. In addition, tumors can produce hormone-like substances that alter nutrient absorption and metabolism. Other substances produced by cancer cells may alter sense of taste, promote anorexia, or contribute to cancer cachexia.

Cancer cachexia is a wasting syndrome marked by weakness and progressive loss of body weight, fat, and muscle. Unlike simple starvation, to which the body adapts by low-

TABLE 21.1 ***Potential Nutritional Impact of Cancer Based on Location***

Cancer Location	Potential Impact on Nutrition
Head and neck	Chewing and swallowing problems
Esophagus	Swallowing problems
Stomach	Fluid and electrolyte imbalance related to vomiting
Small bowel	Maldigestion and malabsorption
	Protein-losing enteropathy related to lymphatic obstruction within the intestinal villi
Liver	Watery diarrhea related to an increase in serotonin, histamines, and other substances
Pancreatic cancer	Maldigestion and malabsorption secondary to altered insulin secretion

ering metabolic rate, the metabolic rate in cachexia is not adaptive and may increase, decrease, or be normal. Other characteristics of cachexia include early satiety, anorexia, anemia, loss of immunocompetence, and severe weight loss, which is defined as a loss of 10% or more of body weight within 6 months or an unintentional weight loss of 2 pounds/week. Cachexia diminishes quality of life, impairs wound healing, and increases the risk of infection. It is estimated to affect half of all people with cancer. Cachexia is responsible for more deaths than is cancer itself.

Cachexia appears to be caused by changes that are induced by the tumor, because removal of the tumor can reverse the cachexia. Although anorexia may contribute to the development of cachexia, neither the incidence nor the severity of cachexia can be related directly to calorie intake (ie, cachexia can develop even if calorie intake is high), nor to tumor weight or tumor cell type. Factors that contribute to cachexia are shown in Figure 21–1. Cancers of the gastrointestinal tract, pancreas, lung, and prostate, as well as some lymph node cancers, are more likely to cause cachexia than are breast cancers or sarcomas.

EFFECT OF CANCER THERAPIES ON NUTRITIONAL STATUS

Cancer may be treated with chemotherapy, radiation, surgery, immunotherapy, or a combination of therapies. Some hematologic cancers are treated by bone marrow transplantation. Each of these treatment modalities can contribute to progressive nutritional deterioration related to systemic or localized side effects that interfere with intake, increase nutrient losses, or alter metabolism. Actual response to each of these therapies depends on the individual and the type and extent of treatment.

Nutritional support that is used as an adjuvant to effective cancer therapy helps sustain the client through adverse side effects and may reduce morbidity and mortality. Nutrition therapy can reverse weight loss, restore or maintain immunocompetence, help restore normal metabolism, enhance tolerance for antineoplastic therapy, maintain body composition during nutritional repletion, and reduce postoperative morbidity. However, for nutritional support to improve the results of cancer therapy, the therapy itself must have a reasonable chance of success. Evidence suggests that aggressive nutritional support may be of little value, or even detrimental, when it is used in conjunction with ineffective cancer treatment.

Chemotherapy

Chemotherapy damages the reproductive ability of both malignant and normal cells, especially rapidly dividing cells such as well-nourished cancer cells and normal cells of the gastrointestinal tract, respiratory system, bone marrow, skin, and gonadal tissue. Cyclic administration of multiple drugs is given in maximum tolerated doses.

The side effects of chemotherapy vary with the type of drug or combination of drugs used, dose, rate of excretion, duration of treatment, and individual tolerance. Chemotherapy side effects generally are more widespread than those associated with

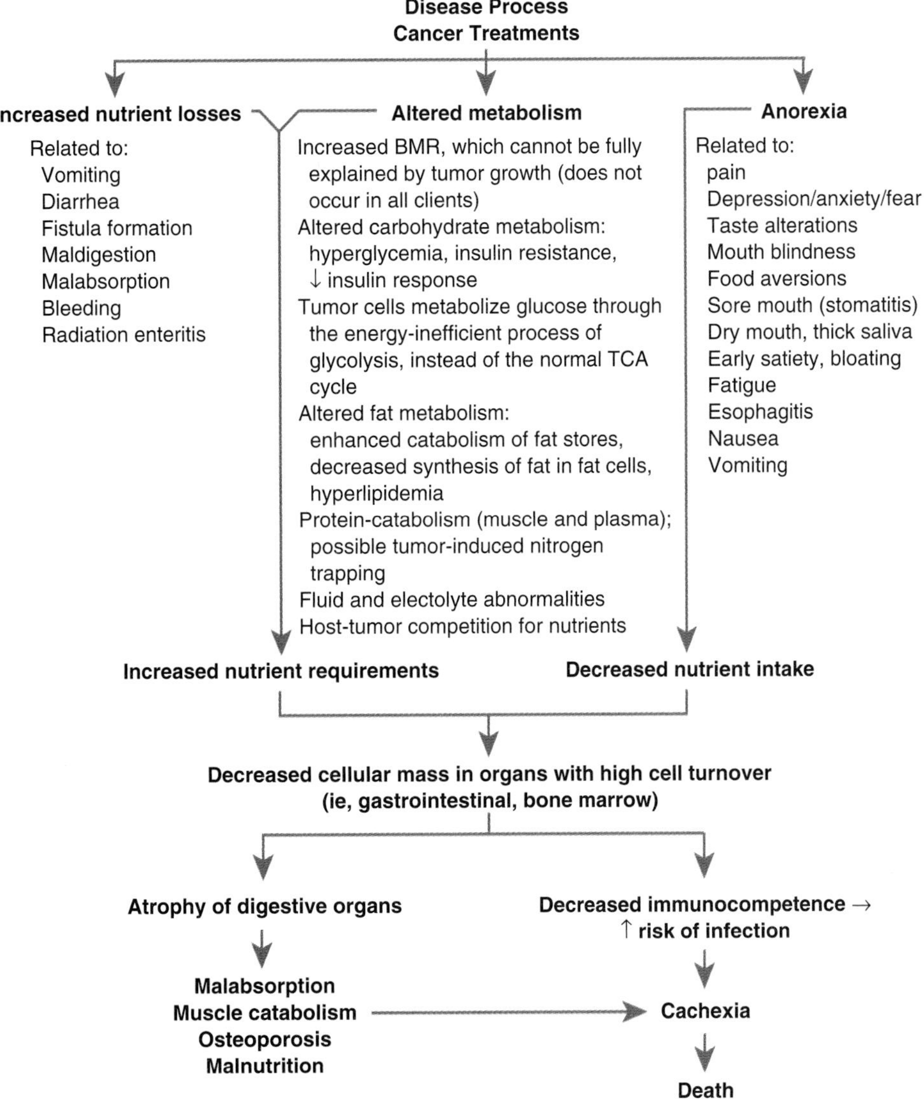

FIGURE 21-1 The causes of cachexia.

other forms of treatment. Symptoms that affect nutrition and last longer than 2 weeks are particularly important. The most frequent side effects are fatigue, anorexia, nausea and vomiting, taste alterations or aversions, sore mouth or throat, diarrhea, constipation, and infectious complications. Some combinations of chemotherapeutic drugs may produce severe and long-lasting gastrointestinal complications. Table 21–2 lists side effects of various chemotherapeutic drugs.

TABLE 21.2 *Side Effects of Various Chemotherapeutic Drugs*

Drug	Anorexia	Nausea and Vomiting	Mucositis/Stomatitis	Diarrhea	Abdominal Pain	Nephrotoxic	Intestinal Ulceration	Constipation	Other
Anastrozole		✓✓		✓✓		✓✓			
Asparaginase	✓✓	✓✓				✓✓			
Azacitidine	✓✓	✓✓		✓✓					
Bleomycin	✓	✓✓	✓✓						
Carboplatin		✓✓		✓✓				✓✓	
Carmustine	✓	✓✓				✓			
Chlorambucil									May cause liver damage
Cisplatin	✓	✓✓		✓✓		✓✓			May cause Mg++ and K+ depletion
Cyclophosphamide	✓	✓✓		✓✓					Heartburn and gastrointestinal pain common
Cytarabine	✓	✓✓	✓	✓✓					
Dacarbazine	✓	✓✓							Restrict food 4–6 h before dose
Dactinomycin	✓	✓✓	✓	✓✓					
Docetaxel		✓✓		✓✓					May need low-sodium diet
Doxorubicin		✓							Heartburn common
Emcyt	✓✓	✓✓		✓✓					Dairy products and other Ca++ sources may ↓ drug absorption
Estramustine phosphate sodium	✓✓	✓✓		✓✓					Dairy products and other Ca++ sources may ↓ drug absorption Decreases glucose tolerance
Etoposide	✓✓	✓✓	✓						
Fluorouracil	✓✓	✓✓	✓✓	✓✓					
Hydroxyurea	✓✓	✓✓	✓✓						
Idarubicin	✓	✓	✓						
Ifosfamide	✓✓	✓✓	✓✓						
Interferon alpha	✓✓	✓✓		✓✓					May need low-sodium diet
Irinotecan HCl	✓✓	✓✓		✓✓					Diarrhea may be severe and cause significant electrolyte imbalance
Mercaptopurine	✓	✓		✓					
Methotrexate	✓	✓✓	✓✓	✓✓	✓	✓✓	✓		
Mitomycin	✓✓	✓✓	✓						May need low-sodium diet
Paclitaxel		✓✓	✓	✓✓					May need low-sodium diet
Pegaspargase		✓✓		✓					May alter glucose metabolism May need low-sodium diet
Pentostatin	✓✓	✓✓		✓✓		✓✓			
Procarbazine	✓	✓✓	✓						
Streptozocin	✓	✓✓				✓✓	✓		
Teniposide	✓✓	✓✓	✓	✓✓					
Topotecan HCl	✓✓	✓✓	✓	✓✓				✓✓	May need increased fiber and fluids
Vinblastine	✓	✓	✓	✓				✓✓	May need increased fiber and fluids
Vincristine		✓✓		✓✓	✓			✓✓	
Vinorelbine		✓✓		✓✓					

✓, low potential; ✓✓, moderate to high potential.

Fatigue is one of the most distressing side effects of both chemotherapy and radiation. It differs from fatigue in healthy people in that it is more intense, persists longer, and it is not relieved by sleep. It tends to peak within a few days after chemotherapy and then declines until the next treatment, when the cycle repeats itself. Fatigue significantly impairs quality of life by decreasing mental activity, work capacity, and activities of daily living. Recognizing their decline in function, clients may feel hopelessness and despair. Clients are often too tired to eat, and food purchasing and preparation may be exhausting. Fatigue impairs intake, and poor intake exacerbates fatigue.

Radiation

Radiation causes cell death; particles of radioactive energy break chemical bonds, disrupting reproductive ability. Although radiation injures all rapidly dividing cells, it is most lethal for the poorly differentiated and rapidly proliferating cells of cancer tissue. Recovery from sublethal doses of radiation occurs in the interval between the first dose and subsequent doses. Normal tissue appears to recover more quickly from radiation damage than cancerous tissue does.

Side effects are specific for the area irradiated, usually develop within 1 to 2 days after treatment is given, and may last for 2 weeks. The type and intensity of radiation side effects depend on the type of radiation used, the site, the volume of tissue irradiated, the dose of radiation, the duration of therapy, and individual tolerance. The rapidly growing cells of the gastrointestinal mucosa, skin, and bone marrow are particularly vulnerable. General weakness, fatigue, and anorexia are common side effects, regardless of the site, amount, and duration of therapy. Radiation to the abdomen or pelvis can produce nausea, vomiting, diarrhea, enteritis, proctitis, or fistula formation. Delayed side effects can develop years after radiation is completed. Surgical and nutritional intervention may be required to alleviate progressive diarrhea, malabsorption, and malnutrition. Potential complications of radiation are shown in Table 21–3.

Surgery

Surgery may be better tolerated (shorter postoperative hospital stay and fewer complications) by people who have good nutritional status before treatment. Postsurgical nutritional requirements increase for protein, calories, vitamin C, B vitamins, and iron to replenish losses and promote healing. Actual side effects and complications incurred depend on the location and extent of surgery (Table 21–4).

Immunotherapy

Immunotherapy seeks to enhance the body's immune system to help control cancer. Potential adverse effects include fever, which may increase protein and calorie requirements, and fatigue and weakness, which may impair appetite and intake.

TABLE 21.3 *Potential Complications of Radiation*

Area	Potential Complications
Head and neck	Altered or loss of taste ("mouth blindness") Decreased salivary secretions → dry mouth Thick salivary secretions Difficulty swallowing and chewing Loss of teeth
Lower neck and midchest	Acute: esophagitis with dysphagia Delayed: fibrosis → esophageal stricture → difficulty swallowing
Abdomen and pelvis	Extensive radiation to upper or middle abdomen → nausea and vomiting Acute or chronic bowel damage → cramps, steatorrhea, malabsorption, disaccharidase deficiency, protein-losing enteropathy, bowel constriction, obstruction, or fistula formation Chronic blood loss from intestine and bladder Pelvic radiation → increased urinary frequency, urgency, and dysuria

Bone Marrow Transplantation

Bone marrow transplantation is used primarily to treat hematologic cancers and experimentally to treat solid tumors such as breast cancer. Bone marrow transplantation is preceded by high-dose chemotherapy and total-body irradiation to suppress immune function and destroy cancer cells. Immunosuppressants are given before and after the procedure. Although cancer cells are killed, the preparation renders the client unable to resist infection.

Treatments given before transplantation commonly cause anorexia, taste alterations, nausea, vomiting, and inflammation of the mucous membranes lining the gastrointestinal tract. Post-transplantation complications include delayed mucositis, stomatitis, esophagitis, and intestinal damage that causes severe diarrhea and malabsorption. Oral intake often is not an option. Total parenteral nutrition (TPN) may be needed for 1 to 2 months after bone marrow transplantation.

ASSESSING THE NUTRITIONAL NEEDS OF CLIENTS WITH CANCER

Because a "typical" cancer client does not exist, nutrition therapy must be individualized and continually monitored and revised according to the client's assessment data.

Historical Data

What is the client's usual, current, and ideal weight? Does the client have fluid retention that masks true weight status?

TABLE 21.4 *Potential Complications of Surgery*

Type	Potential Complications
Head and neck resection	Difficulty chewing and swallowing Tube feeding dependency
Esophagectomy or esophageal resection	Early satiety Regurgitation Fistula formation Stenosis Vagotomy → decreased stomach motility, decreased gastric acid production, diarrhea, steatorrhea
Gastric resection	"Dumping syndrome": crampy diarrhea that develops quickly after eating, accompanied by flushing, dizziness, weakness, pain, distention, and vomiting Hypoglycemia Malabsorption Achlorhydria Vitamin B_{12} malabsorption related to lack of intrinsic factor
Intestinal resection	Malnutrition related to generalized malabsorption Fluid and electrolyte imbalance Diarrhea Hyperoxaluria → increased risk of renal oxalate stone formation and increased excretion of calcium Calcium and magnesium deficiency Steatorrhea and malabsorption of fat-soluble vitamins
Massive bowel resection	Steatorrhea Malnutrition related to severe generalized malabsorption Metabolic acidosis Dehydration
Ileostomy or colostomy	Fluid and electrolyte imbalance
Pancreatic resection	Generalized malabsorption Diabetes mellitus

Is the client following a special diet? Is the usual intake adequate? What dietary changes has the client made in response to symptoms or side effects of cancer or cancer treatment? Which foods are best and least tolerated? Does the client have food allergies or intolerances? Does the client do the shopping and cooking? What is the client's attitude about the role of nutrition in cancer and recovery? What nutritional supplements does the client use and for what purpose?

What cancer treatments is the client undergoing? Does the client have side effects that interfere with intake or metabolism, such as nausea, vomiting, anorexia, diarrhea, alterations in taste, dry or sore mouth, pain, or fatigue? If so, determine the onset, frequency, duration, severity, interventions attempted, and results. Does the client have preexisting conditions that require nutrition therapy, such as diabetes, heart disease, renal impairments, or a liver disorder? What cultural, religious, or ethnic influences affect the client's food choices? What over-the-counter and prescribed medications does the client use? What is the client's emotional state? Does the client participate in physical activity? Are there outside support systems?

Physical Findings

Does the client exhibit signs of malnutrition, such as skin changes, edema, ascites, easy fatigability, loss of subcutaneous fat, and tissue wasting? Does the client have signs of fluid and electrolyte imbalance? Is the client able to perform the activities of daily living?

Laboratory Data

Because cancer and cancer therapies can cause low values for hemoglobin, hematocrit, and total lymphocyte count, these tests are not valid indicators of poor nutritional status in cancer clients. Criteria to look at include:

- Protein status, as indicated by serum albumin, serum transferrin, thyroxine-bound prealbumin, and retinol-binding protein
- Nitrogen balance, if available
- Serum electrolytes and minerals (calcium, magnesium, sodium, potassium)
- Other abnormal laboratory values

NUTRITION THERAPY

The needs of cancer clients change as they move along the continuum of recovery. For instance, clients in the first phase, the initial period after diagnosis that may include surgery, do not need specific information about what to eat. They may not have experienced any side effects of cancer that interfere with intake or nutritional status. Advice that may or may not be needed in 6 months is inappropriate for a client who feels overwhelmed by the task of coming to terms with a cancer diagnosis. Side effects appear in the next phase as the client undergoes chemotherapy or radiation. During this phase, some clients believe there is nothing food or nutrition therapy can do to help them feel better. At the other end of the spectrum are clients who believe dietary changes can cure, arrest, or treat their disease. The goal is to get clients to the middle ground, where they feel empowered with the sense that they can take an active role in their own recovery. Finally, the long-term recovery phase begins as the client resumes a normal intake. Acute care needs transition into long-term goals of optimal nutrition for health and well-being.

Nutrition therapy objectives and interventions are based on the client's treatment goals. For instance, nutrition therapy for clients who are receiving aggressive treatment to arrest or cure the disease differs from that for clients who are receiving palliative care for comfort and improved quality of life. For all cancer clients, the overall goal of nutrition therapy is to keep the client out of the hospital whenever possible.

Nutrition Therapy for Clients Aggressively Treated for Cancer

Used as an adjunct to cancer treatment, aggressive nutritional support may reduce morbidity and mortality by stimulating weight gain, reversing negative nitrogen balance, preventing or correcting nutritional deficiencies, improving immunocompetence, and increasing the sense of well-being. Because cachexia is easier to prevent than to treat, nutritional support should be initiated before the downward spiral of malnutrition develops. However, because it is likely that some characteristics of cachexia are not caused simply by an inadequate intake, some cachectic clients may not respond to aggressive nutritional support.

Minimizing Side Effects

Alleviating eating problems is key to promoting an adequate intake. Modifications in texture, temperature, and eating schedule, as well as administering medications to control side effects, are options for promoting intake.

ANOREXIA

Anorexia, which may be continuous or sporadic, is among the most common symptoms in people with cancer. Appetite is often best in the morning and deteriorates gradually throughout the day. A major cause of anorexia is food odor. To limit the client's exposure to food odors in the hospital, remove the tray cover before the tray is placed in front of the client so that food odors can dissipate. The following tips may help manage anorexia:

- Overeat during "good" days.
- Eat a high-protein, high-calorie, nutrient-dense breakfast if appetite is best in the morning.
- Eat small, frequent meals (eg, every 1 to 2 hours by the clock).
- Limit low-calorie and empty-calorie items such as carbonated beverages.
- Increase the nutrient density of foods by adding butter, skim milk powder, peanut butter, cheese, honey, or brown sugar.
- Limit liquids with meals to avoid early satiety and bloating at mealtime.
- Use liquid supplements (instant breakfast mixes, milk shakes, commercial supplements) in place of meals when appetite deteriorates or the client is too tired to eat.
- Taste-test a variety of different commercial supplements.
- Enhance appetite with light exercise, a glass of wine or beer if not contraindicated, and the use of appetite stimulants.
- Make eating a pleasant experience by eating in a bright, cheerful environment, playing soft music, and enjoying the company of friends or family.
- Experiment with recipes, flavorings, spices, and the consistency of food. Preferences may change daily.
- Avoid strong food odors if they contribute to anorexia. Cook outdoors on a grill, serve cold foods rather than hot foods, or use takeout meals that do not need to be prepared at home.
- Use appropriate medications to control pain, nausea, and depression.

NAUSEA AND VOMITING

Nausea and vomiting occur as a result of cancer and cancer therapies, especially chemotherapy. Acute nausea and vomiting can develop within 2 hours after drug administration and may last up to 24 hours. Some drugs can produce delayed nausea and vomiting beyond the day of chemotherapy, which may last for 3 to 5 days or even up to 3 weeks. Rarely, nausea and vomiting persist from one cycle of chemotherapy to the next. Clients who have poor control of emesis may experience **anticipatory nausea and vomiting,** defined as nausea and vomiting that occur before or during chemotherapy, at a time when symptoms normally would not be expected. Nausea may persist even after vomiting is controlled, and it can have a more devastating impact on quality of life. Long-term survival may be affected if the client refuses or postpones chemotherapy treatments because of nausea and vomiting.

The following tips may help manage nausea:

- Eat foods served cold or at room temperature, because hot foods may contribute to nausea.
- Eat high-carbohydrate, low-fat foods, such as toast, crackers, yogurt, sherbet, cooked cereal, soft or canned fruits, watermelon, bananas, fruit juices, and angel food cake.
- Avoid fatty, greasy, fried, or strongly seasoned foods.
- Keep track of foods that cause nausea so that they can be avoided.
- Avoid eating 1 to 2 hours before chemotherapy or radiotherapy to decrease the likelihood of nausea.
- Take antiemetics as prescribed, even when symptoms are absent.

FATIGUE

Cancer fatigue may appear suddenly, can be overwhelming, is not relieved by rest, and can continue after treatment ends. It impairs quality of life. Fatigue leads to poor intake, and poor intake contributes to fatigue. Encourage a good breakfast, because fatigue may worsen as the day progresses. The following tips may help manage fatigue:

- Engage in regular exercise, if possible.
- Consume easy-to-eat foods that can be prepared with a minimal amount of effort.
- Drink commercially prepared oral supplements, such as Ensure or Boost, to increase protein and calorie intake with a minimum of effort. High-nitrogen and high-calorie variations of both products are available.
- Use convenience foods and labor-saving appliances (eg, blender, Crock-Pot, toaster oven, microwave oven, dishwasher).
- Drink adequate fluids, because chronic dehydration contributes to fatigue.
- Assistance may be available from Meals On Wheels or other community services.

TASTE CHANGES

Taste changes may result from cancer or cancer treatments. Radiation-induced taste alterations usually develop by the third week of therapy and return to normal within 1 year.

Clients who experience taste changes are more likely to lose weight. Conversely, clients who lose weight may be more likely to develop taste alterations. Elemental zinc has been shown to correct taste abnormalities. If prescribed, zinc should be taken with food or milk to decrease the risk of gastrointestinal irritation. The most common taste changes are a decreased threshold for urea (bitter) and an increased threshold for sucrose (sweet). The following tips may help manage taste changes:

- Suck on hard candy during therapy if chemotherapy causes a bitter or metallic taste.
- Use plastic utensils and dishes.
- Tart foods such as citrus juices, cranberry juice, pickles, or relishes may help overcome metallic taste.
- Practice good oral hygiene before eating to eliminate unpleasant tastes.
- Experiment with a variety of seasonings, especially if the oral mucosa is not impaired.
- Avoid anything that tastes unpleasant.
- If red meats (beef and pork) have a "bad," "rotten," or "fecal" taste, eat other high-protein foods, such as eggs, cheese, mild fish, nuts, and dried peas and beans. If those sources are not tolerated, milk shakes, eggnogs, puddings, ice cream, and commercial supplements can provide sufficient protein and calories.
- Add the juice from half of a freshly squeezed lemon to commercial supplements to lessen excessive sweetness and bitter aftertaste that affects people with cancer.
- Meats may be better tolerated if served cold or at room temperature or if highly flavored with strong seasonings, sweet marinades, or sauces.
- Serve attractively presented food in a bright, cheerful environment.

FOOD AVERSIONS

Food aversions may be intermittent or may worsen as the day progresses. To avoid learned aversions, instruct the client to avoid his or her favorite foods or fast completely before receiving radiation or chemotherapy. If nausea and vomiting tend to occur at about the same time each day, withholding food beforehand may help avoid learned aversions.

SORE MOUTH (STOMATITIS)

Stomatitis may produce taste alterations, mouth blindness, or the association between eating and pain. Topical anesthetics may help relieve discomfort. Stomatitis also increases susceptibility to *Candida albicans* infections, which may cause ulcerated white or yellow patches on the oral mucosa and further diminish taste sensation. The following tips may help manage stomatitis:

- Practice good oral hygiene (thorough cleaning with a soft-bristle toothbrush or cotton swabs plus frequent mouth rinses with normal saline and water or baking soda and water). Commercial mouthwashes containing alcohol may irritate and burn the oral mucosa.
- Cut food into small portions.

- Avoid spices, acidic foods, coarse foods, alcohol, and smoking, which can aggravate an already irritated oral mucosa.
- Eat a soft or liquid bland diet, drink plenty of fluids, and avoid hot foods and beverages. Try mashed potatoes, macaroni and cheese, scrambled eggs, and cooked cereals.
- Cold items may help numb the oral mucosa. Try frozen bananas, applesauce, canned fruit, watermelon, cottage cheese, yogurt, ice cream, puddings, custards, and instant breakfast mixes.
- Straws may ease swallowing.
- Avoid wearing ill-fitting dentures.

DRY MOUTH OR THICK SALIVA

Clients with decreased saliva production are susceptible to dental caries. Encourage good oral hygiene, frequent mouth rinsing, and the avoidance of concentrated sweets. Provide mouth care immediately before mealtime for added moisture. The following tips may help manage dry mouth:

- Take small bites and chew food thoroughly.
- Avoid dry, coarse foods.
- Eat soft or moist foods (eg, foods with gravies or sauces).
- Avoid foods that stick to the roof of the mouth, such as peanut butter.
- Drink high-calorie, high-protein liquids in between meals.
- Use ice chips and sugar-free hard candies and gum between meals to relieve dryness.
- Artificial saliva and the use of straws may facilitate swallowing. Petroleum jelly applied to the lips may help prevent drying.

Protein and Calories

Actual nutrient requirements vary with the type and severity of the cancer, the treatments used, and the client's nutritional status. Usually, a high-protein diet of 1.5 to 2.0 g/kg is prescribed to prevent body protein catabolism. Calorie needs range from 25 to 35 cal/kg for weight maintenance to 40 to 50 cal/kg to replenish body stores. Although it is commonly assumed that all cancer clients develop anorexia and cachexia, weight gain is a common side effect of chemotherapy for breast cancer. The cause of this weight gain is unclear, but it may be related to decreased physical activity. Calories and protein should be adjusted to meet the individual's needs (see Chapter 16 for methods of determining calorie and protein requirements).

Vitamins and Minerals

Clients with poor intakes and increased losses (eg, vomiting, malabsorption) are at risk for vitamin and mineral deficiencies. Individual assessment of intake and requirements is needed to determine who may benefit from multivitamin and mineral supplements.

Method of Feeding

For both physiologic and psychological reasons, an oral diet is preferred whenever possible. Small, frequent meals and nutrient-dense supplements help maximize intake. When oral intake is inadequate or contraindicated, enteral feedings are the next best choice, if the gastrointestinal tract is functional.

Parenteral nutrition is not used routinely because its risks and cost are hard to justify in view of the fact that aggressive nutritional support has not been proven to improve survival or treatment success. Parenteral nutrition is generally indicated when:

- The gastrointestinal tract is nonfunctional due to:
  - Temporary problems lasting longer than 10 days, especially when a nutritional problem is identified
  - Obstruction or other mechanical problems that are expected to be resolved by cancer treatment or surgery
  - Multiple and/or noncorrectable obstructive problems associated with an inactive cancer
- There is severe short-bowel syndrome related to surgical resection, radiation enteritis, high gastrointestinal fistula, or inability to maintain weight and body composition with enteral support
- There is severe and/or continuing nutritional deterioration in which malnutrition, not cancer, is the primary problem

Beyond the Nutritional Value of Food

Loss of dignity and control, change in sexuality and body image, and loss of appetite can create a frustrating, seemingly hopeless situation for the client, and food may be used to express anger and resentment. Allow the client and family to verbalize feelings, and emphasize a positive, supportive, team-effort approach. Although the client may need the encouragement and support of family and friends, putting them in a position of "force-feeding" the client may add tension to an already stressful situation.

Nutritional support is one area of treatment in which the client can be an active participant. The client and the health care team may "contract" for an acceptable amount of weight loss. As long as the client does not lose more weight than was agreed on, the client is in charge of his or her own nutritional care. The client's rights and preferences should be respected at all times.

Nutrition Therapy for Clients Receiving Palliative Care

For clients whose prognosis is terminal, the value of nutritional support is a controversial ethical issue. No benefit is derived from aggressively feeding a client whose cancer is not being treated, because both body weight gain and tumor growth are stimulated. Instead, enteral nutrition should be maintained as an integral component of palliative care, with the goals of providing comfort and improving the quality of life. Eating should be encouraged as a source of pleasure, not as an adjunct to treatment. The client's requests and preferences are more important than the nutritional quality of the diet. Important supportive measures include:

- Controlling unpleasant side effects, such as pain, constipation, nausea, vomiting, and heartburn, with medication
- Respecting the client's wishes regarding the level of nutritional support desired
- Providing adequate mouth care to control dryness and thirst
- Respecting the client's personal tastes and preferences
- Ensuring a pleasant eating environment and serving attractive food
- Serving food of appropriate textures
- Using a team approach that includes physician, dietitian, and nurse

ALTERNATIVE NUTRITIONAL THERAPIES

Distrust of traditional medicine, inadequate medical insurance coverage, increasing ethnic populations that traditionally use herbs, and the appeal of a more "natural" approach to health care have contributed to the dramatic increase in sales of herbal and nutritional supplements. Adding to the interest in supplements is growing evidence that chemicals in plants may help protect against cancer. Important drugs such as paclitaxel (Taxol), aspirin, and digoxin are derived from plants. However, because of the life-threatening nature of cancer, self-diagnosis and self-treatment are dangerous. Supplements and diets that people with cancer may be using are summarized in this section.

Echinacea

Echinacea, also known as coneflower, has been used since the 1800s to treat a variety of conditions ranging from colds to syphilis. Because it is promoted as an immune system booster, many people take it today to prevent or treat colds and flu. Echinacea does have compounds that appear to stimulate the production and activity of white blood cells. It may also reduce inflammation and increase production of cytokines, chemicals that help control immune system activity. Researchers are investigating whether echinacea has potential to treat cancer. Not enough is known about echinacea to establish dosage levels or identify potential toxic effects.

Shark Cartilage

Shark cartilage, available in capsule and powder forms, is extracted from between the heads and fins of sharks. During the 1970s and 1980s, researchers discovered that shark cartilage contains certain proteins that block the development of new blood vessels. In theory, these substances could cause cancerous tumors to shrink or disappear by depriving them of an adequate blood supply. However, it is not known which proteins in shark cartilage have these antiangiogenic effects. Also, the protein molecules are too large to be absorbed through the human gastrointestinal tract. Many people take shark cartilage by enema because the recommended dose is high (60–90 g/day) and because it has an offensive taste and may cause nausea and diarrhea.

There is no evidence that shark cartilage can prevent or cure cancer. It is not appropriate for pregnant women, children, or people recovering from surgery. Not only is shark cartilage not efficacious in treating cancer patients, but there are also problems with purity. In 1994 the National Cancer Institute halted its study on shark cartilage because all of the samples submitted for testing were found to be contaminated.

Astragalus membranaceus (Huang ch'i)

Astragalus membranaceus has been used for thousands of years throughout the Orient to stimulate the immune system. It has been shown to stimulate the production of interferon, reduce the duration of the common cold, and promote macrophage activity. However, it may also act like a diuretic and trigger low blood pressure, causing dizziness and fatigue. Large doses may suppress the immune system. Many Chinese medical practitioners prescribe *Astragalus membranaceus* with other herbs during chemotherapy and radiation treatments. It appears to help reduce the side effects of cancer therapies and may promote immune system function.

Vitamin C

In 1979 Linus Pauling published a book entitled *Cancer and Vitamin C*, which promoted the idea that large doses of vitamin C are useful in preventing and treating cancer. He claimed that terminal cancer patients who took 10 g/day of vitamin C had significantly longer survival times than cancer patients who were not treated with vitamin C. However, his study has been refuted by researchers at the National Cancer Institute, and subsequent studies have found that vitamin C not only does not increase survival time but may actually promote tumor formation by damaging proteins and nucleic acids. Although research on vitamin C continues, there is presently little substantive evidence to indicate that it is effective for treating cancer.

Hoxsey Herbal Treatment

The Hoxsey treatments consist of external and internal components. The external remedies, promoted for external cancers, include several herbs plus arsenic sulfide, which are corrosive enough to destroy body tissues on contact. These chemicals do not distinguish between normal cells and cancer cells and have no value in cancer treatment.

The internal tonic for internal cancers is a liquid mixture that contains potassium iodide plus a variety of herbs said to be individually adjusted for each client. Hoxsey claimed that the internal formula normalizes body fluids, restores normal acid-base balance, and "deals with the DNA." Hoxsey's former head nurse opened a clinic called the Bio-Medical Center in Tijuana, Mexico, after repeated battles with the U.S. Food and Drug Administration forced Hoxsey to stop practicing in the United States. There is no acceptable evidence that Hoxsey's internal herbal formula is effective against cancer, and some of the herbs it contains have toxic side effects. Ironically, Hoxsey himself died of prostate cancer.

Gerson Diet

Proponents of the Gerson diet claim that cancer can be cured only if toxins are eliminated from the body. The basic treatment includes "detoxification" of the body with frequent coffee enemas and a special diet that enables the body to "heal itself." The diet contains very low amounts of sodium or fat and little animal protein; is high in potassium and rich in carbohydrates; and includes more than a gallon of juice daily made from fruits, vegetables, and raw calf's liver. Additional protocols include liver extract injections, dehydrated defatted liver capsules, linseed oil, ozone enemas, "live cell therapy," thyroid tablets, royal jelly capsules, castor oil enemas, clay packs, laetrile, and vaccines made from the flu virus and dead *Staphylococcus aureus* bacteria. This method of treatment is available only at a clinic near Tijuana, Mexico.

No studies published in peer-reviewed literature provide reasonable evidence that the Gerson therapy is effective against cancer. In fact, the Gerson method has significant potential to cause harm. A number of Gerson patients have been treated for *Campylobacter fetus* sepsis, believed to be caused by the liver injections. Low serum sodium has been blamed for inducing coma in five Gerson patients. Serious infections and deaths from electrolyte imbalance related to the use of coffee enemas have been reported.

Macrobiotic Diet

The Zen-macrobiotic diet is an extreme type of vegetarian diet based on metaphysical beliefs, not nutritional science. In a series of ten steps, the macrobiotic diet advances from meat-containing meals to a highly restrictive intake consisting mainly of brown rice, which is supposedly the "ultimate food." The higher macrobiotic diet levels can cause severe malnutrition.

NURSING PROCESS

Karen is a 59-year-old reformed smoker who now calls herself a "health nut." She was recently diagnosed with lung cancer. She had surgery to remove her right lung and is now receiving chemotherapy for cancerous "spots" on the left lung and stomach. She has lost 28 pounds and complains of nausea, vomiting, and a bad taste in her mouth. Because she has followed an "anticancer" diet for years, she is reluctant to now change her eating habits and eat more protein, fat, and calories. She eats mostly fruit, sherbet, and skim milk.

Assessment

Obtain clinical data:

- Height, current weight, body mass index (BMI), usual weight, rate of weight loss
- Medical history, such as diabetes, heart disease, or hypertension
- Types of drugs the client is receiving through chemotherapy; other prescribed medications that affect nutrition
- Physician's goals and plan of treatment
- Laboratory data: serum albumin, serum transferrin, thyroxine-bound prealbumin, retinol-binding protein, serum electrolytes, and other abnormal values. Nitrogen balance study, if available.
- Fluid intake and output

Interview the client to assess:

- Usual 24-hour intake, portion sizes, frequency and pattern of eating, food aversions, daily fluid intake
- Pattern of nausea and vomiting. Determine how the client has coped with nausea, vomiting, and taste changes.
- Understanding of increased nutritional needs related to cancer and cancer therapies
- Willingness to change her attitudes toward food and nutrition
- Cultural, religious, and ethnic influences on eating habits
- Psychosocial and economic issues, such as financial status, employment, and outside support system
- Usual activity patterns
- Use of vitamins, minerals, and nutritional supplements. Determine what, how much, and why the client is using each.
- Use of alcohol and nicotine

Nursing Diagnosis

Altered Nutrition: Less Than Body Requirements, related to nausea, vomiting, and taste changes secondary to cancer/cancer therapy.

Planning and Implementation

CLIENT GOALS

The client will:

- Eat six to eight times daily
- Verbalize the importance of consuming adequate protein and calories and the role of fat in providing required calories
- Switch from skim milk to 2% milk
- Drink at least 16 ounces of a high-calorie, high-protein supplement daily
- Practice ways to increase protein and calorie density of foods consumed

Maintain present weight until chemotherapy is completed
List interventions she will try at home to help relieve nausea and taste alterations

NURSING INTERVENTIONS

Nutrition Therapy

Provide a high-protein house diet as ordered.
Provide 8 ounces of Boost Plus three times daily between meals.

Client Teaching

Instruct the client:

That an adequate nutritional status reduces the side effects of treatment, may make cancer cells more receptive to treatment, improves quality of life, and may increase survival rate. Poor nutritional status may potentiate chemotherapeutic drug toxicity.

That a preventative eating style is no longer appropriate. Consuming adequate protein and calories (even fat calories) is the major priority.

On eating plan essentials, including:

- Protein sources the client may tolerate despite nausea and taste changes, such as eggs, cheese, mild fish, nuts, dried peas and beans, milk shakes, eggnogs, puddings, ice cream, instant breakfast mixes, and commercial supplements
- How to increase the protein and calorie density of foods eaten
- To eat small, frequent "meals" to help maximize intake but to avoid eating 12 hours before chemotherapy
- To drink ample fluids 1 to 2 days before and after chemotherapy to enhance excretion of the drugs and to decrease the risk of renal toxicity

On interventions to minimize nausea, such as:

- Eating foods served cold or at room temperature
- Eating high-carbohydrate, low-fat foods, such as toast, crackers, yogurt, sherbet, cooked cereal, soft or canned fruits, watermelon, bananas, fruit juices, and angel food cake
- Avoiding fatty, greasy, fried, and strongly seasoned foods

On behavior matters to help maximize intake, including:

- Viewing food as a medicine, rather than a social pleasure, that must be "taken" even when the desire to eat is lacking
- Keeping track of foods that cause nausea so that they can be avoided
- Taking antiemetics as prescribed, even when symptoms are absent
- Sucking on hard candy during chemotherapy and using plastic utensils and dishes to mitigate the "bad taste" in her mouth
- Avoiding anything that tastes unpleasant

On where to find additional information (Box 21–1)

Evaluation

The client:

Eats six to eight times daily

BOX 21.1

Where to Get Additional Cancer Information

National Cancer Institute, Cancer Information Center
31 Center Drive
MSC 2580, Building 31, Room 10A-17
9000 Rockville Pike
Bethesda, MD 20892
800-422-6237
www.nci.nih.gov

American Cancer Society
1599 Clifton Road NE
Atlanta, GA 30329
800-227-2345
www.cancer.org

American Institute for Cancer Research
1759 R Street NW
Washington, DC 20009
800-843-8114
www.aicr.org/aicr.htm

Verbalizes the importance of consuming adequate protein and calories and the role of fat in providing required calories
Switches from skim milk to 2% milk
Drinks at least 16 ounces of a high-calorie, high-protein supplement daily
Practices ways to increase protein and calorie density of foods consumed
Maintains present weight until chemotherapy is completed
Lists interventions she will try at home to help relieve nausea and taste alterations

Nutrition and Immunodeficiency

Nutritional status and immunity are interrelated. Clearly, malnutrition itself impairs immune system function and the ability to fight infection. Conversely, infection increases the risk for malnutrition. Although the relation between malnutrition and the progression of human immunodeficiency virus (HIV) disease is not clearly understood, nutrition status may play a role.

PATHOGENESIS OF HIV/AIDS

AIDS is an end-stage immune disorder that is caused by infection with the retrovirus known as HIV. HIV is transmitted through direct exchange of infected body fluids from one person to another, such as through sexual intercourse, from use of contaminated needles or blood products, or from mother to infant during pregnancy, delivery, or lactation.

The clinical course of HIV disease may begin with an acute, mononucleosis-like illness with variable and nonspecific symptoms. The middle phase is called symptomatic HIV infection, or **AIDS-related complex (ARC)**. Weight loss, diarrhea, and enlarged lymph glands occur. Other symptoms include fatigue, seborrhea, eczema, intermittent fever, muscle pain, and night sweats. AIDS is diagnosed by a blood test positive for HIV antibodies and at least one of the following:

- An opportunistic infection, which is an infection caused by microorganisms found in the environment that normally do not cause infection, such as *Pneumocystis carinii* pneumonia or candidiasis of the esophagus
- An AIDS-related cancer. The malignancies that commonly develop include Kaposi's sarcoma (cancer of the connective tissues that support blood vessels) and T-cell lymphoma of the skin.
- Fewer than 200 CD4+ T lymphocyte cells per microliter (μL) of blood. Normal helper T-cell count ranges from 800 to 1000/cells/μL.

As yet, there is no cure for AIDS. Treatment focuses on forestalling the onset of AIDS symptoms, preserving independence, and maintaining quality of life. Drugs are used to inhibit HIV replication and to prevent and treat infections. Chemotherapeutic drugs may be used to combat any malignancies that develop (Table 21–1). Improved treatment methods have greatly prolonged survival, which has led to the view that HIV is a chronic process.

EFFECT OF HIV AND AIDS ON NUTRITIONAL STATUS

HIV has a devastating and progressive impact on nutritional status. In the early stages of HIV, subclinical signs of malnutrition may exist, but they are frequently overlooked. Deficiencies in thiamine, riboflavin, vitamin B_6, vitamin B_{12}, folate, magnesium, selenium, and zinc have been reported in asymptomatic clients, as well as a decline in body cell mass. Symptoms of nutrient deficiencies, such as neuropathy, fatigue, depression, and diarrhea, may exacerbate HIV symptoms. As the process advances, the cumulative effect of more numerous and severe infections, malignancies, and therapies, combined with unmet nutritional needs, promotes the downward spiral of weight loss that may be as much as 30% to 50% of pre-illness weight. As many as 88% of HIV-infected clients develop malnutrition.

The HIV wasting syndrome is diagnosed when unintentional weight loss reaches 10% or more of usual body weight. A prominent difference between normal weight loss from dieting and weight loss through HIV wasting is that there is a disproportionate loss of lean body mass compared to the amount of fat lost. Wasting exacerbates illness and is associated with significant morbidity, such as fatigue, weakness, and reduced quality of

DRUG ALERT

Drug	Effect on Appetite	Effect on Weight	Nausea and Vomiting	Heartburn/Gastrointestinal Pain	Diarrhea	Mouth or Esophageal Ulcers	Altered Taste	Other Nutritional Considerations
Protease Inhibitors								
Invirase (saquinavir)			✓	✓	✓			Loss of appetite and taste changes may occur
Norvir (ritonavir)	↓	↓		✓	✓		✓	Mix with milk chocolate, Ensure, or Adverta to improve taste
Crixivan (indinavir)	↑↓						✓	Increase fluid to at least 1.5 L/d to help prevent kidney stones
Viracept (nelfinavir)			✓	✓	✓			Mix powder with water, milk, or formula
Reverse Transcriptase Inhibitors								
AZT (zidovudine)	↓		✓	✓	✓		✓	May cause decrease in serum B_{12} and folate
DDI (didanosine)		↓		✓	✓	✓		May cause thirst and dry mouth. Each 100-mg buffered tablet contains 264 mg Na^+. May need decreased-sodium diet.
DDC (zalcitabine)		↓	✓	✓	✓	✓		Contains lactose as an inactive ingredient
D4T (stavudine)	↓	↓		✓	✓			Contains lactose as an inactive incredient
3TC (lamivudine)		↓	✓	✓	✓			Maintain adequate hydration
Nonnucleoside Reverse Transcriptase Inhibitors								
Viramune (nevirapine)			✓					Contains lactose as an inactive ingredient
Rescriptor (delavirdine)			✓		✓			May cause anorexia and gastrointestinal pain

life. The amount of wasting, rather than the specific cause of weight loss, has been shown to be the primary determinant of death in AIDS.

Like cancer cachexia, the cause of malnutrition in AIDS is multifactorial and varies among individuals. Metabolism is accelerated because of infection, fever, cancer, and/or drug-induced reactions; this increases energy and nutrient requirements. Nutrient malabsorption occurs secondary to intestinal infections, drug therapy, low serum albumin, gastrointestinal malignancies, and AIDS enteropathy (diarrhea caused by no diagnosable pathogen). Uncorrected, malabsorption can rapidly lead to malnutrition, wasting, and impaired quality of life. Intake is poor because of infection, fatigue, mouth ulcers, depression, anxiety, nausea, vomiting, impaired swallowing, impaired taste, esophageal ulcerations, and/or shortness of breath. Inadequate oral intake appears to be the most important factor contributing to weight loss.

Evidence suggests that weight loss and malnutrition are not inevitable consequences of HIV. Rather, it may be that malnutrition evolves from nutritional assaults that occur so frequently that the client is not able to replenish nutritional losses before the next challenge develops. Malnutrition can be prevented and reversed with current therapies, including nutrition therapy. Management of HIV-related wasting represents a major challenge.

ASSESSING NUTRITIONAL NEEDS OF CLIENTS WITH HIV INFECTION

Nutritional assessment should occur as soon as HIV infection is diagnosed, and it should be repeated periodically.

Historical Data

What is the client's usual weight and BMI? Has there been recent weight loss and, if so, what percentage of usual weight has been lost?

Is the client's usual intake adequate? Does the client have symptoms that interfere with eating, such as nausea, vomiting, diarrhea, dysphagia, altered taste, difficulty chewing, or shortness of breath? If so, determine the onset, frequency, severity, interventions attempted, and results. What dietary changes has the client made in response to symptoms (eg, foods avoided, foods preferred)? Does the client use unorthodox or unproved dietary remedies to combat HIV/AIDS and, if so, what is their potential impact on nutritional status? What types and doses of vitamins and minerals does the client take? What is the client's usual intake of alcohol?

Is the client being treated with chemotherapy or radiation? What prescription and over-the-counter medications does the client use? What physical complaints or complications does the client have? Does the client use tobacco or recreational drugs? Is the client employed? Is the client's food budget adequate? What cultural, religious, and ethnic influences affect the client's food choices? What is the client's emotional status?

Physical Findings

What are the client's vital signs, especially temperature? Does the client have muscle wasting? Can the client perform self-care activities, including cooking and eating? Does the client have edema or other signs of fluid and electrolyte imbalance? Does the client have alterations in skin and mucous membranes, including decreased turgor and ulcerations? Are neurologic impairments evident, such as the tendency to choke and forgetfulness? Are there enlarged lymph nodes?

Laboratory Data

Assess:

- Protein status, as indicated by low albumin, prealbumin, and retinol-binding protein
- Serum cholesterol. Hypocholesterolemia is associated with adverse clinical outcomes.
- Other abnormal laboratory values

NUTRITION THERAPY

If initiated soon after the diagnosis of HIV infection is made, nutrition therapy may help prevent or delay wasting and loss of lean body mass. The ultimate goal of nutrition therapy is to provide a balanced, nutrient-dense diet to help preserve the client's independence (eg, allowing the client to stay at home), maintain quality of life, and possibly slow the progression of AIDS. Nutrition therapy should begin before the client exhibits any symptoms of HIV disease, even if intake appears adequate, because once the client is ill enough to need hospital care, the effectiveness of nutrition therapy may be limited.

Clinical trials are currently underway to test the effectiveness of certain nutrition therapies (eg, whole versus partially hydrolyzed proteins, long-chain versus medium-chain fatty acids) in the treatment of HIV wasting. For now, nutrition therapy focuses on providing adequate calories and protein and minimizing side effects (eg, anorexia, diarrhea) that impair nutrient intake and use.

Calories

Although exact nutrient requirements for patients with HIV/AIDS have not yet been established, calorie needs are increased, even in the absence of malabsorption, possibly related to altered metabolism. It is recommended that calorie intake be 35 to 45 cal/kg. Calorie requirements are higher when fever is present.

Protein

Protein requirements are also increased, especially for clients with serum protein depletion and loss of lean body tissue. Increase protein intake to 1.0 to 2.0 g/kg to replenish losses and help maintain lean body mass.

Fat

Clients with malabsorption may need to limit fat intake and use supplemental medium-chain triglyceride (MCT) oil for additional calories. MCT oil does not require pancreatic lipase or bile for digestion and absorption and therefore can be absorbed easily by people with impaired digestion or absorption.

Vitamins and Minerals

Vitamin and mineral requirements for clients with HIV/AIDS are not known, but poor intake and altered nutrient absorption and metabolism place the client at high risk for nutrient deficiencies. It is recommended that fat-soluble vitamins be taken at Recommended Dietary Allowance (RDA) levels and that water-soluble vitamins be taken in amounts two to five times the RDA. Trace element and antioxidant supplements may also be prescribed. Clients should be advised to avoid large doses of iron and zinc because they can impair immune function.

Minimizing Side Effects

Clients with HIV/AIDS may experience problems with appetite and intake similar to those of cancer clients (see earlier discussion). Encourage clients to eat small feedings frequently (eg, six to nine times daily), even when appetite is lacking. Liquid commercial supplements are frequently used because they tend to leave the stomach quickly, are easy to consume, and provide significant quantities of calories and protein. Intake-enhancing drugs approved by the U.S. Food and Drug Administration for treatment of HIV wasting are megestrol acetate (Megace) and dronabinol (Marinol, which contains the active ingredient in marijuana). Controlling diarrhea and malabsorption can substantially improve quality of life. Although diarrhea may seem to be triggered by eating, clients need to understand that limiting food intake to control diarrhea only exacerbates wasting. Antidiarrheals should be used shortly before a meal. Foods high in pectin and other soluble fibers, such as oatmeal, cooked carrots, bananas, peeled apples, and applesauce, may help slow transit time. Clients with diarrhea related to lactose intolerance should avoid milk or use lactose-reduced milk.

Method of Feeding

Clients who are unable to consume an adequate oral intake may require tube feeding for supplemental or complete nutrition. Because many formulas have the potential to cause diarrhea, the client's tolerance should be closely monitored. Advera and Impact are commercial formulas designed for clients with impaired immune function.

DRUG ALERT

Appetite Stimulants Used for Cancer and HIV/AIDS

Megace (megestrol acetate) has been shown to stimulate appetite, promote weight gain, increase lean body mass, and improve sense of well-being. It may take 8 to 12 weeks to experience maximum appetite improvement. Adverse side effects include diarrhea, impotence, rash, flatulence, and pain. Hyperglycemia that occurs may resolve when the drug is discontinued.

Marinol (dronabinol) contains the marijuana ingredient tetrahydrocannabinol (THC). It stimulates the appetite and promotes weight gain, but heartburn, nausea, vomiting, dry mouth, drowsiness, and feeling "high" are common side effects. Clients must avoid alcohol. Psychological and physical dependence can occur, as can withdrawal syndrome when the drug is discontinued.

Clients with intractable vomiting, severe secretory diarrhea, or bowel obstruction, and those at risk for aspiration may be candidates for TPN. However, the use of TPN is controversial because it may not be able to stop progressive wasting in clients who have systemic infections. Some studies have found that TPN increases body fat without increasing body cell mass. The client should be counseled on the potential risks and benefits of both tube feedings and parenteral nutrition.

ALTERNATIVE NUTRITION THERAPIES USED BY CLIENTS WITH HIV/AIDS

Because a cure for AIDS does not currently exist, clients are susceptible to unorthodox therapies. Some alternative nutrition therapies used for patients with cancer are also promoted for those with HIV/AIDS. None of the following commonly used alternative ther-

DRUG ALERT

Nutritional Supplements Formulated Specifically for Patients With HIV/AIDS

Advera (Ross Laboratories) is a high-calorie, high-protein, low-fat liquid supplement that contains n-3 fatty acids. It is fortified with beta carotene; vitamins E, C, B_6, and B_{12}; and folic acid. Fiber is added. One 240-mL can provides 303 cal, 14.2 g protein, and 5.4 g fat. It may be used as a supplement or as a total oral diet. Chocolate and vanilla flavors are available.

Immun-Aid is a high-protein powdered formula enriched with arginine, glutamine, and branched-chain amino acids. Canola oil provides n-3 fatty acids. It may be used orally or via tube. Because some of the nutrients in Immun-Aid lose their potency, it should be prepared no longer than 24 hours before it is consumed. A 500-mL serving (16.7 oz) provides 500 cal, 40 g protein, and 11 g fat, half of which is in the form of MCT oil.

apies can stop the progression of HIV disease, and some are potentially harmful. Be aware of the potential complications, and "work around" the therapy whenever possible to ensure an adequate intake.

Cat's Claw

Cat's claw comes from the woody vine *Uncaria tomentosa,* which is grown in South America. Although it is used by Amazonians as treatment for a variety of conditions, including tumors, the Natural Products Branch of the National Cancer Institute has determined that there is insufficient activity to warrant further research on cat's claw. It has been demonstrated to contain substances that stimulate immune function. However, cat's claw appears in nature in two different varieties, which have different chemical patterns that are antagonistic toward one another, so that mixing them would be unsuitable for immunotherapy. Although cat's claw does not appear to be hazardous, it is not recommended because there are no clinical trials supporting its efficacy as an immune system enhancer.

Blue-Green Algae

Blue-green algae is also known as spirulina. It comes from microscopic plants grown mainly in brackish ponds and lakes throughout the world. Proponents claim it boosts energy and immunity and detoxifies the body. In reality, it contains protein, beta carotene, and small amounts of minerals that are obtained much more economically and safely from foods. Blue-green algae may contain toxins that are harmful to the liver.

Yeast-Free Diet

Based on the rationale that limiting yeast will help prevent candidiasis and other infections, foods that contain yeast and high concentrations of simple sugars are eliminated. This diet can compromise calorie intake and thereby promote weight loss.

Macrobiotic Diet

The macrobiotic diet is based on yin and yang ideology and the belief that AIDS is caused by an imbalance in the body. It purports to maintain balance and thus cure AIDS. This highly restrictive diet is composed of brown rice and other whole grains, vegetables, seaweed, legumes, miso, soup, and a little fish. The macrobiotic diet is likely to be deficient in calories, complete protein, iron, calcium, vitamin D, vitamin B_{12}, folic acid, riboflavin, and vitamin C.

Kombucha Tea

Kombucha tea is an herbal product that is also known as mushroom tea, Japanese tea fungus, kargasok, kvass tea, and kwassan. It is purported to cure AIDS. In reality, the benefits have not been proven, and there are reports of liver damage, gastrointestinal upset, and death. It also has the potential to cause allergic reactions.

Cleansing Rituals

Fasting and starvation are promoted to "starve" the infection. Unfortunately, the body is also starved. Enemas may be used with the idea that they cleanse the bowel and body by removing toxins and bacteria, but they can compound problems with malabsorption and alter fluid and electrolyte balance.

NUTRITION COUNSELING

The nutritional care of most HIV-infected clients is poor or nonexistent. Many clients do not see a dietitian until severe nutrition problems are evident. Some physicians do nutrition counseling themselves, but lack of time and the perception that clients do not want or need nutrition counseling limits their impact. Nurses are in an ideal position to provide nutrition counseling when appropriate and to recommend referrals to the dietitian as needed. Counseling may include:

- Information on food and water safety to reduce the risk of foodborne illness. Stress the importance of refrigerating foods immediately after purchase, washing fruits and vegetables thoroughly, cooking meats thoroughly, refrigerating leftovers immediately, discarding leftovers after a couple of days, avoiding cross-contamination by using separate cutting boards and work surfaces for raw meats, keeping work surfaces clean, and maintaining personal hygiene.
- How to cope with side effects, such as anorexia, nausea, and vomiting
- Guidelines for evaluating nutritional supplements and products. Remind clients that there are no supplements or diets that cure HIV/AIDS and that some therapies are potentially harmful. Advise clients to be skeptical when they hear the words "breakthrough," "magical cure," and "new discovery." Likewise, "detoxify," "purify," and "energize" are nonscientific jargon, not medical terms.
- The benefits of using high-protein supplements. Products such as Boost High Protein, Boost Plus, Ensure HN, and Ensure Plus provide quick and easy protein and calories.
- The benefits of comfort foods. Clients with HIV disease may experience anger, depression, and anxiety. Comfort foods may provide some consolation and may be appealing when other foods are not. Even if the nutritional value of comfort foods is small, their emotional value is important.

BOX 21.2

Where to Get Additional HIV/AIDS Information

HIV InfoWeb
www.infoweb.org

AIDS Education Global Information System (AEGIS)
949-248-5843
www.aegis.com

Centers for Disease Control and Prevention
Division of HIV/AIDS Prevention Homepage
www.cdc.gov/nchstp/hiv-aids/dhap.htm

- The recommendation to periodically keep food records so that intake can be monitored and problems can be identified
- Information on food and drug interactions (see Drug Alerts)
- Information about home-delivered meals that may be available from a local AIDS service provider
- Where to get more information (Box 21–2)

KEY CONCEPTS

- Without early and aggressive nutritional interventions, cancer and HIV/AIDS can have profound and devastating effects on nutritional status, often resulting in wasting and malnutrition.
- Cancer alters metabolism by increasing energy expenditure, increasing protein catabolism, increasing fat catabolism, and increasing the use of fat for energy.
- Neither the incidence nor the severity of cachexia can be related directly to calorie intake or tumor weight.
- Nutrition therapy cannot cure cancer or HIV/AIDS, but it may improve tolerance to therapies and promote quality of life.
- In general, the nutrition therapy for cancer and for HIV/AIDS is similar: minimize side effects that interfere with nutrient intake and use and increase protein and calorie intake.
- For most people undergoing chemotherapy, fatigue and nausea and vomiting are the most distressing side effects.
- Increasing the calorie and protein density of the diet is generally more acceptable than increasing the volume of food served.
- No benefit is derived from force-feeding a client whose cancer is not being aggressively treated.
- As many as 88% of clients with HIV/AIDS have malnutrition, which may speed the progression from HIV disease to AIDS.
- Nutrient requirements for people with HIV/AIDS have not been determined, but it appears that calorie, protein, and micronutrient needs are increased.

- Clients with cancer or HIV/AIDS are susceptible to nutritional "cures" and may use unorthodox diets or supplements that may be detrimental to their health.

Focus on Critical Thinking

Irene is a 58-year-old woman who was recently diagnosed with colon cancer with metastasis to the liver. After surgical removal of part of her colon, she began chemotherapy, which was to be given for 30 minutes each day for 7 days, followed by 21 days off. This cycle was to be repeated for 3 months.

Irene lost 12 pounds while hospitalized for her surgery. When she began chemotherapy, she weighed 128 pounds; she is 5 feet 5 inches tall. Within days after beginning chemotherapy, Irene developed stomatitis and stopped eating. She has always been fearful of nausea and believes fasting is the most effective approach to avoiding nausea. She is complaining of tremendous mouth pain, and she told her daughter that she will not continue with chemotherapy if these problems persist. Because her mother is so fatigued, Irene's daughter brought her a large pot of homemade vegetable soup that she could simply heat up when she was too tired to cook.

How many calories and grams of protein should Irene be consuming to meet her estimated requirements while undergoing chemotherapy? What types of food should you encourage Irene to eat in order to meet her nutritional requirements, keeping in mind that she has mouth pain and nausea? Plan a day's menu that Irene could follow.

In counseling Irene about the importance of eating, what important points should you stress?

Was homemade soup a good choice for premade meals? Why or why not? Name foods that you would encourage her daughter to make for Irene.

ANSWER KEY

1. **FALSE** Even cancers that have not metastasized can cause generalized nutritional effects.
2. **TRUE** Cachexia is estimated to affect half of all people with cancer. It is responsible for more deaths than cancer itself.
3. **FALSE** Although anorexia can contribute to the development of cachexia, neither the incidence nor the severity of cachexia can be related directly to calorie intake.
4. **FALSE** Appetite of cancer patients is generally better in the morning and tends to deteriorate as the day progresses.
5. **TRUE** The cancer patient should avoid eating 1 to 2 hours before chemotherapy or radiation therapy to decrease the likelihood of nausea.
6. **TRUE** Taste alteration may be caused by cancer treatment, and if roast beef has a "bad" or "rotten" taste, a cheese sandwich is a high-protein alternative.
7. **FALSE** Not all cancer patients develop cachexia and anorexia. Weight gain is a common side effect of breast cancer chemotherapy. Calorie and protein requirements should be evaluated on an individual basis.
8. **FALSE** Evidence suggests that weight loss and malnutrition are not inevitable consequences of HIV infection. Malnutrition can be prevented and reversed with therapy, including nutritional intervention.

9. **TRUE** Patients with HIV/AIDS may well experience problems related to appetite and intake similar to those of cancer patients.

10. **TRUE** The risk of foodborne infections in patients with HIV/AIDS can be reduced by educating them on food and water safety, such as the importance of refrigerating foods, washing fruit and vegetables, and cooking meats thoroughly.

REFERENCES

American Cancer Society. (1993). *Questionable nutritional therapies*. Atlanta: Author.

American Cancer Society. Popular herbs under alternative and complementary therapies. [On-line]. Available: www.cancer.org/alt-therapy/pupherbs.html. Accessed November 12, 1999.

American Dietetic Association. (2000). Position of the American Dietetic Association and the Canadian Dietetic Association: Nutrition intervention in the care of persons with human immunodeficiency virus infection. *Journal of the American Dietetic Association*, *100*(6), 708–717.

Bass, F., & Cox, R. (1995). The need for dietary counseling of cancer patients as indicated by nutrient and supplement intake. *Journal of the American Dietetic Association*, 95, 1319–1321.

Chlebowski, R., Grosvenor, M., Lillington, L., Sayre, J., & Beall, G. (1995). Dietary intake and counseling, weight maintenance, and the course of HIV infection. *Journal of the American Dietetic Association*, 95, 428–432, 435.

Haller, D. (1994). Weight gain in patients with AIDS-related cachexia: Is bigger better? *Annals of Internal Medicine*, *121*, 462–463.

Henkel, J. (1999). Attacking AIDS with a "cocktail" therapy. *FDA Consumer Magazine*. [On-line]. Available: www.fda.gov/fdac/features/1999/499_aids.html. Accessed November 12, 1999.

Karch, A. (1999). *1999 Lippincott's Nursing Drug Guide*. Philadelphia: Lippincott-Raven Publishers.

McKinley, M., Goodman-Block, J., Lesser, M., & Salbe, A. (1994). Improved body weight status as a result of nutrition intervention in adult, HIV-positive outpatients. *Journal of the American Dietetic Association*, 94, 1014–1017.

National Institute of Allergy and Infectious Diseases, National Institutes of Health. (1997). *Fact sheet: HIV wasting syndrome*. U.S. Department of Health and Human Services, Public Health Service. [On-line]. Available: www.niaid.nih.gov/factsheets/hivwasting.htm. Accessed November 12, 1999.

National Institutes of Health, PDQ Supportive Care for Health Professionals, Nutrition. [On-line]. Available: Cancernet.nci.nih.gov.clinpdq/supportive/Nutrition-Physician.html. Accessed November 8, 1999.

Rabeneck, L., Palmer, A., Knowles, J., Seidehamel, R., Harris, Ch., Merkel, K., Risser, J., & Akabawi, S. (1998). A randomized controlled trial evaluating nutrition counseling with or without oral supplementation in malnourished HIV-infected patients. *Journal of the American Dietetic Association*, 98, 434–438.

Robbers, J., & Tyler, V. (1999). *Tyler's herbs of choice*. Binghamton, NY: The Haworth Press.

Roche-Dudek, M., & Roche-Klemma, K. (1998). *Drug-nutrient resource: Part of the Drug-Nutrient Intervention System* (3rd ed.). Riverside, IL: Roche Dietitians, LLC.

Salomon, S., Jung, J., Voss, T., Suguitan, A., Rowe, W., & Madsen, D. (1998). An elemental diet containing medium-chain triglycerides and enzymatically hydrolyzed protein can improve gastrointestinal tolerance in people infected with HIV. *Journal of the American Dietetic Association*, 98, 460–462.

Spaulding-Albright, N. (1997). A review of some herbal and related products commonly used in cancer patients. *Journal of the American Dietetic Association*, *97*(Suppl. 2), S208–S215.

Timbo, B., & Tollefson, L. (1994). Nutrition: A cofactor in HIV disease. *Journal of the American Dietetic Association*, *94*, 1018–1022.

U.S. Department of Health and Human Services. (1992). *Eating defensively: Food safety advice for persons with AIDS*. (DHHS Publication No. 92-2232). Public Health Service, U.S. Food and Drug Administration. [On-line]. Available: www.hivatis.org/leatdef.html. Accessed November 12, 1999.

Wilkes, G. (2000). Nutrition: The forgotten ingredient in cancer care. *American Journal of Nursing*, *100*(4), 46–54.

Young, J. (1997). HIV and medical nutrition therapy. *Journal of the American Dietetic Association*, *97*(Suppl. 2), S161–S166.

Appendices

APPENDIX 1

Food and Nutrition Board, Institute of Medicine-National Academy of Sciences—Dietary Reference Intakes: Recommended Levels for Individual Intake[a]

Life-stage group	Calcium (mg/d)	Phosphorus (mg/d)	Magnesium (mg/d)	Vitamin D[b,c] (μg/d)	Fluoride (mg/d)	Thiamine (mg/d)	Riboflavin (mg/d)	Niacin[d] (mg/d)	Vitamin B_6 (mg/d)	Folate[e] (μg/d)	Vitamin B_{12} (μg/d)	Pantothenic Acid (mg/d)	Biotin (μg/d)	Choline[f] (mg/d)	Vitamin C[j] (mg/d)	Vitamin E[k] (mg/d)	Selenium (μg/d)
Infants																	
0–6 mo	210*	100*	30*	5*	0.01*	0.2*	0.3*	2*	0.1*	65*	0.4*	1.7*	5*	125*	40*	4*	15*
7–12 mo	270*	275*	75*	5*	0.5*	0.3*	0.4*	4*	0.3*	80*	0.5*	1.8*	6*	150*	50*	6*	20*
Children																	
1–3 y	500*	460	80	5*	0.7*	0.5	0.5	6	0.5	150	0.9	2*	8*	200*	15	6	20
4–8 y	800*	500	130	5*	1*	0.6	0.6	8	0.6	200	1.2	3*	12*	250*	25	7	30
Males																	
9–13 y	1,300*	1,250	240	5*	2*	0.9	0.9	12	1.0	300	1.8	4*	20*	375*	45	11	40
14–18 y	1,300*	1,250	410	5*	3*	1.2	1.3	16	1.3	400	2.4	5*	25*	550*	75	15	55
19–30 y	1,000*	700	400	5*	4*	1.2	1.3	16	1.3	400	2.4	5*	30*	550*	90	15	55
31–50 y	1,000*	700	420	5*	4*	1.2	1.3	16	1.3	400	2.4	5*	30*	550*	90	15	55
51–70 y	1,200*	700	420	10*	4*	1.2	1.3	16	1.7	400	2.4[g]	5*	30*	550*	90	15	55
>70 y	1,200*	700	420	15*	4*	1.2	1.3	16	1.7	400	2.4[g]	5*	30*	550*	90	15	55
Females																	
9–13 y	1,300*	1,250	240	5*	2*	0.9	.09	12	1.0	300	1.8	4*	20*	375*	45	11	40
14–18 y	1,300*	1,250	360	5*	3*	1.0	1.0	14	1.2	400[h]	2.4	5*	25*	400*	65	15	55
19–30 y	1,000*	700	310	5*	3*	1.1	1.1	14	1.3	400[h]	2.4	5*	30*	425*	75	15	55
31–50 y	1,000*	700	320	5*	3*	1.1	1.1	14	1.3	400[h]	2.4	5*	30*	425*	75	15	55
51–70 y	1,200*	700	320	10*	3*	1.1	1.1	14	1.5	400	2.4[g]	5*	30*	425*	75	15	55
>70 y	1,200*	700	320	15*	3*	1.1	1.1	14	1.5	400	2.4[g]	5*	30*	425*	75	15	55

Pregnancy																	
≤18 y	1,300*	**1,250**	**400**	5*	3*	**1.4**	**1.4**	**18**	**1.9**	**600**[i]	**2.6**	6*	30*	450*	**80**	**15**	**60**
19–30 y	1,000*	**700**	**350**	5*	3*	**1.4**	**1.4**	**18**	**1.9**	**600**[i]	**2.6**	6*	30*	450*	**85**	**15**	**60**
31–50 y	1,000*	**700**	**360**	5*	3*	**1.4**	**1.4**	**18**	**1.9**	**600**[i]	**2.6**	6*	30*	450*	**85**	**15**	**60**
Lactation																	
≤18 y	1,300*	**1,250**	**360**	5*	3*	**1.5**	**1.6**	**17**	**2.0**	**500**	**2.8**	7*	35*	550*	**115**	**19**	**70**
19–30 y	1,000*	**700**	**310**	5*	3*	**1.5**	**1.6**	**17**	**2.0**	**500**	**2.8**	7*	35*	550*	**120**	**19**	**70**
31–50 y	1,000*	**700**	**320**	5*	3*	**1.5**	**1.6**	**17**	**2.0**	**500**	**2.8**	7*	35*	550*	**120**	**19**	**70**

[a]Recommended Dietary Allowances (RDAs) are presented in bold type and Adequate Intakes (Als) in ordinary type followed by an asterisk (*). RDAs and Als may both be used as goals for individual intake. RDAs are set to meet the needs of almost all (97% – 98%) individuals in a group. For healthy breast-fed infants, the Al is the mean intake. The Al for other life-stage and gender groups is believed to cover needs of all individuals in the group, but lack of data or uncertainty in the data prevent being able to specify with confidence the percentage of persons covered by this intake. Source: The National Academy of Sciences. ©2000.

[b]As cholecalciferol. 1 μg cholecalciferol=40 IU vitamin D.

[c]In the absence of adequate exposure to sunlight.

[d]As niacin equivalent (NE). 1 mg niacin=60 mg tryptophan; 0 to 6 mo=preformed niacin (not NE).

[e]As dietary folate equivalent (DFE). 1 DFE=1 μg food folate=0.6 μg folic acid (from fortified food or supplement) consumed with food=0.5 μg synthetic (supplemental) folic acid taken on an empty stomach.

[f]Although Als have been set for choline, there are few data to assess whether a dietary supply of choline is needed at all stages of the life cycle, and it may be that the choline requirement can be met by endogenous synthesis at some of these stages.

[g]Because 10% to 30% of older people may malabsorb food-bound vitamin B_{12}, it is advisable for those older than 50 years to meet their RDA mainly by consuming foods fortified with vitamin B_{12} or a supplement containing vitamin B_{12}.

[h]In view of evidence linking folate intake with neural tube defects in the fetus, it is recommended that all women capable of becoming pregnant consume 400 μg synthetic folic acid from fortified foods and/or supplements in addition to intake of food folate from a varied diet.

[i]It is assumed that women will continue consuming 400 μg folic acid until their pregnancy is confirmed and they enter prenatal care, which ordinarily occurs after the end of the periconceptional period—the critical time for formation of the neural tube.

[j]Smokers need an additional 35 mg vit C/day.

[k]As mg of α-tocopherol. α-tocopherol includes RRR-α-tocopherol; the only form of α-tocopherol that occurs naturally in foods, and the 2R-stereoisomeric forms of α-tocopherol (RRR-, RSR-, and RRR-α-tocopherol) that occur in fortified foods and supplements. It does not include the 25-stereoisomeric forms of α-tocopherol (SRR-, SSR-, and SSS-α-tocopherol) also found in fortified foods and supplements.

APPENDIX 2

Tolerable Upper Intake Levels[a] (ULs) for Certain Nutrients[b]

Life-stage group	Calcium (g/d)	Phosphorus (g/d)	Magnesium[c] (mg/d)	Vitamin D (µg/d)	Fluoride (mg/d)	Niacin[d] (mg/d)	Vitamin B_6 (mg/d)	Synthetic folic acid[d] (µg/d)	Choline (g/d)	Vitamin C (mg/d)	Vitamin E (mg/d)	Selenium (µg/d)
0–6 mo	ND[e]	ND	ND	25	0.7	ND	ND	ND	ND	ND	ND	45
7–12 mo	ND	ND	ND	25	0.9	ND	ND	ND	ND	ND	ND	60
1–3 y	2.5	3	65	50	1.3	10	30	300	1.0	400	200	90
4–8 y	2.5	3	110	50	2.2	15	40	400	1.0	650	300	150
9–13 y	2.5	4	350	50	10	20	60	600	2.0	1200	600	280
14–18 y	2.5	4	350	50	10	30	80	800	3.0	1800	800	400
19–70 y	2.5	4	350	50	10	35	100	1,000	3.5	2000	1000	400
>70y	2.5	3	350	50	10	35	100	1,000	3.5	2000	1000	400
Pregnancy												
≤18 y	2.5	3.5	350	50	10	30	80	800	3.0	1800	800	400
19–50 y	2.5	3.5	350	50	10	35	100	1,000	3.5	2000	1000	400
Lactation												
≤18 y	2.5	4	350	50	10	30	80	800	3.0	1800	800	400
19–50 y	2.5	4	350	50	10	35	100	1,000	3.5	2000	1000	400

[a]UL = the maximum level of daily nutrient intake that is unlikely to pose any risk of adverse effects. Unless otherwise specified, the UL represents total intake from food, water, and supplements. Due to lack of suitable data, ULs could not be established for thiamine, riboflavin, vitamin B_{12}, pantothenic acid, or biotin. In the absence of ULs, extra caution may be warranted in consuming levels above recommended intakes.

[b]Source: references 1 and 5.

[c]The UL for magnesium represents intake from a pharmacological agent only and does not include intake from food and water.

[d]The ULs for niacin and synthetic folic acid apply to forms obtained from supplements, fortified foods, or a combination of the two.

[e]ND: Not determinable due to lack of data on adverse effects in this age group and concern with regard to lack of ability to handle excess amounts. Food should be the only source of intake in order to prevent high levels of these vitamins.

APPENDIX 3

Food and Nutrition Board, National Academy of Sciences—National Research Council Recommended Dietary Allowances, Revised 1989 (Abridged)—Designed for the Maintenance of Good Nutrition of Practically All Healthy People in the United States*

							Fat-Soluble Vitamins		Minerals		
Category	Age (years) or Condition	Weight† (kg)	Weight† (lb)	Height† (cm)	Height† (in)	Protein (g)	Vitamin A (μg RE)‡	Vitamin K (μg)	Iron (mg)	Zinc (mg)	Iodine (μg)
Infants	0.0–0.5	6	13	60	24	13	375	5	6	5	40
	0.5–1.0	9	20	71	28	14	375	10	10	5	50
Children	1–3	13	29	90	35	16	400	15	10	10	70
	4–6	20	44	112	44	24	500	20	10	10	90
	7–10	28	62	132	52	28	700	30	10	10	120
Males	11–14	45	99	157	62	45	1,000	45	12	15	150
	15–18	66	145	176	69	59	1,000	65	12	15	150
	19–24	72	160	177	70	58	1,000	70	10	15	150
	25–50	79	174	176	70	63	1,000	80	10	15	150
	51+	77	170	173	68	63	1,000	80	10	15	150
Females	11–14	46	101	157	62	46	800	45	15	12	150
	15–18	55	120	163	64	44	800	55	15	12	150
	19–24	58	128	164	65	46	800	60	15	12	150
	25–50	63	138	163	64	50	800	65	15	12	150
	51+	65	143	160	63	50	800	65	10	12	150
Pregnant						60	800	65	30	15	175
Lactating	1st 6 months					65	1,300	65	15	19	200
	2nd 6 months					62	1,200	65	15	16	200

(Reprinted with permission from the National Academy of Sciences, Washington, DC.)

*The allowances, expressed as average daily intake over time, are intended to provide for individual variations among most normal persons as they live in the United States under usual environmental stresses. Diets should be based on a variety of common foods in order to provide other nutrients for which human requirements are less well defined.

†Weights and heights of Reference Adults are actual medians for the U.S. population of the designated age, as reported by NHANES II. The median weights and heights of those under 19 years of age were taken from Hamill, et al. (1979). The use of these figures does not imply that the height-to-weight ratios are ideal.

‡Retinol equivalents. 1 retinol equivalent = 1 μg retinol or 6 μg β-carotene.

APPENDIX 4

*Estimated Safe and Adequate Daily Dietary Intakes of Selected Vitamins and Minerals**

Category	Age (years)	Trace Elements† Copper (mg)	Manganese (mg)	Chromium (μg)	Molybdenum (μg)
Infants	0–0.5	0.4–0.6	0.3–0.6	10–40	15–30
	0.5–1	0.6–0.7	0.6–1.0	20–60	20–40
Children and Adolescents	1–3	0.7–1.0	1.0–1.5	20–80	25–50
	4–6	1.0–1.5	1.5–2.0	30–120	30–75
	7–10	1.0–2.0	2.0–3.0	50–200	50–150
	11+	1.5–2.5	2.0–5.0	50–200	75–250
Adults		1.5–3.0	2.0–5.0	50–200	75–250

(Food and Nutrition Board, National Research Council. [1989]. *Recommended dietary allowances* [10th ed]. Washington DC: National Academy Press.)

*Because there is less information on which to base allowances, these figures are not given in the main table of RDAs and are provided here as ranges of recommended intakes.

†Since the toxic levels for many trace elements may be only several times the usual intakes, the upper levels for the trace elements given in this table should not be habitually exceeded.

APPENDIX 5

*Estimated Minimum Requirements of Sodium, Chloride, and Potassium for Healthy Persons**

Age	Weight (kg)*	Sodium (mg)†	Chloride (mg)*†	Potassium (mg)‡
Months				
0–5	4.5	120	180	500
6–11	8.9	200	300	700
Years				
1	11.0	225	350	1,000
2–5	16.0	300	500	1,400
6–9	25.0	400	600	1,600
10–18	50.0	500	750	2,000
>18§	70.0	500	750	2,000

(Food and Nutrition Board, National Research Council. [1989]. *Recommended dietary allowances* [10th ed]. Washington DC: National Academy Press.)

* No allowance has been included for large, prolonged losses from the skin through sweat.

†There is no evidence that higher intakes confer any health benefit.

‡Desirable intakes of potassium may considerably exceed these values (~3,500 mg for adults).

§No allowance included for growth. Values for those below 18 years assume a growth rate at the 50th percentile reported by the National Center for Health Statistics and averaged for males and females.

APPENDIX 6

CDC Growth Charts: United States

CDC Growth Charts: United States

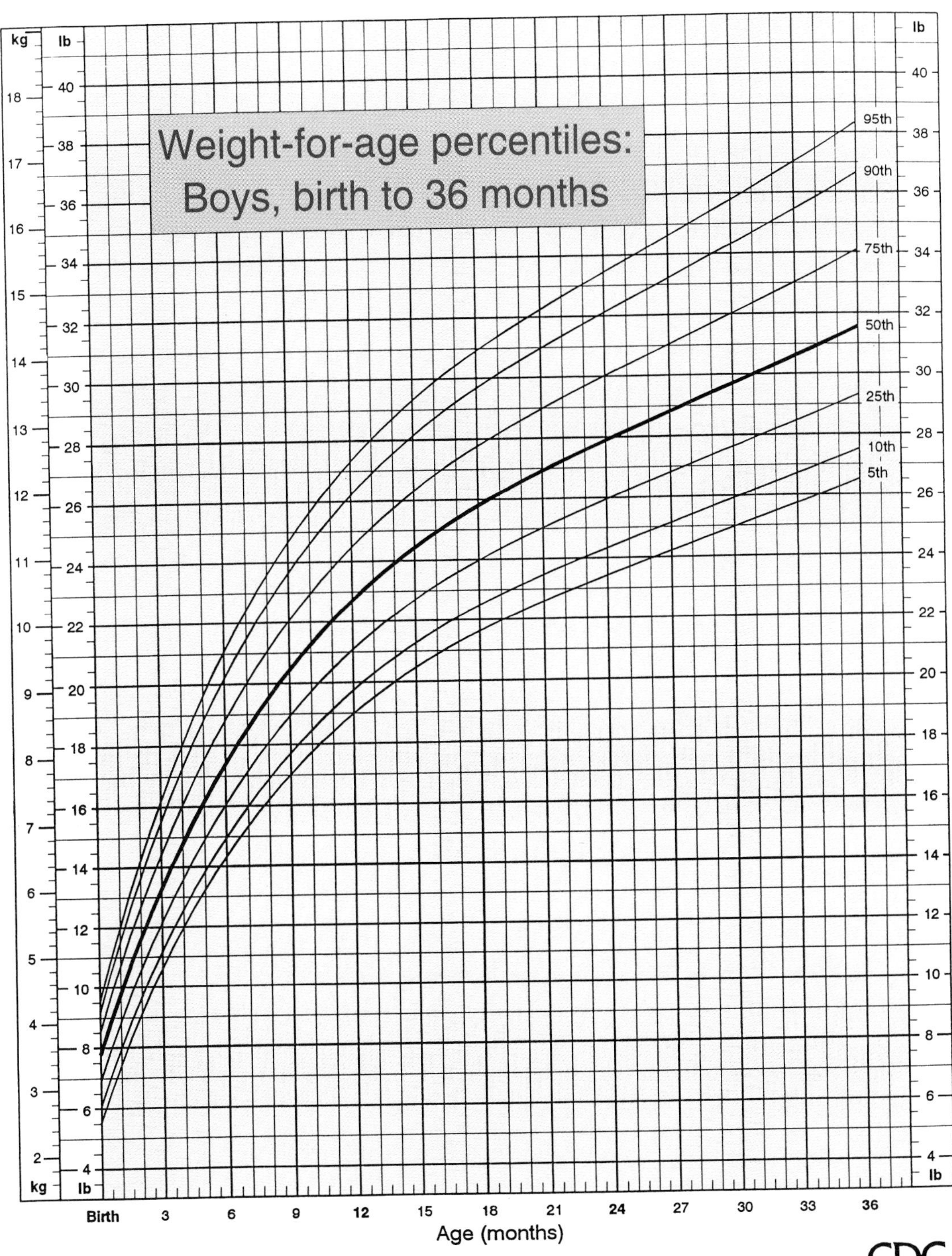

SOURCE: Developed by the National Center for Health Statistics in collaboration with the National Center for Chronic Disease Prevention and Health Promotion (2000).

CDC

CDC Growth Charts: United States

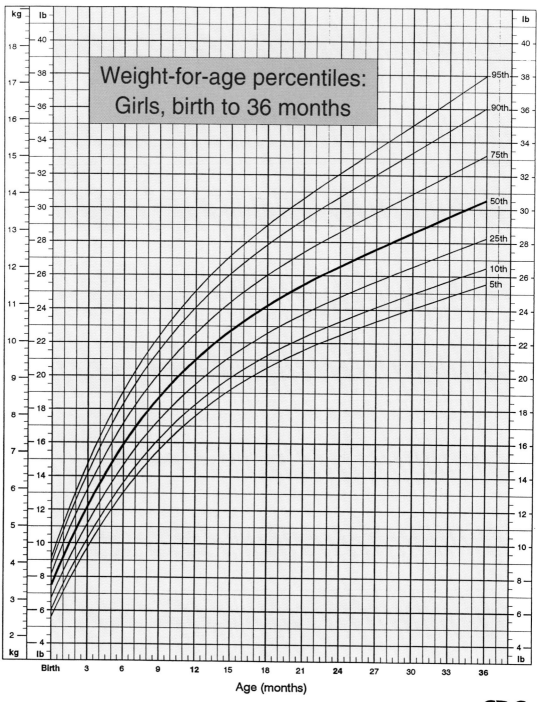

Weight-for-age percentiles: Girls, birth to 36 months

kg | lb

95th
90th
75th
50th
25th
10th
5th

Birth 3 6 9 12 15 18 21 24 27 30 33 36

Age (months)

SOURCE: Developed by the National Center for Health Statistics in collaboration with the National Center for Chronic Disease Prevention and Health Promotion (2000).

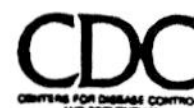

CDC Growth Charts: United States

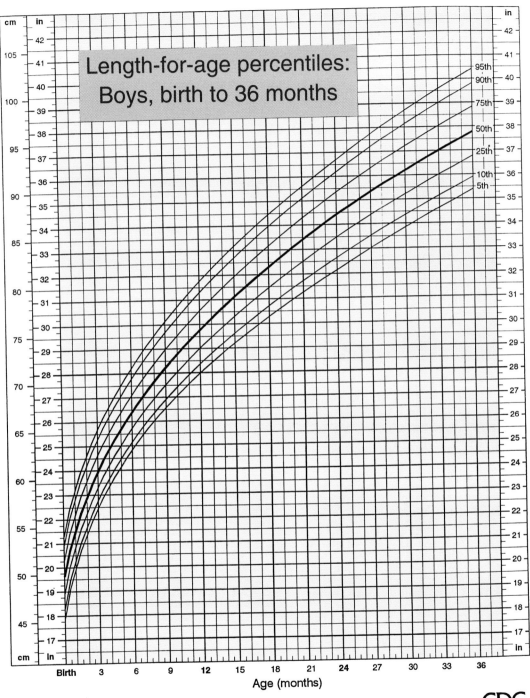

Length-for-age percentiles: Boys, birth to 36 months

cm: 45, 50, 55, 60, 65, 70, 75, 80, 85, 90, 95, 100, 105

in: 17, 18, 19, 20, 21, 22, 23, 24, 25, 26, 27, 28, 29, 30, 31, 32, 33, 34, 35, 36, 37, 38, 39, 40, 41, 42

95th
90th
75th
50th
25th
10th
5th

Birth 3 6 9 12 15 18 21 24 27 30 33 36

Age (months)

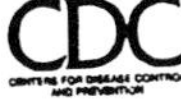

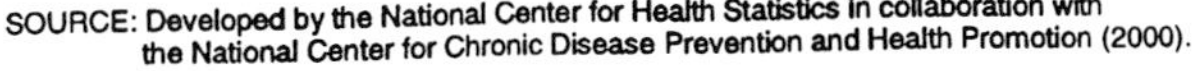
SOURCE: Developed by the National Center for Health Statistics in collaboration with the National Center for Chronic Disease Prevention and Health Promotion (2000).

CDC Growth Charts: United States

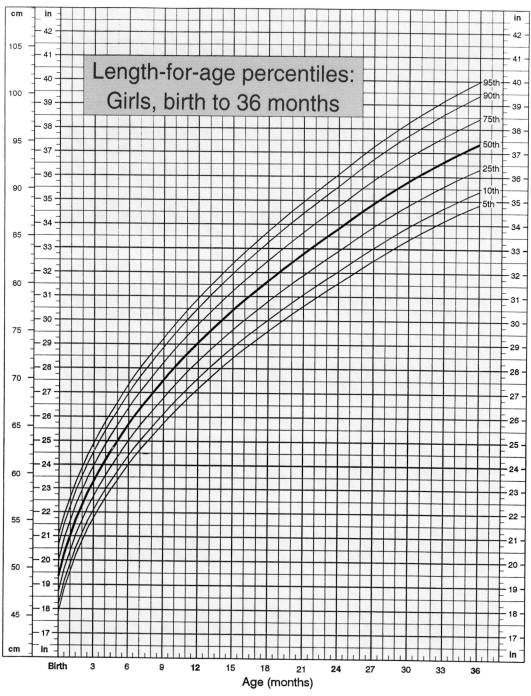

Length-for-age percentiles: Girls, birth to 36 months

cm: 105, 100, 95, 90, 85, 80, 75, 70, 65, 60, 55, 50, 45

in: 42, 41, 40, 39, 38, 37, 36, 35, 34, 33, 32, 31, 30, 29, 28, 27, 26, 25, 24, 23, 22, 21, 20, 19, 18, 17

95th
90th
75th
50th
25th
10th
5th

Birth 3 6 9 12 15 18 21 24 27 30 33 36

Age (months)

SOURCE: Developed by the National Center for Health Statistics in collaboration with the National Center for Chronic Disease Prevention and Health Promotion (2000).

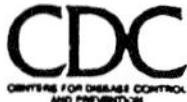

CDC Growth Charts: United States

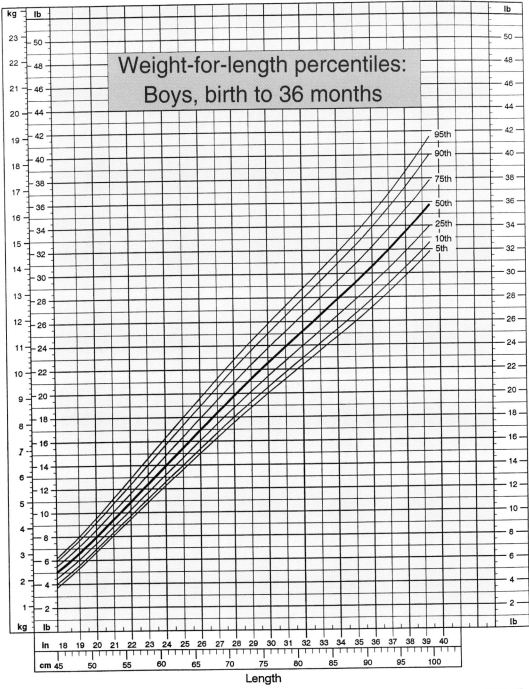

Weight-for-length percentiles: Boys, birth to 36 months

kg | lb | lb

95th
90th
75th
50th
25th
10th
5th

in 18 19 20 21 22 23 24 25 26 27 28 29 30 31 32 33 34 35 36 37 38 39 40

cm 45 50 55 60 65 70 75 80 85 90 95 100

Length

SOURCE: Developed by the National Center for Health Statistics in collaboration with the National Center for Chronic Disease Prevention and Health Promotion (2000).

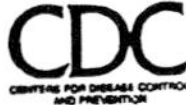

CDC Growth Charts: United States

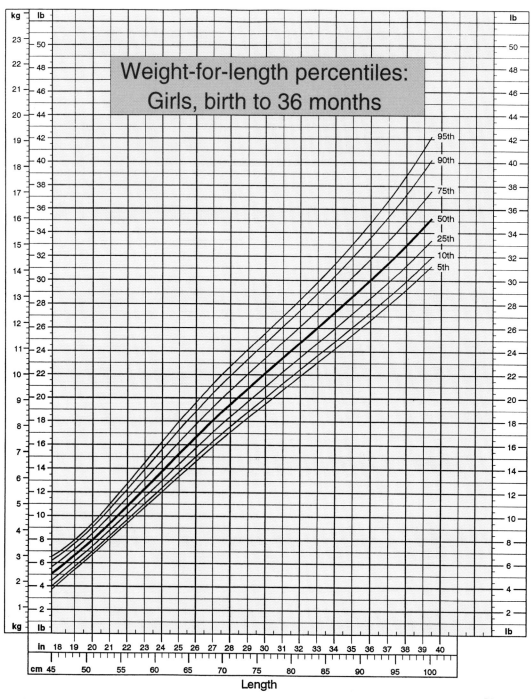

Weight-for-length percentiles: Girls, birth to 36 months

SOURCE: Developed by the National Center for Health Statistics in collaboration with the National Center for Chronic Disease Prevention and Health Promotion (2000).

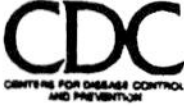

CDC Growth Charts: United States

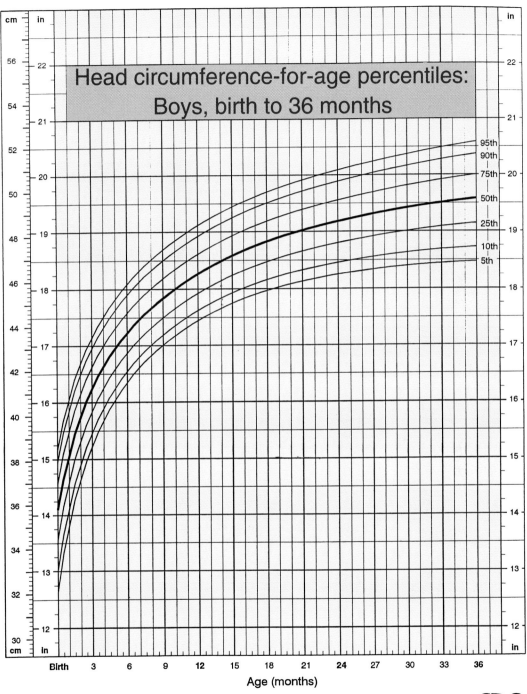

Head circumference-for-age percentiles: Boys, birth to 36 months

cm | in

56 | 22
54 | 21
52 | 20
50 | 19
48
46 | 18
44 | 17
42 | 16
40
38 | 15
36 | 14
34 | 13
32
30 | 12

cm | in

95th
90th
75th
50th
25th
10th
5th

in: 22, 21, 20, 19, 18, 17, 16, 15, 14, 13, 12

Birth 3 6 9 12 15 18 21 24 27 30 33 36

Age (months)

SOURCE: Developed by the National Center for Health Statistics in collaboration with the National Center for Chronic Disease Prevention and Health Promotion (2000).

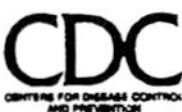

CDC Growth Charts: United States

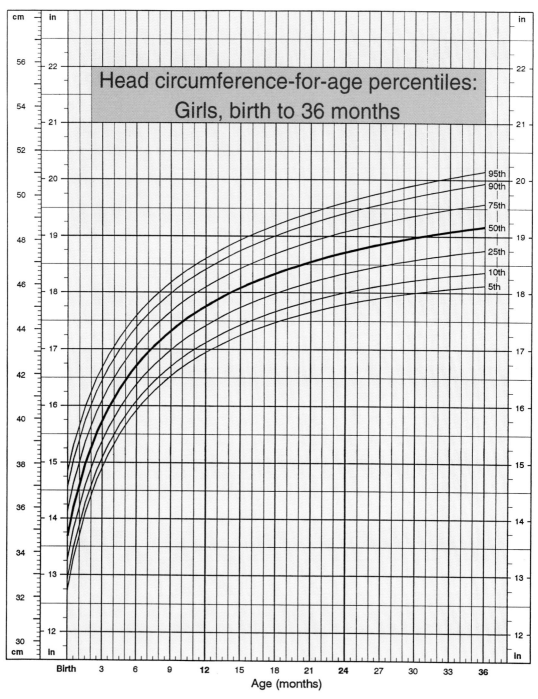

Head circumference-for-age percentiles: Girls, birth to 36 months

cm | in

56 | 22
54 | 21
52 | 20
50 |
48 | 19
46 | 18
44 | 17
42 |
40 | 16
38 | 15
36 | 14
34 | 13
32 |
30 | 12
cm | in

95th
90th
75th
50th
25th
10th
5th

in: 22, 21, 20, 19, 18, 17, 16, 15, 14, 13, 12, in

Birth 3 6 9 **12** 15 18 21 **24** 27 30 33 **36**

Age (months)

SOURCE: Developed by the National Center for Health Statistics in collaboration with the National Center for Chronic Disease Prevention and Health Promotion (2000).

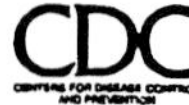

CDC Growth Charts: United States

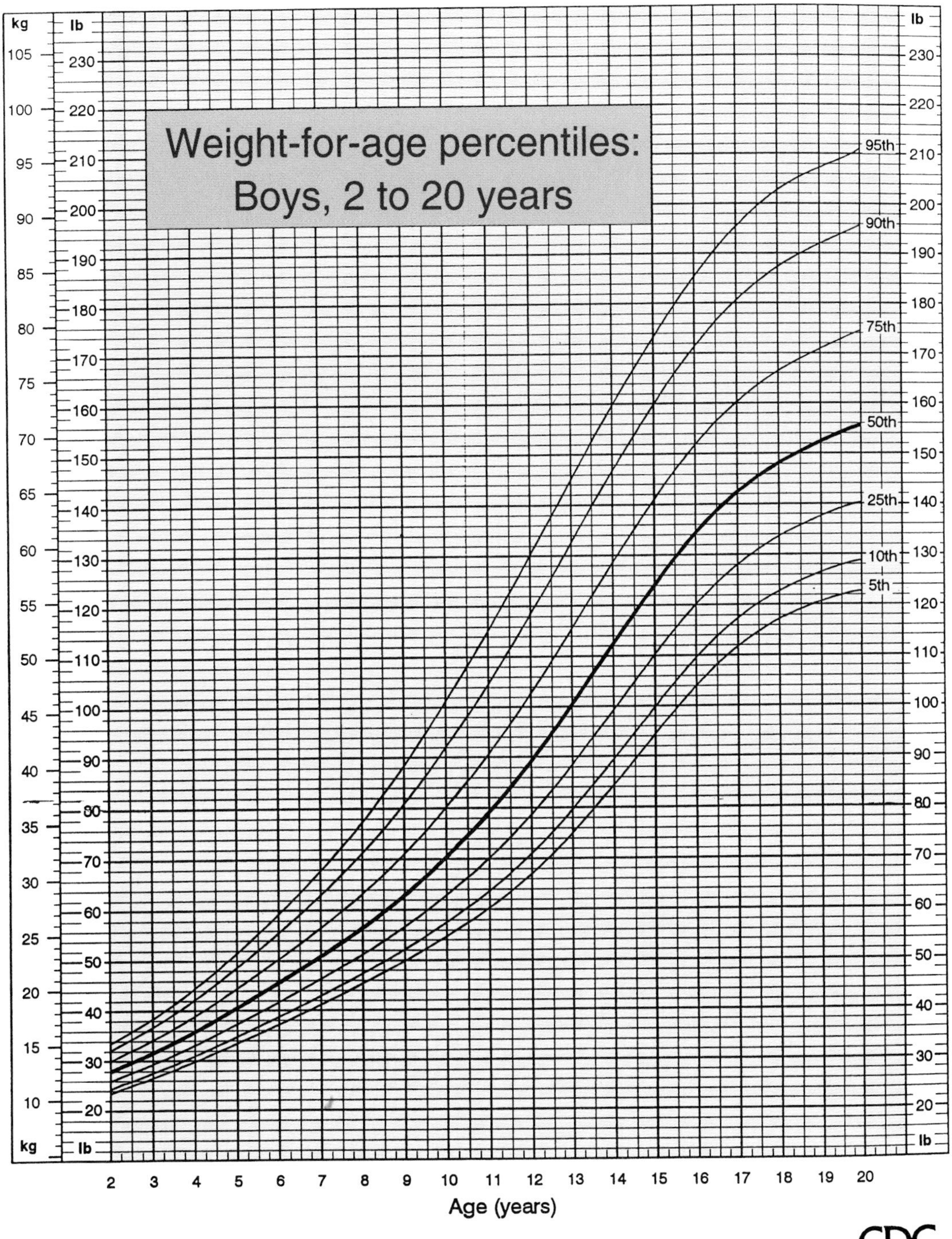

Weight-for-age percentiles: Boys, 2 to 20 years

kg lb

95th
90th
75th
50th
25th
10th
5th

Age (years)

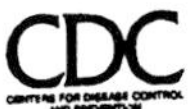

SOURCE: Developed by the National Center for Health Statistics in collaboration with the National Center for Chronic Disease Prevention and Health Promotion (2000).

CDC Growth Charts: United States

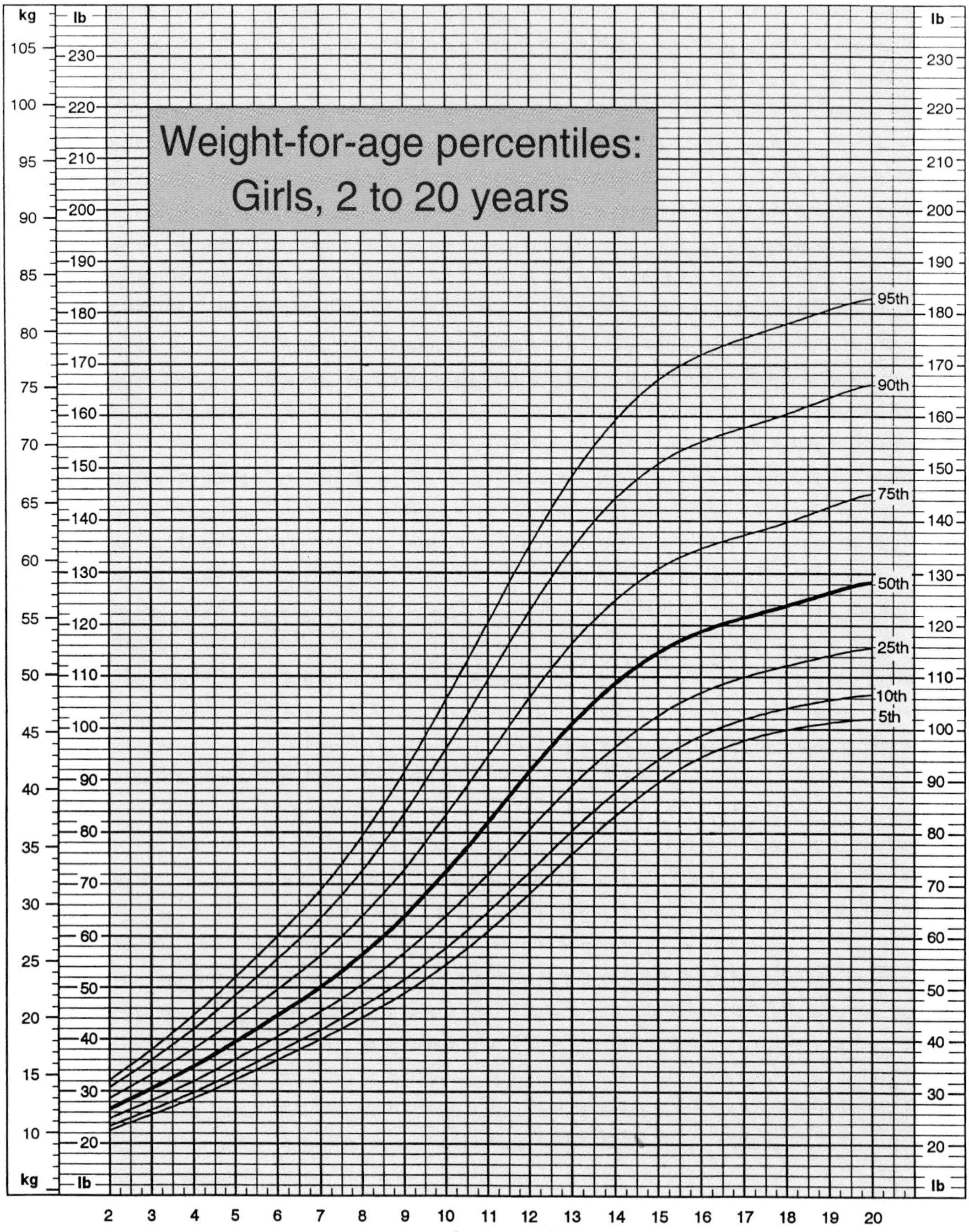

Weight-for-age percentiles: Girls, 2 to 20 years

kg | lb

105 | 230
100 | 220
95 | 210
90 | 200
85 | 190
80 | 180
75 | 170
70 | 160
65 | 150
60 | 140
55 | 130
50 | 120
45 | 110
40 | 100
35 | 90
30 | 80
25 | 70
20 | 60
15 | 50
10 | 40

30

20

kg | lb

95th
90th
75th
50th
25th
10th
5th

lb: 230, 220, 210, 200, 190, 180, 170, 160, 150, 140, 130, 120, 110, 100, 90, 80, 70, 60, 50, 40, 30, 20, lb

2 3 4 5 6 7 8 9 10 11 12 13 14 15 16 17 18 19 20

Age (years)

SOURCE: Developed by the National Center for Health Statistics in collaboration with the National Center for Chronic Disease Prevention and Health Promotion (2000).

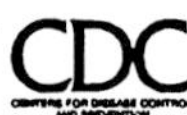

CDC Growth Charts: United States

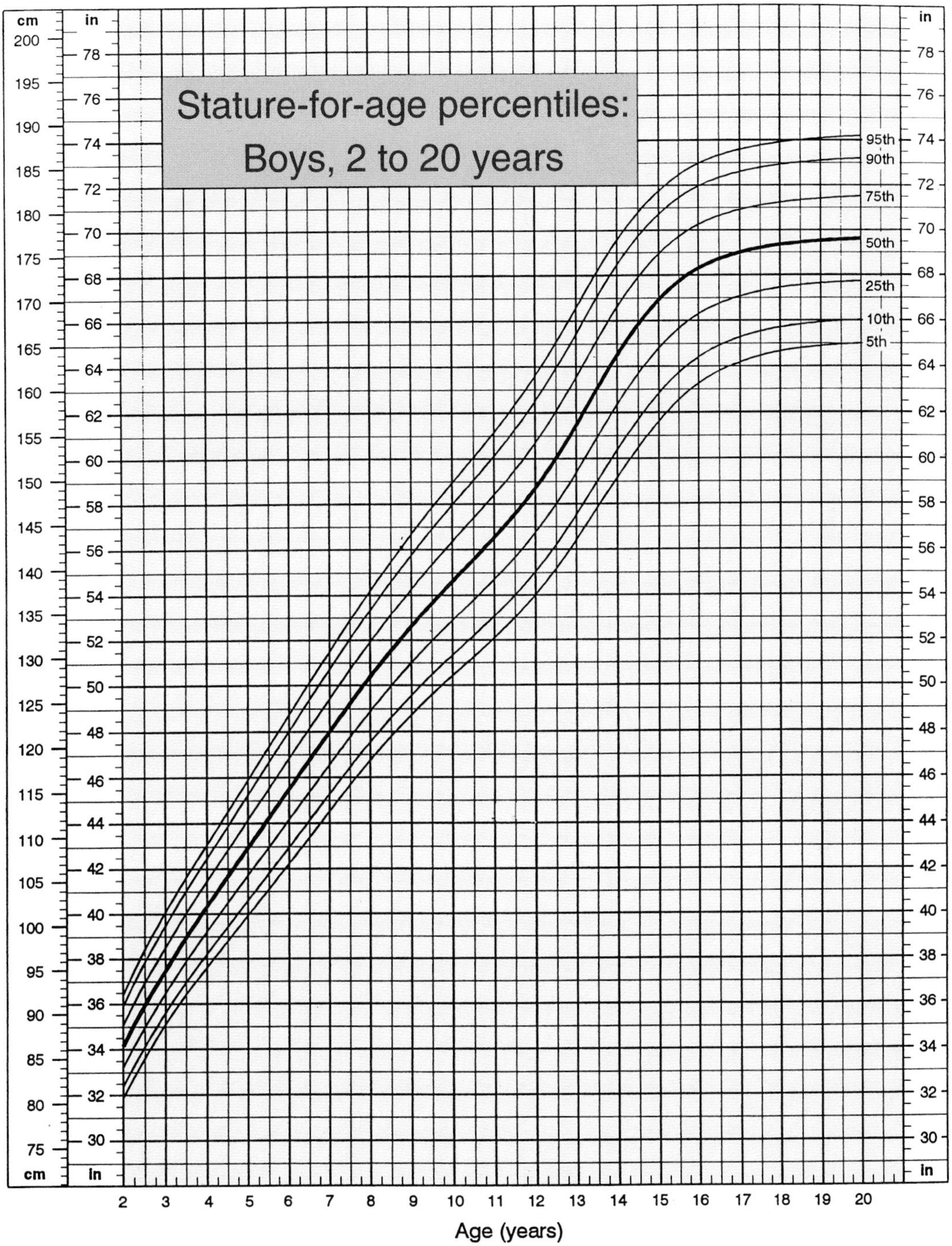

Stature-for-age percentiles: Boys, 2 to 20 years

cm | in

95th
90th
75th
50th
25th
10th
5th

Age (years)

2 3 4 5 6 7 8 9 10 11 12 13 14 15 16 17 18 19 20

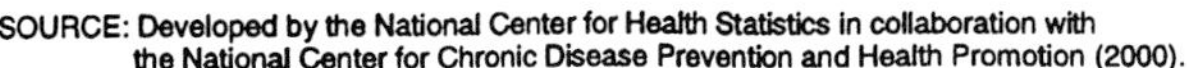
SOURCE: Developed by the National Center for Health Statistics in collaboration with the National Center for Chronic Disease Prevention and Health Promotion (2000).

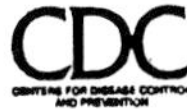

CDC Growth Charts: United States

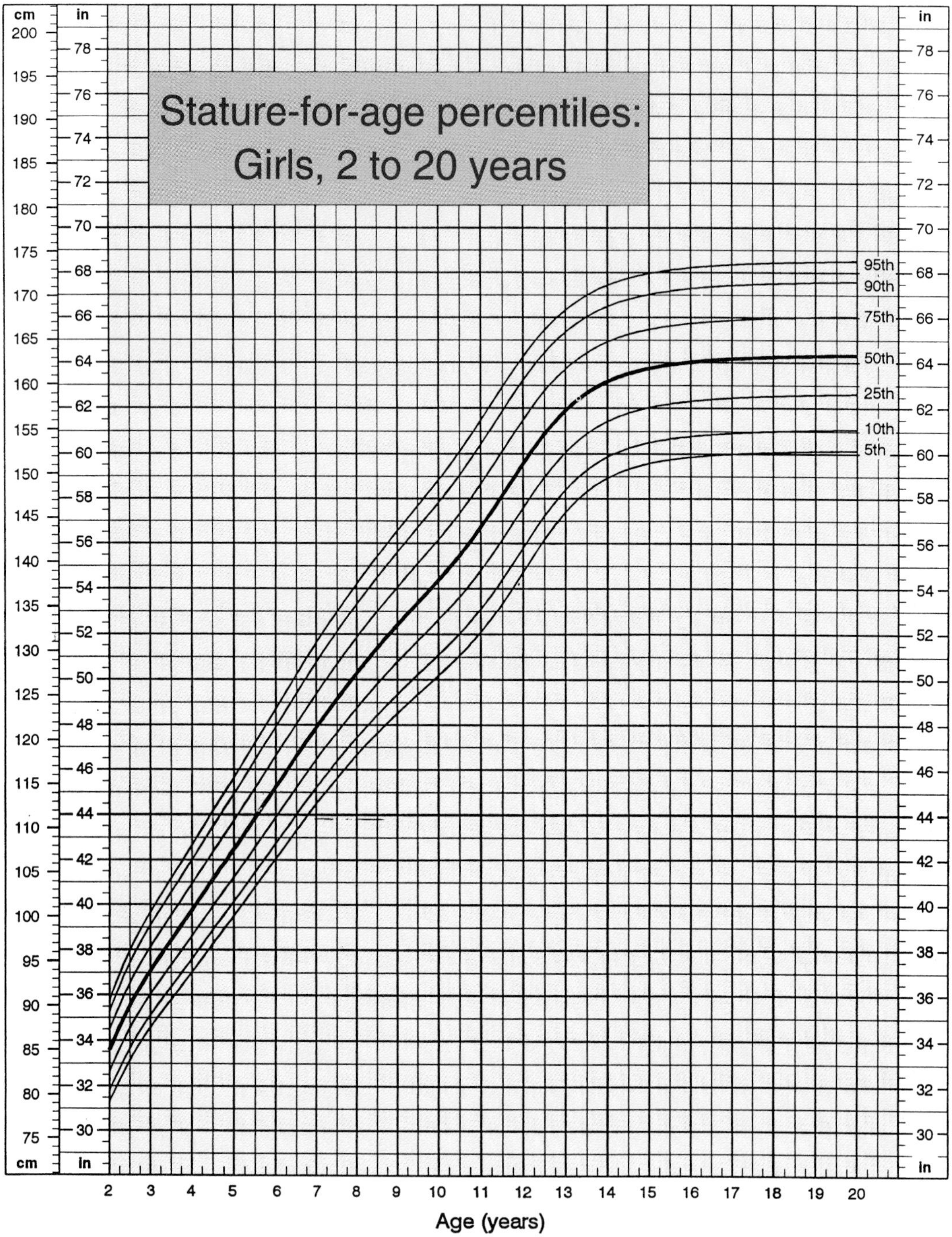

Stature-for-age percentiles: Girls, 2 to 20 years

cm 200 195 190 185 180 175 170 165 160 155 150 145 140 135 130 125 120 115 110 105 100 95 90 85 80 75 cm

in 78 76 74 72 70 68 66 64 62 60 58 56 54 52 50 48 46 44 42 40 38 36 34 32 30 in

95th
90th
75th
50th
25th
10th
5th

2 3 4 5 6 7 8 9 10 11 12 13 14 15 16 17 18 19 20

Age (years)

SOURCE: Developed by the National Center for Health Statistics in collaboration with the National Center for Chronic Disease Prevention and Health Promotion (2000).

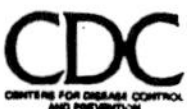

CDC Growth Charts: United States

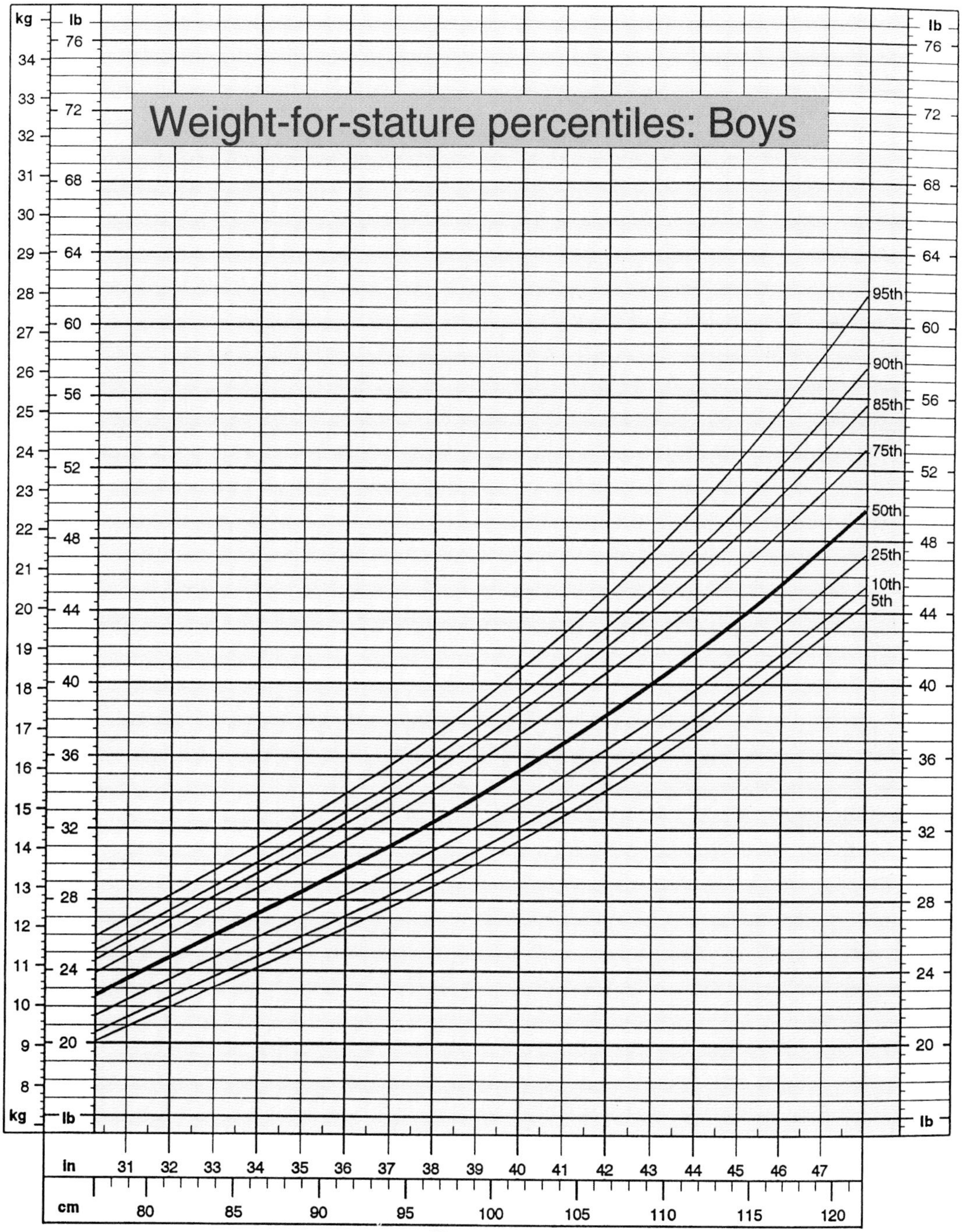

Weight-for-stature percentiles: Boys

kg: 8, 9, 10, 11, 12, 13, 14, 15, 16, 17, 18, 19, 20, 21, 22, 23, 24, 25, 26, 27, 28, 29, 30, 31, 32, 33, 34

lb: 20, 24, 28, 32, 36, 40, 44, 48, 52, 56, 60, 64, 68, 72, 76

95th
90th
85th
75th
50th
25th
10th
5th

in: 31, 32, 33, 34, 35, 36, 37, 38, 39, 40, 41, 42, 43, 44, 45, 46, 47

cm: 80, 85, 90, 95, 100, 105, 110, 115, 120

Stature

SOURCE: Developed by the National Center for Health Statistics in collaboration with the National Center for Chronic Disease Prevention and Health Promotion (2000).

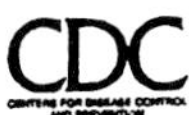

CDC Growth Charts: United States

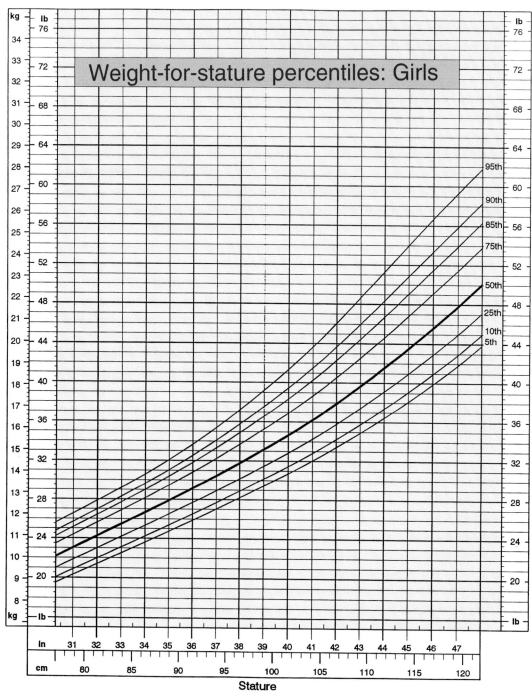

Weight-for-stature percentiles: Girls

SOURCE: Developed by the National Center for Health Statistics in collaboration with the National Center for Chronic Disease Prevention and Health Promotion (2000).

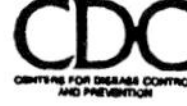

CDC Growth Charts: United States

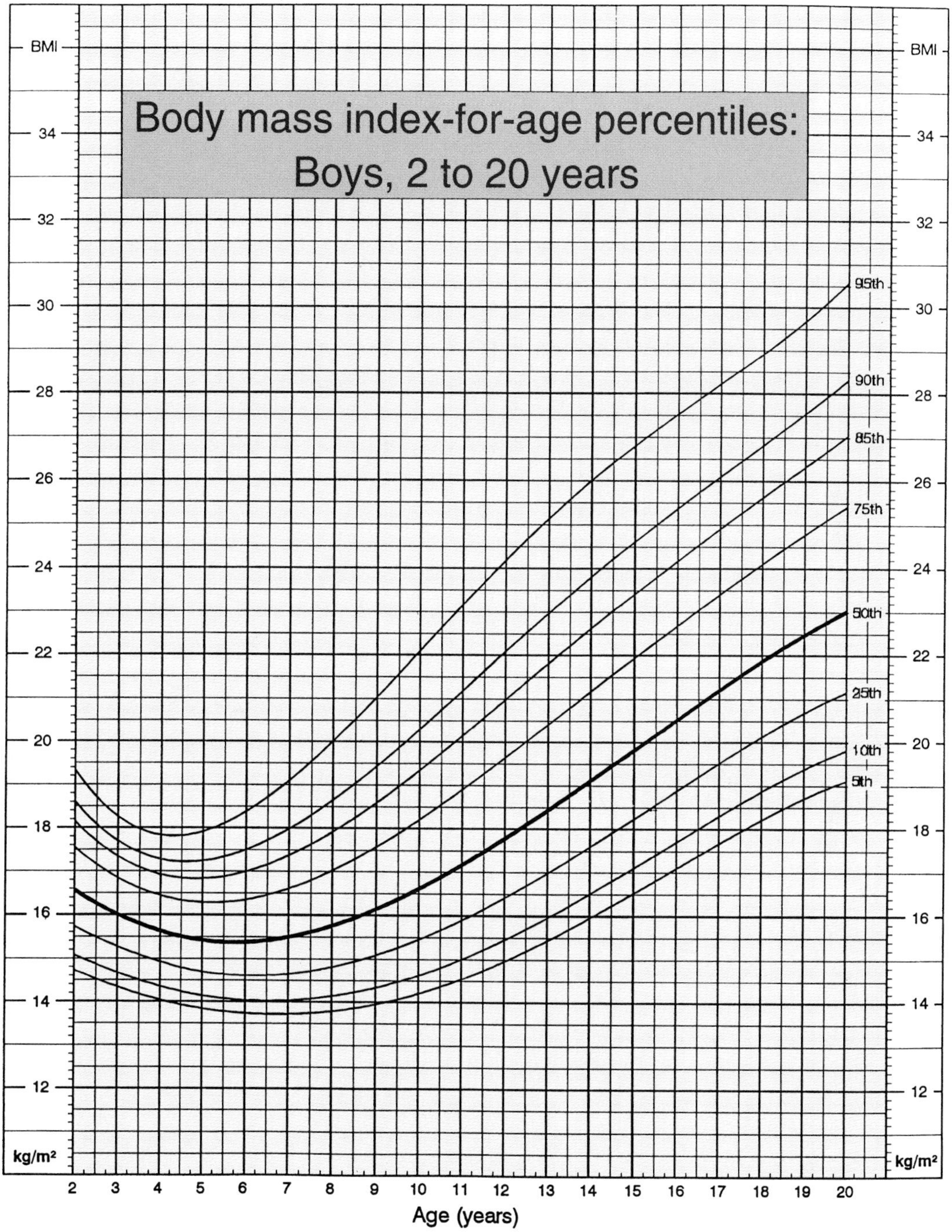

SOURCE: Developed by the National Center for Health Statistics in collaboration with the National Center for Chronic Disease Prevention and Health Promotion (2000).

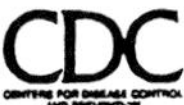

CDC Growth Charts: United States

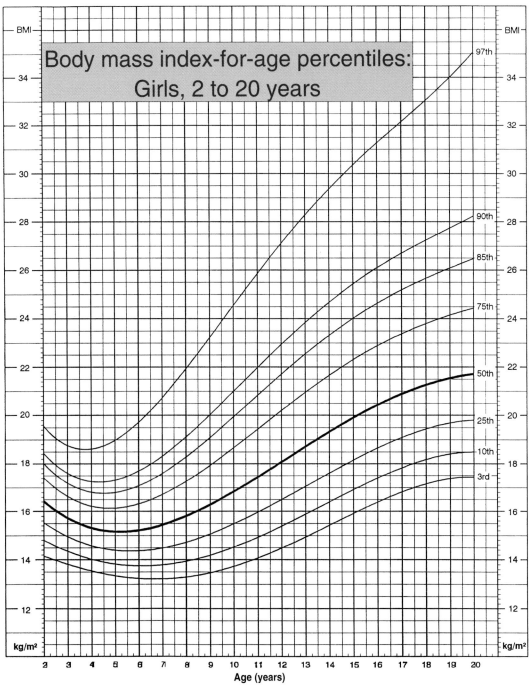

Body mass index-for-age percentiles: Girls, 2 to 20 years

BMI

34
32
30
28
26
24
22
20
18
16
14
12

kg/m²

97th
90th
85th
75th
50th
25th
10th
3rd

2 3 4 5 6 7 8 9 10 11 12 13 14 15 16 17 18 19 20

Age (years)

SOURCE: Developed by the National Center for Health Statistics in collaboration with the National Center for Chronic Disease Prevention and Health Promotion (2000).

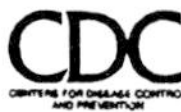

APPENDIX 7

Diet and Drugs

Many drugs have the potential to affect and be affected by nutrition. Sometimes, drug-nutrient interactions are the intended action of the drug. At other times, alterations in nutrient intake, metabolism, or excretion may be unfortunate side effects of drug therapy.

Well-nourished individuals on short-term drug therapy may easily withstand the negative effects of drug-nutrient interactions. Patients who are malnourished or on long-term drug regimens may experience significant nutrient deficiencies and decreased tolerance to drug therapy. Although potential and actual drug-nutrient interactions vary considerably among specific drugs, clients at greatest risk for developing drug-induced nutrient deficiencies include those

- Whose diets are chronically inadequate.
- Who have increased nutritional needs, such as infants, adolescents, and pregnant and lactating women.
- Who are elderly.
- Who have chronic illnesses.
- Who are on long-term or multiple drug regimens.
- Who self-medicate.
- Who are substance abusers.

The common nutritional side effects of selected drugs and possible nutrition interventions are highlighted below.

Drug Classification and Examples	Common Nutritional Side Effects	Possible Nutrition Interventions
Analgesics		
Narcotic: codeine, meperidine, morphine sulfate	N/V, gastrointestinal upset, constipation, lethargy	May need increased fiber and fluids.
Nonnarcotic: aspirin, ibuprofen, naproxen	N/V, gastrointestinal upset, gastrointestinal bleeding, constipation	Avoid Gastrointestinal irritants with long-term use, such as pepper, caffeine, and alcohol. Increase intake of foods rich in folic acid, vitamin C, and iron.
Antacids		
Aluminum hydroxide	Constipation	May need increased vitamin A, folacin, iron, thiamine, and riboflavin.
Calcium-containing	Constipation, chalky taste	

continued

Drug Classification and Examples	Common Nutritional Side Effects	Possible Nutrition Interventions
Magnesium hydroxide	N/V, gastrointestinal distress, diarrhea, chalky taste	Increase fiber and fluids.
Antianxiety agents		
Alprazolam	N/V, diarrhea, constipation, drowsiness, dry mouth	Take with food. Avoid alcohol.
Buspirone hydrochloride	N/V, gastrointestinal distress, diarrhea, dry mouth	Avoid alcohol.
Lorazepam	Drowsiness	Limit caffeine to <500 mg/d.
Antiarrhythmic		
Betapace	N/V, gastrointestinal distress, diarrhea, dry mouth, altered taste, edema, drowsiness	Food decreases absorption. Avoid alcohol.
Antibiotics		
Amoxicillin	N/V, diarrhea	Take with food.
Ampicillin	N/V, diarrhea	
Azithromycin	N/V, gastrointestinal distress, diarrhea	Take 1 h before or 2 h after full meal.
Ciprofloxacin	N/V, gastrointestinal distress, diarrhea	Maintain adequate hydration. Do not take with antacids or supplements containing magnesium, aluminum, or calcium. Do not take with iron, zinc, or multivitamin supplements containing minerals.
Clarithromycin	N/V, gastrointestinal distress, diarrhea, altered taste	Avoid alcohol.
Dirithromycin	N/V, gastrointestinal distress, diarrhea	Take with food. May need low-potassium diet.
Erythromycin	N/V, gastrointestinal distress	Take with food.
Lomefloxacin	N/V, gastrointestinal distress, diarrhea, constipation, altered taste, dry mouth	Avoid caffeine. Increase fluids. May need high-fiber, low-potassium, low-sodium diet.
Penicillin	Diarrhea	Maintain hydration.
Timentin	Hypokalemia	May need low-sodium, high-potassium diet.
Trimethoprim with sulfamethoxazole	N/V, diarrhea, gastrointestinal distress, drowsiness, anorexia	Maintain adequate hydration. May need folacin supplement.
Zosyn	N/V, gastrointestinal distress, diarrhea, constipation	May need low-sodium diet.
Anticoagulants		
Ticlopidine	N/V, gastrointestinal upset, diarrhea	Take with or immediately after food.
Warfarin	Nausea	Maintain consistent vitamin K intake.
Anticonvulsants		
Carbamazepine	N/V, diarrhea, drowsiness	Take with food. Avoid alcohol. May deplete sodium.
Clonazepam	Dry mouth, drowsiness	Take with food. Avoid alcohol.

continued

Drug Classification and Examples	Common Nutritional Side Effects	Possible Nutrition Interventions
Ethosuximide	N/V, gastrointestinal distress, diarrhea	Avoid alcohol.
Felbamate	N/V, gastrointestinal distress, diarrhea, constipation, drowsiness, edema, altered taste, dry mouth	May need low-sodium diet. Do not crush or chew.
Phenobarbital	Drowsiness	Causes vitamin D deficiency, low calcium absorption. May need vitamin D, B_{12}, and folacin supplements with long-term use.
Phenytoin	N/V, constipation, drowsiness	Increase foods rich in vitamin D, vitamin K, and folacin.
Valproic acid	N/V, gastrointestinal distress	Avoid alcohol.
Antidepressants		
Amitriptyline	Constipation, altered taste	Avoid caffeine and alcohol.
Aventyl	Constipation, drowsiness	Take with food. Avoid alcohol.
Bupropion HCl	N/V, gastrointestinal distress, constipation, edema, dry mouth	Take with food. Avoid alcohol. Avoid GI irritants with long-term use: pepper, caffeine, potassium supplements.
Clomipramine HCl	N/V, gastrointestinal distress, diarrhea, constipation, dry mouth	Take with food. May need high fiber, high fluids.
Fluoxetine HCl	N/V, gastrointestinal distress, diarrhea, dry mouth	Tryptophan supplements increase side effects.
Imipramine	N/V, constipation, dry mouth	Take with food. Avoid caffeine and alcohol. High fiber may decrease drug effectiveness. Causes increased urinary losses of riboflavin.
Mirtazapine	N/V, constipation, dry mouth, appetite changes	Take at bedtime. Avoid alcohol.
Nefazodone	Gastrointestinal distress, dry mouth	Do not take with food. Avoid alcohol.
Paroxetine	N/V, diarrhea, constipation, drowsiness, edema	No tryptophan supplements. Avoid alcohol.
Phenelzine sulfate	Gastrointestinal distress, constipation, drowsiness, edema, dry mouth	Avoid caffeine, alcohol, and foods high in tyramine. May need vitamin B_6 supplement.
Sertraline HCl	N/V, gastrointestinal distress, diarrhea, constipation, altered taste, thirst, dry mouth, drowsiness	Take with food. Avoid alcohol.
Antidiabetics		
Acarbose	Flatulence, diarrhea, hypoglycemia	Take 3 times daily with the first bite of each meal.
Chlorpropamide	N/V, diarrhea	Avoid alcohol.
Glipizide	N/V, Gastrointestinal distress, diarrhea, constipation, hypoglycemia	Diet important. Avoid alcohol.

continued

Drug Classification and Examples	Common Nutritional Side Effects	Possible Nutrition Interventions
Glyburide	N/V, gastrointestinal distress, hypoglycemia	Diet important. Avoid alcohol.
Tolbutamide	N/V, diarrhea, constipation, drowsiness	Diet important. Avoid alcohol.
Antidiarrheals		
Diphenoxylate HCl with atropine sulfate	Gastrointestinal distress, constipation	Take with food. Avoid alcohol.
Octreotide acetate	N/V, gastrointestinal distress, diarrhea	Maintain adequate hydration.
Antifungals		
Amphotericin	N/V, anorexia, gastrointestinal distress	Maintain adequate hydration. Increase potassium and magnesium intake.
Fluconazole	N/V, gastrointestinal distress, diarrhea	May need high-potassium diet.
Ketoconazole	N/V	Separate from antacids and histamine blockers by 2 hours.
Antigout		
Allopurinol	N/V, diarrhea	High fluid intake to prevent renal stones. No high doses of vitamin C.
Colchicine	N/V, gastrointestinal distress, diarrhea	Avoid alcohol. May decrease absorption of protein, fat, vitamin A, carotene, iron, calcium, sodium, and potassium.
Antihistamine		
Astemizole	N/V, gastrointestinal distress, diarrhea	Take on empty stomach or 2 hours after meals.
Antihypertensives		
ACE inhibitors: benazepril, captopril, fosinopril	Hyperkalemia, altered taste, dry mouth	No licorice. May need low-sodium, low-calorie diet. No potassium supplement.
Aldactazide	Gastrointestinal distress, dry mouth, constipation	Take with food. Avoid alcohol. May need low-sodium, low-calorie diet. No licorice. Avoid high potassium foods.
Amiodinpine besylate	N/V, edema	Take with food. May need low-sodium, low-calorie diet. No licorice.
Atenolol	N/V, diarrhea, dry mouth, drowsiness	Take separately from calcium supplements and antacids. No licorice.
Bisoprolol fumarate	N/V, gastrointestinal distress, diarrhea, constipation	May need low-sodium, low-potassium, low-calorie, low-fat, high-fiber diet.
Clonidine	N/V, dry mouth, constipation, drowsiness	May need low sodium, low calorie diet. No licorice. Avoid alcohol.
Doxazosin mesylate	N/V, dry mouth, diarrhea	May need low-sodium diet.
Guanfacine	N/V, dry mouth, diarrhea, constipation	Take with food. May need high-fiber, high-fluid diet.

continued

Drug Classification and Examples	Common Nutritional Side Effects	Possible Nutrition Interventions
Hydralazine HCl	N/V, altered taste, diarrhea	Take consistently either with or without food. May need low-sodium, low-calorie diet. No licorice. May need vitamin B_6 supplement to avoid nerve damage in hands and feet.
Isradipine	N/V, gastrointestinal distress, diarrhea, constipation	Take with food. May need low-sodium, high-fiber, high-fluids.
Iosartan potassium	N/V, gastrointestinal distress, diarrhea, edema	May need low-sodium diet.
Methyldopa	N/V, diarrhea, constipation, edema, dry mouth, drowsiness	May need low-sodium, low-calorie diet. No licorice. Increase B_{12}. Take iron supplement 2 h before or after drug.
Metoprolol tartrate	N/V, gastrointestinal distress, diarrhea, constipation, edema, altered taste	Take with food. May need low-sodium, low-calorie diet. No licorice.
Minoxidil	N/V, edema	May need low-sodium, low-calorie diet. No licorice.
Nifedipine	N/V, gastrointestinal distress, diarrhea, constipation, drowsiness, edema	May need low-sodium, low-calorie diet. No licorice. No calcium supplement.
Prazosin HCL	N/V, diarrhea, constipation, drowsiness, edema, dry mouth	May need low-sodium, low-calorie diet. No licorice. Avoid alcohol.
Antinausea		
Chlorpromazine HCl	Constipation, dry mouth, drowsiness	Take with food. Avoid caffeine and alcohol. Separate B_{12} and magnesium supplements by 2 hours.
Dronabinol	N/V, gastrointestinal distress, drowsiness	Avoid alcohol.
Granisetron HCl	Diarrhea, constipation, altered taste	May need high-fiber, high-fluid diet.
Ondansetron HCl	Constipation, gastrointestinal distress	
Antineoplastic		
Anastrozole	N/V, gastrointestinal distress, diarrhea, constipation	May need low-sodium diet.
Busulfan	N/V	
Carboplatin	N/V, gastrointestinal distress, diarrhea, constipation	May need high-fiber, high-fluid, high-potassium diet.
Carmustine	N/V	Avoid alcohol.
Cisplatin	N/V, diarrhea, altered taste	Maintain adequate hydration. May need mineral supplement due to increased urinary excretion of magnesium, potassium, calcium, zinc, and copper.
Cyclophosphamide	N/V, gastrointestinal distress, diarrhea	
Cytarabine	N/V, diarrhea	
Dacarbazine	N/V	
Dactinomycin	N/V, gastrointestinal distress, diarrhea	

continued

Drug Classification and Examples	Common Nutritional Side Effects	Possible Nutrition Interventions
Docetaxel	N/V, diarrhea	
Doxorubicin	Gastrointestinal distress	
Emcyt	N/V, gastrointestinal distress, diarrhea, drowsiness, edema	Take separately from dairy products and sources of calcium.
Estramustine phosphate sodium	N/V, gastrointestinal distress, diarrhea, drowsiness, edema, decreased appetite	Take separately from dairy products and sources of calcium.
Etoposide	N/V	
Fluorouracil	N/V, gastrointestinal distress, diarrhea	May need vitamin B_6.
Irinotecan HCl	N/V, diarrhea	Electrolyte imbalances may occur from severe diarrhea.
Melphalan	N/V, gastrointestinal distress, diarrhea	
Methotrexate	N/V, diarrhea, drowsiness, anorexia	Folate antagonist. Folate deficiency may increase drug toxicity. May decrease absorption of fat, vitamin B_{12}, and calcium.
Paclitaxel	N/V, diarrhea	May need low-sodium diet.
Vinblastine sulfate	Constipation	
Vinorelbine tartrate	N/V, diarrhea	
Antiparkinson		
Benztroopine mesylate	Constipation, increased risk of dental problems	Take with food. Avoid alcohol.
Bromocriptine mesylate	N/V, gastrointestinal distress, diarrhea, constipation, dry mouth	Take with food. May need high-fiber, high-fluids.
Levodopa	N/V, gastrointestinal distress, dry mouth, altered taste	Do not take with high-protein foods, amino acids, or protein hydrolysates. Do not take with high-fiber meals. Limit vitamin B_6 to < 5 mg/d.
Selegiline	Drowsiness	If >10 mg drug/d, avoid high-tyramine foods.
Antiprotozoan		
Atovazuone	N/V, gastrointestinal distress, diarrhea, constipation, altered taste	Take with high-fat meal or snack.
Metronidazole	N/V, gastrointestinal distress, altered taste, anorexia	May need fluid and electrolyte replacement if stools are liquid.
Antipsychotic		
Haloperidol	N/V, gastrointestinal distress, diarrhea, constipation, drowsiness, dry mouth	Do not mix concentrate with coffee, tea, or fruit juice (drug may precipitate). Take with food. Avoid caffeine and alcohol.
Thioridazaine HCl	Constipation, drowsiness, dry mouth	Take with food. Avoid caffeine and alcohol.
Antivirals		
Acyclovir	N/V	Maintain adequate hydration.

continued

Drug Classification and Examples	Common Nutritional Side Effects	Possible Nutrition Interventions
Didanosine (DDI)	Gastrointestinal distress, diarrhea, dry mouth, thirst	Take on empty stomach. May need low-sodium diet.
Famiciclovir	N/V, gastrointestinal distress, diarrhea, constipation	May need high-fiber, high-fluid diet.
Foscarnet sodium	N/V, gastrointestinal distress, diarrhea, constipation, altered taste, dry mouth	Maintain adequate hydration. Monitor for low calcium.
Indinavir sulfate	Altered taste	Take on empty stomach. Need adequate fluid to avoid renal stones.
Lamivudine	N/V, gastrointestinal distress, diarrhea, drowsiness	Maintain adequate hydration.
Nelfinvir mesylate	N/V, gastrointestinal distress, diarrhea	Mix with water, milk, or formula.
Ritonavir	N/V, gastrointestinal distress, diarrhea, altered taste	Mix with chocolate milk, Ensure, or Advera to improve taste.
Saquinavir mesylate	N/V, gastrointestinal distress, diarrhea	Take within 2 h of full meal.
Stavudine (D_4T)	N/V, gastrointestinal distress, diarrhea, constipation	Maintain adequate hydration.
Zalcitabine	N/V, gastrointestinal distress, diarrhea	Do not take within 2 h of magnesium-containing antacids.
Zidovudine (AZT)	N/V, gastrointestinal distress, diarrhea, altered taste	Monitor for anemia.
Bronchodilators		
Albuterol sulfate	N/V, gastrointestinal distress, dry mouth, altered taste, hypertension	Take with food. Avoid caffeine.
Aminophylline	N/V, constipation, drowsiness, anorexia	Avoid caffeine. Maintain consistent intake of protein and carbohydrate for consistent drug levels.
Ipratropium bromide	N/V, gastrointestinal distress, dry mouth	Not appropriate for people with allergies to soy lecithin, soybeans, or peanuts.
Theophylline	N/V, constipation, anorexia	Take with food. High-protein, low carbohydrate diet causes decreased blood levels of drug.
Corticosteroid		
Dexamethasone	N/V, gastrointestinal distress	May need low-sodium, high-protein diet. May need increased potassium; calcium; vitamins A, C, D, B_6; and folacin.
Diuretic		
Bimetanide	N/V	Increase potassium; may need supplement. Take with food. Avoid alcohol.
Chlorothiazide	Hypokalemia	Take with food. Avoid alcohol. May need potassium and magnesium supplement. No licorice.

continued

Drug Classification and Examples	Common Nutritional Side Effects	Possible Nutrition Interventions
Spironolactone	N/V, gastrointestinal distress, diarrhea, thirst, dry mouth	Take with food. Maintain adequate hydration. No licorice. Avoid high-potassium intake.
Hypnotic		
Flurazepam HCl	N/V, gastrointestinal distress, diarrhea, constipation, drowsiness	Take at bedtime. Avoid alcohol. May need high-fiber, high-fluid diet.
Zolpidem tartrate	N/V, gastrointestinal distress, diarrhea, constipation, anorexia, dry mouth	Food decreases and delays drug absorption.
Immunosuppressant		
Artithymocyte globin	N/V, gastrointestinal distress, diarrhea	May need low-calorie diet. Maintain hydration.
Azathioprine	N/V	Take after meals.
Cyclosporine	N/V, gastrointestinal distress, diarrhea, hyperkalemia	May need low-fat, low-potassium, low-calorie diet.
Muromonab	N/V, gastrointestinal distress, diarrhea, drowsiness	Maintain adequate hydration.
Lipid lowering		
Atorvastatin calcium	Gastrointestinal distress, constipation	Need low-fat diet. May need increased fiber and fluids.
Cholestryamine	N/V, gastrointestinal distress, constipation	May need supplements of calcium, magnesium, iron, zinc, folacin, B_{12}, and fat-soluble vitamins due to decreased absorption.
Clofibrate	N/V, gastrointestinal distress, diarrhea, drowsiness	Low-fat, low-cholesterol diet important.
Colestipol	N/V, gastrointestinal distress, diarrhea, constipation	Low-fat, low-cholesterol diet important. May need multivitamin with mineral supplement.
Fluvastatin	N/V, gastrointestinal distress, diarrhea, constipation	Need low-fat, low-cholesterol diet.
Lovastatin	N/V, gastrointestinal distress, diarrhea, constipation	May need low-fat, low-cholesterol, low-calorie diet. Do not take fiber, pectin, or oat bran within 3 h of dosage.
Niacin	N/V, gastrointestinal distress, diarrhea	Need low-fat, low-cholesterol, low-calorie diet.
Simvastatin	N/V, gastrointestinal distress, diarrhea, constipation	Need low-fat, low-cholesterol, low-calorie diet. Avoid alcohol.

N/V = nausea and vomiting

Monoamine oxidase inhibitors (MAOIs) are antidepressants that potentiate the cardiovascular effect of tyramine and other vasoactive amines in food. A hypertensive crisis may occur within several hours after foods containing tyramine are infected with MAOIs. Signs and symptoms include increased blood pressure, headache, pallor, nausea, vomiting, restlessness, dilated pupils, sweating palpitations, angina, and fever. Death caused by intracranial bleeding occurs rarely. Tyramine-containing foods that are contraindicated during MAOI therapy include the following:

Aged, dried, fermented, salted, smoked, and pickled meat and fish, including processed meats and luncheon meats such as bacon, sausage, liverwurst, hot dogs, corned beef, pepperoni, salami, bologna, and ham
All aged and mature cheese, such as blue, Boursault, brick, Brie, Camembert, cheddar, Emmentaler, gruyère, mozzarella, parmesan, processed American, provolone, Romano, Roquefort, and Stilton
Broad beans and pods
Certain alcoholic beverages, such as beer, Chianti wine, burgundy, sherry, vermouth, and ale
Fermented soybean products including miso and some tofu products
Overripe and spoiled fruit
Sauerkraut
Sourdough and homemade yeast breads
Yeast extracts and meat extracts, which can be found in soups, gravies, stews, and sauces

The following foods should be limited to ½ cup or 4 oz or less per day during MAOI therapy:

Buttermilk
Caviar
Certain fruits, such as bananas, avocados, canned figs, raisins, red plums, raspberries
Chocolate and products containing chocolate
Coffee
Other wines and distilled spirits
Sour cream
Soy sauce, teriyaki sauce
Yogurt

REFERENCES

Karch, A. (1999). *Lippincott's nursing drug guide*. Philadelphia: Lippincott-Raven Publishers.

Roche-Dudek, M., & Roche-Klemma, K. (1998). *Drug-nutrient resource* (3rd ed). Riverside, IL: Roche Dietitians, L.L.C.

APPENDIX 8

Exchange Lists for Meal Planning*

CARBOHYDRATE LISTS

Starch List

One starch exchange equals 15 grams carbohydrate, 3 grams protein, 0–1 gram fat, and 80 calories.

BREAD

Bagel	½ (1oz)	Pita, 6 in across	½
Bread, reduced-calorie	2 slices (1½ oz)	Roll, plain, small	1 (1 oz)
Bread, white, whole wheat, pumpernickel, or rye	1 slice (1oz)	Raisin bread, unfrosted	1 slice (1 oz)
Bread sticks, crisp, 4 in × ½ in	2 (⅔ oz)	Tortilla, corn, 6 in across	1
English muffin	½	Tortilla, flour, 7–8 in across	1
Hot dog or hamburger bun	½ (1 oz)	Waffle, 4½-in square, reduced-fat	1

CEREALS AND GRAINS

Bran cereals	½ cup	Millet	¼ cup
Bulgur	½ cup	Muesli	¼ cup
Cereals	½ cup	Oats	½ cup
Cereals, unsweetened, ready-to-eat	¾ cup	Pasta	½ cup
Cornmeal (dry)	3 tbsp	Puffed cereal	1½ cups
Couscous	⅓ cup	Rice milk	½ cup
Flour (dry)	3 tbsp	Rice, white or brown	⅓ cup
Granola, low-fat	¼ cup	Shredded wheat	½ cup
Grape-Nuts	¼ cup	Sugar-frosted cereal	½ cup
Grits	½ cup	Wheat germ	3 tbsp
Kasha	½ cup		

STARCHY VEGETABLES

Baked beans	⅓ cup	Plantain	½ cup
Corn	½ cup	Potato, baked or boiled	1 small (3 oz)
Corn on cob, medium	1 (5 oz)	Potato, mashed	½ cup
Mixed vegetables with corn, peas, or pasta	1 cup	Squash, winter (eg, acorn, butternut)	1 cup
Peas, green	½ cup	Yam or sweet potato, plain	½ cup

* = 400 mg or more sodium per exchange.

CRACKERS AND SNACKS

Animal crackers	8	Pretzels	¾ oz
Graham crackers, 2½-in square	3	Rice cakes, 4 in across	2
Matzoh	¾ oz	Saltine-type crackers	6
Melba toast	4 slices	Snack chips, fat-free (tortilla, potato)	15–20 (¾ oz)
Oyster crackers	24	Whole wheat crackers, no fat added	2–5 (¾ oz)
Popcorn (popped, no fat added or low-fat microwave)	3 cups		

DRIED BEANS, PEAS, AND LENTILS

(Count as 1 starch exchange, plus 1 very lean meat exchange.)

Beans and peas (garbanzo, pinto, kidney, white, split, black-eyed)	½ cup	Lima beans	⅔ cup
		Lentils	½ cup
		Miso*	3 tbsp

STARCHY FOODS PREPARED WITH FAT

(Count as 1 starch exchange, plus 1 fat exchange.)

Biscuit, 2½ in across	1	Popcorn, microwave	3 cups
Chow mein noodles	½ cup	Sandwich crackers, cheese or peanut butter filling	3
Corn bread, 2-in cube	1 (2 oz)	Stuffing, bread (prepared)	⅓ cup
Crackers, round butter type	6	Taco shell, 6 in across	2
Croutons	1 cup	Waffle, 4½-in square	1
French fries	16–25 (3 oz)	Whole wheat crackers, fat added	4–6 (1 oz)
Granola	¼ cup		
Muffin, small	1 (1½ oz)		
Pancake, 4 in across	2		

Fruit List

One fruit exchange equals 15 grams of carbohydrates and 60 calories. The weight includes skin, core, seeds, and rind.

FRUIT

Apple, unpeeled, small	1 (4 oz)	Figs, dried	1½ cup
Applesauce, unsweetened	½ cup	Fruit cocktail	½ cup
Apples, dried	4 rings	Grapefruit, large	½ (11 oz)
Apricots, fresh	4 whole (5½ oz)	Grapefruit sections, canned	¾ cup
Apricots, dried	8 halves	Grapes, small	17 (3 oz)
Apricots, canned	½ cup	Honeydew melon	1 slice (10 oz) or 1 cup cubes
Banana, small	1 (4 oz)	Kiwi	1 (3½ oz)
Blackberries	¾ cup	Mandarin oranges, canned	¾ cup
Blueberries	¾ cup	Mango, small	½ fruit (5½ oz) or ½ cup
Cantaloupe, small	⅓ melon (11 oz) or 1 cup cubes	Nectarine, small	1 (5 oz)
Cherries, sweet, fresh	12 (3 oz)	Orange, small	1 (6½ oz)
Cherries, sweet, canned	½ cup	Papaya	½ fruit (8 oz) or 1 cup cubes
Dates	3	Peach, medium, fresh	1 (6 oz)
Figs, fresh	1½ large or 2 medium (3½ oz)		

FRUIT (continued)

Peaches, canned	½ cup	Prunes, dried	3
Pear, large, fresh	½ (4 oz)	Raisins	2 tbsp
Pears, canned	½ cup	Raspberries	1 cup
Pineapple, fresh	¾ cup	Strawberries	1¼ cup whole berries
Pineapple, canned	½ cup	Tangerines, small	2 (8 oz)
Plums, small	2 (5 oz)	Watermelon	1 slice (13½ oz) or 1¼ cup cubes
Plums, canned	½ cup		

FRUIT JUICE

Apple juice/cider	½ cup	Grapefruit juice	½ cup
Cranberry juice cocktail	⅓ cup	Orange juice	½ cup
Cranberry juice cocktail, reduced-calorie	1 cup	Pineapple juice	½ cup
Fruit juice blends, 100% juice	⅓ cup	Prune juice	⅓ cup
Grape juice	⅓ cup		

Milk List

One milk exchange equals 12 grams carbohydrate and 8 grams protein.

SKIM AND VERY-LOW-FAT MILK (0–3 GRAMS FAT PER SERVING)

Skim milk	1 cup	Nonfat dry milk	⅓ cup dry
½% milk	1 cup	Plain nonfat yogurt	¾ cup
1% milk	1 cup	Nonfat or low-fat fruit-flavored yogurt sweetened with aspartame or with a nonnutritive sweetener	1 cup
Nonfat or low-fat buttermilk	1 cup		
Evaporated skim milk	½ cup		

LOW-FAT (5 GRAMS FAT PER SERVING)

2% milk	1 cup	Sweet acidophilus milk	1 cup
Plain low-fat yogurt	¾ cup		

WHOLE MILK (8 GRAMS FAT PER SERVING)

Whole milk	1 cup	Goat's milk	1 cup
Evaporated whole milk	½ cup	Kefir	1 cup

Other Carbohydrates List

One exchange equals 15 grams carbohydrate, or 1 starch, or 1 fruit, or 1 milk.

Food	*Serving Size*	*Exchanges Per Serving*
Angel food cake, unfrosted	1/12th cake	2 carbohydrates
Brownie, small, unfrosted	2-in square	1 carbohydrate, 1 fat
Cake, unfrosted	2-in square	1 carbohydrate, 1 fat
Cake, frosted	2-in square	2 carbohydrates, 1 fat
Cookie, fat-free	2 small	1 carbohydrate
Cookie or sandwich cookie with creme filling	2 small	1 carbohydrate, 1 fat
Cupcake, frosted	1 small	2 carbohydrates, 1 fat
Cranberry sauce, jellied	¼ cup	2 carbohydrates
Doughnut, plain cake	1 medium (1½ oz)	1½ carbohydrates, 2 fats

Food	Serving Size	Exchanges Per Serving
Doughnut, glazed	3¾ in across (2 oz)	2 carbohydrates, 2 fats
Fruit juice bars, frozen, 100% juice	1 bar (3 oz)	1 carbohydrate
Fruit snacks, chewy (pureed fruit concentrate)	1 roll (¾ oz)	1 carbohydrate
Fruit spreads, 100% fruit	1 tbsp	1 carbohydrate
Gelatin, regular	½ cup	1 carbohydrate
Gingersnaps	3	1 carbohydrate
Granola bar	1 bar	1 carbohydrate, 1 fat
Granola bar, fat-free	1 bar	2 carbohydrates
Hummus	⅓ cup	1 carbohydrate, 1 fat
Ice cream	½ cup	1 carbohydrate, 2 fats
Ice cream, light	½ cup	1 carbohydrate, 1 fat
Ice cream, fat-free, no sugar added	½ cup	1 carbohydrate
Jam or jelly, regular	1 tbsp	1 carbohydrate
Milk, chocolate, whole	1 cup	2 carbohydrates, 1 fat
Pie, fruit, 2 crusts	⅙ pie	3 carbohydrates, 2 fats
Pie, pumpkin or custard	⅛ pie	1 carbohydrate, 2 fats
Potato chips	12–18 (1 oz)	1 carbohydrate, 2 fats
Pudding, regular (made with low-fat milk)	½ cup	2 carbohydrates
Pudding, sugar-free (made with low-fat milk)	½ cup	1 carbohydrate
Salad dressing, fat-free*	¼ cup	1 carbohydrate
Sherbert, sorbet	½ cup	2 carbohydrates
Spaghetti or pasta sauce, canned*	½ cup	1 carbohydrate, 1 fat
Sweet roll or Danish	1 (2½ oz)	2½ carbohydrates, 2 fats
Syrup, light	2 tbsp	1 carbohydrate
Syrup, regular	1 tbsp	1 carbohydrate
Syrup, regular	¼ cup	4 carbohydrates
Tortilla chips	6–12 (1 oz)	1 carbohydrate, 2 fats
Yogurt, frozen, low-fat, fat-free	⅓ cup	1 carbohydrate, 0–1 fat
Yogurt, frozen, fat-free, no sugar added	½ cup	1 carbohydrate
Yogurt, low-fat with fruit	1 cup	3 carbohydrates, 0–1 fat
Vanilla wafers	5	1 carbohydrate, 1 fat

Vegetable List

One vegetable exchange equals 5 grams carbohydrate, 2 grams protein, 0 grams fat, and 25 calories. In general, one vegetable exchange is ½ cup cooked vegetables or vegetable juice or 1 cup raw vegetables.

Artichoke
Artichoke hearts
Asparagus
Beans (green, wax, Italian)
Bean sprouts
Beets
Broccoli
Brussels sprouts
Cabbage
Carrots
Cauliflower
Celery
Cucumber
Eggplant
Green onions or scallions
Greens (collard, kale, mustard, turnip)
Kohlrabi
Leeks
Mixed vegetables (without corn, peas, or pasta)
Mushrooms
Okra
Onions
Pea pods
Peppers (all varieties)
Radishes
Salad greens (endive, escarole, lettuce, romaine, spinach)
Sauerkraut*
Spinach
Summer squash
Tomato
Tomatoes, canned
Tomato sauce*
Tomato/vegetable juice*
Turnips
Watercress
Zucchini

MEAT AND MEAT SUBSTITUTES LIST

Very Lean Meat and Substitutes List

One exchange equals 0 grams carbohydrate, 7 grams protein, 3 grams fat, and 55 calories. One very lean meat exchange is equal to any one of the following items:

Poultry: Chicken or turkey (white meat, no skin), Cornish hen (no skin)	1 oz
Fish: Fresh or frozen cod, flounder, haddock, halibut, trout; tuna, fresh or canned water	1 oz
Shellfish: Clams, crab, lobster, scallops, shrimp, imitation shellfish	1 oz
Game: Duck or pheasant (no skin), venison, buffalo, ostrich	1 oz
Cheese with 1 gram or less fat per ounce:	
Nonfat or low-fat cottage cheese	¼ cup
Fat-free cheese	1 oz
Other: Processed sandwich meats with 1 gram or less fat per ounce, such as deli-thin, shaved meats, chipped beef,* turkey ham	1 oz
Egg whites	2
Egg substitutes, plain	¼ cup
Hot dogs with 1 gram or less fat per ounce*	1 oz
Kidney (high in cholesterol)	1 oz
Sausage with 1 gram or less fat per ounce	1 oz
(Count as one very lean meat and one starch exchange.)	
Dried beans, peas, lentils (cooked)	½ cup

Lean Meat and Substitutes List

One exchange equals 0 grams carbohydrate, 7 grams protein, 3 grams fat, and 55 calories. One lean meat exchange is equal to any one of the following items:

Beef: USDA Select or Choice grades of lean beef trimmed of fat, such as round, sirloin, and flank steak; tenderloin; roast (rib, chuck, rump); steak (T-bone, porterhouse, cubed); ground round	1 oz
Pork: Lean pork, such as fresh ham; canned, cured, or boiled ham; Canadian bacon;* tenderloin; center loin chip	1 oz
Lamb: Roast, chop, leg	1 oz
Veal: Lean chop, roast	1 oz
Poultry: Chicken, turkey (dark meat, no skin), chicken (white meat with skin), domestic duck or goose (well drained of fat, no skin)	1 oz
Fish:	
Herring (uncreamed or smoked)	1 oz
Oysters	6 medium
Salmon (fresh or canned), catfish	1 oz
Sardines (canned)	2 medium
Tuna (canned in oil, drained)	1 oz
Game: Goose (no skin), rabbit	1 oz
Cheese:	
4.5%-fat cottage cheese	¼ cup
Grated Parmesan	2 tbsp
Cheese with 3 grams or less fat per ounce	1 oz

* = 400 mg or more sodium per exchange.

Other:

Hot dogs with 3 grams or less fat per ounce*	1½ oz
Processed sandwich meat with 3 grams or less fat per ounce, such as turkey pastrami or kielbasa	1 oz
Liver, heart (high in cholesterol)	1 oz

Medium-Fat Meat and Substitutes List

One exchange equals 0 grams carbohydrate, 7 grams protein, 5 grams fat, and 75 calories. One medium-fat meat exchange is equal to any one of the following items:

Beef: Most beef products fall into this category (ground beef, meat loaf, corned beef, short ribs, prime grades of meat trimmed of fat, such as prime rib)	1 oz
Pork: Top loin, chip, Boston butt, cutlet	1 oz
Lamb: Rib roast, ground	1 oz
Veal: Cutlet (ground or cubed, unbreaded)	1 oz
Poultry: Chicken (dark meat with skin), ground turkey or ground chicken, fried chicken (with skin)	1 oz
Fish: Any fried fish product	1 oz
Cheese: With 5 grams or less fat per ounce	
Feta	1 oz
Mozzarella	1 oz
Ricotta	¼ cup (2 oz)
Other:	
Egg (high in cholesterol, limit to 3 per week)	1
Sausage with 5 grams or less fat per ounce	1 oz
Soy milk	1 cup
Tempeh	¼ cup
Tofu	4 oz or ½ cup

High-Fat Meat and Substitutes List

One exchange equals 0 grams carbohydrate, 7 grams protein, 8 grams fat, and 100 calories.

Remember these items are high in saturated fat, cholesterol, and calories and may raise blood cholesterol levels if eaten on a regular basis. One high-fat meat exchange is equal to any one of the following items.

Pork: Spareribs, ground pork, pork sausage	1 oz
Cheese: All regular cheeses, such as American,* cheddar, Monterey jack, Swiss	1 oz
Other: Processed sandwich meats with 8 grams or less fat per ounce, such as bologna, pimento loaf, salami	1 oz
Sausage, such as bratwurst, Italian, knockwurst, Polish, smoked	1 oz
Hot dog (turkey or chicken)*	1 (10/lb)
Bacon	3 slices (20 slices/lb)
(Count as one high-fat meat plus one fat exchange.)	
Hot dog (beef, pork, or combination)*	1 (10/lb)
Peanut butter (contains unsaturated fat)	2 tbsp

* = 400 mg or more sodium per exchange.

FAT LIST

Monounsaturated Fats List

One fat exchange equals 5 grams fat and 45 calories.

Avocado, medium	⅛ (1 oz)
Oil (canola, olive, peanut)	1 tsp
Olives: ripe (black)	8 large
green, stuffed*	10 large
Nuts	
almonds, cashews	6 nuts
mixed (50% peanuts)	6 nuts
peanuts	10 nuts
pecans	4 halves
Peanut butter, smooth or crunchy	2 tsp
Sesame seeds	1 tbsp
Tahini paste	2 tsp

Polyunsaturated Fats List

One fat exchange equals 5 grams fat and 45 calories.

Margarine: stick, tub, or squeeze	1 tsp
lower-fat (30% to 50% vegetable oil)	1 tbsp
Mayonnaise: regular	1 tsp
reduced-fat	1 tbsp
Nuts (walnuts, English)	4 halves
Oil (corn, safflower, soybean)	1 tsp
Salad dressing: regular*	1 tbsp
reduced-fat	1 tbsp
Miracle Whip® salad dressing: regular	2 tsp
reduced-fat	1 tbsp
Seeds (pumpkin, sunflower)	1 tbsp

Saturated Fats List†

One fat exchange equals 5 grams of fat and 45 calories.

Bacon, cooked	1 slice (20 slices/lb)
Bacon, grease	1 tsp
Butter: stick	1 tsp
whipped	2 tsp
reduced-fat	1 tbsp
Chitterlings, boiled	2 tbsp (½ oz)
Coconut, sweetened, shredded	2 tbsp
Cream, half and half	2 tbsp
Cream cheese: regular	1 tbsp (½ oz)
reduced-fat	2 tbsp (1 oz)
Fatback or salt pork, see below‡	
Shortening or lard	1 tsp
Sour cream: regular	2 tbsp
reduced-fat	3 tbsp

FREE FOOD LISTS

A *free food* is any food or drink that contains less than 200 calories or less than 5 grams of carbohydrate per serving. Foods with a serving size listed should be limited to 3 servings per day. Be sure to spread them out throughout the day. If you eat all 3 servings at one time, it could affect your blood glucose level. Food listed without a serving size can be eaten as often as you like.

Fat-Free or Reduced-Fat Foods

Cream cheese, fat-free	1 tbsp
Creamers, nondairy, liquid	1 tbsp
Creamers, nondairy, powdered	2 tsp
Mayonnaise, fat-free	1 tbsp

* = 400 mg or more sodium per exchange.

†Saturated fats can raise blood cholesterol levels.

‡Use a piece 1 in × 1 in × ¼ in if you plan to eat the fatback cooked with vegetables. Use a piece 2 in × 1 in × ½ in when eating only the vegetables with the fatback removed.

Mayonnaise, reduced-fat	1 tbsp	Salad dressing, fat-free	1 tbsp
Margarine, fat-free	4 tbsp	Salad dressing, fat-free, Italian	2 tbsp
Margarine, reduced-fat	1 tsp	Salsa	¼ cup
Miracle Whip®, nonfat	1 tbsp	Sour cream, fat-free, reduced-fat	1 tbsp
Miracle Whip®, reduced-fat	1 tsp	Whipped topping, regular or light	1 tbsp
Nonstick cooking spray			

Sugar-Free or Low-Sugar Foods

Candy, hard, sugar-free	1 candy	Jam or jelly, low-sugar or light	2 tsp
Gelatin dessert, sugar-free		Sugar substitutes§	
Gelatin, unflavored		Syrup, sugar-free	2 tbsp
Gum, sugar-free			

Drinks

Bouillon, broth, consommé*		Club soda	
Bouillon or broth, low-sodium		Diet soft drinks, sugar-free	
Carbonated or mineral water		Drink mixes, sugar-free	
Cocoa powder, unsweetened	1 tbsp	Tea	
Coffee		Tonic water, sugar-free	

Condiments

Ketchup	1 tbsp	Pickles, dill*	1½ large
Horseradish		Soy sauce, regular or light*	
Lemon juice		Taco sauce	1 tbsp
Lime juice		Vinegar	
Mustard			

Seasonings

Be careful with seasonings that contain sodium or are salts, such as garlic or celery salt, and lemon pepper.

Flavoring extracts	Pimento	Tabasco or hot pepper sauce	Wine, used in cooking
Garlic	Spices		Worcestershire sauce
Herbs, fresh or dried			

* = 400 mg or more of sodium per choice.

§Sugar substitutes, alternatives, or replacements that are approved by the U.S. Food and Drug Administration (FDA) are safe to use. Common brand names include:

Equal (aspartame)
Sprinkle Sweet (saccharin)
Sweet One (acesulfame-K)
Sweet-10 (saccharin)
Sugar Twin (saccharin)
Sweet 'N Low (saccharin)

COMBINATION FOODS LIST

Many of the foods we eat are mixed together in various combinations. These combination foods do not fit into any one exchange list. Often it is hard to tell what is in a casserole dish or baked food item. This is a list of exchanges for some typical combination foods. This list will help you fit these foods into a meal plan. Ask your dietitian for information about any combination foods you would like to eat.

Food	*Serving Size*	*Exchanges Per Serving*
ENTREES		
Tuna noodle casserole, lasagna, spaghetti with meatballs, chili with beans, macaroni and cheese*	1 cup (8 oz)	2 carbohydrates, 2 medium-fat meats
Chow mein (without noodles or rice)	2 cups (16 oz)	1 carbohydrate, 2 lean meats
Pizza, cheese, thin crust*	¼ of 10 in (5 oz)	2 carbohydrates, 2 medium-fat meats, 1 fat
Pizza, meat topping, thin crust*	¼ of 10 in (5 oz)	2 carbohydrates, 2 medium-fat meats, 1 fat
Pizza, meat topping, thick crust*	¼ of 10 in (5 oz)	2 carbohydrates, 2 medium-fat meats, 2 fats
Pot pie*	1 (7 oz)	2 carbohydrates, 1 medium-fat meat, 4 fats
FROZEN ENTREES		
Salisbury steak with gravy, mashed potato*	1 (11 oz)	2 carbohydrates, 3 medium-fat meats, 3–4 fats
Turkey with gravy, mashed potato, dressing*	1 (11 oz)	2 carbohydrates, 2 medium-fat meats, 2 fats
Entree with less than 300 calories*	1 (8 oz)	2 carbohydrates, 3 lean meats
SOUPS		
Bean*	1 cup	1 carbohydrate, 1 very lean meat
Cream (made with water)*	1 cup (8 oz)	1 carbohydrate, 1 fat
Split pea (made with water)*	½ cup (4 oz)	1 carbohydrate
Tomato (made with water)*	1 cup (8 oz)	1 carbohydrate
Vegetable beef, chicken noodle, or other broth-type*	1 cup (8 oz)	1 carbohydrate
FAST FOODS†		
Burritos with beef*	2	4 carbohydrates, 2 medium-fat meats, 2 fats
Chicken nuggets*	6	1 carbohydrate, 2 medium-fat meats, 1 fat
Chicken breast and wing, breaded and fried*	1 each	1 carbohydrate, 4 medium-fat meats, 2 fats
Fish sandwich/tartar sauce*	1	3 carbohydrates, 1 medium-fat meat, 3 fats
French fries, thin	20–25	2 carbohydrates, 2 fats

* = 400 mg or more sodium per exchange.

†Ask your fast food restaurant for nutrition about your favorite fast foods.

Food	*Serving Size*	*Exchanges Per Serving*
Hamburger, regular	1	2 carbohydrates, 2 medium-fat meats
Hamburger large*	1	2 carbohydrates, 3 medium-fat meats, 1 fat
Hot dog with bun*	1	1 carbohydrate, 1 high-fat meat, 1 fat
Individual pan pizza*	1	5 carbohydrates, 3 medium-fat meats, 3 fats
Soft-serve cone	1 medium	2 carbohydrates, 1 fat
Submarine sandwich*	1 sub (6 in)	3 carbohydrates, 1 vegetable, 2 medium-fat meats, 1 fat
Taco, hard shell*	1 (6 oz)	2 carbohydrates, 2 medium-fat meats, 2 fats
Taco, soft shell*	1 (3 oz)	1 carbohydrate, 1 medium-fat meat, 1 fat

* = 400 mg or more of sodium per exchange.

The Exchange Lists are the basis of a meal-planning system designed by a committee of the American Diabetes Association and The American Dietetic Association. While designed primarily for people with diabetes and others who must follow special diets, the Exchange Lists are based on principles of good nutrition that apply to everyone.

Index

NOTE: A *t* following a page number indicates tabular material, an *f* following a page number indicates a figure, and a *b* following a page number indicates boxed material. Drugs are listed under their generic names. When a drug trade name is listed, the reader is referred to the generic name.

A

C

E

G

I

O

T

U

V

W

X

Y

Z